Diagnostic Evaluation of the RESPIRATORY SYSTEM

Diagnostic Evaluation of the RESPIRATORY SYSTEM

Claudio Sorino MD PhD
Associate Medical Director
Respiratory Pathophysiology Unit
Department of Pulmonary and Critical Care Medicine
S. Anna Hospital
Como, Italy
Assistant Professor
Biomedical Department of Internal and Specialistic Medicine
Cardiorespiratory Section
University of Palermo
Palermo, Italy
and
Department of Epidemiology and Biostatistics
Mel and Enid Zuckerman College of Public Health
University of Arizona
Tucson, Arizona, USA

Foreword
Nicola Scichilone MD PhD

JAYPEE The Health Sciences Publisher
New Delhi | London | Panama

Jaypee Brothers Medical Publishers (P) Ltd

Headquarters

Jaypee Brothers Medical Publishers (P) Ltd
4838/24, Ansari Road, Daryaganj
New Delhi 110 002, India
Phone: +91-11-43574357
Fax: +91-11-43574314
Email: jaypee@jaypeebrothers.com

Overseas Offices

J.P. Medical Ltd
83, Victoria Street, London
SW1H 0HW (UK)
Phone: +44 20 3170 8910
Fax: +44 (0)20 3008 6180
Email: info@jpmedpub.com

Jaypee-Highlights Medical Publishers Inc
City of Knowledge, Bld. 235, 2nd Floor, Clayton
Panama City, Panama
Phone: +1 507-301-0496
Fax: +1 507-301-0499
Email: cservice@jphmedical.com

Jaypee Brothers Medical Publishers (P) Ltd
17/1-B Babar Road, Block-B, Shaymali
Mohammadpur, Dhaka-1207
Bangladesh
Mobile: +08801912003485
Email: jaypeedhaka@gmail.com

Jaypee Brothers Medical Publishers (P) Ltd
Bhotahity, Kathmandu, Nepal
Phone +977-9741283608
Email: kathmandu@jaypeebrothers.com

Website: www.jaypeebrothers.com
Website: www.jaypeedigital.com

Inquiries for bulk sales may be solicited at: jaypee@jaypeebrothers.com

Diagnostic Evaluation of the Respiratory System

First Edition: 2017

ISBN 978-93-86056-00-9

Printed at

Dedication

To my wife and children,

the reason for my life.

To my mother,

she taught me how to keep my dreams alive.

To my father,

he taught me how to fall and get up.

To Arthur Miles,

an artist, a patient, a friend.

To all the people who fight against respiratory diseases,

never stop doing it, all things are possible for those who believe.

Contributors

Sergio Agati MD
Associate Medical Director
Bronchology Unit
Department of Pulmonary and Critical Care Medicine
S. Anna Hospital
Como, Italy

Zeid Al-Ani MBChB MRCP
Radiology Specialist Registrar
Department of Radiology
North Manchester General Hospital
Manchester, UK

Benfante Alida MD
Pulmonologist
University of Palermo
Palermo, Italy

Hamdan Al-Jahdali MD FRCPC FCCP
Associate Professor
King Saud bin Abdulaziz University for Health Sciences
Riyadh, Saudi Arabia
Adjunct Professor
McGill University
Montreal, Canada

Carolyn Allen MD
Consultant Radiologist and
Radiology Clinical Director
Department of Radiology
The Pennine Acute Hospitals NHS Trust
North Manchester General Hospital
Manchester, UK

Ross Arena MD
Professor and Head
Department of Physical Therapy
Interim Head
Department of Kinesiology and Nutrition
College of Applied Health Sciences (AHS)
University of Illinois at Chicago
Chicago, Illinois, USA

Sixto Arias MD
Assistant of Medicine
Department of Pulmonology
Section of Interventional Pulmonology
Johns Hopkins Medical Institutions
Baltimore, Maryland, USA

Giuseppe Augugliaro MD
Pulmonologist
Ministero della Difesa (Ministry of Defense)
Vicenza, Italy

Diego Bagnasco MD
Pulmonologist
Department of Allergy and Respiratory Diseases
Azienda Ospedaliera Universitaria
Istituto di Ricovero e Cura a Carattere Scientifico (IRCCS)
San Martino, Genova, Italy

Marika Bajc MD PhD
Associate Professor
Skåne University Hospital
Department of Clinical Physiology
Lund University
Lund, Sweden

Debabrata Bandyopadhyay MD
Pulmonologist
Department of Pulmonary Allergy and Critical Care Medicine
Cleveland Clinic
Cleveland, Ohio, USA

Salvatore Battaglia MD PhD
Assistant Professor
Biomedical Department of Internal and Specialistic Medicine
Cardiorespiratory Section
University of Palermo
Palermo, Italy

Maria Bellia MD PhD
Radiologist
Department of Biotechnology and Legal Medicine
Division of Radiological Sciences
University of Palermo
Palermo, Italy

Vincenzo Bellia MD PhD FCCP
Full Professor
Pulmonology and Past Director
Department of Medicine, Pulmonology, Physiology and
Human Nutrition
University of Palermo
Palermo, Italy

Maria Rosaria Bonsignore MD PhD
Associate Professor
Biomedical Department of Internal and Specialistic Medicine
Cardiorespiratory Section
University of Palermo
Assistant Professor
Institute of Biomedicine and
Molecular Immunology
National Research Council
Palermo, Italy

Fulvio Braido MD PhD
Full Professor
Department of Respiratory Diseases
University of Genoa
Associate Medical Director
Department of Allergy and Respiratory Diseases
Azienda Ospedaliera Universiatria
Istituto di Ricovero e Cura a Carattere Scientifico (IRCCS)
Milan, Italy

Robert H Brown MD PhD MPH
Professor
Department of Anesthesiology and
Critical Care Medicine
Environmental Health Sciences
Division of Physiology
Medicine
Division of Pulmonary Medicine and Radiology
The Johns Hopkins University School of Medicine
Baltimore, Maryland, USA

Angelo Maria Calati MD
Chief of Thoracic Surgery Service
Division of Vascular and Thoracic Surgery
S. Anna Hospital
Como, Italy

Claudia Calogero MD
Associate Medical Director
Unit of Respiratory Medicine
Department of Pediatrics
Anna Meyer University Hospital for Children
University of Florence
Florence, Italy

Fabio Cannizzaro MD
Radiologist
Department of Radiology
University of Palermo
Palermo, Italy

Tiziana Cappelletti MD
Associate Medical Director
Intermediate Respiratory Intensive Care Unit
Department of Pulmonary and
Critical Care Medicine
S. Anna Hospital
Como, Italy

Roberto Caronno MD
Director
Division of Vascular and Thoracic Surgery
S. Anna Hospital
Como, Italy

Roberta Catania MD
Pulmonologist
University of Palermo
Palermo, Italy

Angelo Corsico MD PhD
Associate Professor
Department of Pulmonology
Division of Respiratory Diseases
Istituto di Ricovero e Cura a Carattere Scientifico (IRCCS)
S Matteo Hospital
University of Pavia
Pavia, Italy

Harvey O Coxson PhD
Associate Professor
Department of Radiology
University of British Columbia
Principal Investigator
Centre for Heart Lung Innovation
St. Paul's Hospital
Vancouver, Canada

Adriano Di Paco MD
Pulmonologist
Pulmonary Rehabilitation and Weaning Center
Auxilium Vitae Volterra Spa
Volterra, Italy

David Feller-Kopman MD
Associate Professor of Medicine
Section of Interventional Pulmonology
Division of Pulmonary and Critical Care Medicine
Johns Hopkins University
Baltimore, Maryland, USA

Giuliana Ferrante MD
Pediatrician
Department of Science for Health Promotion and Mother and Child
University of Palermo
Palermo, Italy
Assistant Professor
Allergologic Pulmonary Pediatrics Unit
CNR Institute of Biomedicine and Molecular Immunology
Palermo, Italy

Daniel Forman MD
Professor of Medicine
University of Pittsburgh
Chair
Geriatric Cardiology Section
University of Pittsburgh Medical Center
Director
Cardiac Rehabilitation
VA Pittsburgh Healthcare System
Pittsburgh, Pennsylvania, USA

Mario Galli MD
Medical Director
Cardiovascular Interventional Unit
Cardiology Department
S. Anna Hospital
Como, Italy

Stefano Gasparini MD FCCP
President
Italian Association of Hospital Pulmonologists
Associate Professor, Department of Pulmonology
Polytechnic University of Marche
Director, Pulmonary Diseases Department
Ospedali Riuniti Hospital
Ancona, Italy

Thomas R Gildea MD MS FCCP FACP
Head
Section of Bronchoscopy
Department of Pulmonary Allergy and Critical Care Medicine
Cleveland Clinic's Respiratory Institute
Cleveland, Ohio, USA

Johannes Gossner MD
Radiologist
Department of Clinical Radiology
Evangelisches Krankenhaus Göttingen
Göttingen, Lower Saxony, Germany

Ann M Granchelli MD
Internist Pulmonologist
University of Utah Hospitals and Clinics
Salt Lake City, Utah, USA

Massimo Guglielmetti MD
Associate Medical Director
Thoracic Surgery Service
Division of Vascular and Thoracic Surgery
S. Anna Hospital
Como, Italy

Robert G Hamilton MD PhD
Professor of Medicine and Pathology
Johns Hopkins University School of Medicine
Director
Dermatology, Allergy and Clinical Immunology (DACI)
Johns Hopkins Asthma & Allergy Center
Baltimore, Maryland, USA

Riccardo Inchingolo MD PhD
Pulmonologist
Department of Pulmonary Medicine
Fondazione Policlinico Universitario A Gemelli
Catholic University of Sacred Heart
Rome, Italy

Klaus L Irion PhD FRCR
Consultant Radiologist and
Medical Director
Cardiothoracic Centre
Liverpool NHS Trust
The Royal Liverpool University Hospitals
Liverpool, UK

Dhruv Joshi MD
Pulmonary and Critical Care Fellow
Cleveland Clinic Foundation
Cleveland, Ohio, USA

Richard Kanner MD PhD
Professor of Medicine
University of Utah Health Sciences Center
Salt Lake City, Utah, USA

Ali Nawaz Khan MD
Honorary Professor and
Consultant Radiologist
North Manchester General Hospital
Manchester, UK

Danai Khemasuwan MD MBA
Pulmonologist
Department of Pulmonary Allergy and Critical Care Medicine
Cleveland Clinic
Cleveland, Ohio, USA

Miranda Kirby PhD
Fellow
Canadian Institutes of Health Research (CIHR) Banting
Postdoctoral Research
Centre for Heart Lung Innovation
St. Paul's Hospital
Vancouver, Canada

Dilip Kumar MP MD
Senior Resident
Department of Radiodiagnosis
Sanjay Gandhi Postgraduate Institute of
Medical Sciences
Lucknow, Uttar Pradesh, India

Stefania La Grutta MD PhD
Assistant Professor
Institute of Biomedicine and Molecular Immunology
National Research Council
Palermo, Italy

Caterina Lambiase MD
Pediatrician
Department of Pediatrics
Sapienza University of Rome
Rome, Italy

Hans Lee MD
Assistant Professor
Medicine
Director
Pleural Disease Services
Interventional Pulmonology Section
Johns Hopkins Medical Institutions
Baltimore, Maryland, USA

Theodore G Liou MD
Director
Intermountain Adult Cystic Fibrosis Center
Salt Lake City, Utah, USA
Associate Professor
Internal Medicine and
Adjunct Associate Professor
Pediatrics Division of Respiratory, Critical Care and
Occupational Pulmonary Medicine
University of Utah
Salt Lake City, Utah, UK

Andrew S Liteplo MD RDMS FACEP
Director
Emergency Ultrasound Fellowship
Massachusetts General Hospital
Assistant Professor
Department of Surgery
Harvard Medical School
Boston, Massachusetts, USA
Assistant Professor
Department of Emergency Medicine
Kings County, California, USA

Enrico Lombardi MD
Assistant Professor
Departmental Unit of Pediatric Pulmonology
Anna Meyer Pediatric University-Hospital
Florence, Italy

Damiano Magrì MD PhD
Researcher
Department of Clinical and Molecular Medicine
Sapienza University of Rome
Rome, Italy

Simona Maida MD PhD
Associate Medical Director
Thoracic Surgery Service
Division of Vascular and Thoracic Surgery
S. Anna Hospital
Como, Italy

Oreste Marrone MD
Assistant Professor
Institute of Biomedicine and Molecular Immunology
National Research Council
Palermo, Italy

Anna Rosa Maspero MD
Medical Director
Department of Pulmonary and Critical Care Medicine
S. Anna Hospital
Como, Italy

Atul C Mehta MB BS FACP FCCP
Vice Chairman
Pulmonary, Allergy and Critical Care Medicine
Medical Director
Lung Transplantation
Head
Bronchology Section
Cleveland Clinic
Cleveland, Ohio, USA

Keith Meyer MD MS
Professor of Medicine
University of Wisconsin School of Medicine and Public Health
Madison, Wisconsin, USA

Giuseppe Milani MD
Associate Medical Director
Intermediate Respiratory Intensive Care Unit
Department of Pulmonary and Critical Care Medicine
S. Anna Hospital
Como, Italy

Zafar Neyaz MD
Assistant Professor
Department of Radiodiagnosis
Sanjay Gandhi Postgraduate Institute of Medical Sciences
Lucknow, Uttar Pradesh, India

Giada Oliviero MD
Cardiology Fellow
Department of Clinical and Molecular Medicine
Sapienza University
Rome, Italy

Ricardo Ortiz BS
Research Coordinator
Interventional Pulmonology Section
Johns Hopkins Medical Institutions
Baltimore, Maryland, USA

Grace Parraga PhD
Scientist
Robarts Research Institute
Professor and Graduate Chair
Department of Medical Biophysics
The University of Western Ontario
Ontario, Canada

Claudio Pedone MD PhD MPH
Associate Professor
Chair of Geriatrics
University Campus Bio-Medico
Rome, Italy
Associate Medical Director
Center for Gerontology and Health Care Research
Brown University
Providence, Rhode Island, USA

Giorgio Piacentini MD
Associate Professor
Pediatrics Section
Department of Life and Reproduction Sciences
GB Rossi Polyclinic
University of Verona
Verona, Italy

Riccardo Pistelli MD
Associate Professor
Department of Pulmonology School of Medicine
Catholic University of the Sacred Heart
Associate Medical Director
Respiratory Pathophysiology Unit
Columbus-Gemelli University Hospital
Rome, Italy

Francesca Puggioni MD PhD
Assistant Professor
Department of Allergy and Respiratory Diseases
Istituto di Ricovero e Cura a Carattere Scientifico (IRCCS)
Istituto Clinico Humanitas
Milan, Italy

Koteyar Shyamsunder Radhakrishna MD FRCR
Consultant Radiologist
North Manchester General Hospital
Manchester, UK

Prabhakar Rajiah MBBS MD FRCR
Assistant Professor
Cardiothoracic Imaging
Case Western Reserve University
University Hospitals of Cleveland
Cleveland, Ohio, USA

Filippo Russo MD
Associate Medical Director
Cardiovascular Interventional Unit
Department of Cardiology
S. Anna Hospital
Como, Italy

Durr-e-Sabih MBBS MSc (Nuclear Medicine) FRCP Edinburgh FANMB
Director
Multan Institute of Nuclear Medicine and Radiotherapy
Multan, Punjab, Pakistan

Nicola Scichilone MD PhD
Associate Professor of Pulmonology
Biomedical Department of Internal and Specialistic Medicine
Cardiorespiratory Section
University of Palermo
Palermo, Italy

Laura Serafino-Agrusa MD
Pulmonologist
Biomedical Department of Internal and Specialistic Medicine
Cardiorespiratory Section
University of Palermo
Palermo, Italy

Simona Soresi MD
Pulmonologist
Department of Lung Failure and Transplant Medicine
Royal Brompton and Harefield NHS Foundation Trust
London, UK

Claudio Sorino MD PhD
Associate Medical Director
Respiratory Pathophysiology Unit
Department of Pulmonary and Critical Care Medicine
S. Anna Hospital
Como, Italy
Assistant Professor
Biomedical Department of Internal and Specialistic Medicine
Cardiorespiratory Section
University of Palermo
Palermo, Italy
and
Department of Epidemiology and Biostatistics
Mel and Enid Zuckerman College of Public Health
University of Arizona
Tucson, Arizona, USA

Mario Spatafora MD PhD
Associate Professor of Pulmonology and Director
Biomedical Department of Internal and Specialistic Medicine
Cardiorespiratory Section
University of Palermo
Palermo, Italy

Syahminan Suut MBChB FRCR
Consultant Radiologist
Salford Royal Foundation NHS Trust
Greater Manchester, UK

Giancarlo Tancredi MD
Associate Professor
Department of Pediatrics
Sapienza University
Rome, Italy

Daniele Trevisan MD
Associate Medical Director
Thoracic Surgery Service
Division of Vascular and Thoracic Surgery
S. Anna Hospital
Como, Italy

Giovanni Viegi MD PhD
Director
Institute of Biomedicine and Molecular Immunology
National Research Council
Palermo, Italy

Lonny Brett Yarmus MD DO FCCP
Clinical Director
Division of Pulmonary and Critical Care
Fellowship Director
Section of Interventional Pulmonology
Assistant Professor of Medicine
Johns Hopkins Medical Institutions
Baltimore, Maryland, USA

Kazuhiro Yasufuku MD PhD
Director
Interventional Thoracic Surgery Program
Associate Professor
Department of Surgery
University of Toronto
Division of Thoracic Surgery
Toronto General Hospital
University Health Network
Toronto, Canada

Foreword

Life is not so short but that there is always time enough for courtesy.

—Ralph Waldo Emerson

I was just asked by the leading author whether I was willing to write a short introduction to the book, and I immediately accepted, in a hot Saturday afternoon of July in Palermo, Italy. I asked myself why I should have done this instead of taking a stroll on the beach or taking my kids to the park. I know why: I know the author, I know his devotion to work, I know his devotion to family, I know his devotion to life. I first met Dr Claudio Sorino about 15 years ago, when he was a student, and I was immediately impressed by his scientific personality and his clear-thinking attitude. He soon showed how work can be exciting when you combine research skills with the ability to solve clinical issues.

I was a member of the Committee on the day of his medical degree with honors and I was his tutor during his specialization in Respiratory Medicine and his PhD in Clinical and Experimental Pulmonology. Today, Dr Sorino is a prominent scientific leader, certainly a rising star in respiratory medicine. When he shared with me his willingness to coordinate the writing of a book on respiratory medicine, I admit I was skeptical about it, but I soon realized that nothing would have stopped him from doing it! Therefore, encouraging him was just an easy task. Now that I have the opportunity to see the final product, I am astonished by the high quality of the book. The practical approach to the diseases, with the scientific rationale always behind it, and the constant presence of the necessary hints make this book a valuable help for young physicians and those who 'feel young'. Indeed, Dr Sorino's experience led him to think that physicians want and need practical information, but they also require solid scientific basis. Therefore, the decision to write such a book was the most appropriate. Moreover, he was never in a hurry to finish it and now I understand why: he wanted to be sure that everything was clear and was in place. I read somewhere—I apologize with the authors for not recalling—a sentence that fully applies to this project: "*Don't start vast projects with half-vast ideas*". If you read this book, I am confident you will enjoy doing it and, most important, profit from it.

Nicola Scichilone MD PhD
Associate Professor of Pulmonology
Biomedical Department of Internal and Specialistic Medicine
Cardiorespiratory Section
University of Palermo
Palermo, Italy

Preface

The idea of creating a guide on the diagnostics of the respiratory system originated from the analysis of needs arising from the undertaking of daily medical activities.

Modern technological progress has made available several diagnostic tests, which may be relatively sophisticated. Some are specific for the respiratory system (e.g. pulmonary function tests), others are more generic (e.g. blood tests, radiological and nuclear medicine tests).

Despite these innovations, clinical hypothesis is based on the adequate collection of medical history and physical examination, which remain the cornerstone of the diagnostic process. The first therapeutic decisions and the request for further investigation arise from this preliminary evaluation. Clinical reasoning and interpretation of symptoms and signs are, therefore, a key element in avoiding confusion and reducing the risk of diagnostic delays and therapeutic mistakes, as well as reducing the waste of resources: time, energy and money. Indeed, many tests are often performed without a specific clinical basis, with the consequent acquisition of a large amount of data not necessarily relevant to patient symptoms and which can sometimes be misleading.

In the light of this common experience, we have conceived this book with the intention of providing an essential tool for medical practice, including clear, practical and useful suggestions, following evidence-based medical criterion. Key information from the most updated and authoritative guidelines have been included for every topic, in the attempt of providing all the elements needed to make the appropriate choices in each circumstance.

The book has been divided into four major sections: 1. Respiratory system assessment; 2. Evaluation of respiratory function; 3. Diagnostic imaging; 4. Invasive diagnostic procedures. These sections are further divided into chapters, each focusing on the comprehensive needs related to diagnostic technique. Where necessary, pathophysiological aspects have been added to clarify when and how to perform a diagnostic test and how to interpret the results.

Another aspect that this book has addressed is the quality of diagnostic tests and procedures, both in terms of execution and interpretation. Indeed, in order for some diagnostic tests to be as safe as possible, particularly when considering invasive procedures, careful assessment is required regarding not only indications and contraindications, but also their execution. Moreover, the consequences of badly effectuated or misinterpreted tests can be worse than a test which has never been carried out, as it can lead to diagnostic misunderstandings and errors concerning the subsequent treatment plan. The quality of execution is particularly important for tests in which the role of the performer and/or the cooperation of the patient are crucial, such as pulmonary function tests, ultrasound, and invasive diagnostic procedures.

The book aims to be a valuable aid for medical students, pulmonologists and nonrespiratory physicians, who may refer to it for quick answers about the most appropriate choice of investigation in different clinical situations, as well as the correct interpretation of each symptom and test.

We have tried to make the chapters as clear and direct as possible, using a wide iconography and numerous diagrams and algorithms so as to ease understanding and the storage of information.

Our hope is that this book will become a practical guide for physicians and students, stimulating their clinical reasoning in the diverse circumstances they encounter while exercising the medical profession.

The book has been enriched by the contribution and hard work of over 40 international authors. I wish to thank them all. Special thanks are given to Professor Vincenzo Bellia for his suggestions and constant encouragement, Christine Sanders for her language support, Luca Badalamenti for his technical assistance in the creation of images, and the publisher for his support throughout the production process of this book.

Last, but not least, I would like to thank my wife, Maria Rita for her understanding and love during the preparation of the book.

Claudio Sorino MD PhD

Acknowledgments

Kerstin Brauer for her excellent technical assistance in the preparation of the chapter on SPECT.

Domenico Santoro and **Chiara Colombo** from the Division of Infectious Diseases, S. Anna Hospital, Como for their suggestions on the chapter on Tuberculosis Diagnostics.

Raffaella Acconcia from the University of Insubria for the pictures on arterial blood gas analysis.

Radiometer Medical ApS, Denmark for the material supplied to the chapter on Arterial Blood Gas.

Olympus Europe SE & CO. KG for the pictures of the section on Invasive Diagnostic Procedures.

Patrick Morgan for the images in the chapters on Lung Function Testing in Preschool Children.

COSMED for the images in the chapters on Lung Volumes and Cardiopulmonary Exercise Testing.

Pietro Quaretti and **Lorenzo Moramarco** from the Unit of Interventional Radiology, IRCCS Policlinico San Matteo Foundation, Pavia, Italy for the pictures in the chapter on Conventional Pulmonary Angiography.

We would like to thank Mr Jitendar P Vij (Group Chairman), Mr Ankit Vij (Group President), Ms Chetna Malhotra Vohra (Associate Director–Content Strategy), Mr Umar Rashid (Development Editor), and the production team of Jaypee Brothers Medical Publishers (P) Ltd, New Delhi, India for their cooperation in publishing this book.

Contents

Section 2: Evaluation of Respiratory Function

Section 4: Invasive Diagnostic Procedures

Section 1

Respiratory System Assessment

Chapter

1

Signs, Symptoms, and Medical History in Respiratory Medicine

Claudio Sorino, Vincenzo Bellia

HISTORY OF PRESENT ILLNESS (HPI)

The first step in the clinical evaluation of a patient is to obtain a description of the symptoms that he/she experienced [*history of present illness* (HPI)]. This should include a chronological narration, as detailed as possible, of the development of the current health problems from their onset to the present. It is preferable that the description is made by the patient with his own words if the clinical condition allows him/her to do so. For older people, and for patients with cognitive decline or confusion, it is necessary to consult family members or caregivers.

Certain symptoms should always be investigated during a pneumological examination: dyspnea, chest pain, cough and hemoptysis (coughing up blood). Other symptoms may be helpful for the diagnosis of a respiratory disease, such as fever, hoarseness, elevated blood pressure and heart rate, sweating, flushing, hand flaps, confusion, and lethargy (see below).

PAST MEDICAL HISTORY (PMH)

The clinical history of a patient includes prior illnesses, their treatments and consequences. It can provide decisive information in the diagnostic process when a person has problems that affect the respiratory system as well as any other extrapulmonary disorder. For example, a lesion evident on chest radiograph in a patient diagnosed with cancer in other parts of the body is highly suspicious for metastatic involvement of the lung. In addition, the clinical history may suggest that a lesion evident on chest radiographs is a result of a previous lung disease. It is very useful to view previous radiologic images, when available, and compare them with the recent findings. Information relating the quality of *nocturnal sleep*, as well as the presence of daytime sleepiness are important in patients with suspected *obstructive sleep apnea syndrome (OSAS)*, especially when other risk factors are present (e.g. obesity, alcohol intake, smoking). A simple acronym to recall the aspects of sleep to be queried is "BEAR": Bedtime problems (e.g. snoring, nightmares, nicturia), Excessive daytime sleepiness, Awakenings at night, Regularity and duration of sleep. The main aspects to be investigated in context of a PMH are listed in Table 1.1.

Among the various aspects of medical history, the exposure to *tobacco smoke* has a major role in clinical care, since it is a risk factor for several diseases including *lung cancer* and *chronic obstructive pulmonary disease (COPD)*.

The physician should always assess whether the patient is a lifelong nonsmoker, current or former smoker. In the last two cases, it is important to ask the number of cigarettes smoked per day and the number of years the person has smoked. The *pack-year* is an index useful to quantify the overall degree of exposure to active cigarette smoke in subjects who have smoked over a long period of time. It is calculated according to the following formula: number of cigarettes smoked daily multiplied by the number of years the person has smoked, divided by 20. For example, 1 *pack-year* can correspond to 20 cigarettes (1 pack) smoked per day for 1 year, or 10 cigarettes per day for 2 years. In case of former smokers, it is also important to know how long it has been since he quit smoking. Also the exposure to secondhand smoke can be important, especially if prolonged and in small environments such as home, workplace, car.

Table 1.1: Main questions to be asked while collecting a past medical history.
Past illnesses with the approximate date of onset
Hospitalizations and their causes
Injuries or accidents
Surgeries with possible complications
Quality of sleep: bedtime problems (snoring, nightmares, nicturia), excessive daytime sleepiness, awakenings at night, regularity and duration of sleep
Current and past drugs and/or alternative therapies (e.g. acupuncture, herbal medicine, homeopathy).
Food and/or inhalant allergies with the type of reaction (e.g. rash, itching, edema of the glottis, anaphylaxis)
Gynecologic history (if female) with reproductive status (fertility, menopause), total number of pregnancies, related problems or abortions.
Diet, nutritional status, changes in body weight
Bowel regularity
Urinary disorders
Substance abuse: alcohol, tobacco, illicit drugs
Immunizations (exanthematous disease of childhood, antipneumococcal and seasonal flu vaccine)
Birth history, growth, and development
Sexual habits and related problems

DRUG HISTORY (DH)

Patients should always be asked about the use of drugs, with name, dosage, frequency of intake of each medication. Many clinical symptoms may be the side effects of therapies. Examples of respiratory diseases associated with drugs include pulmonary infections in patients receiving *immunosuppressants*, respiratory failure due to excessive use of *sedatives*, lipoid pneumonia in people taking nasal drops or laxatives containing an oil base, interstitial lung disease caused by the administration of amiodarone, bleomycin, minocycline, methotrexate or nitrofurantoin.

Another aspect of the DH is adherence to the prescriptions, with a focus on the understanding and application of proper technique of inhalation therapy with a special emphasis on different devices including metered dose and dry powder inhalers. A fundamental, though obvious, consideration is that *"Drugs do not work in patients who do not take them"*. Therefore, in case of persistence of respiratory symptoms a careful check of the effective drug intake is needed before concluding that the treatment is ineffective.

FAMILY HISTORY

The family history (FH) comprises the main current diseases or cause of death of parents, grandparents, brothers, sisters and offspring. In the respiratory field, the family history plays an important role in infectious diseases like tuberculosis or *severe acute respiratory syndrome (SARS)*, hereditary disorders (e.g. *cystic fibrosis*, alpha-1 antitrypsin deficiency), and illness with possible familiarity such as bronchial asthma. Since the incidence of cancer is higher in certain families, familiarity for lung cancer should also be asked.

OCCUPATIONAL HISTORY (OH)

The information on the types of current or past job, as well as of customarily performed leisure activities, may indicate an exposure to physical, chemical, or biological agents and/or other possible conditions that are potentially responsible for diseases. Two wide groups of occupational lung illnesses can be identified: diseases related to a specific occupation, such as *pneumoconiosis* and *hypersensitivity pneumonitis*, and diseases which are not occupation-specific, but are aggravated at work, such as *occupational asthma*.

Pneumoconiosis is a disease caused by the accumulation of inhaled dust into the lungs and by the subsequent non-neoplastic reaction of the tissues to it.

Most of the dusts causing pneumoconiosis are inorganic, and they are inhaled in the environment or the workplace. The risk for pneumoconiosis exists in workers who breathe for a long time certain mineral dusts: *carbon* (responsible for *anthracosis*, also known as *coal worker's pneumoconiosis, miner's lung* or *black lung*), *silica* (for *silicosis*, also known as *grinder's disease* or *Potter's rot*), *beryllium* (for *berylliosis*), *iron* (for *siderosis*), *cotton* (for *byssinosis*), *bauxite* (for *bauxite fibrosis*), and *asbestos* (responsible for *asbestosis*).

Some inorganic dusts are *biologically inert* (e.g. iron, tin, barium); they can accumulate within alveolar macrophages and produce radiological abnormalities, but often have minimal functional or clinical consequences. Other dusts have *fibrosing action* and induce a pulmonary damage; this can be initially localized and nodular (as in silicosis or black lung) or diffuse (as in asbestosis). Finally, other dusts induce a noncaseating granulomatous reaction (e.g. beryllium), with clinical and radiological consequences similar to sarcoidosis.

Currently, more attention should be paid to three forms of pneumoconiosis: silicosis, because its prevalence is still high; asbestosis, because it is frequently associated with pleural mesothelioma; and berylliosis, because it can be difficult to distinguish from sarcoidosis.

An occupational history should always include the history of exposure to all commercial *asbestos* fiber types, since they have been associated with high rates of lung cancer and mesothelioma, as well as the above mentioned asbestosis. For nearly one century, asbestos was one of the most commonly used materials in industries such as construction, shipbuilding and manufacturing. According to the National Institute for Occupational Health and Safety, more than 75 occupational groups are considered works with significant exposure to asbestos (Table 1.2). It should be noted that a risk of asbestos-related illnesses exists, though smaller, in subjects who have been in contact with the exposed workers or their clothes (especially the wives or other family members).

Hypersensitivity pneumonitis (HP), also called *extrinsic allergic alveolitis (EAA),* is a complex disease due to an immunologic reaction to repeatedly inhaled organic substances. The two most common types of HP are the *farmer's lung* (caused by moldy hay) and the *poultry worker's lung* (or *bird-breeder's lung*, caused by feathers and bird droppings). Other forms of HP are listed in Table 1.3.

DYSPNEA

Dyspnea (most often referred to as breathlessness or shortness of breath) is an uncomfortable sensation of difficulty in breathing. It is a subjective symptom variable in type and intensity, often reported by patients as a greater effort required to breathe, inability to take a deep breath or chest tightness. Less frequently the symptom is described as tiredness or fatigue. Dyspnea can occur together with *tachypnea* (rapid breathing), but the two words should not be confused.

The cardiopulmonary and neuromuscular systems account for the great majority of the causes of dyspnea. Other possible causes include physical deconditioning, anemia, and psychogenic factors. Frequently pathogenesis is multifactorial.

We can identify different types of dyspnea, depending on its features, the chronology (rapidity of onset, duration, progression), the circumstances in which it occurs, the position that provokes it. In case of obstruction of the upper airways (for example due to larynx spasm, edema of glottis) the passage of air can generate a *laryngeal stridor,*

Table 1.2: Occupations and job sites associated with the highest risk of asbestos exposure and popular products known for containing asbestos.

Occupations		*Job sites*	*Products*
Army veterans	Plumbers	Shipyards	Car brakes
Military service	Welders	Power plants	Drywall
Drywall tapers	Miners	Metal works	Ceiling tiles
Electricians	Painters	Chemical plants	Floor tiles
Firefighters	Roofers	Oil refineries	Insulation
Auto mechanics	Railroad workers	Schools	Cements
Ship builders	Cement finishers		Paint
Navy personnel	Construction workers		

Table 1.3: Main types of hypersensitivity pneumonitis (HP) and causative agents.

HP type	*Responsible agent*
Farmer's lung	Moldy hay, straw, and grain
Poultry worker's lung (or bird fancier's lung)	Feathers and bird droppings
Bagassosis	Moldy bagasse (pressed sugarcane)
Cephalosporium HP	Contaminated basements (from sewage)
Coffee worker's lung	Coffee bean dust
Chemical worker's lung	Paints, resins, polyurethane foams, plastics
Cheese-washer's lung	Cheese casings
Compost lung	Compost
Detergent worker's disease	Detergent
Familial HP (or domestic HP)	Contaminated walls
Hot tub lung	Mist from hot tubs
Humidifier lung	Mist generated humidifiers, heating systems, or air conditioners from standing water
Japanese summer house HP	Damp wood and mats
Laboratory worker's lung	Laboratory rats
Lycoperdonosis	Spore dust from mature puffballs
Malt worker's lung	Moldy barley
Maple bark disease	Moldy maple bark
Metalworking fluids HP	Mist from metal-working fluids
Miller's lung	Dust-contaminated grain
Mollusc shell HP	Mollusc shell dust
Mushroom worker's lung	Mushroom compost
Peat moss worker's lung	Peat moss
Pituitary snuff taker's lung	Medication
Sauna worker's lung	Contaminated sauna water
Sequoiosis	Redwood bark, sawdust
Streptomyces HP	Contaminated fertilizer
Suberosis	Moldy cork dust
Tap water HP	Contaminated tap water
Thatched roof disease	Dried grass
Tobacco worker's lung	Moldy tobacco
Wine-grower's lung	Moldy grapes
Woodworker's lung	Wood pulp, dust

and dyspnea is mainly *inspiratory*. Conversely, an obstruction involving the distal airways (for example, due to bronchoconstriction in asthma) causes a breathlessness which is mainly *expiratory*. When dyspnea is of *acute* onset (24–48 hours), the number of options at differential diagnosis is greatly reduced, including pulmonary embolism, acute asthma, *pneumothorax, congestive heart failure, myocardial infarction,* or *cardiac tamponade. Chronic* dyspnea is the most common cause of respiratory limitation of activity in patients with pulmonary or cardiac disease, being responsible for economic and social disabilities. Tables 1.4 and 1.5 list the most frequent causes of acute and chronic dyspnea and the main findings associate with them. Flowchart 1.1 shows a possible algorithm for the evaluation of chronic dyspnea. Besides any instrumental and laboratory investigations, in certain circumstances the choice of an empirical treatment can be useful for diagnostic purposes. For example, if bronchial asthma is suspected, a significant clinical benefit during a trial with bronchodilator therapy can be considered a valuable support to the diagnosis.

According to its *onset*, dyspnea can occur at rest or on exertion. Dyspnea *at rest* is usually expression of higher clinical severity. Dyspnea *on exertion* must be distinguished from exertional fatigue and weakness. It can reveal an exercise-induced asthma, especially when it occurs in a young person. Moreover, it is recommended to evaluate other possible precipitating factors of dyspnea, such as occupational or environmental exposures, and emotional state.

According to the *position* that provokes dyspnea we can distinguish orthopnea, trepopnea and platypnea. *Orthopnea* is the sensation of breathlessness in the recumbent position, that is relieved by sitting or standing in the upright position. *Trepopnea refers* to dyspnea that occurs in one lateral decubitus position and is relieved in the other. It can result from disorders of one lung or major bronchus, or from congestive heart failure. Patients with trepopnea from unilateral lung disease prefer to lie with their healthy lung down, since the gravitation increases blood perfusion of the lower lung with consequent improvement of oxygenation. Patients with congestive heart failure usually prefer to have their right side down, to enable a better blood return, whereby cardiac output is augmented. *Platypnea* refers to shortness of breath that worsens when sitting or standing up, and is relieved when lying down. It is the opposite of orthopnea. *Paroxysmal nocturnal dyspnea* refers to attacks of severe shortness of breath and coughing that generally occur at night. Differently from orthopnea,

Table 1.4: Main causes of acute and chronic dyspnea.

Acute dyspnea	*Chronic dyspnea*
	Cardiac causes
Acute pulmonary edema	Left ventricular failure
Acute myocardial infarction	Valvular heart disease
Acute heart arrhythmia	Chronic heart arrhythmias
Pericarditis and pericardial effusion	Pericardial disease
	Pulmonary causes
Respiratory infection (e.g. acute bronchitis, pneumonia)	Not well-controlled asthma
Pneumothorax	Chronic obstructive pulmonary disease (COPD)
Pulmonary embolism	Interstitial lung diseases
Asthma attack	Pleural effusion
COPD exacerbation	Primary or secondary lung malignancy
Foreign body aspiration	Bronchiectasis
Anaphylaxis	
	Other causes
Pain	Severe anemia
Diabetic ketoacidosis	Thyroid diseases (hypothyroidism or hyperthyroidism)
Thyroid diseases (Thyrotoxicosis)	Obesity
Drugs, e.g. aspirin overdose	Dehydration
Psychogenic (e.g. panic attack)	Psychogenic (e.g. anxiety)
Acute mountain sickness	Neuromuscular diseases (e.g. myasthenia gravis, Guillain-Barré syndrome)

Table 1.5: Main symptoms and clinical findings associated with principal causes of dyspnea.

Diagnosis	*Common presenting symptoms*	*Frequent findings*
Pulmonary embolism	Pleuritic chest pain, sudden onset dyspnea, syncope, hemoptysis	Acute hypoxic-hypocapnic respiratory failure, wheezing, pleural friction rub, signs of deep venous thrombosis
Acute myocardial ischemia	Radiating chest pain or tightness, diaphoresis, acute dyspnea	Tachycardia, signs of heart failure
Congestive heart failure	Dyspnea on exertion, orthopnea, paroxysmal nocturnal dyspnea	Peripheral edema, jugular venous distension, heart murmurs, S3 or S4 heart sounds, hepatojugular reflux, tachycardia, hypertension, diaphoresis, wheezing, basilar crackles or rales at chest examination
Pneumothorax	Sudden onset pleuritic chest pain, dyspnea not relieved with oxygen	Absent breath sounds, chest hyperesonance, jugular venous distension, tracheal deviation, hypoxia, hypotension
Asthma	Cough often dry, expiratory dyspnea relieved with bronchodilator, chest tightness	Wheezing, reduced peak of expiratory flow, use of accessory muscles
COPD	Productive cough, smoke exposure, expiratory dyspnea relieved with bronchodilator	Barrel chest, clubbing, decreased breath sounds, pulsus paradoxus, use of accessory muscle, hypoxic-hypercapnic respiratory failure
Pneumonia	Productive cough, dyspnea	Fever, crackles, increased fremitus

in a patient with paroxysmal nocturnal dyspnea, coughing and wheezing often persist even by sitting or standing up.

It can be assumed that a sensation of respiratory discomfort (dyspnea) occurs when the mechanical response of the respiratory system (changes in respiratory pressure, airflow, or movement of the lungs and chest wall) are not appropriate for the outgoing motor command. The rate and depth of breathing increase in case of metabolic acidosis, pontine lesions of the central nervous system, anxiety, aspirin poisoning, hypoxemia and pain. On the contrary, a decrease in ventilation can be observed in metabolic alkalosis, cerebrum lesions, myasthenia gravis, narcotic overdoses and severe obesity.

Pathophysiology of Dyspnea

The main pathophysiological mechanisms of dyspnea include:

1. *Increased ventilatory demand*: It can be observed both in normal and pathologic conditions. For instance, lung parenchymal and pulmonary vascular disease with enlarged dead space requires increases in ventilation. Hypoxemia due to respiratory disease or altitude stimulates arterial chemoreceptors and increases respiratory motor activity. Physical deconditioning due to prolonged inactivity causes an early and enhanced lactic acid production by skeletal muscles during exercise; the raised blood levels of lactic acid provoke an additional respiratory stimulus, thus increasing the ventilation at a given level of effort. Dyspnea from deconditioning often causes a reduction in the activity, which in turn triggers and maintains a cycle that leads to a progressive functional decline and worsening of exercise tolerance (Fig. 1.1).
2. *Weakness or mechanical inefficiency of the respiratory muscles*: This can occur in neuromuscular diseases or chronic respiratory diseases. For example, in *COPD* an excessive inflation of the lung and expansion of the thorax is often observed. This causes an alteration of the length-tension properties of diaphragm, with consequent reduction of its force-generating capacity and respiratory muscle fatigue. Moreover patients with COPD usually undergo a dynamic hyperinflation, which worsens dyspnea particularly during exercise. The reduction in exercise dynamic hyperinflation can explain a large part of the relief of dyspnea with inhaled bronchodilators.
3. *Greater ventilatory impedance*: It can be due to the narrowing of airways in chronic obstructive respiratory diseases such as bronchial asthma and COPD or to reduced compliance of lung parenchyma in interstitial lung diseases and other conditions that cause restrictive ventilatory abnormalities (e.g. the

Flowchart 1.1: Algorithm for the evaluation of chronic dyspnea.

History

Smoking: Increases probability of COPD
Orthopnea: Suggests CHF
Dyspnea on exertion: Aspecific, consider CHF, COPD, ILD, exercise-induced asthma
Inspiratory dyspnea: Suggests obstruction of the upper airways
Exposure to chemicals: Consider ILD and side effects of drugs

Physical examination

Jugular venous distention: Suggests CHD
Peripheral edema: Suggests CHD
Decreased breath sounds or wheezing: Suggest COPD or asthma
Pleural rub: Common in pleurisy, penumonia, pulmonary embolism
Clubbing: Aspecific, consider lung cancer, COPD, ILD
Pallor: Suggests anemia
Plethoric face: Suggests chronic hypoxemia and secondary polycythemia

If the diagnosis is not clear ↓

First-level tests

Pulse oximetry: Can reveal desaturation
Spirometry: Can show restrictive or obstructive pulmonary diseases
Chest X-ray: Can reveal pleural or parenchimal lesions; shows the cardiac size
Electrocardiography: Can reveal left ventricular hyperthrophy or arytmyas
Complete blood count: Can reveal anemia or high hematocrit due to chronic hypoxemia

↓

Second-level tests

Arterial blood gas analysis: Can revel respiratory or metabolic acidosis or alcalosis: in case of hypoxemia with respiratory alcalosis consider pulmonary embolism
Brain natriuretic peptide: Low levels help exclude CHF
D-dimer: Low levels help exclude pulmonary embolism

↓

Third-level tests

Chest CT: High resolution if an ILD is suspected, contrast if cancer is suspected
Echocardiography: Gives information on heart's structure and function and an estimate of pulmonary artery pressure
Right heart catheterization: Is the gold standard for the diagnosis of pulmonary hypertension
Cardiopulmonary exercise testing: Evaluates cardiac or respiratory limit to the exercise and deconditioning
DLCO: A reduction suggests parenchymal lung disease (ILD, emphysema) or pulmonary hypertension

(COPD: Chronic obstructive pulmonary disease; CHF: Congestive heart failure; ILD: Interstitial lung diseases; DLCO: Diffusing capacity of the lung for carbon monoxide).

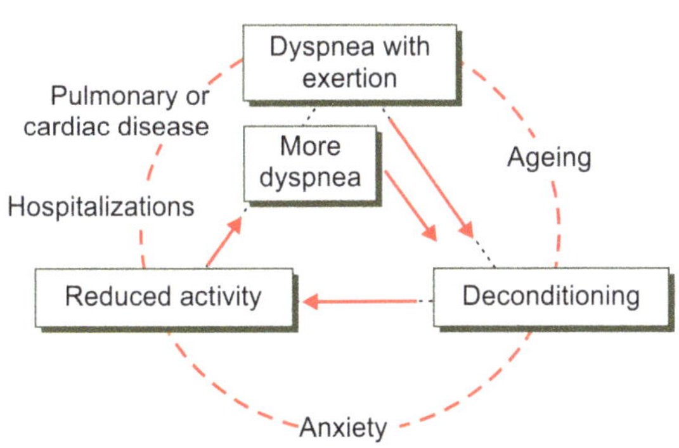

Fig. 1.1: The dyspnea cycle and the factors affecting it.

infiltration of the lungs by neoplastic or inflammatory processes, interstitial or alveolar pulmonary edema).

4. *Abnormal breathing patterns*: It is supposed that a reflex response to the stimulation of pulmonary vagal receptors can cause the rapid shallow breathing often observed in some diseases of lung parenchyma such as pulmonary edema, pulmonary embolism. Pursed lip breathing observed in patients with emphysema (particularly in the so called *pink puffer phenotype*) is considered a way to increase intrabronchial pressure to prevent airway collapse; at the same time this way of breathing should reduce dyspnea intensity through a prolongation of expiratory time, reduction in respiratory frequency, changes in the pattern of ventilatory muscle recruitment, and larger tidal volumes.

5. *Blood-gas abnormalities*: Hypoxemia and hypercapnia cause an increase of the respiratory motor activity mainly through the stimulation of central and peripheral chemoreceptors. However, in many patients blood-gas abnormalities poorly correlate with dyspnea. The effect of pCO_2 on ventilation is largely mediated by changes in hydrogenion concentration (consequently of pH) at the chemoreceptor level. In patients with chronic hypercapnia, the ventilatory responses are limited because of a reduced sensitivity of these chemoreceptors and a metabolic compensation which minimizes the rising of hydrogenion concentration. Changes in hydrogenion concentration due to metabolic conditions such as diabetic ketoacidosis and renal insufficiency can be also responsible for dyspnea.

Measurement Tools for Dyspnea

The quantification of dyspnea is useful in estimating the severity of the underlying disease. Nevertheless, since dyspnea, is a subjective symptom (like pain), it can be influenced by the cognitive or mood status of the patient, and a discrepancy between severity of disease and intensity of breathing discomfort is quite frequent. Several tools have been proposed to evaluate the degree of dyspnea. They can provide the average estimates over a period of time or be referred to a precise point in time, e.g. upon waking in the morning or after exercise. Such instruments can be *unidimensional* [*e.g. Visual Analogue Scales (VAS), Numerical Rating Scales (NRS),* the *modified Borg scale,* the *Medical Research Council (MRC) scale*], or *multidimensional,* such as the *Chronic Respiratory Disease Questionnaire (CRQ).*

The VAS is a horizontal or vertical line, usually 100 mm long that is widely used in the measurement of symptoms such as breathlessness and pain. Precise limits are defined at each end of the VAS such as "no breathlessness at all" to "breathlessness as bad as it can be" (Fig. 1.2). The patient indicates his/her level of dyspnea through a mark on the line. The VAS is particularly suitable for evaluating the trend of dyspnea over time in the same subject. Similarly, the NRS allows to rate shortness of breath from 0 to 10, with 0 being no shortness of breath and 10 shortness of breath as bad as can be. NRS has been shown to be more repeatable and easier to use for people than VAS. The *modified Borg scale* is a categorical scale similar to a NRS but with descriptive terms (severe, moderately severe, etc.). The *MRC scale* is a simple and widely used categorical scale grading the effect of breathlessness on daily activities. As shown in Table 1.6, it comprises of five statements that describe almost the entire range of respiratory disability from none (Grade 1) to almost complete incapacity (Grade 5). It can be either self-reported or interviewer-administered.

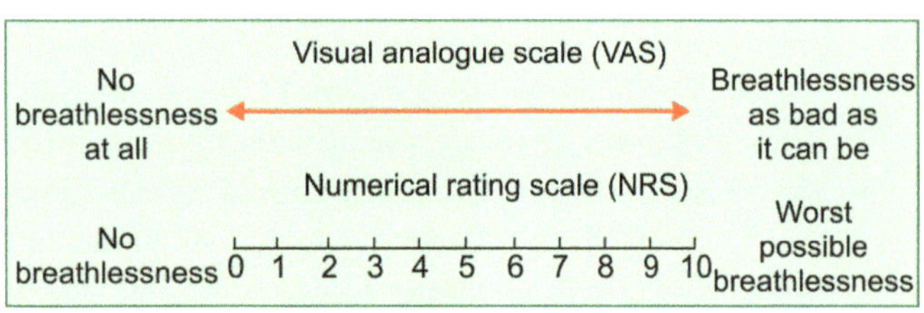

Fig. 1.2: Examples of visual analogue scale (VAS) and numerical rating scale (NRS) for dyspnea.

Multidimensional tools assess the impact of breathlessness on various domains such as activities of daily living, mood, social relationships or other person related outcomes. *Dyspnea Management Questionnaire (DMQ)* is a multidimensional tool recently proposed to evaluate specifically the impact of dyspnea on everyday life. It consists of five theoretically derived dyspnea dimensions: dyspnea intensity, dyspnea anxiety, activity avoidance, activity self-efficacy and satisfaction with strategy use. Other multidimensional questionnaires such as the *St. George's Respiratory Questionnaire (SGRQ),* the *CRQ,* and the *Seattle Obstructive Lung Disease Questionnaire (SOLQ)* allow to assess the impact that various symptoms, including dyspnea, have on quality of life.

CHEST PAIN

Chest pain is often a difficult symptom to be evaluated because of the many possible variables involved. All

Table 1.6: Medical Research Council (MRC) dyspnea scale for grading the degree of a patient's breathlessness.

Grade	
1	Not troubled by breathlessness except on strenuous exercise
2	Short of breath when hurrying or walking up a slight hill
3	Walks slower than people of the same age on the level ground because of breathlessness, or has to stop for breath when walking at own pace
4	Stops for breath after about 100 yds or after a few minutes on the level ground
5	Too breathless to leave the house, or breathless when dressing or undressing

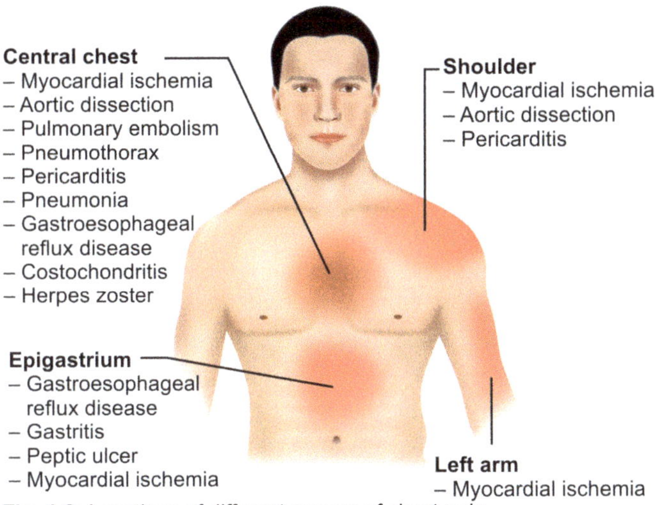

Fig. 1.3: Locations of different causes of chest pain.

structures within the thorax are sensitive to pain, except the lung parenchyma and visceral pleura which have no sensory innervation. For this reason, a lung disease may progress to advanced stages without giving thoracic pain. Schematically, chest pain may originate mainly from three sites: mediastinum, pleura and chest wall. Furthermore, chest pain can also come from extrathoracic sites. Figure 1.3 shows the most frequent locations of different causes of chest pain.

Central or Mediastinal Pain

The mediastinum is the central compartment of the thorax, between the two pleural cavities. It contains the heart, esophagus, trachea, aorta and the other great vessels of the heart, nerves, lymph nodes of the central chest and fat. Any disease involving these structures may result in chest pain in the mediastinal region, often called central or retrosternal pain.

Myocardial ischemia is a major cause of retrosternal pain for both frequency and importance of the disease. This pain is typically associated with a sensation of pressure, fullness or tightness of the chest, and may extend to the left arm or both arms, the neck, jaw, or teeth. It is usually accentuated by exertion and relieved by rest; it is often associated with dyspnea, sometime with sudden nausea or vomiting, dizziness, flushing, or cold sweat. In most cases patient with ischemic heart disease have risk factors such as old age, hypertension, diabetes, hypercholesterolemia, smoke exposure, male gender. However, as many as 25% of patients with myocardial ischemia present with nontypical symptoms and no risk factors. In the differential diagnosis of chest pain suspected for a myocardial origin, it is mandatory to obtain an electrocardiogram, the dosage of markers of myocardial injury (*Cardiac Troponin T and I, MB isoenzymes of creatine kinase: CK-MB*). It is also very useful to evaluate the response to the administration of sublingual nitroderivatives (nitroglycerin), which are usually effective in relieving the pain caused by myocardial ischemia (*angina*).

A central chest pain can be also evoked by other serious conditions such as massive *pulmonary embolism, dissecting aortic aneurysm, pneumothorax,* and *acute pericarditis.*

Patients with *pulmonary embolism* usually present with sudden onset of breathlessness, chest pain, tachycardia, ipoxiemia and ipocapnia (the latter due to hyperventilation). They may have a history of *deep venous thrombosis (DVT)* of lower *extremity* or one or more risk factors for *venous thromboembolic diseases* (e.g. prolonged bed rest, malignancy, older age, recent orthopedic surgery, obesity, congestive heart failure, childbirth, use of oral contraceptives).

Aortic dissection may present with sudden onset of tearing chest pain which can radiate to the inter-scapular region. It is always a medical emergency and can be rapidly fatal as a result of decreased blood supply to other organs, cardiac failure, and sometimes rupture of the aorta with circulatory collapse or bleeding into the mediastinum that can cause *cardiac tamponade.* Measurement of blood pressure is important since severe hypotension at presentation is an ominous prognostic indicator, pointing out pericardial tamponade, aortic insufficiency or thoracic aortic rupture. The patient is usually in advanced age (male over 50 female over 70), may have history of atherosclerosis, hypertension or be known to have an aortic aneurysm. It is more frequent in patients with diseases that affect blood vessel wall integrity such as *Marfan syndrome* and the vascular subtype of *Ehlers-Danlos syndrome.* Immediate diagnostic investigations include: computed tomography (CT), aortic angiography, transthoracic and transesophageal echocardiography. Magnetic resonance imaging (MRI) can also be performed, but it requires a much longer execution time than a CT scan and is not easily feasible with unstable patients.

Tension pneumothorax is also a medical emergency presen ting with sudden onset of dyspnea and chest pain. The examination reveals a tympanic hyperresonance on percussion of the chest wall. A chest X-ray can be sufficient to confirm the diagnosis.

The *gastroesophageal reflux disease (GERD)* is responsible for a burning pain that is accentuated when the person lies down and gets better when the patient gets up. In other disorders of the esophagus (tumors, ulcers, diverticulitis, infectious esophagitis) pain is usually related to the ingestion of food.

Pleuritic Pain

Unlike the visceral pleura, the parietal pleura is highly sensitive to pain, because of its rich innervation which can be stimulated by inflammatory processes or stretch. In normal conditions, between visceral and parietal pleura there is a very small amount of liquid that allows them to move relative to one another during respiration. If the pleura layers are inflamed, damaged or dry, they can no longer move smoothly. Consequently, every time the lungs expand to breathe in air, they rub against each other rather than sliding, thus evoking pleuritic pain.

Pleuritic pain is often described as a sharp or stabbing pain and is often felt only on one side, with an increased intensity at a specific site corresponding to the affected pleura. It is usually exacerbated by deep inspiration, coughing or sneezing. As a consequence, the patient often takes only shallow breaths to reduce the pain.

The irritation of the central region of the diaphragm (sometimes involved in abdominal diseases such as subphrenic abscesses or hiatus hernia), as well as the mediastinal and diaphragmatic pleura, can cause a pain that is perceived in the neck and shoulder. This occurs because the central diaphragm and the mediastinal and diaphragmatic pleura are innervated through the phrenic nerve by the same cervical spinal segments (third and fourth) that supply the skin and muscles of the neck and shoulder. In contrast, the pain due to the involvement of the peripheral part of the diaphragm or the parietal pleura is perceived locally.

It should be noted that a pleuritic pain may be the indicator of serious cardiac or pulmonary diseases. For example it can occur in *pericarditis* (due to the extension of inflammation from pericardium to the pleura) or in other diseases in which the pleura can be affected by an inflammatory process, such as pulmonary embolism, lung neoplasms and abscesses. Pain arising from the pericardium is characteristically positional: it increases on lying down (supine). A pleuritic pain can also occur in the early stages of congestive heart failure, as a consequence of pleural effusion; usually the pain tends to subside as the fluid builds up.

Chest Wall Pain

A pain referred at the chest wall that is not caused by irritation of the parietal pleura can be due to a muscle, nerve, bone or skin disorder.

Differently from a pain that originates from the parietal pleura, a pain related to muscle damage worsens with cough or thoracic movement, but not during deep inspiration, and is inducible with palpation of the affected area.

A radicular pain is usually caused by compression of the posterior roots of the spinal nerves (for example, due to herniation of the intervertebral disc or malignancy involving the vertebrae or spinal cord). It occurs along the distribution of the specific intercostal nerve. *Herpes zoster* can also be the cause of a pain that originates at the root of the intercostal nerves.

Chest pain originated from bone tissue can be caused by a trauma with rib fracture (sometimes by severe and repeated episodes of cough in patients with osteoporosis), by inflammatory or neoplastic diseases (often metastatic). In the latter case, the symptom may appear before a mass is radiologically appreciable.

Costochondritis (an inflammation of the cartilage joining the ribs to the breastbone) can cause tenderness at the junction of the ribs and the breastbone, which increases with movement and deep breathing. The reproducibility of the pain by a pressure on the affected area usually confirms the diagnosis. In uncertain cases, other tests such as electrocardiogram and chest X-ray may be useful to rule out other more serious conditions. Costochondritis can be associated with an injury to the rib cage with unusual physical activity, a recent respiratory illness (e.g. cold or flu). Moreover, it is more frequent in people with *fibromyalgia, systemic lupus erythematosus,* and *ankylosing spondylitis.*

Intercostal neuralgia can be due to several conditions in which a suffering of intercostals nerves occurs (including infections, inflammation, trauma, malignancy, thoracic surgery). The pain is usually spasmodic and intermittent, may wrap around the chest or radiate from the back toward the front of chest or *vice versa*. In relation to the location of the area of innervation, the pain can be exacerbated by motions such as breathing, laughing or sneezing. Continuous nerve pain may also be felt. The skin can be painful to the touch.

Chest Pain Radiating from Extrathoracic Sites

A chest pain can be radiated from an abdominal disease: the painful symptoms extend for continuity and contiguity from the place of origin (which can be identified in this way) to the adjacent chest. Thus in meteoric syndromes (entrapment of gas) the pain extends easily from the affected site (stomach, liver or splenic flexure) to the lower areas of the chest.

Pain from *GERD, diffuse esophageal spasm (DES),* and *peptic ulcer disease* is usually experienced in the epigastrium but it may appear as central lower chest wall pain. *Gallbladder disease* is another possible cause of chest pain from abdominal cause. It often involves the upper right quadrant of the abdomen, may spread to right upper back or shoulder blade area and usually gets worse by eating.

The diagnostic approach to chest pain may vary depending on the clinical circumstances. Acute clinical situations require a quick analysis aimed at confirming or excluding severe cardiorespiratory diseases such as heart attack, pulmonary embolism, and dissecting aneurysm of the aorta. In addition, the most severe circumstances may require an immediate treatment before a precise diagnostic definition has been made.

An approach to chest pain may be to first exclude the most severe and life-threatening causes:

1. Ischemic heart disease (IHD)
2. Pulmonary embolism
3. Pneumothorax
4. Ruptured aortic aneurysm.

Subsequently, it is affordable to analyze the features of chest pain for identifying the causes with a typical clinical presentation. For example, the increase on inspiration suggests pleuritic pain; changes with position suggest *pericarditis* or, less frequently, pleuritic and musculoskeletal diseases; a tenderness elicited by touching the site of pain suggests a chest wall disease such as *costochondritis* and other musculoskeletal diseases; the history of trauma, muscle strain or sprain suggests musculoskeletal causes; a dermatomal distribution suggests a *spinal disease* that affects the nerve radicles or *Herpes zoster* infection; a referred chest pain from the neck can indicate a disease of the cervical vertebrae such as *spondylosis*; chest pain associated with food intake usually recognize gastrointestinal causes. A *psychogenic* chest pain can be considered after excluding all the possible organic causes. It is more commonly seen in women and those with a history of psychological illness. Figure 1.4 is an illustration of the main causes of chest pain.

On the basis of the clinical suspicion, a number of tests may be performed. X-rays of the chest is usually the first imaging test used to help diagnose many conditions involving the chest wall, lungs, heart, and great

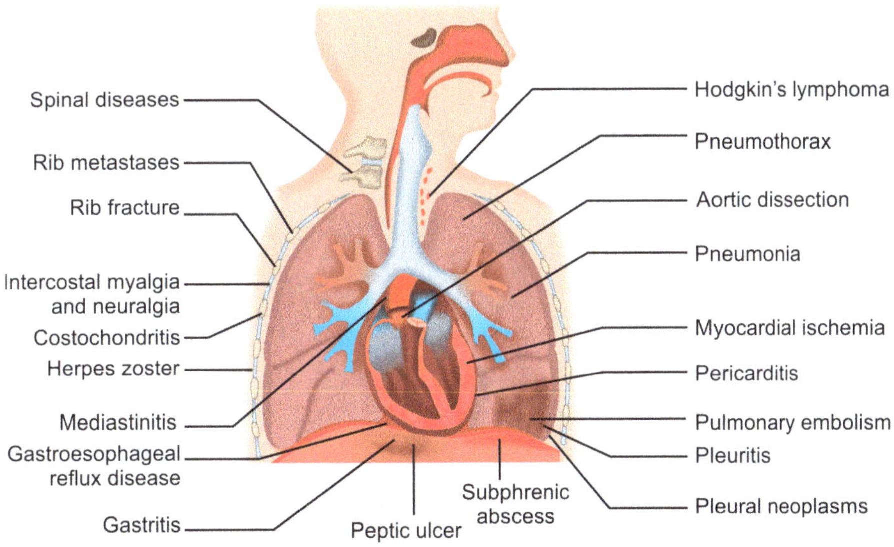

Fig. 1.4: Main causes of chest pain.

vessels. Electrocardiogram and indexes of myocardial damage (Troponin I or T, MB fraction of Creatine kinase) are essential if myocardial ischemia is suspected. The determination of plasma D-dimer levels is useful if pulmonary embolism is a possible cause (due to its high negative predictive value), whereas CT pulmonary angiogram or V/Q scintigraphy are needed if such a suspicion is high. More details about such examinations are provided in other chapters of the book.

COUGH

Cough is a sudden noisy expulsion of air from the lungs. This symptom occurs whenever the mucous membranes of the respiratory tract are irritated; it is aimed at clearing them from secretions, irritants, foreign particles, and microbes.

The cough receptors are located mainly on the posterior wall of the trachea, carina, and pharynx. Some structures situated near the airways, such as the pericardium, the esophagus, diaphragm and stomach also have receptors that can trigger a cough.

The cough may be caused by more than 100 diseases, mainly affecting the respiratory system. However, only three (alone or in combination), account for more than 80% of the cases: *postnasal drip syndrome (PNDS)*, also termed *upper airway cough syndrome* (UACS), *GERD)* and *bronchial asthma*.

Less frequently described in literature are the *cough-variant asthma (CVA)* and the *eosinophilic bronchitis (EB)*. The latter condition is very similar to the CVA, but it is distinguished by three characteristics: negative methacholine challenge test, absence of *peak expiratory flow (PEF)* variability and sensitivity to glucocorticoids but not to beta2-agonist bronchodilator.

Cough can be classified according to its duration and the presence or absence of sputum. According to the first criterion, we distinguish an *acute cough* that lasts less than 3 weeks, a *subacute cough*, lasting between 3 and 8 weeks (it remains even after a cold or other respiratory infection is over), and a *chronic cough*, lasting more than 8 weeks.

Common cold or other infections of the upper and lower respiratory tract, including flu, are the most frequent causes of acute cough. A subacute cough is often due to the persistence of irritation of the respiratory tract after cold or other respiratory infections. Bronchial inflammation caused by cigarette smoking and obstructive lung diseases (COPD, asthma) is the leading causes of chronic cough.

Lesions that compress the upper airway such as retrotracheal masses or arteriovenous malformations, may present with chronic cough, too.

Chronic cough can also be a symptom of *tracheobronchomalacia*, resulting from the softening or damage of rigid cartilaginous support of the large airways, which collapse during inspiration. This is often seen in combination with COPD in patients with a history of cigarette smoking.

Persistent *modifications* in the characteristics of cough in a smoker should put the suspicion of lung cancer.

A *dry cough* (or nonproductive) can be due to several diseases, including respiratory infections, asthma, irritation to the lungs or trachea from smoke, exposure to polluted or very dry air, cancerous growth in the lungs. A foreign body in the throat can also cause coughing as an attempt to expel the occluding object. GERD can also cause a dry cough, since the refluxed gastric content irritates receptors in the lower esophagus. Less commonly, tiny particles of the acid are aspirated into the trachea and lungs, triggering a cough to expel the unwanted substance. In the case of cough due to GERD, the symptom is usually persistent and worsens at night, after meals or when the patient is lying down.

A dry cough is a known side effects of *angiotensin converting enzyme* (ACE) inhibitors, occurring in up to 15% of patients treated with these agents. The pathogenetic mechanism commonly hypothesized is the stimulation of afferent C-fibers in the airway by bradykinin, which is normally degraded in part by ACE, and may accumulate due to ACE inhibitors. Cough does not appear to occur with increased frequency in patients treated with angiotensin II receptor antagonists (which do not increase kinin levels), consistently with the kinin hypothesis.

PNDS is a frequent cause of chronic cough, due to mucus dripping down the back of the throat. Many acute respiratory illnesses can cause short bouts of postnasal drip. Chronic postnasal drip is usually the result of a sinus infection (sinusitis) or allergies. The expression *UACS* is today preferred over PNDS, and indicates cough that is associated with several conditions that affect the upper airway, including the nose, sinuses, or throat. Such conditions may stimulate cough nerve endings by a combination of post nasal drip and inflammation of the tissues. UACS is considered the most common cause of chronic cough in nonsmoking adults and has a prevalence of up to 40% in the American population.

Bronchial asthma is one of the most common causes of chronic cough. It is usually dry, tends to be worse at night, and often occurs together with *wheezing*. However, cough may also be productive and may be the only or the predominant symptom of the disease *(CVA)*. The mechanisms of cough in asthma are complex and presumably multifactorial. Coughing in asthma may be the consequence of narrowing of the airways caused by broncho-constriction and by their plugging with mucus.

Expectoration or *sputum production* is the act of coughing up and spitting out the material produced in the respiratory tract. This occurs when the respiratory secretions are beyond the ability of the mucociliary mechanism to remove them from the airways. Since the patient can swallow the sputum raised to the level of the pharynx, the absence of expectoration is not necessarily indicative of a dry cough. The sound of the cough can help in ascertaining its productive or dry nature. It is very useful to ask the patient about the *f*requency of sputum production, as well as the *main* features of the sputum including the amount produced with each cough and in the whole day, color, consistency, difficulty of its expectoration, taste, and smell.

Mucous sputum contains only few of microscopic elements and appears clear and viscous. *Purulent sputum* is usually opaque, with a whitish, yellowish or greenish color, as a result of the presence of numerous white blood cells, mainly neutrophilic granulocytes. In asthmatic subjects, the sputum may look purulent due to the abundance of eosinophils. The presence of blood in the sputum may occur with its uniform or streaky red coloration.

Chronic production of purulent sputum suggests the presence of *bronchiectasis*.

Sudden expectoration of foul-smelling and bad tasting sputum indicates anaerobic infection and suggests a *lung abscess* (usually in febrile patients).

If the sputum contains carbon particles, it can appear gray (e.g. in cigarette smokers) or black (e.g. in coal miners).

The presence of productive cough occurring on most days for at least 3 months of the year and for at least two consecutive years is the most accepted criterion for defining chronic bronchitis. Patients with chronic bronchitis are often accustomed to cough daily, but they notice when the characteristics of their cough and sputum production change. The most frequent cause for this change is the intercurrence of a respiratory infection, but the possible occurrence of a malignancy should never be ignored.

It is generally recommended not to use cough sedatives until the cause has been found. In fact, these could mask the symptom, allowing dangerous underlying diseases (such as asthma or lung cancer) to progress inadvertently, Moreover, in the case of productive cough, antitussives would compromise the effectiveness of bronchial secretions removal.

HEMOPTYSIS (COUGHING UP BLOOD)

The term hemoptysis indicates the expectoration of blood that originates from the respiratory tract (larynx, trachea, bronchi, or lungs). The amount of such a blood expectoration may range from blood-streaked sputum to gross blood without associated sputum.

A bleeding that exceeds 300 mL in 24 hours may be referred to as *massive hemoptysis*, which, though rare, is a potentially life-threatening condition. The risk for life is related to asphyxia following flooding of tracheobronchial tree rather than to hypovolemia or hemodynamic deterioration.

About 95% of lung blood supply circulates through pulmonary circulation, whereas a small part flows through the bronchial circulation. However, the source of bleeding is more frequently from bronchial arteries (which have systemic pressure) rather than pulmonary arteries (which have low pressure and may produce usually small-volume hemoptysis), except when pulmonary arteries are damaged by trauma, by neoplastic erosion or by granulomatous or calcified lymph nodes).

After confirming the presence of blood, an initial task is to understanding the origin of bleeding and differentiating hemoptysis from the spitting of blood that comes from extrapulmonary sites, including nasopharynx, oropharynx (pseudohemoptysis) and upper gastrointestinal tract (hematemesis).

The blood coming from the lungs is generally bright red, often frothy and usually causing cough. It can be mixed with mucus or purulent secretions. In contrast, the blood coming from the esophagus or stomach is usually dark red or black, can be associated with nausea or vomiting and can be mixed with food particles.

Diagnosis is particularly difficult when the coughed blood is swallowed or, conversely, when the vomited blood is aspirated into the airway.

Endoscopic inspection of the rhinopharynx, larynx, and airways may be indicated along with esophagogastric endoscopy when the etiology is obscure to distinguish hemoptysis, pseudo hemoptysis and hematemesis.

Frothy pink sputum suggests pulmonary edema from congestive heart failure or mitral stenosis.

All patients with hemoptysis, even if mild, should have *chest X-ray*, which can localize infiltrates or masses, whereas pulse oximetry is indicated in more severe cases to evaluate the presence of respiratory failure.

In many cases sputum microscopy and culture for *Mycobacterium tuberculosis* should be also performed, as well as cytology with looking for malignant cells.

Patients with normal radiographic results can be submitted to prolonged observation or undergo empiric antibiotic treatment if clinical history and physical examination are consistent with low respiratory-tract infection.

In case of persistent or recurrent hemoptysis, it is useful to perform high resolution CT with contrast, which may reveal pulmonary lesions that are not apparent on the chest X-ray and can help locate lesions increasing the yield of bronchoscopy and biopsy. Moreover, CT is the best method for diagnosing other causes of hemoptysis such as bronchiectasis, broncholith or arteriovenous malformation, aspergilloma.

Patients with abnormal results of chest X-ray and patients with risk factors for cancer (*smoking, age over 40 years, recurrent hemoptysis or bleeding lasting longer than one week)* should undergo chest CT and bronchoscopy.

Bronchoscopy, performed with either a rigid or a flexible endoscope, is useful in diagnosing active hemorrhage and in controlling the airway in patients with devastating hemorrhage. However, its capacity to localize the site of bleeding and detect underlying disease is not higher than that of CT. The probability of identifying the bleeding site is three times greater if bronchoscopy is done within 48 hours.

Ventilation/perfusion scanning or CT angiography can confirm the diagnosis of pulmonary embolism. CT and pulmonary angiography can also detect pulmonary arteriovenous fistulas. Flowchart 1.2 shows a possible algorithm for the evaluation of nonmassive hemoptysis.

MISCELLANEOUS SYMPTOMS

Confusion, irritability, lethargy; and even *coma* may result from pathological processes that affect the lungs, especially in elderly patients. Several diseases can be the underlying causes, including pneumonia, pulmonary embolism, pulmonary edema and lung cancer. In these conditions the nervous system may suffer as a result of a reduced oxygenation or an increase in carbon dioxide blood levels. The same symptoms can also occur due to metabolic abnormalities such as hyponatremia or hypercalcemia or a direct involvement of the central nervous system, such as metastatic neoplastic disease, fat embolism, cryptococcosis, neurosarcoidosis, and disseminated aspergillosis. Other sign that may occur in case of carbon dioxide retention

Flowchart 1.2: Algorithm for the evaluation of nonmassive hemoptysis.

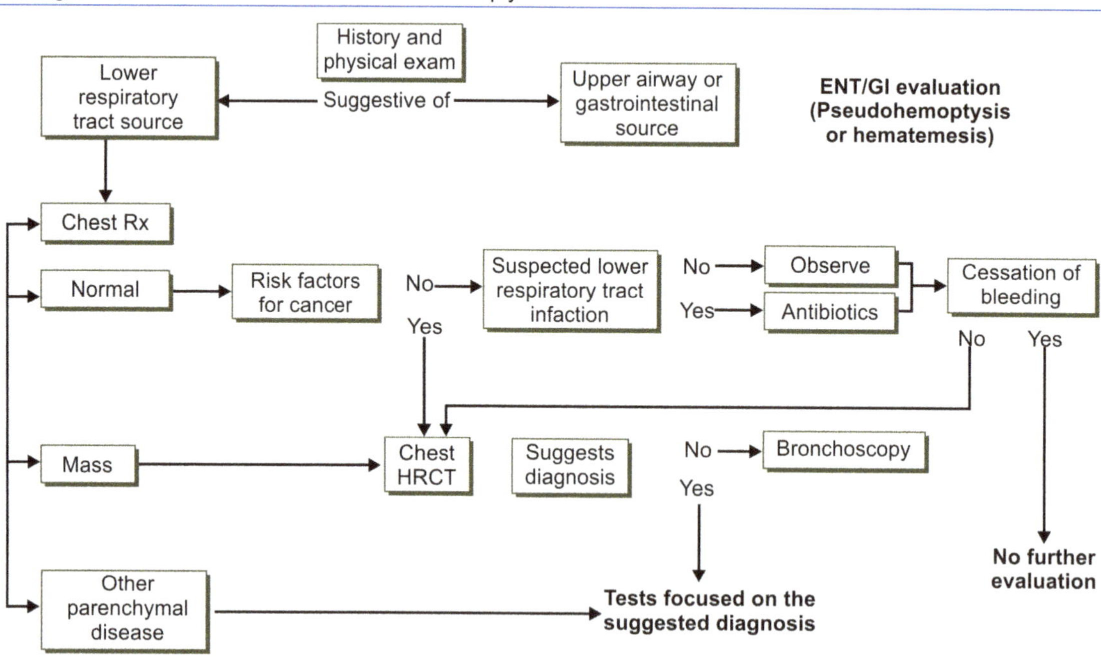

[ENT: Ear, nose, and throat (otorhinolaryngologic); GI: Gastrointestinal; HRCT: High resolution computed tomography].

include *flapping tremor* of the hands, muscle twitches, flushed skin, and dyspnea. Moreover, hypercapnia can increase cardiac output with consequent elevation of arterial blood pressure, full pulse and susceptibility toward extrasystoles or other arrhythmias.

Hoarseness indicates a coarse or rough quality of the voice, whereas *dysphonia* is defined as an alteration in the production of voice that impairs communication or reduces voice-related quality of life. However, the two terms are frequently used as synonyms. They are often caused by benign or self-limited conditions, but they may also be the presenting symptom of more serious or progressive diseases.

Sudden onset of hoarseness almost always indicates an intrinsic laryngeal disease (acute laryngitis), often as a result of a viral infection, trauma, allergic edema or inhaled irritants.

The endoscopic visualization of the larynx (*laryngoscopy*) can be a useful tool in the global evaluation for voice disorders and it is mandatory in cases of chronic hoarseness. Laryngoscopy is the main investigation for the diagnosis of cancer of the larynx, and allows to evaluate laryngeal patency and vocal folds mobility.

In patients with dysphonia subsequent surgery or intubation, a laryngoscopy can be performed at the bedside to identify vocal folds immobility or intubation trauma.

Laryngoscopy is crucial in the evaluation of laryngeal patency after laryngeal trauma, enabling to assess if surgical intervention is required and to follow patients in whom immediate surgery is not necessary.

Unexplained vocal fold paralysis found on laryngoscopy imposes a diagnostic imaging test (CT or MRI) of the skull base and chest for the evaluation of the entire course of the inferior laryngeal nerves. These nerves, called "recurring" (because they loop around the arch of the aorta on the left and the subclavian artery on the right), are the main nerves deputed to the phonatory function, as they innervate all the endolaryngeal muscles responsible for the vocal cords motility. The lesion of a recurring laryngeal nerve (e.g. for cancer or metastasis in one of the lung apices) makes the ipsilateral vocal fold fixed in the paramedian position, with a reduction of the respiratory space and a characteristic dysphonia (bitonal voice). If the lesion is bilateral, both vocal cords are arranged in paramedian position, reducing the space and causing dyspnea.

Hoarseness is also common in patients who use high-dose corticosteroids for the treatment of asthma, as a result of myopathy or mycosis at the level of the vocal folds.

Fever is usually suggestive of an infectious process. If this originates from the respiratory system (or involves it), fever occurs along with symptoms such as cough and dyspnea, as well as laboratory findings like as leukocytosis and increased inflammatory indices. The suspicion of pneumonia can be confirmed by a chest radiograph. If the fever is very high and accompanied by *shaking chills*, it is very likely that the cause is *Streptococcus pneumoniae* (also known as pneumococcus), which usually causes an alveolar opacity at chest radiograph.

Some types of pneumonia, in particular those caused by *intracellular* bacteria (such as *Mycoplasma pneumoniae, Chlamydia species, Legionella pneumophila, Coxiella burnetii)* or viruses, can occur with mild symptoms and low grade fever, while chest radiographic can show significant and variable features. These include, in order of frequency, peribronchial and perivascular interstitial infiltrates, airspace consolidation, reticulonodular opacification, nodular or mass-like opacification, sometimes with pleural effusion and hilar lymphadenopathy. For these reasons they are commonly defined "*atypical*" pneumonia, but none of the radiologic patterns is pathognomonic. Further laboratory tests (e.g. specific antibodies, urinary antigens for *Legionella pneumophila* and pneumococcus) and imaging (chest CT) may facilitate the differential diagnosis.

It should be recalled that a lung infection may overlap with a cancerous growth. Therefore, in case of risk factors for lung cancer, a lung opacity deserves an additional radiological study (by chest CT with contrast or further chest X-ray) after antibiotic therapy, in order to ascertain its resolution.

BIBLIOGRAPHY AND FURTHER READING

1. Alfakih K, Plein S. The NICE guidelines on the assessment of chest pain. J R Soc Med. 2012;105(5):192-4.
2. Boer LM, Asijee GM, van Schayck OC, Schermer TR. How do dyspnoea scales compare with measurement of functional capacity in patients with COPD and at risk of COPD? Prim Care Respir J. 2012;21(2):202-7.
3. Chung KF, Pavord ID. Prevalence, pathogenesis, and causes of chronic cough. Lancet. 2008;371:1364-74.
4. Gigliotti F. Mechanisms of dyspnea in healthy subjects. Multidiscip Respir Med. 2010;5(3):195-201.
5. Gruettner J, Henzler T, Sueselbeck T, Fink C, Borggrefe M, Walter T. Clinical assessment of chest pain and guidelines for imaging. Eur J Radiol. 2012;81(12):3663-8.
6. Guyatt, GH, Berman LB, Townsend M, Pugsley SO, Chambers LW. A measure of quality of life for clinical trials in chronic lung disease. Thorax. 1987;42:773-8.

7. Hwang IC, Kim YJ, Kim KH, Shin DH, Lee SP, Kim HK, et al. Diagnostic yield of coronary angiography in patients with acute chest pain: role of noninvasive test. Am J Emerg Med. 2014;32(1):1-6.
8. Irwin RS, Baumann MH, Bolser DC, Boulet LP, Braman SS, Brightling CE, et al. Diagnosis and management of cough executive summary: ACCP evidence-based clinical practice guidelines. Chest. 2006;129(1 Suppl):1S-23S.
9. Johnston BC, Thorlund K, Schünemann HJ, Xie F, Murad MH, Montori VM, et al. Improving the interpretation of quality of life evidence in meta-analyses: the application of minimal important difference units. Health Qual Life Outcomes. 2010;8:116.
10. Jones PW, Quirk FH, Baveystock CM, Littlejohns P. A self-complete measure of health status for chronic airflow limitation. The St. George's Respiratory Questionnaire. Am Rev Respir Dis. 1992;145:1321-7.
11. Lougheed MD, Turcotte SE, Fisher T. Cough variant asthma: lessons learned from deep inspirations. Lung. 2012;190(1):17-22.
12. McCool FD. Global physiology and pathophysiology of cough: ACCP evidence-based clinical practice guidelines. Chest. 2006;129(1 Suppl):48S-53S.
13. Migliore Norweg A, Whiteson J, Demetis S, Rey M. A new functional status outcome measure of dyspnea and anxiety for adults with lung disease: The dyspnea management questionnaire (DMQ-30). J Cardiopulm Rehabil. 2006;26:395-404.
14. Morice AH, Fontana GA, Belvisi MG, Birring SS, Chung KF, Dicpinigaitis PV, et al. ERS guidelines on the assessment of cough. Eur Respir J. 2007;29:1256-76.
15. Moscato G, Pala G, Cullinan P, Folletti I, Gerth van Wijk R, Pignatti P, et al. EAACI position paper on assessment of cough in the workplace. Allergy. 2014;69:292-304.
16. Norweg A, Jette A, Ni P, Whiteson J, Kim M. Outcome Measurement for COPD: reliability and validity of the Dyspnea Management Questionnaire. Respir Med. 2011;105:442-53.
17. Oga T, Tsukino M, Hajiro T. Analysis of longitudinal changes in dyspnea of patients with chronic obstructive pulmonary disease: an observational study. Respir Res. 2012;13(1):85.
18. Scano G, Stendardi L, Grazzini M. Understanding dyspnoea by its language. Eur Respir J. 2005;25(2):380-5.
19. Tu SP, McDonell MB, Spertus JA, Steele BG, Fihn SD. A new self-administered questionnaire to monitor health-related quality of life in patients with COPD. Ambulatory Care Quality Improvement Project (ACQUIP) Investigators. Chest. 1997;112:614-22.
20. Turcotte SE, Lougheed MD. Cough in asthma. Curr Opin Pharmacol. 2011;11(3):231-7.

Chapter

2

Respiratory Examination

Claudio Pedone, Giuseppe Augugliaro, Claudio Sorino

OVERVIEW OF THE SEMEIOTICS OF THE RESPIRATORY SYSTEM

Physical examination of the chest is a crucial element of respiratory system assessment. Together with the medical history, it provides an important aid in determining the correct diagnosis, often before the laboratory and instrumental examinations are available.

Similarly to what is done for other parts of the body, chest examination includes four phases: (1) inspection, (2) palpation (feeling with the hands), (3) percussion (tapping with the fingers), and (4) auscultation (listening). The examination should be carried out in a quiet, well-lit room; no instruments are required but a phonendoscope. A marking pen and a tape measure can help when pathological changes are observed. For every section of the chest examination, right and left findings should be always compared. Natural landmarks and artificial lines are important in order to locate organs within the chest and to document the location of respiratory assessment findings. Most common thoracic landmarks are described in Box 2.1 and shown in Figures 2.1 and 2.2.

Box 2.1: Most common thoracic landmarks.

Natural landmarks

- *Jugular (or suprasternal) notch*: Between the clavicles, above the manubrium sterni
- *Intercostal spaces*: The space between two adjacent ribs; they are identified starting from the angle of Louis (the sternal angle, formed by the conjunction of the sternum and the manubrium sterni) that corresponds to the second rib
- *Infraclavicular fossae*: It is a triangular depression below the clavicle, at the angle formed by the great pectoral and the deltoid muscle
- *Supraclavicular fossae*: The depression between the clavicle and the anterior margin of the trapezius muscles
- *Suprascapular region*: Above the upper margin of the scapula (or the acromion), between the posterior midline and the lateral margin of the trapezius muscle
- *Scapular region*: The area over the scapula (between the second and the seventh rib), it is divided in supraspinous and infraspinous regions
- *Interscapular region*: The region between the medial borders of the two scapulae

Artificial vertical lines

- *Midsternal line (or anterior middle line)*: From the jugular notch to the xiphoid process (also known as "anterior midline")
- *Marginosternal (or lateral sternal) lines*: Parallel to the midsternal line, run along the vertical edges margins of the sternum
- *Midclavicular lines*: Parallel to the midsternal line, passing from the clavicular midpoint
- *Anterior axillary lines*: Parallel to the midsternal line, passing from the anterior axillary fold
- *Middle axillary line*: Parallel to the midsternal line, passing from the uppermost point of the axillary pit
- *Posterior axillary line*: Parallel to the midsternal line, passing from the posterior axillary fold
- *Scapular lines*: Running down the inferior angle of the scapulae as the arm is in the neutral position, parallel to the spine
- *Paravertebral lines*: Vertical line parallel to the spine running about 1-inch medially to the scapular lines, over the tip of the transverse processes of the vertebrae
- *Midspinal line*: Runs vertically through the posterior spinal processes

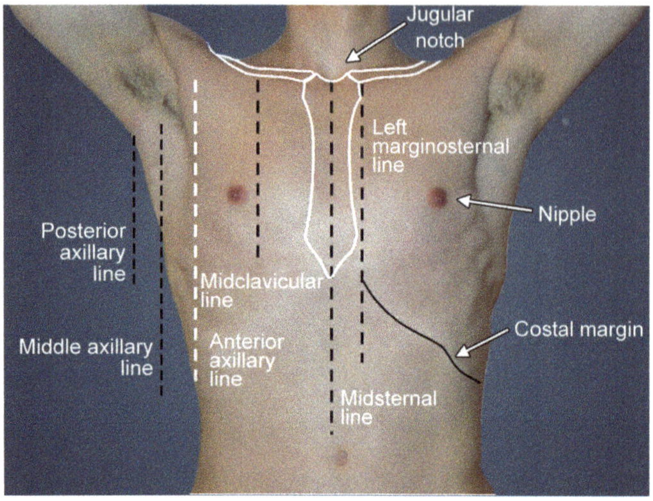

Fig. 2.1: Main landmarks on the anterior chest.

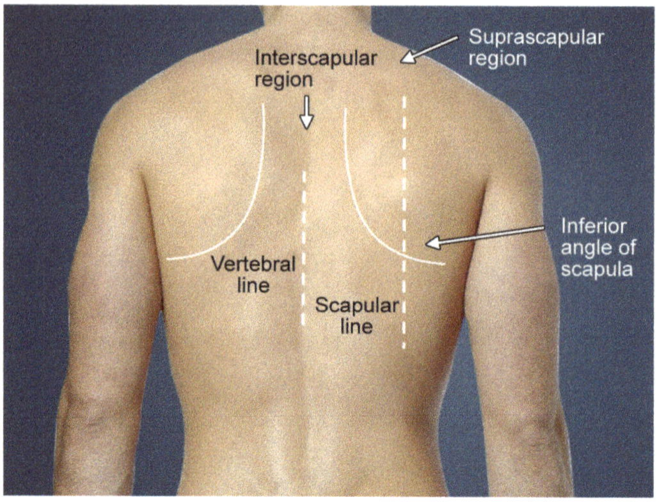

Fig. 2.2: Main landmarks on the posterior chest.

On the chest surface, both pulmonary apices project in the supraclavicular fossa. The upper lobes project mainly on the anterior surface, as well as the middle lobe, while the basal lobes project on the posterior surface. On the anterior thoracic surface, the right upper lobe projects in the region between the clavicula and the fourth intercostal space, while the middle lobe projects between the fourth intercostal space and the diaphragm, that is about at the sixth intercostal space on the parasternal line and at the eighth intercostal space on the middle axillary line. The upper left lobe projects anteriorly on the whole thoracic wall. The posterior projection of the two lungs is similar: the upper lobes project in the right interscapular region above the third thoracic vertebra, while the lower lobes occupy the space from the third thoracic vertebra to the diaphragm, at the ninth intercostal space. Figures 2.3A to D shows the projection of the lungs on anterior, posterior and lateral chest surface.

CHEST INSPECTION

Inspection consists in a methodical, accurate and complete observation of the patient.

In a patient with suspected respiratory disease, it should not be limited to chest, whereas it should include the evaluation of some general aspects, such as the appearance or expression of the face of the patient ("facies"), the preferred posture, the use of accessory respiratory muscles, the presence of nasal flaring, cyanosis.

At inspection, the general *shape* and *symmetry* of the thorax must be evaluated. The patient should be sited, if possible without support, unclothed to the waist. Normally, the ratio between the sagittal diameter (also known as anteroposterior diameter) and coronal (or transverse) diameter of the thorax ranges between 0.5 and 0.7. An increase in the ratio is seen in people with *hyperkyphosis* (exaggerated anterior curvature of the thoracic spine due to posture or vertebral fractures). It is also observed in subjects with *barrel chest*, where the ribs are horizontal, and the increased anteroposterior diameter results in a cylindrical shape of the thorax. Barrel chest can be a feature of severe emphysema, but is also common in elderly people with weight loss and increased thoracic kyphosis (Fig. 2.4).

Asymmetry of the thorax is frequently due to vertebral deformities (scoliosis) that cause an enlargement of the side of vertebral convexity with lung hyperexpansion, and a reduction in volume of the contralateral side, with consensual reduction of lung volume. Other thoracic deformities include:

Pectus carinatum (pigeon chest): It is a deformity characterized by a protrusion of the distal portion of the sternum, with increased anteroposterior diameter and reduction of the vertical diameter. The ribs adjacent to the protruding chest are depressed. This condition can be congenital, but is also seen in rachitic patients.

Pectus excavatum (funnel chest): It is a condition caused by the abnormal growth of ribs and sternum, causing a concavity most evident at the distal sternum. It is the most common congenital chest wall abnormality.

Flail chest: It is characterized by a paradoxical inward movement of a section of the thorax during inspiration and

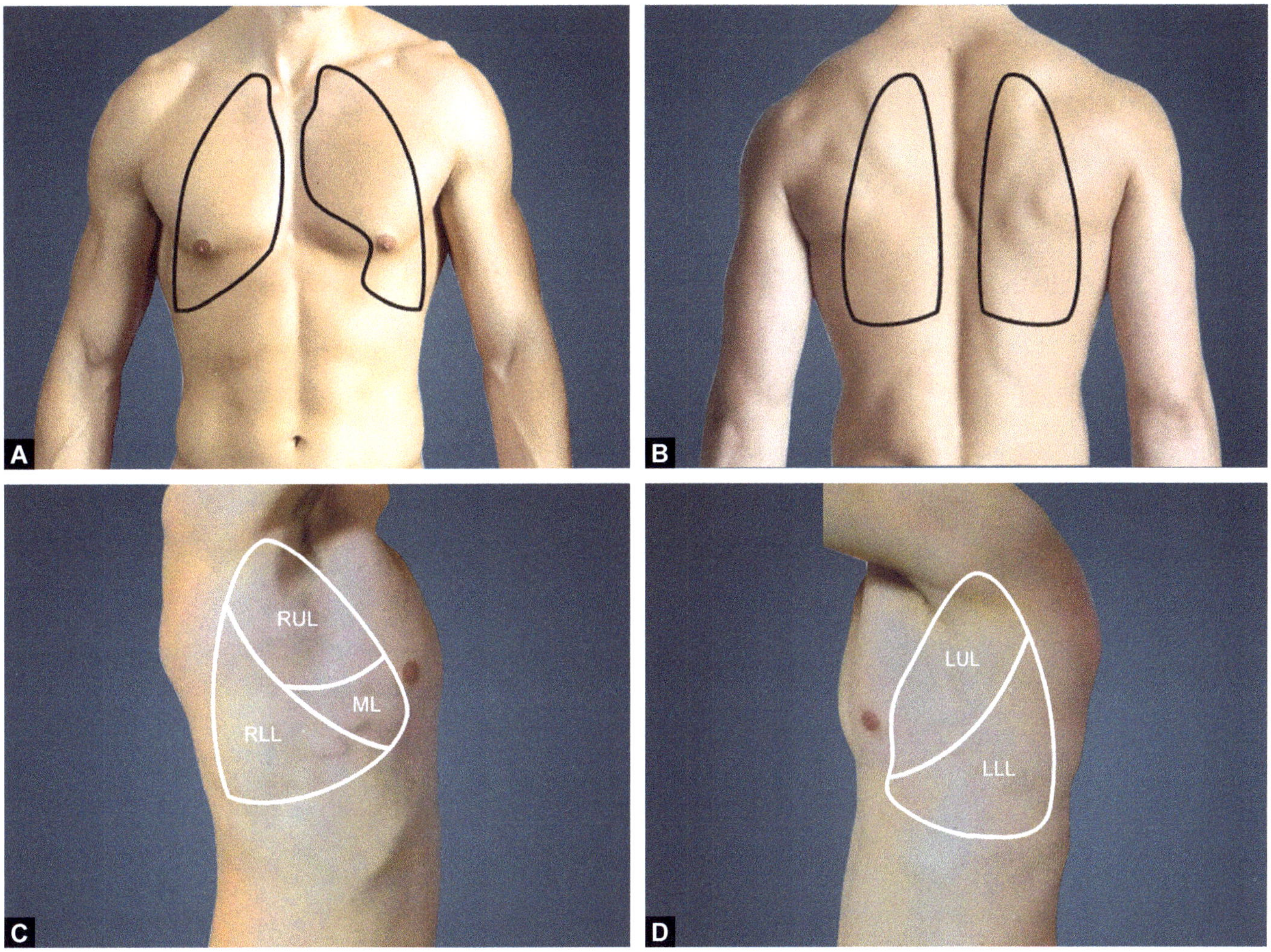

Figs. 2.3A to D: Projection of the lungs on (A) anterior, (B) posterior, and (C and D) lateral chest surfaces. (RUL: Right upper lobe; RLL: Right lower lobe; ML: Middle lobe; LUL: Left upper lobe; LLL: Left lower lobe).

outward movement during expiration. It is due to severe blunt trauma that causes both posterior and anterior fractures of three or more ribs.

Bulging or retraction of the intercostal spaces should be recorded. Uniform bulging of one side of the thorax can be seen in patients with massive pleural effusion, pneumothorax, or severe emphysema. Uniform retraction of one side of the thorax may be due to fibrothorax, atelectasis, or may be the consequence of demolitive lung surgery. Retraction of the intercostal spaces during inspiration can be observed in patients with obstruction to the free inward flux of air.

The *respiratory frequency* should always be recorded by observing the chest movements. It is of fundamental importance to evaluate the respiratory dynamics. The normal respiratory rate is 10–14 per minute, with slightly higher rates in women and infants. The use of accessory muscles should be noted. During normal breathing, muscular effort is required only during inspiration to expand the rib cage while expiration is passive due to the elastic recoil of the lungs. The most important inspiratory muscle is the diaphragm that moves downward during inspiration, causing an outward movement of the abdominal wall that is best seen in men compared to women. An increased length of the expiratory phase with contraction of accessory expiratory muscles (internal intercostal muscles, abdominal wall muscles) may be seen in patients with bronchospasm, while the use of accessory inspiratory muscles (sternocleidomastoid, scalene muscles) may be due to obstruction of the extrathoracic airways or to increased stiffness of the thorax or of the lung (pulmonary fibrosis). An inward motion of the abdominal wall

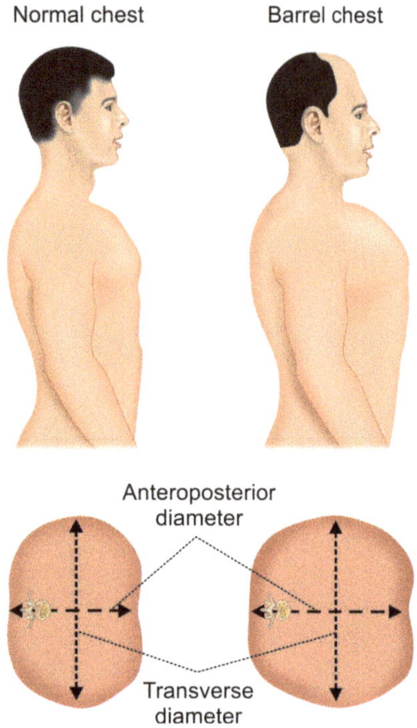

Fig. 2.4: Anteroposterior and transverse diameters in normal and barrel chests.

during inspiration indicates a severe dysfunction of the diaphragm that moves passively upward due to decreased thoracic pressure.

Abnormalities of the respiratory rhythm and pattern should be considered.

Cheyne-Stokes respiration is characterized by a progressive increase in tidal volume, followed by a progressive decrease and an apneic phase, and indicates an increased central hypercapnic ventilatory responsiveness. In *Kussmaul respiration*, seen in severe metabolic acidosis, the respiratory rate decreases with deep respiratory acts. *Biot's respiration* is characterized by irregular breathing with prolonged phases of apnea. It is seen in patients with increased intracranial pressure or lesion of the brain stem.

Asymmetry of thoracic movements during respiration can be due to both pleural and pulmonary diseases. Pleural effusions or pneumothorax can cause a reduction in the movements of the affected size. Complete pneumothorax or massive atelectasis can also cause changes in the size of the affected hemithorax.

Inspection of the thorax should include the observation of skin abnormalities such as scars or eruptions (e.g. vesicular eruption caused by *herpes zoster virus*). The superficial thoracic veins are normally scarcely visible, but may become evident when the vena cava (either inferior or superior) is occluded and collateral circulation is activated. The blood flow in thoracic varicose veins is downward when the superior vena cava is occluded and upward when the inferior vena cava is occluded. The causes of the occlusion of the superior vena cava include thrombosis, mediastinal masses, pericarditis and thoracic aortic aneurisms.

Inspection of the neck should complement the inspection of the thorax. As mentioned above, activation the sternocleidomastoid and scalene muscles can be seen when ventilation is markedly increased, and can also be seen in patients with severe chronic obstructive pulmonary disease (COPD). Distension of the neck veins can be seen in superior vena cava syndrome, in which it is associated with edema of the neck, shoulders and face. It can also be due to increased right atrium pressure in patients with heart failure.

A thorough inspection must also include the evaluation of extrathoracic manifestations of pulmonary diseases. Cyanosis is the appearance of a bluish discoloration of the skin or mucous membranes. It is due to excessive amounts of deoxygenated hemoglobin (*deoxyhemoglobin*) in the blood of the superficial capillaries and venules that become blue-colored. Usually cyanosis is apparent when deoxyhemoglobin is 5 g/dL or greater.

Since the presence of cyanosis depends on the absolute quantity of deoxyhemoglobin, the bluish color is more readily apparent in subjects with high hemoglobin counts than in those with anemia.

In some patients, a bluish tinge to the skin can result from increased amounts of methemoglobin or sulfhemoglobin.

We can distinguish two main forms of cyanosis: (1) central and (2) peripheral.

Central cyanosis is due to desaturation of central arterial blood resulting from cardiac and respiratory disorders that do not allow the venous blood to be oxygenated adequately before flowing into the systemic circulation (shunt effect).

Peripheral cyanosis is caused by decreased local circulation and increased extraction of oxygen in the peripheral tissues. It may occur in conditions associated with peripheral vasoconstriction and stasis of blood in the extremities, which are usually cold (e.g. congestive heart failure, circulatory shock, exposure to cold temperatures, abnormalities of the peripheral circulation). Peripheral cyanosis is often most evident in nail beds, while the mucous membranes of the oral cavity are usually spared. It may resolve just with warming of the extremity.

Pseudocyanosis, on the contrary, refers to a permanent bluish discoloration caused by deposition of blue pigments in the skin.

Nail clubbing is characterized by enlargement of the distal segment of the fingers, with decreased (< 165°) of the angle between the made at the meeting of the nail fold and the nail plate. It can be associated with different lung diseases: lung cancer, bronchiectasis, mesothelioma, lung abscesses. *Peripheral edema* is commonly associated with reduced oxygen saturation and therefore can be seen in patients with respiratory failure, regardless of the coexistence of heart failure.

A *plethoric facies* (i.e. a face too red) may be the expression of elevated red blood cell count (polycythemia), which in turn may be secondary to a chronic respiratory failure. Polycythemia is considered when the hematocrit (HCT) is greater than 48% in women and 52% in men, or when the hemoglobin level is greater than 16.5 g/dL in women or greater than 18.5 g/dL in men.

It can be divided into two categories: (1) primary polycythemia, due to inherent problems in the process of red blood cell production and (2) secondary polycythemia that generally occurs as a response to other factors or underlying conditions promoting red blood cell production.

An example of the latter condition is the upregulation in erythropoietin secretion as a response to prolonged low oxygen levels in the blood (hypoxia).

CHEST PALPATION

The anterior surface of the chest is palpated by placing the palm of both arms flat on the chest wall with the thumbs touching on the midline while the patient is taking deep breaths. The hands are placed first at the angle of Louis, then on the fourth or fifth intercostal space, and finally at the lower costal margin. The posterior chest surface can also be palpated with the patient sitting, by putting the thumbs on the paravertebral lines and the other fingers each on a different intercostal space (Fig. 2.5A). The expansion of the apices can be appreciated by putting the palm of the hand flat on the supraclavicular fossa. The position of the trachea can be determined by placing the thumb and index finger on the lateral aspects of the trachea over the jugular notch. Lateral deviation of the trachea can be caused by mediastinal shift.

During anterior palpation, attention should be paid to the cardiac impulse, usually palpable at the anterior axillary line, at fourth or fifth intercostal space. Although it is not palpable in a large proportion of normal people, lack a palpable apex beat may be a sign of pulmonary emphysema. Palpation of the thorax also is important for the detection of enlarged axillary or supraclavicular lymph nodes. It can also disclose the presence of subcutaneous emphysema.

Most of the alteration of respiration dynamic suspected at inspection can be confirmed by palpation. Attention should be paid to the amplitude and symmetry of the movements, and to the presence of retraction of the costal margin at the end of inspiration, that indicates severe air trapping. Palpation is also of aid in detecting contractions of auxiliary respiratory muscles, by putting the hand on the sternocleidomastoid or on the abdominal wall, and to evaluate the presence of thoracoabdominal dyssynchrony, by putting on hand in the midline on the middle chest and the other on the upper abdomen. During this phase of the physical examination, an end-inspiratory retraction of the costal margin can be appreciated (*Hoover's sign*), indicating pulmonary hyperinflation.

While the subject is speaking, the lung parenchyma and the chest wall normally transmit a palpable vibration known as tactile fremitus. It should be assessed by placing the ulnar aspect of both hands firmly on the posterior chest wall while the patient says the word "ninety-nine". For comparison, both sides should be palpated simultaneously and symmetrically, using one hand quick alternating between the two sides (Fig. 2.5B). The vibration is best appreciated in the region close to the tracheal bifurcation (e.g. the interscapulovertebral region) and in people with low-pitched voice. The tactile fremitus is reduced when an obstruction of the airways block its transmission to the chest wall (e.g. endobronchial neoplasm) or lung elasticity is reduced (e.g. emphysema, pulmonary edema). Tactile fremitus is also reduced or absent in the area over a pleural effusion, but the lung parenchyma above the superior margin of the effusion may be compressed and hence transmits a reinforced vibration. Another cause of reduction or absence of tactile fremitus is pneumothorax. Tactile fremitus is better transmitted by consolidated lung parenchyma, provided that the bronchi are patent, and it is also reinforced in the presence of bronchiectasis or lung excavations.

Palpation of the thorax can also disclose enlarged lymph nodes, especially those of the supraclavicular region and of the axillary region. *Supraclavicular lymph nodes* are best appreciated at the insertion of the sternocleidomastoid on the clavicula. Lymph nodes of the right supraclavicular fossa may be enlarged in patients with pulmonary or intrathoracic diseases; while, because

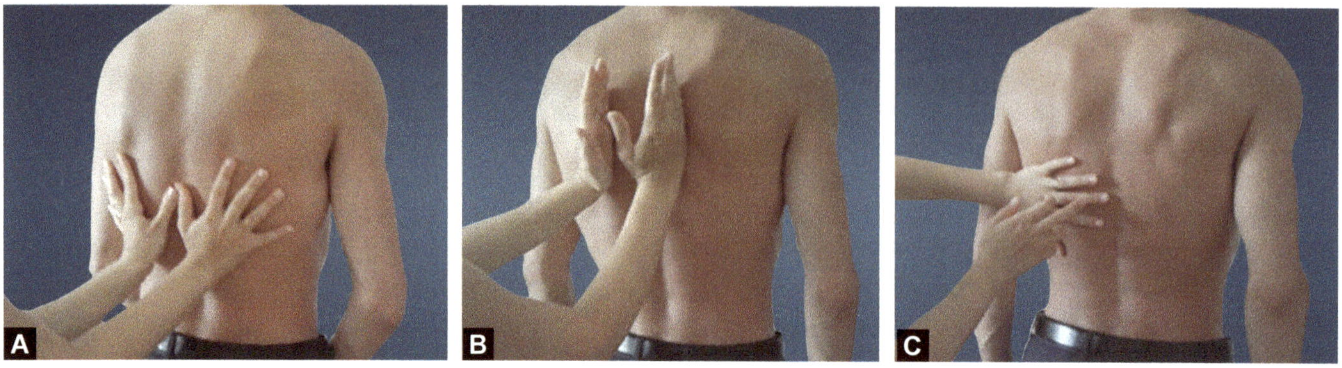

Figs. 2.5A to C: (A) Posterior palpation; (B) Tactile fremitus; (C) Percussion.

the subdiaphragmatic lymphatic drainage enters the venous circulation in the left subclavian vein, nodes in the left supraclavicular fossa may also be enlarged in patients with metastatic neoplasms of the stomach, gallbladder, kidney, ovarium, or testicle (*Virchow-Troisier's lymph node*). Lymph nodes of this region can also be enlarged in patients with tubercular peritonitis. Palpation of these lymph nodes should be performed while the patient is sitting in a neutral position; in particular the head should not be extended or rotated let the gland is compressed by the overlying skin. The characteristics (size, firmness, mobility) of the lymph node should be evaluated by compressing it between the fingers or against the underlying solid structure (e.g. bone), if present.

Axillary lymph nodes are divided into five groups. The lateral axillary nodes receive lymph from the arm and also from the posterior axillary group that drains the posterior chest wall. Anterior axillary lymph nodes drain lymph from the anterior chest wall and the breast. All axillary nodes eventually drain into the central and then apical (subclavian) groups that can be enlarged in pulmonary or mediastinal diseases. Palpation of the axillary lymph nodes is performed while the patient is sitting, with the arm abducted between 45° and 90°.

Moreover, chest palpation can also disclose the presence of a *crepitus*, a crackling sensation, can be heard and palpated under the skin during palpation. It indicates air in the subcutaneous tissue from rupture somewhere in the respiratory system or by infection with a gas-producing organism. Subcutaneous emphysema usually affects the neck or thorax, but it may also be found in the supraclavicular regions, abdominal wall, perineal region, or upper or lower limbs. In every circumstance, the *crepitus* requires attention.

CHEST PERCUSSION

There are two types of chest percussion: (1) direct and (2) indirect. "Direct" percussion of the thorax is usually used to explore the apexes and is performed by rapping with the tip of the middle finger on the middle third of the clavicles. "Indirect" percussion is performed rapping the middle finger of the dominant hand (plexor) on the distal interphalangeal joint of the index or middle finger of the opposite hand (pleximeter) that is firmly put flat on the region of interest (Fig. 2.5C). The pleximeter should not be placed directly on the ribs but rather on the intercostal spaces; the plexor should be promptly removed from the pleximeter to allow the propagation of the sound. During this phase of physical examination, the patient should be sitting with the arms crossed and the hands on the opposite shoulder, in order to move the scapulae laterally and clear as much as possible the region over the apexes. The percussion of the posterior thorax should begin in the region between the scapulae and the spine, proceeding from the top downward. The normal lung parenchyma produces a "resonant" sound that is a relatively loud and low pitched. It should be distinguished from other sounds such as the dull sound (normally heard percussing the area over the liver) or the hyperresonant sound that is louder and with a lower pitch compared to the resonant sound. Since the lung is contiguous with solid organs (heart, liver, spleen), it is possible to identify the borders of the lung by examining the changes in the sound elicited by percussion (*topographic percussion*).

The pulmonary apices can be delimited by identifying the Kronig's area: putting the pleximeter finger perpendicular to the superior border of the trapezius muscle and on the scapular line, and performing the percussion moving both medially and laterally, an area of resonant sound between two areas of dull sound caused by the muscles can be appreciated. It is usually 4–5 cm in width. The anterior pulmonary border can be delimited by following the resonant sound produced by a light percussion over the anterior chest wall. The percussion should begin on the midclavicular line at the second intercostal space and then proceeding medially and downward. On the horizontal line, the resonant sound is usually present up to the parasternal line. On the vertical line, on the right, the resonant sound is usually appreciated from the second to the sixth intercostal space, then the presence of the liver cause the sound to become more dull. On the left, the resonant sound is appreciated from the second to the fourth intercostal space, then the presence of the heart cause the sound to become more dull. Hence, the border of the lung can be followed moving the pleximeter laterally and then again downward to delimit the lingula. The area of resonant sound thus delimited becomes smaller in patients with cardiomegaly, mediastinal masses, or pulmonary sclerosis, while becomes larger in patients with pulmonary emphysema.

The inferior border of the lung is identified by light percussion along the vertical lines. Normally, the border between the resonant sound and the area of dullness due to surrounding organs is at the sixth intercostal space on the hemidiaphragm, on the seventy or eight intercostal space on the middle axillary line and on the tenth intercostal space on the paravertebral lines. The *Traube's space* is an area of hyperresonant sound due to the gastric bubble that is delimited by the sixth rib superiorly, the left costal margin inferiorly and the anterior axillary line laterally. Loss of this area of hyperresonance is seen in left pleural effusions.

A dull sound is appreciated in conditions that cause a reduction of the air content of the lung (e.g. atelectasis), or when air is substituted with fluid or solid tissue (e.g. flogosis, neoplasm). Dullness can also be present when there is liquid between the lung and the chest wall, as is the case in pleural effusions. Pleural effusions are typically appreciated at the base of the lungs; when the liquid is rich in protein (exudate), the upper margin of the area of dullness is convex with the highest point on the posterior axillary line. Because of a contralateral shift of the mediastinum caused by the effusion, a triangle of dullness can be present on the other side, delimited by the spine and the diaphragm. Diseases that increase the air content of the lung, such as pneumothorax, emphysema or excavations, cause the sound to become hyperresonant. See Table 2.1 for a list of causes of changes in pulmonary resonance.

Table 2.1: Causes of abnormal findings at percussion.

Dullness	Pleural effusion
	Pneumonia
	Atelectasis
	Neoplasm
	Marked pleural thickening
Hyperresonance	Pneumothorax
	Cavitation (e.g. tuberculosis, abscesses)
	Pulmonary emphysema

Percussion is fundamental to evaluate diaphragmatic mobility. The diaphragm is usually higher on the right than on the left because it sits over the bulk of the liver. In order to measure diaphragmatic excursion, the patient should take a deep breath and hold it. The percussion should be done along the scapular line until the lower limit of lungs, a point marked by a change in note from resonance to dullness. This point could be marked with a skin pencil at the scapular line. Now the patient is allowed to breathe, the percussion is repeated. The whole procedure could be repeated on the other side. The distance in centimeters between the marks on each side is recorded. Normally, the diaphragm shifts about 3–5 cm downward during inspiration. When percussion is performed over the posterior thoracic wall, an area of "relative" dullness can be appreciated where the lung parenchyma overlaps the liver or the spleen, about at the eight intercostal space, and of dullness two intercostal spaces below that line, because there is no more lung parenchyma between the chest wall and the solid organs. During maximal inspiration, the line between the resonant sound and the relative dullness shifts downward of about 2 cm. Causes of reduction of diaphragmatic movement are:

- Pulmonary fibrosis, in which the fibrotic lung parenchyma attracts the diaphragm, with an upward shift of the dullness line and loss or reduction of change in the dullness area due to reduced lung expansion
- Pulmonary emphysema, with downward shift of the diaphragm due to pulmonary hyperinflation and loss or reduction of change in the dullness area
- Ascites, liver or spleen enlargement, abdominal masses, subphrenic abscesses cause an upward shift of the diaphragm
- Diaphragmatic paralysis, with asymmetric upward shift of the affected hemidiaphragm.

Suspected abnormalities of the diaphragmatic position should be confirmed by a chest X-ray, while diaphragmatic mobility can be studied by ultrasonography.

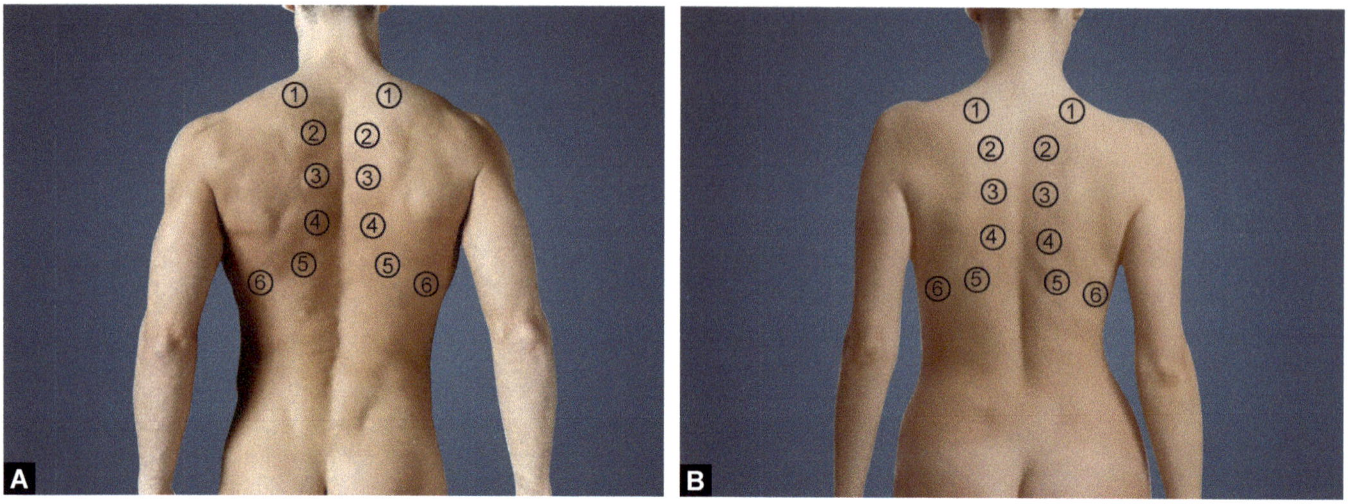

Figs. 2.6A and B: Sites of posterior chest auscultation.

CHEST AUSCULTATION

Auscultation provides information on the airways and the lung parenchyma. It can be performed either with the membrane or the bell of the stethoscope; sounds with higher frequency are best heard with the former, sound with lower frequency with the latter. During auscultation, the patient should be breathing deeply with the mouth open, in order to increase the flux of air in the airways. When the individual breath sound is being evaluated, there should be no movement of patient or stethoscope except for the respiratory excursion. Even if most of the pathological findings are usually found at the auscultation of patient's posterior chest walls (Figs. 2.6A and B), the auscultation of anterior chest is also recommended during physical examination.

Normally, the lung parenchyma produces a *vesicular murmur* sound that is best heard during inspiration, while the bronchi produce a louder, higher pitched sound that is typically heard over the trachea. The bronchial sound is not normally heard elsewhere. The intensity of the vesicular sound is proportional to the airflow in the region being examined, thus it is louder at the bases than at the upper lobes. A reduction or abolition of the vesicular sound indicates a consolidation of the lung parenchyma due to infection or neoplasm, or the presence of air (e.g. pneumothorax) or fluid (e.g. pleural effusions) between the lung and the thoracic wall. In these situations, the bronchial sound can usually be heard over the affected area. In people with reduced alveolar ventilation without alveolar consolidation, a reduced vesicular sound is heard along with the bronchial sound, resulting in what is sometimes referred to as *bronchovesicular* sound. This sound can also be heard at the apex of the right lung, where the alveolar component is normally minimal.

Vocal resonance is evaluated in the same way as the tactile fremitus is, by asking the patient to say the word "ninety-nine". Normally, the word is less loud and clear when heard through the stethoscope on the chest wall. In the presence of parenchymal consolidation without bronchial obstruction, vocal resonance is increased in both loudness and clarity (*bronchophony*). In some cases, usually when the consolidation is accompanied by a small pleural effusion, the vocal resonance is not only increased, but also has a "bleating" or nasal quality, with the vowel "E" heard as "A" (*egophony*).

During auscultation, additional sounds can be appreciated (Table 2.2):

Rhonchi: Low-pitched sounds that resemble snoring. They are usually caused by thick exudate in the larger bronchi and are typically heard in patients with inflamed bronchial walls (e.g. acute or chronic bronchitis).

Crackles: They are best heard during inspiration and occur when fluid is present in the airways. The crackles are fine when the air opens alveoli that are filled with fluid, e.g. in the early and final phases of pneumonia, and in pulmonary edema. In this latter case, crackles are first present at the basis because of gravity, then they spread to the upper pulmonary fields. Fine crackles with a characteristic "Velcro" sound are present in patients with interstitial

Table 2.2: Causes of adventitious pulmonary sounds.

Rhonchi	Acute or chronic inflammation of the airways
Crackles	Acute pulmonary edema
	Heart failure
	Pneumonia (only at onset or during resolution)
	Pulmonary fibrosis ("Velcro" sounds)
Wheezes	Bronchospasm (asthma, exacerbated chronic obstructive pulmonary disease, acute bronchitis)
	Acute pulmonary edema ("cardiac asthma")
Stridor	Laryngeal stenosis (inflammation, neoplasm, foreign body)
	Tracheal stenosis (flogosis, neoplasm, foreign body, scars, tracheomalacia)
Pleural rubs	Pleuritis
	Pericarditis

lung disease. In such cases, idiopathic pulmonary fibrosis should be considered. When the sound originates from the airways, it becomes coarser as the size of the affected airways increases.

Wheezes: High-pitched sounds best heard during expiration that are caused by the passage of air through narrowed airways, as is typical during asthma attacks or exacerbated chronic bronchitis.

Stridor: it is similar to wheezes in quality, but tends to be louder and is usually heard during inspiration. It is often associated with the use of accessory inspiratory muscles and intercostal retraction. It is often due to laryngeal stenosis caused by foreign bodies, laryngeal edema or spasm, croup, or neoplasm. It can also be caused by tracheal stenosis, either fixed (e.g. scars, neoplasm, goiter) or dyna mic (tracheomalacia).

Pleural rubs: the sound is similar to the rubbing of leather, and is due to the friction between the inflamed and roughened visceral and parietal pleurae. Pleural rubs are present during both inspiration and expiration, and are synchronous with respiration. Rubs that are not synchronous with respiration and that are present also during apnea are due to inflammation of pericardial membranes.

BIBLIOGRAPHY AND FURTHER READING

1. Cottin V, Cordier JF. Velcro crackles: the key for early diagnosis of idiopathic pulmonary fibrosis? Eur Respir J. 2012;40:519-21.
2. Dalmay F, Antonini MT, Marquet P, et al. Acoustic properties of the normal chest. Eur Respir J. 1995;8:1761-9.
3. Meslier N, Charbonneau G, Racineux JL. Wheezes. Eur Respir J. 1995;8:1942-8.
4. Pasterkamp H, Brand PLP, Everard M, et al. Towards the standardisation of lung sound nomenclature. Eur Respir J. 2016;47:724-32
5. Piirilä P, Sovijärvi AR. Crackles: recording analysis and clinical significance. Eur Respir J. 1995;8:2139-48.
6. Simpson H. Respiratory assessment. Br J Nurs. 2006 May 11-24;15(9):484-8.
7. Sovijärvi AR, Dalmasso F, Vanderschoot J, et al. Definition of terms for applications of respiratory sounds. Eur Respir Rev. 2000;10:597-610.

Chapter

3

Clinical Utility and Interpretation of Laboratory Tests in Respiratory Medicine

Damiano Magrì, Giada Oliviero, Giuseppe Milani, Claudio Sorino

OVERVIEW OF LABORATORY TESTS IN RESPIRATORY MEDICINE

Several laboratory tests on blood samples are used to support the diagnosis and monitor the treatment of respiratory diseases. Most of them are useful tools in the evaluation of infectious diseases [e.g. blood count and marker of systemic inflammation such as C-reactive protein (CRP), erythrocyte sedimentation rate (ESR), and procalcitonin (PCT)]. They are not specific for a respiratory tract involvement, but constitute valid indicators of the severity of disease and may represent early warnings of possible complications including sepsis and septic shock. Some limitations in their use exist, related to logistical factors (e.g. unavailability of the required test) or confounding factors (e.g. multiple diseases or advanced age of the patients), so that they should always be correlated to the clinical findings.

A few antigen and antibody assays on blood or urine samples are available to help the etiologic diagnosis of certain acute respiratory infections. Each diagnostic test has limitations with respect to sensitivity, and/or specificity and/or speed of execution and obtaining the result. In addition, despite the use of such tests in combination with cultural examinations, the etiologic agent is not found in the majority of cases. Consequently, the empirical approach is still the most widespread practice in acute respiratory tract infections.

Other laboratory tests are useful in the differential diagnosis of acute and chronic dyspnea [e.g. D-dimer and brain natriuretic peptide (BNP)], while other blood substances, known as tumor markers, are measured to help diagnosis, prognosis and monitoring of neoplastic diseases.

BLOOD COUNT

A complete blood count (CBC) gives a lot of information, including the number and quality of erythrocytes [or red blood cells (RBCs)], leukocytes [or white blood cells (WBCs)], and platelets (Table 3.1). Despite both hemoglobin and erythrocytes can vary during respiratory tract infections, the main target of blood count analysis in such a suspicion is WBC count. Indeed, most infections occur with an increase in total leukocytes (leukocytosis). The extent of the increased number of leukocytes is relative to both the underlying pathogen and the efficiency of the host immune system.

White blood cell differential count is usually included as part of a CBC. It provides absolute value and relative percentage of each type of WBC, namely neutrophils, lymphocytes, monocytes, eosinophils and basophils. Since neutrophils represent the largest quote of leukocytes, they have the greatest influence on the variations of total WBC count.

Normal values for WBC and differential count are age-related. WBC count is highest in children under 1 year of age (mainly in the lymphocyte population) and then decreases somewhat until adulthood. Table 3.2 shows the normal ranges for differential WBC count in adults. It should be noted that the reference ranges may vary according to the population studies, laboratory, instruments and methods.

Neutrophils are one of the most important types of WBC in fighting infections. Thus, leukocytosis due to infections usually consists mainly of neutrophils, with bacterial infections being more likely to give increased leukocytes counts than viral infections. This can occur in minutes or

Table 3.1: Information included in a complete blood count.

Parameter	Meaning
Red blood cells (RBC) count	Total number of RBC per microliter of blood
White blood cells (WBC) count	Total number of WBC per microliter of blood
Hemoglobin (Hb) level	Total amount of hemoglobin in the blood
Hematocrit (Hct)	Fraction of the blood made up of RBC
Mean corpuscular volume (MCV)	Average RBC size
Mean corpuscular hemoglobin (MCH)	Average amount of Hb per RBC
Mean corpuscular Hb concentration (MCHC)	Average concentration of Hb per RBC
Platelet count	Number of platelets per microliter of blood
WBC differential count	Different types of WBC expressed as a percentage

Table 3.2: Reference ranges for differential white blood cell count in normal adults.

Cells	Absolute values	Percentage (%)
All leukocytes	4,500–11,000/µL	
Neutrophils	2.0–7.0 × 10^9/L	40–80
Lymphocytes	1.0–3.0 × 10^9/L	20–40
Monocytes	0.2–1.0 × 10^9/L	2–10
Eosinophils	0.02–0.5 × 10^9/L	1–6
Basophils	0.02–0.1 × 10^9/L	0–2

hours from the beginning of the infection. Neutrophils are released from bone marrow as immature forms called "bands", whose number increases in circulating blood as a consequence of bacterial infections. The two compartments where immature and activated neutrophils can be found include the circulating compartment and the marginal compartment (attached to the endothelium of blood vessels). WBC count reflects the leukocytes present within the blood and not those in the bone marrow, tissue or attached to the endovascular lining of blood vessels. Severe infections may lead to an enhanced neutrophil utilization at the site of infection, with depletion of the marrow's storage pool and peripheral neutropenia rather than neutrophilia. Accordingly, neutropenia can facilitate infection but can also be the consequence of infection.

The interpretation of leukocytes values is harder in elderly people than in adults. Due to the wide variability of normal WBC count, punctual values could give little information, if not compared to previous data. An elevation above 25,000 cells/µL is more likely to be associated with acute severe infections, and a high leukocyte count has been demonstrated to be related with higher death rate.

A WBC count higher than 50,000 cells/µL due to causes other than leukemia is named *leukemoid reaction*. Infections and the administration of hematopoietic growth factors or all-trans retinoic acid are the major causes of a leukemoid reaction.

In the absence of an increase in total leukocyte count, a relative increase in neutrophils can help find an infection, whereas a relative increase in eosinophils or lymphocytes can be associated with other specific conditions.

A relative reduction of eosinophils (eosinopenia) can be induced by stress reactions, Cushing's syndrome, or the use of corticosteroids. It may also occur in acute infections and is considered a negative prognostic factor, being associated to worse outcomes, mainly in certain conditions as acute exacerbations of chronic obstructive pulmonary disease (COPD).

Cigarette smoking has been positively linked to an increase in neutrophils, with a strong relation between pack/years and leukocytes increase. They may reset to normal values in 1 or 2 years after smoking cessation, but longer periods of increased leukocytes in blood count are reported.

Several medications and noninfectious conditions may affect the WBC count (Box 3.1). The treatment with glucocorticoids (e.g. methylprednisolone, prednisone, dexamethasone) or catecholamines (e.g. epinephrine) causes an increase of polymorphonuclear leukocytes in blood. This is mainly due to WBCs shifting from the marginated to circulating pools (increased rate of entrance from marrow and a decreased rate of removal from the vascular), as a result of downregulation of adhesion molecule expression. As a consequence, patients with acute exacerbation of COPD treated with systemic corticosteroids may have an improvement of clinical conditions and inflammation markers, whereas a transitory increase in WBC count may be observed.

On the contrary, the number of lymphocytes, eosinophils, monocytes and basophils decreases after administration of glucocorticoids.

An elevated WBC count may also occur in allergy, systemic illness, inflammation, tissue injury and leukemia (Box 3.2). A low number of WBC (leukopenia) may occur in some viral infections, immunodeficiency states, and bone marrow failure (Box 3.3). The lower the number of neutrophils, the higher is the risk of infection.

Box 3.1: Medications able to modify white blood cell (WBC) count.

Drugs that may increase WBC count:

- Beta-adrenergic agonists (e.g. albuterol)
- Corticosteroids
- Epinephrine
- Granulocyte colony-stimulating factor
- Heparin
- Lithium

Drugs that may lower WBC count:

- Antibiotics
- Anticonvulsants
- Antithyroid drugs
- Arsenicals
- Captopril
- Chemotherapy drugs
- Chlorpromazine
- Clozapine
- Diuretics
- Histamine-2 blockers
- Sulfonamides
- Quinidine
- Terbinafine
- Ticlopidine

Box 3.2: Causes of high white blood cell count (leukocytosis).

- Anemia
- Some drugs or medications
- Cigarette smoking
- Infections, especially those caused by bacteria
- Inflammatory disease (e.g. rheumatoid arthritis or allergy)
- Leukemia
- Intense mental or physical stress
- Tissue damage (e.g. burns)

Box 3.3: Causes of low white blood cell count (leukopenia).

- Bone marrow deficiency or failure (e.g. due to infection, tumor, or abnormal scarring)
- Cancer treating drugs, or other medicines
- Some autoimmune disorders (e.g. systemic lupus erythematosus)
- Disease of the liver or spleen
- Radiation treatment for cancer
- Some viral diseases (e.g. mononucleosis)
- Cancers that damage the bone marrow
- Very severe bacterial infections

Neutropenia, defined as an absolute neutrophils count less than 1,500 cell/μL, may be the expression of severe sepsis and septic shock, and it is a predictor of worse outcome in patients with respiratory infection. The evaluation of circulating inflammation markers such as CRP and PCT (*see* below) is recommended when a leukocyte reduction is observed in the absence of clinical improvement, to monitor the possible evolution toward sepsis.

For the same reason, blood count should be repeated at regular intervals to allow a correct evaluation of the evolving disease. Exact timing depends on many factors, both related to the clinical and logistical situation.

Chronic inflammatory disorders, be they of respiratory (like bronchiectasis or cystic fibrosis) or systemic nature [like rheumatoid arthritis (RA)], have been linked to a chronic increase in leukocytes count. Relative increase in leukocytes subsets, which can appear without an increase in the total number of leukocytes (relative leukocytosis), is linked to other diagnostic hypotheses. For example, an increase in eosinophils can be seen in some acute and chronic respiratory diseases such as eosinophilic pneumonia, eosinophilic granulomatosis with polyangiitis (also known as Churg-Strauss disease) or in extrinsic allergic alveolitis. Eosinophilia may also be associated with allergy, helminth infections, neoplasia and the hypereosinophilic syndromes.

Eosinophilia can be classed as mild greater than 500 cells/μL, moderate greater than 500 cells/μL but less than 1,500 cells/μL, or severe greater than 1,500 cells/μL. Note that eosinophilia refers to an absolute eosinophil count in peripheral blood. A mild-to-moderate eosinophilia may be observed in patients with asthma, while a severe eosinophilia should direct toward different diagnostic hypothesis, including malignancy.

An increase in lymphocytes can be related to acute viral infections (e.g. mononucleosis). An increase in monocytes can be found in various diseases including sepsis, tuberculosis, sarcoidosis. Moreover, lymphocytic or monocytic leukocytosis raises the suspect of bone marrow malignancy (leukemia). Leukocytosis linked to leukemia in its acute form usually presents with cell counts higher than 50,000 cells/μL, while chronic forms can present with lower values, especially during latency.

C-REACTIVE PROTEIN

More than forty plasma proteins have been defined as *"acute phase proteins"*, based on changes in their circulating concentration of at least 25% after an inflammatory stimulus.

C-reactive protein is a member of the pentraxin family of proteins, which are nonspecific, acute-phase reactant proteins. It is synthesized by the liver in response to a number of acute and chronic inflammatory stimuli, in particular interleukin-6 (IL-6), and then excreted into the bloodstream. Normal serum concentration of CRP in healthy humans is usually lower than 10 mg/L, slightly increasing with aging.

C-reactive protein function is to activate the complement system after binding to the phosphocholine expressed on the surface of dead or dying cells and some bacteria. This promotes phagocytosis by macrophages of necrotic and apoptotic cells and bacteria.

The plasma levels of CPR rise quickly in case of inflammatory conditions such as bacterial, viral, or fungal infections.

The levels of CRP increase within 4–8 hours after the onset of the inflammatory process and reach a peak within 2–3 days, sometimes with values even greater than 500 mg/L (Fig. 3.1). Usually the increase in CRP precedes the classical symptoms of inflammation such as fever and pain. When the inflammation ceases, the values of CRP return to the normal range. Overall, the possible causes of increase in polymerase chain reaction (PCR) include:

- Bacterial and viral infections (except in limited processes such as impetigo, ear infections and cystitis)
- Acute articular rheumatism (AAR)
- Systemic lupus erythematosus (SLE)
- Rheumatoid arthritis
- Malignancies
- Myocardial infarction (MI)
- Abdominal abscesses
- Peritonitis
- Crohn's disease
- Trauma and burns.

The determination of CRP value is also useful for:

- Assessing the effectiveness of anti-inflammatory therapies
- Assessing the occurrence of infections in patients at risk (as in the postoperative)
- Monitoring of chronic inflammatory diseases.

Circulating CRP levels under 10 mg/L have historically been regarded as clinically insignificant. About two-thirds of the general population in most developed countries has plasma CRP levels under 3 mg/L. Recently, several studies have shown an association between slightly elevated CRP plasma levels (between mg/L and 10 mg/L) and the risk of developing cardiovascular disease, metabolic syndrome and colon cancer. This probably reflects a low level of underlying chronic inflammation that occurs in many of these conditions.

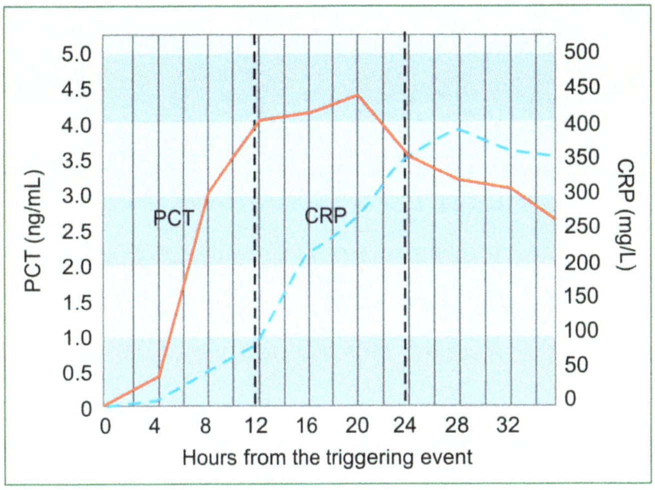

Fig. 3.1: Example of trends in blood levels of CRP and PCT after a major acute inflammatory stimulus.
(CRP: C-reactive protein; PCT: Procalcitonin).

Rapid tests for CRP were introduced into general practice about 20 years ago. CRP levels are frequently increased in association with respiratory tract infections, and CRP levels can be monitored to assess therapy efficacy. Usually, in patients with suspected low respiratory tract infection (LRTI), the administration of antibiotics may be avoided if CRP levels are less than 20 mg/L.

ERYTHROCYTE SEDIMENTATION RATE

The ESR is the rate at which RBCs sediment in a period of 1 hour and is a nonspecific measure of inflammation. Normal ESR values tend to rise with age and are slightly higher in females.

The ESR is usually increased in pregnancy, inflammation, anemia and RA.

It can sometimes be useful in diagnosing some diseases where the ESR may exceed 100 mm/hour such as multiple myeloma, temporal arteritis, polymyalgia rheumatica, various autoimmune diseases, SLE, RA, inflammatory bowel disease and chronic kidney diseases.

It can be reduced in conditions such as polycythemia, sickle cell anemia, hereditary spherocytosis and congestive heart failure.

PROCALCITONIN

Procalcitonin is a peptide precursor of the hormone calcitonin. In healthy individuals (adults and children older

Table 3.3: Conditions associated with an increase of serum procalcitonin (PCT) levels.	
Causes of mild rise (PCT 0.15–2 ng/mL)	*Causes of marked rise (PCT > 2 ng/mL)*
Localized mild-to-moderate bacterial infection	Bacterial sepsis
Noninfectious systemic inflammatory response	Severe localized bacterial infection (e.g. severe pneumonia, meningitis, peritonitis)
Untreated end-stage renal failure	Severe noninfectious inflammatory stimuli (e.g. major burns, severe trauma, acute multiorgan failure, major abdominal or cardiothoracic surgery)
Renal involvement in pediatric urinary tract infections	Medullary thyroid carcinoma (may exceed 10,000 ng/mL)

than 72 hours), the values of serum PCT are commonly below the limit of detection 0.05 ng/mL of clinical assays. The level of PCT rises in a response to several proinflammatory stimuli, especially bacterial infections. In such situations, PCT is produced mainly by the cells of the lung and the intestine (Table 3.3). PCT does not rise significantly with viral or noninfectious inflammations. Noninfectious inflammatory stimuli need to be extremely severe to result in PCT elevations. Levels of PCT higher than 2.0 ng/mL are highly suggestive of systemic bacterial infection, sepsis or severe localized bacterial infection.

Procalcitonin starts to increase faster than CRP, and becomes detectable within 2-4 hours after a triggering event and peaks after 12-24 hours (*see* Fig. 3.1). In serum, PCT has a half-life of 25-30 hours. The high PCT levels produced during infections are not followed by a parallel increase in calcitonin or a decrease in serum calcium levels.

Measurement of PCT can be used as a marker of severe sepsis caused by bacteria and generally grades well with the degree of sepsis. After validation in different trials in the intensive care unit (ICU), PCT has been proposed and tested to assess bacterial infections and to drive diagnosis and treatment in patients outside of intensive care.

Procalcitonin level can help guide antibiotic therapy in patients with suspected or confirmed respiratory low tract infection. Serial testing of PCT levels (daily or every 2 days) may be a successful strategy to monitor the clinical course, adjust the duration of antibiotic therapy and identify nonresponders in severe infections. Serum PCT measurement may not be available in some laboratories.

LABORATORY DIAGNOSIS OF PNEUMONIA

Microbiology

The diagnosis of pneumonia is purely clinical, and is based on the medical history, physical examination and imaging. Only after the diagnosis has been made, laboratory tests may be useful and should be requested in relation to the severity of the disease. A close collaboration between clinicians, radiologists and microbiologists can guide the choice of the most appropriate tests to reach the etiological diagnosis. However, this remains unknown in more than half of the cases of infection of the lower respiratory tract.

Establishing the etiology of a respiratory tract infection is complicated by the frequent presence, at this site, of many microorganisms that are normal flora or commensals.

The finding of *Streptococcus pneumoniae, Klebsiella pneumoniae, Haemophilus influenzae,* and *Moraxella catarrhalis* as the predominant microorganisms in a sample of respiratory secretions from a patient with pneumonia highly suggests its pathogenic role.

The samples of respiratory secretions which can be used for microscopic examination and culturing include expectorated sputum, endotracheal aspirate, bronchial aspirate and bronchoalveolar lavage.

Ideally such samples, as well as blood cultures (at least two sets), should be collected for bacterial culture prior to start antibiotic therapy.

Early morning sputum samples are preferred since they contain pooled overnight secretions where probably the concentration of pathogenic bacteria is higher.

Sputum samples should be carefully collected to reduce contamination by the flora of the oropharynx, through which the sputum passes. The patient should brush his teeth and gargle immediately prior to collection.

If sputum is scant, its collection can be effectively facilitated through the inhalation of nebulized saline. The samples should be processed as soon as possible.

The sensitivity of Gram's stain is quite low (about 10^5 CFU/mL are needed to be positive). A useful quality assurance tool is the comparison of Gram's stain and cultures. If organisms found in the sputum smear do not grow in culture or if organisms that grow in culture are not seen in smear, the results should be reviewed.

If the patient has produced an adequate sputum specimen (not salivary, > 25 neutrophils and < 10 epithelial cells per high-power field), the presence of typical organisms suggestive of either *S. pneumoniae* (Gram-positive diplococci) or *Haemophilus* (small Gram-negative rods) has specificity up to 97–99% in most studies, while sensitivity is 60–80%.

Respiratory samples can also be suitable for respiratory virus detection (influenza, parainfluenza, adenovirus, respiratory syncytial virus and metapneumovirus), particularly, during influenza season. Usually nose/throat swab with influenza PCR is the first exam performed when a viral respiratory infection is suspected. Influenza PCR testing from a nasopharyngeal aspirate or lower tract sample may be repeated in order to confirm a diagnosis in patients with initial negative results from nose/throat.

Mycobacterial Ziehl-Neelsen [acid-fast bacilli (AFB)] stain and culture should be considered in the appropriate clinical circumstance, and is a particular concern in the elderly, immunosuppressed and immigrants from countries with high tuberculosis prevalence (*see* the relevant chapter).

In the presence of significant amount of pleural fluid, this should be aspirated for microscopy, biochemistry and culture (*see* the relevant chapter).

Serology and Urine Antigens

The microbiological diagnosis of acute community-acquired respiratory tract infection does not rely only on culture. For many potential pathogens, such as *Legionella*, *Chlamydia pneumoniae*, *Mycoplasma pneumoniae* and viral pneumonias, culture has either a low sensitivity and/or is time-consuming. Therefore, other methods for antibody and antigen detection, as well as nucleic acid amplification techniques (NATs), have been developed in order to improve sensitivity and detection time.

All patients admitted to ICUs with severe community-acquired pneumonia should be tested for serum *M. pneumoniae* antibodies, and *S. pneumoniae* and *Legionella pneumophila* urine antigens.

Mycoplasma pneumoniae-specific immunoglobulin M (IgM) and immunoglobulin G(lgG) antibodies can be detected in the serum. Positive IgM results are consistent with acute *Mycoplasma* infection, whereas positive IgG result indicates previous immunologic exposure.

Negative results of serum IgM assay for *Mycoplasma* do not rule out an acute infection by such a bacterium if the specimen has been collected too early following primary infection (before the appearance of detectable antibodies). If a *Mycoplasma* infection is clinically indicated, a second specimen should be submitted in 14–21 days.

Urine for *Legionella* and *S. pneumoniae* antigens can be collected up to 1 week post presentation.

The most common urinary antigen test for the detection of *Legionella* recognizes infection by serogroup 1, which is responsible for about 90% of legionellosis, but is not capable to detect infections due to other serogroups.

Legionella urine antigens have a high specificity (94–99% depending on which test systems are used), while sensitivity ranges from about 65–95%.

Interestingly, the degree of positivity correlates with the severity of disease.

It should be noted that delayed seroconversion is the rule in *Legionella* infection, and that antigenuria usually persists for many months after infection, so that diagnosis of legionellosis in patients with a history of recent infection could be difficult. If *Legionella longbeachae* is suspected, a specific request should be done, since routine *Legionella* serology seldom detects this.

Streptococcus pneumoniae urinary antigens also have a high specificity (approximately 95%), while sensitivity is between 50% and 80% in patients without bacteremia and 75–85% in those with bacteremia. The use of concentrated urine by selective ultrafiltration slightly increases the sensitivity of the test. A strong relation between a positive urinary antigen and pneumonia severity has been observed.

Urine antigens are less important and not recommended in hospital-acquired and healthcare-associated pneumonia, due to a lower prevalence of such agents in this kind of diseases, and a higher risk of false positives by previous infections.

Pneumonia as part of a systemic viral infection such as measles or varicella-zoster, or Epstein-Barr virus (EBV) and cytomegalovirus (CMV) (antigen testing, histology, PCR) can be easily recognized by serologic procedures, except for patients with immunodeficiency syndrome.

Nucleic acid amplification techniques are very promising with respect to sensitivity and microbiological specificity, but problems of contamination and consequent specificity are not resolved. Currently there are no tests commercially available for routine use.

D-DIMER

D-dimer is a product of fibrin degradation. Blood D-dimer assessment is used in the diagnostic approach to pulmonary embolism (PE). Its main role is to corroborate further investigations, mainly radiologic tests, when suspecting

PE. Patients with suspected PE can be graded as low, moderate or high probability on the basis of symptoms and medical history (*see* Chapter 1).

A serum value of D-dimer lower than 500 ng/mL is generally considered negative and rule out acute PE in patients with lower risk, due to its high negative predictive value.

In high-risk patients, a negative D-dimer value does not rule out PE, so further tests (e.g. CT pulmonary angiography scan or scintigraphy) are required. In middle risk patients, a negative D-dimer offers some comfort but does not allow to rule out PE.

The blood D-dimer values are positively associated with some conditions which are risk factors for PE (e.g. malignancy, peripheral venous embolism, major surgery and trauma). Moreover, D-dimer values in healthy people tend to increase with age. The combination of pretest clinical probability assessment with age-adjusted D-dimer has been proposed, whereas no validated adjustment of normal values exists for patients with tumors or with recent surgery.

Flowchart 3.1 illustrates a possible algorithm for the diagnosis of PE.

Flowchart 3.1: A possible algorithm for the diagnosis of pulmonary embolism.

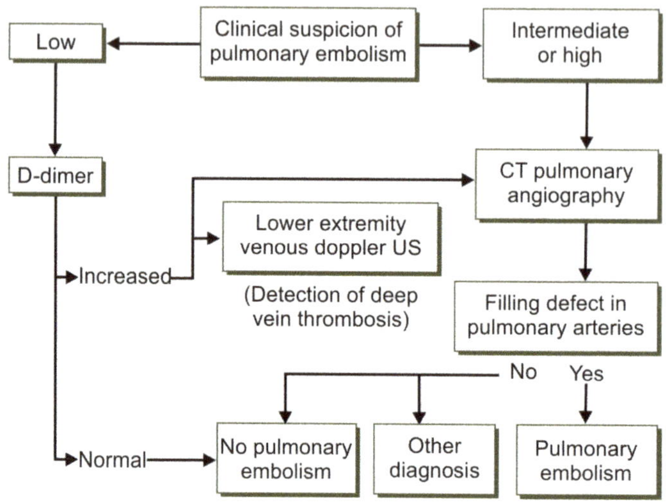

NATRIURETIC PEPTIDES

In 1956, granules in pig atria have been found by Kisch and colleagues; however, only in 1981 de Bold and colleagues conclusively identified the atrial natriuretic peptide (ANP). Indeed, for the first time, the role of the heart not only as a part of circulatory system but also as an endocrine organ has been demonstrated. A subsequent search for possible other related peptides resulted in the discovery by Sudoh and coworkers of a compound from the porcine brain with similar structure and biological function to ANP. This peptide was immediately named BNP and it is still named in such way notwithstanding post hoc studies on human showed that it was mainly synthesized from the heart and, specifically, from ventricular myocytes. Finally, also the C-type natriuretic peptide (CNP) was identified as predominantly synthesized and released by endothelial cells.

B-type natriuretic peptide is a 26 amino acid neurohormone secreted mainly in the cardiac ventricles in response to volume expansion and pressure overload. BNP is firstly synthesized as a 184 amino acid peptide called pre-proBNP and then cosecreted in the bloodstream along with a 76 amino acid N-terminal fragment (NT-proBNP) which is biologically inactive. BNP binds to and activates the atrial natriuretic peptide receptor type A (NPR-A), and to a lesser extent NPR-B, both these receptors linked to guanylyl cyclases. Guanosine 3',5'-cyclic monophosphate (cGMP) will then stimulate cGMP-dependent protein kinase which induces vascular smooth muscle relaxation with a consequent decrease in total peripheral resistance and venous return to the heart. Indeed, the BNP biological properties are definitively opposed to vasoconstriction, sodium retention and to the renin-angiotensin-aldosterone system (Fig. 3.2). Thereafter, BNP will be progressively removed from plasma by proteolytic processes activated through its binding to NPR-C, whereas glomerular filtration will play a marginal role in its removal. NPR-C is widely distributed in human and is mainly expressed on adipocytes For this reason, BNP serum levels may be altered in obese subjects. Conversely, NT-proBNP is predominantly removed by glomerular filtration and, accordingly, the renal function needs to be taken into account in interpreting the NT-proBNP values. Finally, the common reduction in fat distribution and kidney function as well the progressive increase in myocardial stiffness (i.e. diastolic dysfunction) represent all reasonable factors concurring to the described physiological rise in BNP and NT-proBNP plasma levels with aging. The biological half-life of BNP (20 minutes) as well as the one of NT-proBNP (120 minutes), together with their chemical stability, made these two peptides better targets than ANP for diagnostic blood testing reflecting rapid changes in ventricular status.

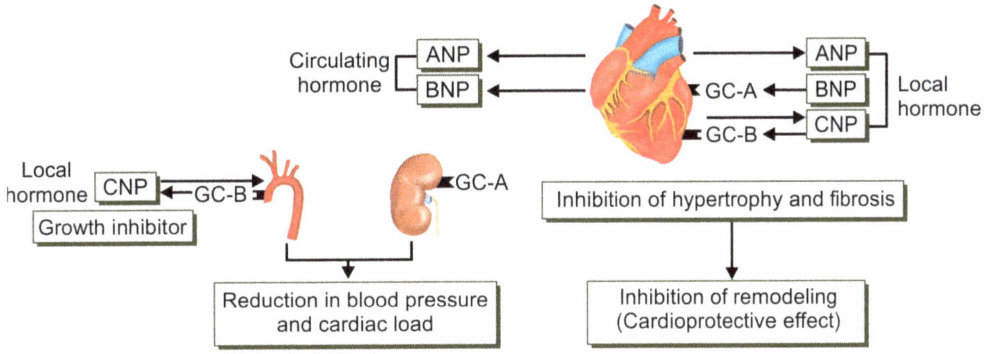

Fig. 3.2: Effects of BNP on heart, kidney and peripheral vascular system.

Role in Diagnosis of Acute Dyspnea

Dyspnea could be defined as an unpleasant difficult breathing or breathless sensation experienced by an individual not only due to pathophysiological but also to social, psychological and environmental factors. Acute dyspnea represents one of the common reasons for emergency department (ED) admission and, in this context, it is understandable how crucial might be to promptly recognize its underlying causes thus managing to start early treatment and improve patients' outcome. Indeed, a number of conditions leading to an acute dyspnea might expose patient to life-threatening events if the correct diagnosis is not established. However, although the differential diagnosis is very broad, acute heart failure (AHF), acute coronary syndrome (ACS) and PE still remain the three syndromes to be excluded for their potential severity and mortality. In ED, besides medical history and clinical evaluation, current literature strongly supports important diagnostic, prognostic and therapeutic implications of several biomarkers used and, particularly, of natriuretic peptides.

Acute Heart Failure

The AHF is routinely defined as the rapid onset of symptoms and signs secondary to abnormal cardiac function in subjects with or without a previous cardiac disease. Indeed, AHF represents one of the leading causes of hospitalization and a significant early readmission rate, as well a high mortality rate, has been reported for those patients discharged following an AHF episode.

The AHF underlying mechanisms vary from systolic to diastolic dysfunction, preload to afterload mismatch and brady- to tachyarrhythmias. Furthermore, concomitant cardiovascular and noncardiovascular diseases are common in these setting of patients and may precipitate the AHF course and/or modify its pathophysiology. Data from several registries demonstrated that nearly most of AHF episodes occur in patients over 70 years old with a previous heart failure diagnosis. These registries even supplied a detailed map of the most important comorbidities. Particularly, two-thirds had a history of coronary artery disease, more than one-half had a hypertension history, one-third suffered from diabetes and/or COPD, and an approximately 20% showed renal dysfunction.

Given the above-described heterogeneous *scenario*, with a large number of variables found to be involved, the AHF represents one of the main challenges in those patients admitted to ED for an acute dyspnea. A prompt recognition of this syndrome will lead to a dedicated and more efficient treatment and, subsequently, to an improvement in patients' outcome (death and rehospitalization). In this acute setting, both BNP and NT-proBNP values might be able to improve the acute dyspnea differential diagnosis. Indeed, it has been extensively shown that if these cardiac biomarkers were part of a first-line evaluation, they yield to a significant reduction in delayed treatment or, even, in wrong diagnosis. As previously mentioned both BNP and NT-proBNP plasma levels are continuous variables, so the higher BNP and NT-proBNP values, the greater the likelihood that dyspnea may be due to AHF. Accordingly, the latest European and American Cardiovascular Society guidelines recommended reasonable cut-off values for these biomarkers to conclude or exclude for AHF in patients referring for an acute dyspnea. As displayed in Flowcharts 3.2 and 3.3, while a BNP lower than 100 pg/mL or an NT-proBNP value below 300 pg/mL makes the AHF diagnosis unlikely, an AHF is almost reasonable for BNP values over 400 pg/mL and NT-proBNP levels higher than

Flowchart 3.2: Use of BNP in the algorithm for the diagnosis of chronic heart failure.

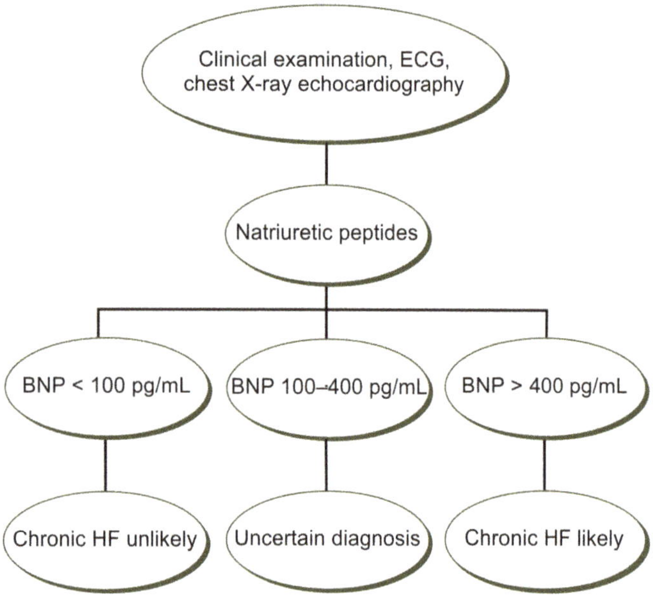

1,800 pg/mL. Noteworthy, both obesity and renal function should be taken into consideration in the natriuretic peptide levels interpretation. Indeed, particularly for BNP, to exclude AHF diagnosis a 55 pg/mL for BNP is recommended in case of moderate-to-severe obesity (body mass index over 35 kg/m^2) as well as a 200 pg/mL in the case of glomerular filtration rate below 60 mL/min/1.73 m^2. Nevertheless, even taking into account all variables, a gray zone of uncertainties still exists both for BNP (100-400 pg/mL) and for NT-proBNP, the latter mainly depending on the patient's age.

Besides helping the diagnostic approach, a significant contribute to risk stratification has been recently demonstrated for natriuretic peptides. Indeed, it has been suggested that natriuretic peptide levels are able to identify the risk of death or readmission within 30 days from discharge. Specifically, it has been shown that admission BNP levels over 1,730 pg/mL three-times were associated to a three-times higher in-hospital mortality rate than that of patients with levels below 430 pg/mL. Similarly, even in-hospital admission NT-proBNP levels higher than 1,000 pg/mL have been strongly associated with a poor outcome. Finally, as expected, subsequent measurements of either BNP or NT-proBNP levels have been shown to provide useful information also in guiding and monitoring the therapeutic approach.

Flowchart 3.3: Use of NT-proBNP in the algorithm for the diagnosis of acute heart failure.

Suspicion of acute heart failure because of symptoms and signs			
Examination, ECG, X-ray and NT-proBNP			
Patient age (years)	NT-pro BNP values (pg/mL)		
< 50 50 – 75 > 75	< 300	300 – 450 300 – 900 300 – 1800	> 450 > 900 > 1800
Interpretation	Acute CHF unlikely	Acute CHF less likely, alternative causes must be considered	Acute CHF likely, consider confounding factors
	NPV = 98%		PPC = 92%

Acute Coronary Syndromes

Notwithstanding the increase in cardiac troponins (I and T) plasma levels remain the gold standard in the laboratory diagnosis of ACS, BNP and NT-proBNP have been demonstrated more sensitive in the detection of acute cardiac chest pain. Indeed, combining natriuretic peptides with cardiac troponins represents a promising approach in the differential diagnosis of patients referring to ED for chest pain. Moreover, NT-proBNP has been suggested as a sensitive marker of myocardial ischemia, and particularly in the non-ST-elevation myocardial infarction (NSTEMI), given that it rises in a faster manner in the earlier phases of these ACS. Besides, the BNP and NT-proBNP plasma values increase could be interpreted per se as a reliable global marker of heart dysfunction due to ACS, thus being an additive prognostic marker in this setting of patients.

Pulmonary Embolism

Natriuretic peptide levels are elevated in most patients with acute PE complicated with right ventricular overload or dysfunction. Accordingly, the combination of NT-proBNP and cardiac troponin I values, together with specific echocardiography signs, are strongly suggested in the acute PE risk stratification (high risk versus low risk). Moreover, both BNP and NT-proBNP plasma levels have been proven to be significantly associated with the severity of pulmonary arterial hypertension as well as with the extension of ventilation-perfusion mismatch areas on scintigraphy. Accordingly, it was even demonstrated that, in patients with acute high-risk PE, a prompt reduction of BNP and cardiac troponin I levels were reliable laboratory indicators of thrombolysis efficacy as well as the reduction in systolic pulmonary arterial pressure.

Table 3.4: Main characteristics of the most used cardiac markers.

Marker	*Troponin I*	*CK-MB*	*Myoglobin*
Cause of increase	Injury to heart	Injury to heart and/or skeletal muscle	Injury to heart and/or skeletal muscle
Time to increase	2–3 hours	4–6 hours	2–4 hours
Peak	24 hours	24 hours	8–12 hours
Time to normalize	7–10 days	48–72 hours	24 hours
Main use	Diagnosis of AMI, assess of damage degree	Diagnosis of reinfarction	Early diagnosis of AMI, in addition to troponin

More in general, in patients with right ventricular pressure overload due to primary pulmonary arterial hypertension and, particularly, in those patients with post-thromboembolic pulmonary arterial hypertension, BNP and NT-proBNP levels are strongly correlated with mean pulmonary artery pressure, right atrial pressure, right ventricular end-diastolic pressure and total pulmonary resistance. Indeed, both these natriuretic peptides could be used in assessing clinical severity of this setting of patients and act as independent predictor of long-term mortality.

Other Applications

Several studies showed that one of the leading causes of death in patients with COPD is cardiac rather than strictly pulmonary. Moreover, pulmonary arterial hypertension as well as *cor pulmonale* also represent important determinant of poor outcome in these patients. It is therefore reasonable that an early detection of a somewhat heart dysfunction in a COPD patient might be fundamental in his clinical management. Accordingly, a significant increase in natriuretic peptide levels has been found in patients with COPD exacerbation particularly in those with a severe right ventricular dysfunction. In this context, again, BNP and NT-proBNP blood levels might be useful in defining therapeutic strategies and monitoring their efficacy.

MARKERS FOR MYOCARDIAL ISCHEMIA

The main markers used when an ACS is suspected include the cardiac troponins (T and I) and creatine kinase-MB (CK-MB) (Table 3.4). The cardiac troponins are today considered the markers of choice to evaluate subjects with ACS, allowing for highly accurate, sensitive and specific determination of myocardial injury in patients with chest pain. Any increase in these markers implies myocardial necrosis and suggests an impaired outcome with increased risk of death for the patient. According to the consensus guidelines from the American College of Cardiology (ACC) and the European Society of Cardiology (ESC), cardiac troponins have a key role in the definition of acute myocardial infarction (AMI). For example, an increase of troponin levels with negative CK-MB values, which was formerly regarded as a sign of unstable angina or minor myocardial injury, is now considered enough to diagnose a *NSTEMI*, even if the electrocardiogram (ECG) does not show diagnostic changes. Moreover, only one elevated troponin level above its upper limit of normal is enough to establish the diagnosis of AMI in subjects with risk factors for ACS and/or coherent symptoms.

It should be noted that cardiac markers have a low sensitivity for acute infarction in the first 6 hours after symptom onset, which represent the timeframe of interest to most emergency physicians in making diagnostic and therapeutic decisions. The increase of cardiac markers is not needed for the diagnosis of MI in subjects with chest pain and diagnostic ECGs with ST-elevation myocardial infarction (STEMI). Such patients may be candidates for immediate reperfusion therapy (thrombolysis or primary angioplasty) and treatment should not be delayed to wait for cardiac marker results.

According to the most recent international guidelines for the management of unstable angina and NSTEMI, cardiac markers should be assessed early when a patient presents to the ED with chest pain and repeated 6-9 hours after presentation. AMI can be ruled out if serial marker results are negative 9 hours after presentation. An increase in cardiac markers after 12-24 hours is unlikely due to AMI unless the patient has ongoing symptoms of ischemia after admission.

Troponins

The term troponins refer to three different subunits (troponin T, troponin I, and troponin C) that constitute the troponin complex. They are regulatory proteins essential for muscle contraction in skeletal and cardiac muscle, but not smooth muscle.

Troponins T and I are also known as cardiac troponins, since an increase in their blood levels has been shown to be a marker of several heart disorders, the most important of which is MI. Raised values of blood cardiac troponins indicate the release of the enzymes into the blood due to injury to the heart with death of cardiac muscle cells (myocytes). The release is prolonged with degradation of actin and myosin filaments. As shown in Figure 3.3, the increase of cardiac troponins after cardiac cell necrosis begins within 2–3 hours, reaches a peak in about 24 hours, and continues for 7–10 days. Beyond AMI, other important cardiac causes of troponin elevation include severe PE with acute right heart overload, congestive heart failure and myocarditis.

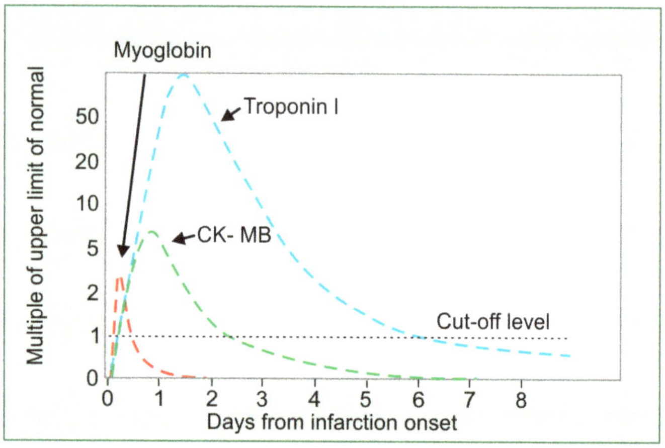

Fig. 3.3: Temporal release patterns of the main cardiac markers after a large acute myocardial infarction without reperfusion. CK-MB often increases 5- to 10-fold above the upper limit of normal, whereas troponins usually increase more than 20 times above the reference range. CK-MB is useful for diagnosing reinfarction since troponins remain elevated for a longer time (up to 7–10 days).

Creatine Kinase

Creatine kinase, also known as creatine phosphokinase (CPK), is an enzyme made of two subunits, which can be either B (brain type) or M (muscle type). Consequently, three different isoenzymes exist: (1) CK-MM, (2) CK-BB, and (3) CK-MB.

The sensitivity and specificity of total CK level are excessively low to allow its use as a test for diagnosing AMI. Conversely, the measurement of CK-MB has a key role in the diagnosis of AMI.

Consequently, CK evaluation may represent just a screening test, and serum of patients with increased total CK values should undergo a CK-MB mass assay. The test is highly specific, and raised value at any time in a patient with chest pain is highly suggestive of an AMI, particularly when CK-MB exceeds 5% of total CK. However, as for other cardiac markers, its value is poor in the first hours following the ischemia onset. In particular, the levels of CK-MB may be normal in one-fourth to one-half of patients with AMI at the time of presentation to the ED.

Figure 3.3 compares the temporal release patterns of troponin I and CK-MB. Blood CK-MB levels usually start to increase 4–6 hours after MI, peak at 24 hours and return to normal within 48–72 hours. Thus, CK-MB measurement is useful not only to diagnose MI but also to monitor for additional cardiac muscle injury over time and the detection of reinfarction.

Myoglobin

Myoglobin is an oxygen-storing protein found in the muscle tissues (skeletal and cardiac). It is released into circulation as early as 1 hour after muscle or myocardial injury. Blood levels typically increase 2–4 hours after onset of myocardial injury, peak at 8–12 hours and normalize within 24 hours. As a consequence, myoglobin is the earliest marker but it is not specific for cardiac damage. If used to diagnose MI, myoglobin measurement should be combined with more cardiac-specific markers such as troponin I. Rapid serial assessment, e.g. every 1–2 hours, can increase the diagnostic yield. Moreover, myoglobin seems to be only slightly more sensitive than CK-MB assays early after symptom onset and less sensitive than CK-MB after 8 hours from beginning of chest pain.

Causes of Elevation Unrelated to Coronary Thrombosis

Several conditions may exert indirect effects on the heart muscle causing the increase of cardiac markers without ACS occurs. For example, troponins are increased in around 40% of patients with critical illnesses such as sepsis. In severe acute anemia, there can also be a mismatch between oxygen demand and supply of the myocardium.

Cardiac markers may rise after chemotherapy due to its toxic effects on the heart, in carbon monoxide poisoning, in dissection of the ascending aorta due to a hemodynamic stress.

Pulmonary embolism, pulmonary hypertension and acute exacerbations of COPD are further possible causes of elevation in cardiac markers due to right ventricular strain with increased wall tension and ischemia. Much attention has to be paid to attribute increased troponin levels to COPD exacerbation, to avoid underestimating a concomitant MI.

Central nervous system disorders (e.g. ischemic or hemorrhagic stroke, generalized seizures) can lead to increased sympathetic tone and/or catecholamine release, which lead to cardiac overstimulation and release of cardiac enzymes in the blood circulation.

Patients with end-stage renal disease can have chronically elevated troponin T levels, whereas troponin I is less likely to be falsely elevated.

Strenuous endurance exercise (e.g. marathons or triathlons) can lead to increased troponin levels in up to one-third of subjects, but it is not linked to adverse health effects in these competitors.

High troponin T levels have also been reported in patients with inflammatory muscle diseases (e.g. polymyositis and dermatomyositis), in rhabdomyolysis, and in hypertensive disorders of pregnancy (pre-eclampsia).

TUMOR MARKERS IN LUNG CANCER

The term *tumor markers* or *oncologic biomarkers* refer to substances that are indicative of the presence of malignancy in the body. They may provide potential information for diagnosis, prognosis or monitoring of the disease during systemic treatment. With regard to lung cancer, a limited number of biomarkers have shown to have such characteristics. They include neuron-specific enolase (NSE) and pro-gastrin-releasing peptide (proGRP) for small cell lung cancer (SCLC), and carcinoembryonic antigen (CEA), cytokeratin 19 fragment (CYFRA 21-1) and squamous cell carcinoma (SCC) antigen for non-small cell lung cancer (NSCLC). More specifically, CEA is sensitive for adenocarcinoma, whereas SCC and CYFRA 21-1 for SCC.

Serum levels of proGRP seem today those that more accurately reflect the disease course of patients with SCLC.

Nucleosomes are cell death markers and have been shown to be useful in the early estimation of chemotherapy response in lung cancer patients, as well as in patients suffering from other solid cancers.

The combination of the biomarkers nucleosomes and CYFRA 21-1 have shown to be valuable in patients with advanced NSCLC treated with chemotherapy for the early estimation of therapy response, which may be helpful already after the application of only one course of cytotoxic therapy.

BIBLIOGRAPHY AND FURTHER READING

1. Adams KF Jr, Fonarow GC, Emerman CL, LeJemtel TH, Costanzo MR, Abraham WT, et al. Characteristics and outcomes of patients hospitalized for heart failure in the United States: rationale, design, and preliminary observations from the first 100,000 cases in the Acute Decompensated Heart Failure National Registry (ADHERE). Am Heart J. 2005;149:209-16.
2. American College of Emergency Physicians; Society for Cardiovascular Angiography and Interventions, O'Gara PT, Kushner FG, Ascheim DD, Casey DE Jr, Chung MK, et al. 2013 ACCF/AHA guideline for the management of ST-elevation myocardial infarction: a report of the American College of Cardiology Foundation/American Heart Association Task Force on Practice Guidelines. J Am Coll Cardiol. 2013;61(4):e78-140.
3. Anderson JL, Adams CD, Antman EM, Bridges CR, Califf RM, Casey DE Jr, et al. ACC/AHA 2007 guidelines for the management of patients with unstable angina/non-ST-elevation myocardial infarction: a report of the American College of Cardiology/American Heart Association Task Force on Practice Guidelines (Writing Committee to Revise the 2002 Guidelines for the Management of Patients With Unstable Angina/Non-ST-Elevation Myocardial Infarction) developed in collaboration with the American College of Emergency Physicians, the Society for Cardiovascular Angiography and Interventions, and the Society of Thoracic Surgeons endorsed by the American Association of Cardiovascular and Pulmonary Rehabilitation and the Society for Academic Emergency Medicine. J Am Coll Cardiol. 2007;50(7):e1-e157.
4. Anderson JL, Adams CD, Antman EM, Bridges CR, Califf RM, Casey DE Jr, et al. 2012 ACCF/AHA focused update incorporated into the ACCF/AHA 2007 guidelines for the management of patients with unstable angina/non-ST-elevation myocardial infarction: a report of the American College of Cardiology Foundation/American Heart Association Task Force on Practice Guidelines. J Am Coll Cardiol. 2013;61(23):e179-347.
5. Andreassen AK, Wergeland R, Simonsen S, Geiran O, Guevara C, Ueland T. N-terminal pro-B-type natriuretic peptide as an indicator of disease severity in a heterogeneous group of patients with chronic precapillary pulmonary hypertension. Am J Cardiol. 2006;98:525-9.
6. Andreeva E, Melbye H. Usefulness of C-reactive protein testing in acute cough/respiratory tract infection: an open cluster-randomized clinical trial with C-reactive protein testing in the intervention group. BMC Fam Pract. 2014;15:80.
7. Bain BJ. The peripheral blood smear. In: Goldman L, Schafer AI (Eds). Goldman's Cecil Medicine, 24th edition. Philadelphia, PA: Saunders Elsevier; 2011.

8. Berliner N. Leukopenia and leukocytosis. In: Goldman L, Schafer AI (Eds). Goldman's Cecil Medicine, 24th edition. Philadelphia, PA: Saunders Elsevier; 2011.
9. Binder L, Pieske B, Olschewski M, Geibel A, Klostermann B, Reiner C, et al. N-terminal pro-brain natriuretic peptide or troponin testing followed by echocardiography for risk stratification of acute pulmonary embolism. Circulation. 2005;112:1573-9.
10. Black S, Kushner I, Samols D. C-reactive protein. J Biol Chem. 2004;279:48487-90.
11. Brown A, George J, Murphy MJ, Struthers A, et al. Could BNP screening of acute chest pain cases lead to safe earlier discharge of patients with non-cardiac causes? A pilot study. QJM. 2007;100:755-61.
12. Carrier M, Righini M, Djurabi RK, Huisman MV, Perrier A, Wells PS, et al. VIDAS D-dimer in combination with clinical pre-test probability to rule out pulmonary embolism. A systematic review of management outcome studies. Thromb Haemost. 2009;101(5):886-92.
13. Cleland JG, Swedberg K, Follath F, Komajda M, Cohen-Solal A, Aguilar JC, et al. The EuroHeart Failure survey programme—a survey on the quality of care among patients with heart failure in Europe. Part 1: patient characteristics and diagnosis. Eur Heart J. 2003;24:442-63.
14. Collinson PO, Gaze DC, thokala p, goodacre s. randomised assessment of treatment using panel assay of cardiac markers—contemporary biomarker evaluation (ratpac cbe). Health Technol Assess. 2013;17(15):v-vi, 1-122.
15. Diercks DB, Mumma BE, Frank Peacock W, Hollander JE, Safdar B, Mahler SA, et al. Incremental value of objective cardiac testing in addition to physician impression and serial contemporary troponin measurements in women. Acad Emerg Med. 2013;20(3):265-70.
16. Enea I, Ceparano G, Mazzarella G, Di Sarno R, Cangiano G, Busino CA. Biohumoral markers and right ventricular dysfunction in acute pulmonary embolism: the answer to thrombolytic therapy. Ital Heart J Suppl. 2004;5:29-35.
17. Fonarow GC, Adams KF Jr, Abraham WT, Yancy CW, Boscardin WJ; ADHERE Scientific Advisory Committee, Study Group, and Investigators. Risk stratification for in-hospital mortality in acutely decompensated heart failure: classification and regression tree analysis. JAMA. 2005;293:572-80.
18. Fonarow GC, Peacock WF, Phillips CO, Givertz MM, Lopatin M; ADHERE Scientific Advisory Committee and Investigators. Admission B-type natriuretic peptide levels and in-hospital mortality in acute decompensated heart failure. J Am Coll Cardiol. 2007;49(19):1943-50.
19. Gruberg L, Sudarsky D, Kerner A, Hammerman H, Kapeliovich M, Beyar R. Troponin-positive, CK-MB-negative acute myocardial infarction: clinical, electrocardiographic and angiographic characteristics. J Invasive Cardiol. 2008;-20(3):125-8.
20. Holdenrieder S, von Pawel J, Dankelmann E, Duell T, Faderl B, Markus A, et al. Nucleosomes and CYFRA 21-1 indicate tumor response after one cycle of chemotherapy in recurrent non-small cell lung cancer. Lung Cancer. 2009;63:128-35.
21. Holdenrieder S, von Pawel J, Dankelmann E, Duell T, Faderl B, Markus A, et al. Nucleosomes, ProGRP, NSE, CYFRA 21-1, and CEA in monitoring first-line chemotherapy of small cell lung cancer. Clin Cancer Res. 2008;14:7813-21.
22. Januzzi JL Jr, Camargo CA, Anwaruddin S, Baggish AL, Chen AA, Krauser DG, et al. The N-terminal Pro-BNP investigation of dyspnea in the emergency department (PRIDE) study. Am J Cardiol. 2005;95:948-54.
23. Maisel A, Mueller C, Adams K Jr, Anker SD, Aspromonte N, Cleland JG, et al. State of the art: using natriuretic peptide levels in clinical practice. Eur J Heart Fail. 2008;10(9):824-39.
24. McMurray JJ, Adamopoulos S, Anker SD, Auricchio A, Böhm M, Dickstein K, et al. ESC guidelines for the diagnosis and treatment of acute and chronic heart failure 2012: the Task Force for the Diagnosis and Treatment of Acute and Chronic Heart Failure 2012 of the European Society of Cardiology. Developed in collaboration with the Heart Failure Association (HFA) of the ESC. Eur Heart J. 2012;33(14):1787-847.
25. Metra M, Zacà V, Parati G, Agostoni P, Bonadies M, Ciccone M, et al. Cardiovascular and noncardiovascular comorbidities in patients with chronic heart failure. J Cardiovasc Med (Hagerstown). 2011;12(2):76-84.
26. Righini M, Van Es J, Den Exter PL, Roy PM, Verschuren F, Ghuysen A, et al. Age-adjusted D-dimer cutoff levels to rule out pulmonary embolism: the ADJUST-PE study. JAMA. 2014;311:1117-24.
27. Stieber P, Hatz R, Holdenrieder S, Molina R, Nap M, von Pawel J, et al. National Academy of Clinical Biochemistry Guidelines for the use of tumor markers in lung cancer. AACC Press. 2006. [online] Available from http://www.nacb.org/lmpg/tumor_LMPG_draft_PDF.stm. [Accessed December, 2015].
28. Thygesen K, Alpert JS, Jaffe AS, Simoons ML, Chaitman BR, White HD, et al. Third universal definition of myocardial infarction. Eur Heart J. 2012;33(20):2551-67.
29. Weintraub NL, Collins SP, Pang PS, Levy PD, Anderson AS, Arslanian-Engoren C, et al. Acute heart failure syndromes: emergency department presentation, treatment, and disposition: current approaches and future aims: a scientific statement from the American Heart Association. Circulation. 2010;122(19):1975-96.
30. Yap LB, Mukerjee D, Timms PM, Ashrafian H, Coghlan JG. Natriuretic peptides, respiratory disease, and the right heart. Chest. 2004;126:1330

Chapter

4

Diagnosis of Respiratory Allergy

Francesca Puggioni, Claudio Sorino, Robert G Hamilton

OVERVIEW OF ALLERGY DIAGNOSIS

In 1921, Prausnitz and Küstner reported an allergic reaction that was induced by injecting a small quantity of serum from a fish allergic individual (Küstner) into the skin of a nonallergic individual (Prausnitz). They subsequently induced an immediate wheal and flare reaction in the skin at the serum injection site following the injection of an extracted fish antigen into the same site. This study demonstrated for the first time that a factor in serum which they termed as an atopic reagin could transfer the tendency of a nonallergic individual to develop atopy. *Atopy* has been defined as an inherited tendency to develop allergic or immediate-type I hypersensitivity to common and generally harmless substances or allergens such as fish. The term *allergy* may be defined as an exaggerated immune reaction to a foreign antigen, regardless of mechanism. An allergen is a substance, usually a glycoprotein, that is released from several hundred biological sources such as weeds, grasses, trees, animal danders, molds, house dust mites, parasites, insect venoms, occupational substances, drugs and foods. In 1967, the atopic reagin was shown to be human immunoglobulin E (IgE). Atopic individuals can develop a spectrum of IgE-mediated diseases including allergic rhinoconjunctivitis, allergic asthma, atopic eczema, IgE-mediated food allergies and in severe cases, systemic anaphylaxis. IgE antibody positivity in an individual is a diagnostic marker of IgE antibody sensitization and a risk factor for the development of allergic disease.

The diagnosis of human allergic disease begins with a thorough clinical history and physical examination. Diagnostic allergy testing should be considered whenever there is the clinical suspicion from the patient's history that an external substance, normally harmless, is the cause of symptoms that are consistent with one of the known allergic diseases. Importantly, the patient's clinical history and physical examination must be the basis upon which the diagnosis of allergic disease is made. Subsequently, so-called "primary confirmatory in vivo and in vitro tests" for allergen-specific IgE antibody provide support to the clinical history by documenting the patient's allergic sensitization status. If there is a mismatch between the history and primary IgE antibody confirmatory tests, then second level provocation testing may be performed to adjudicate the veracity of the history-driven diagnosis. This chapter overviews the principal in vivo and in vitro methods that are used as diagnostic allergy confirmatory tests in the evaluation of humans suspected of having an allergic disease. Second level in vivo provocation tests of the nose, eyes, lung, or gastrointestinal (GI) tract will not be discussed.

IN VIVO (SKIN) TESTS FOR CONFIRMATION OF ALLERGIC SENSITIZATION

Immediate-type hypersensitivity skin testing is an in vivo measure of the presence of allergen-specific IgE. This is an analytically sensitive method to screen for an individual's existing IgE antibody "sensitization" that may be responsible for the manifestation of a spectrum of allergic diseases. An allergen, typically in the form of physiological extract or purified molecule, that is suspected of inducing the allergic response is applied to the skin by either contact, epicutaneous or intradermal techniques. Thus, different skin test modalities are available for the diagnosis of allergic disease. These include *patch testing* (mainly used in the diagnosis of contact dermatitis and, to a lesser extent, food and drug allergy), *skin prick testing* (SPT), and *intradermal skin testing* which is used especially in the diagnosis of allergy to drugs and Hymenoptera venoms.

The SPT is considered the most widely used in vivo examination method in allergy diagnostics. The reasons for the widespread use of the SPT include its ease of performance and interpretation, minimal invasiveness, low risk of side effects, low cost and short time to obtain results. SPT evaluates the presence and magnitude of cutaneous reactivity as a surrogate marker for sensitization that is associated with allergic reactions in target organs such as eyes, nose, lung, gut and skin.

When sensitization exists in an individual, the introduction of relevant allergens into the skin leads to the cross-linking of allergen-specific IgE that is bound to the high affinity surface receptors on mast cells and basophils. This in turn causes these effector cells to degranulate and release histamine and generate other inflammatory mediators. A wheal and flare response is produced which can be quantified. Multiple allergens can be tested simultaneously on the skin because the resultant wheal and flare reaction to a specific allergen is localized to the immediate area of the SPT.

The SPT's distinct advantage over other diagnostic testing methods such as the serological analysis or provocation test is the rapidity with which results can be obtained in 15–20 minutes after the allergen administration to the skin. This enables the physician to obtain evidence of allergic sensitization, make a definitive diagnosis and establish a management plan, often during the initial visit. International societies of allergy have proposed standardized SPT procedures and a reference panel of inhalants allergen specificities (Table 4.1). This list of allergen specificities to be tested can be adjusted to include more local flora and patient history related exposures.

Table 4.1: Illustrative standard prick test panel for inhalant allergens.

Positive control	Histamine dihydrochloride 0.1%
Negative control	NaCl 0.9%
Tree, grass, and weed pollens	Hazel (*Corylus avellana*)
	Alder (*Alnus incana*)
	Birch (*Betula alba*)
	Plane (*Platanus vulgaris*)
	Cypress (*Cupressus sempervirens*)
	Grass mix (smooth meadow grass/*Poa pratensis*, cock's foot grass/*Dactilis glomerata*, perennial rye grass/*Lolium perenne*, timothy grass/*Phleum pratense*, meadow fescue/*Festuca pratensis*, meadow oat grass/*Helictotrichon pretense*)
	Olive (*Olea europaea*)
	Mugwort (*Artemisia vulgaris*)
	Ragweed (*Ambrosia artemisiifolia*)
	Parietaria
Molds	Alternaria (*Alternaria alternata*)
	Cladosporium (*Cladosporium herbarum*)
	Aspergillus (*Aspergillus fumigatus*)
Dander	Cat
	Dog
Dust mites	*Dermatophagoides pteronyssinus*
	Dermatophagoides farinae
Other	German cockroach (*Blattella germanica*)

Precautions and Contraindications

The SPT cannot be performed in subjects with extensive eczema, dermographism, urticaria, or those who cannot stop taking antihistamines or other medications that interfere with the proper interpretation of the test results. Systemic side effects are unlikely when using commercially available aeroallergen extracts. However, since systemic allergic reactions and rare deaths have been reported in association with SPT, a physician or other health care professional and emergency equipment should be immediately available when SPT is performed. Such a recommendation is particularly important when testing for sensitization to a food or drug that on the basis of the patient's history has the potential to induce anaphylaxis. Adverse reactions will usually occur within 30 minutes of SPT application.

Patients who have poorly controlled asthma should postpone their SPT until their disease is more effectively controlled. This will reduce the risk for exacerbation of their disease associated with skin testing. A peak flow of less than 70% in patients with asthma is considered a relative contraindication. Special precautions should be taken in performing the test during the relevant allergy season in which the patient has allergic symptoms, or when baseline tryptase levels are elevated due to a heightened risk of anaphylaxis. Moreover, attention should also be paid to subjects taking a beta-blocker, or less often, angiotensin-converting enzyme (ACE) inhibitor, due to a reduced response to epinephrine that might be needed to treat a systemic allergic reaction. Contraindications for SPT also include pregnancy because of a remote possibility of inducing a systemic allergic reaction with uterine contractions that would require the administration of epinephrine.

Skin Prick Testing Procedure

The SPT is usually performed in the volar aspect of the forearm, at least 2-3 cm from the wrist and the antecubital fossae. The skin on the back is an alternative site, especially in infants. The skin on the back can be more sensitive than the forearm which may result in larger wheals and thus possibly a greater number of positive test results. The site where each allergen is applied should be marked with a pen in order to properly identify the test reading area (Fig. 4.1). Alternatively, a test grid can be used on the forearm to mark the location.

A drop of each test solution (allergen extracts, saline and histamine controls) should be placed on the skin in an identical order for each subject tested and then immediately pricked. Two skin prick tests should be distant from each other by at least 2 cm to prevent overlap and avoid false-positive reactions due to direct contamination of a nearby test site or a secondary axon reflex.

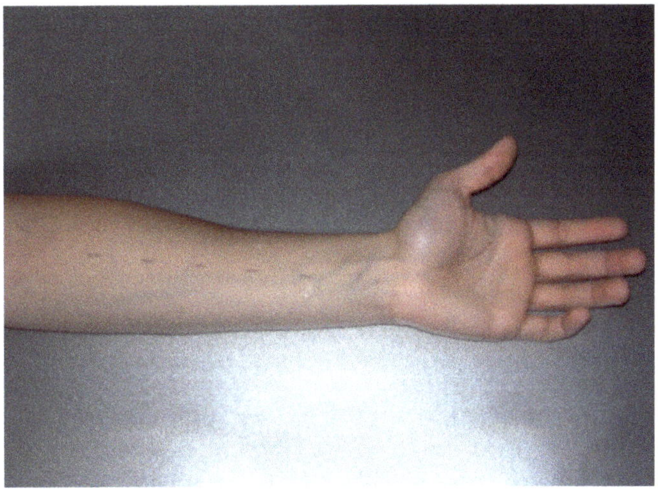

Fig. 4.1: Skin prick testing performed on the inner forearm.

The technique used involves puncturing the skin with a calibrated lancet (1 mm) held vertically. Alternatively, a hypodermic needle or blood lancet can be used at an angle of 45°. The use of a single-head metal lancet or bifurcated needle is recommended as the preferred testing instrument for SPT.

When a positive SPT reaction occurs, the skin becomes itchy within several minutes and then becomes red and swollen. The diameters of the wheal and the erythema are measured to determine the presence of specific IgE antibody positivity of the SPT. However, for some clinicians, only the wheal (papule) is required to confirm positivity. Others use the diameter of the erythema to define positivity. Usually, the largest diameter of the wheal of each allergen tested is measured at 15 minutes. Sometimes the diameter perpendicular to the largest diameter is also measured and a mean diameter is computed. The longest diameter is a better estimate of wheal surface area than the mean perpendicular diameters of a skin prick test above a certain value. The wheal/flare area can be pressed to blanch the erythema so that the size of the wheal can be recorded correctly.

A positive SPT with aeroallergen extracts is an important risk factor for the presence of allergic disease. Together with a positive clinical history, the SPT displays a diagnostic sensitivity of 80-95% and a diagnostic specificity of 75-95% for inhalant allergies. The observed diagnostic

Table 4.2: Examples of interpretative strategies for skin prick testing (SPT).

Wheal size		*Scale*	*Interpretation*
Absolute value (mm)	Percent of what obtained by saline* and histamine†		
< 3	Equal to the negative control	0	Negative
5–10	Smaller than the positive control (from 1/2 to 1/4)	+	Mildly sensitive
11–15	Smaller than the positive control (> 1/4)	++	Moderately sensitive
> 15	Equal to the positive control (or greater but less than double)	+++	Very sensitive
	More than double the positive control or wheal with pseudopod or a satellite	++++	

*Negative control; †Positive control.

sensitivity and specificity of the SPT are typically lower for food allergens. They can range from 30% to 90% and 20% to 60% respectively, depending on the specific allergen, the quality of the allergen extract and the precise SPT method employed. In interpreting the results of SPT, positive (histamine) and negative (diluent or saline) controls should be measured first. The evaluation of the negative control excludes dermographism which, if present, can produce false-positive SPT results. The histamine control should be positive which excludes false-negative results due to the interference of medications that were taken by the individual prior to skin testing.

Wheal diameters of 3 mm or larger are generally considered positive responses and they indicate sensitization (IgE antibody positivity) to the test allergen specificity. Smaller wheals (<3 mm of diameter) are usually not considered significant in clinical studies, while they are considered to be positive in some epidemiological studies. The use of a larger cut-off (5 mm) allows greater specificity but also involves greater false-negative results, thus is not recommended for clinical use.

The skin reaction can be graded by measuring the magnitude of the wheal or flare diameter or it can be expressed as a percentage of the positive histamine control (Table 4.2). When intense reactions occur, the wheal may have pseudopods (lateral extension of the central wheal) or satellite wheals. The size of the wheal does not indicate the severity of the symptoms. It only indicates the degree of patient's sensitization to the specific allergen.

After the puncture skin test has been applied, the clinician should monitor the patient for signs of anaphylaxis. Dyspnea, runny nose and facial itching may be early signs of anaphylaxis, and treatment with epinephrine should be considered. Topical corticosteroids may be applied to alleviate local symptoms at the site of positive reactions. An oral antihistamine may be required for intense local reactions.

IN VITRO (SEROLOGICAL) TESTS FOR ALLERGIC SENSITIZATION

Detection of allergen-specific IgE antibody is viewed as an important risk factor for the presence of allergic disease. Quantification of allergen-specific IgE levels in serum has the advantage over in vivo skin testing methods that its quality is not compromised by antihistamines or other allergy medications. Moreover, serological testing can be performed on patients with affected skin, such as dermatographism or atopic dermatitis. It is also a safe option for the evaluation of patients who are concerned about the risk of anaphylaxis. The discovery of human IgE myelomas in 1967 enabled the production of large quantities of IgE and highly specific antihuman IgE antibodies. These reagents permitted the development of the first immunoassays that could accurately quantify the level of total and allergen-specific IgE antibody concentrations in serum and other body fluids.

Total Serum IgE Autoanalyzers

Clinically, total IgE concentrations in human serum are quantified using computer-driven autoanalyzers that employ solid phase (immobilized) anti-IgE and solution phase enzyme-labeled anti-IgE reagents. These assays are referred to as immunometric or sandwich-type immunoassays. In this assay, human IgE is captured from serum by immobilized IgE-specific antibody. Following a buffer wash to remove unbound proteins, the remaining bound IgE is detected with an enzyme-labeled anti-IgE. Following a second buffer wash, a colorimetric, fluorescent or chemiluminescent substrate is added and the resultant response signal is quantified and is proportional to the amount of human IgE in the original patient's serum.

Total serum IgE concentrations are commonly reported as kilo-international units per liter (kU/L) or nanograms per milliliter (ng/mL), where 1 kU/L = 2.44 ng/mL of IgE. Although the System International (SI) specifies that IgE should be reported as micrograms per liter, this unitage has not been widely adopted by laboratories. The assay is calibrated using human IgE standards that are traceable to the WHO 75/502 international human IgE reference preparation. Use of this internationally-recognized IgE reference preparation has allowed exceptional interlaboratory concordance of clinically measured total serum IgE levels across the world using different assay systems. Precision and reproducibility of the principal autoanalyzers that measure total serum IgE remains excellent, with intra- and inter-assay coefficients of variation typically less than 10% and 15%, respectively. Total serum IgE assays are also extensively quality-controlled internally with low, medium and high IgE controls and laboratories performing total serum IgE measurements must participate in interlaboratory proficiency programs to assess accuracy.

For high total serum IgE, inaccuracies may result due to the so-called *hook effect* where the quantity of IgE exceeds the binding capacity of the assay. This term describes the problem with sera containing very high total IgE concentrations that produce results identical to those of samples with much lower IgE concentrations. If increasing quantities of IgE are added in an assay, there should be a linear rise to a plateau. In some assays, however, the plateau may begin to fall to lower levels as increasing amounts of IgE are added. To avoid this problem, some laboratories analyze sera at two dilutions with the expectation that the more dilute sample will produce a quantitatively lower result. If the more dilute sample does not produce a lower result, the sample needs to be rediluted and reassayed until it is clear that the sample is appropriately diluted. At this point, the concentration of IgE in the unknown can be extrapolated from the linear rising portion of the standard calibration curve. Interdilutional coefficients of variation should remain less than 20% for an assay that maintains parallelism between the reference curve and dilutions of test specimens.

Table 4.3: Reference values of total serum IgE in nonatopic individuals.

Results reported in kU/L

Age	*Mean*	*+1SD*	*+2SD*
0–6 weeks	0.6	2.3	8.8
7 weeks–3 months	1.0	4.1	17.0
4–6 months	1.8	7.3	30.0
7–9 months	2.6	10.0	39.0
10–23 months	3.2	13.0	53.0
2 years	5.7	23.0	93.0
3 years	8.0	32.0	128.0
4 years	10.0	40.0	160.0
5 years	12.0	48.0	192.0
6 years	14.0	56.0	224.0
7 years	16.0	63.0	248.0
8 years	18.0	71.0	280.0
9 years	20.0	78.0	304.0
10 years	22.0	85.0	328.0
Adults	13.2	41.0	127.0

Clinical Use

Measurements of total serum IgE concentration have limited clinical value when used to screen for or predict the risk of allergic disease. This is due to the broad range of overlapping total serum IgE levels among atopic and nonatopic individuals. Importantly, a low total IgE level does not exclude clinically evident allergic symptoms and high levels do not always indicate allergic disease. Table 4.3 displays the age-dependent levels of total serum IgE in nonatopic individuals. The evaluation of patients with suspected allergic bronchopulmonary aspergillosis (ABPA) is one of the few clear indications for measuring serum IgE concentrations. An extremely elevated total serum IgE concentration is found in nearly all patients with ABPA and it is one of the seminal diagnostic hallmarks of the disease. With the licensing of omalizumab for the treatment of allergic asthma, total serum IgE levels are required to insure that the patient is a suitable candidate for anti-IgE therapy. Their total serum IgE level should be between 30 IU/mL and 700 IU/mL to allow proper omalizumab dosing. The predose total serum IgE level is combined with the patient's weight to determine the correct dosing to ensure efficacious reduction of free IgE circulating in blood. At present, there is no validated assay that measures the level of circulating IgE that is free or unbound with omalizumab to confirm the effectiveness of the dosing regimen.

Circulating levels of IgE are often abnormal in patients with congenital immunodeficiencies, but these abnormalities are rarely diagnostic. The primary exception to this statement is the syndrome of hyper-IgE, eczematous dermatitis and recurrent pyogenic infections. Nonspecific elevation of total serum IgE levels is also observed in the Wiskott-Aldrich, ataxia telangiectasia, DiGeorge, and Omenn syndromes. Patients with acquired forms of immunodeficiency may have altered total levels of IgE, but these alterations are not diagnostic. Recent literature shows that total IgE level is altered in patients with human immunodeficiency virus (HIV) infection. Thus, there may be a correlation between the elevation in total serum IgE levels and the clinical course or state of the HIV disease.

Some cases of IgE myeloma may have been misdiagnosed as light chain disease because of failure to measure serum IgE concentrations. Since the course of IgE myeloma is distinct from that of light chain disease and other myelomas, IgE should be measured in patients with clinical symptoms suggestive of myeloma and in whom myelomas of other isotypes have been ruled out. Total serum IgE concentrations are also abnormally high in a variety of diseases. In drug-induced interstitial nephritis or graft-versus-host disease, there may be a relationship among the course of the disease, response to therapy, and the IgE level, but none of these relationships are firm enough to recommend total IgE as part of the clinical evaluation of these diseases.

Allergen-specific IgE Antibody Immunoassays

Three commercially available autoanalyzers are used clinically to measure allergen-specific IgE in human serum. These are produced by Thermofisher Scientific/Phadia (ImmunoCAP), Siemens Healthcare (Immulite) and Hycor Biomedical (HyTec 288). Each of these systems binds specific antibody to immobilized allergen (typically in the form of an extracted allergen preparation). Following a buffer wash to remove unbound serum proteins, bound IgE is detected with an enzyme labeled antihuman IgE reagent. Following a second buffer wash, substrate is added and the response signal is proportional to the amount of IgE antibody in the original test serum. The specific IgE antibody assays employ a heterologous total serum IgE reference curve which is calibrated back to the WHO 75/502 human IgE reference serum. This provides a uniform system of reporting quantitative specific IgE antibody data in kUa/L. This contrasts with the calibration strategy that was used in the 1967 radioallergosorbent test (RAST) that interpolated allergen-specific IgE values from IgE antibirch pollen reference curve. The term RAST is outdated and should not be used because radioisotopic assays are no longer employed in routine IgE antibody testing. Moreover, instead of using arbitrary class and grading schemes for reporting IgE antibody data, the quantitative kUa/L level generated by the autoanalyzer should be provided to the clinician.

Clinical Use

While the diagnostic sensitivity and specificity of the various allergen-specific IgE assays when compared with prick/puncture skin tests have been reported from less than 50% to more than 90%, they are known to vary among the different assays and with different allergen specificities. Thus, because it is not possible to accurately define the allergic status of subjects participating in studies examining in vitro and in vivo IgE antibody assay performance, the presence of IgE antibody needs to be viewed as only one of the "risk factors" for predisposing an individual to allergic disease. When viewed within the context of the patient's clinical history, IgE antibody positivity as assessed by either the skin test or IgE antibody serology can provide confirmation of sensitization and susceptibility of treatment with allergen specific immunotherapy.

Plasma Tryptase

Tryptase (molecular weight, 134,000 kDa) is a neutral serine esterase with trypsin-like substrate specificity. It is present in relatively large quantities in mast cells (approximately 10 pg per lung mast cell and up to 135 pg per skin mast cell). Mast cells activated during an IgE-mediated hypersensitivity reaction release tryptase along with pre-stored histamine and newly generated vasoactive mediators into surrounding soft tissue.

It is stored in the secretory granules and several forms have been described (I, IIβ, IIIα, T) and all are found in mast cells. Only the β form (also referred to as mature tryptase), and, less frequently, α species (referred to as total tryptase) are considered clinically relevant. When dissociated from heparin, tryptase rapidly degrades into its monomers and loses enzymatic activity. Since low amounts of tryptase are present in basophils (< 1% of the level present in mast cells), circulating levels of mature tryptase in the blood are considered to be a good clinical marker of mast cell activation.

Clinical Use

Immunoreactive total tryptase levels in serum of healthy adults are less than 5 g/L. Elevated levels of tryptase (10 g/L) as measured by immunoassay can be detected in serum from 1 hour to 4 hours after the onset of systemic anaphylaxis with hypotension. Thus, the timing of the serum collection is important and it should span 30 minutes to 4 hours after the onset of the acute event. In some cases, tryptase may reach levels as high as 1 mg/L. An elevated tryptase has also been detected, usually within 15–30 minutes, after an allergen challenge, levels decline with an approximate half-life of 2 hours. This is in contrast to histamine, which peaks more quickly within 5–10 minutes after an event and may return to baseline levels in less than 1 hour. Tryptase can be elevated in mastocytosis patients involving a high mast cell burden. Quantification of tryptase provides an indication of mast cell activation by specific allergen. Most commercial laboratories report tryptase results as a combination of total-α and mature-β forms.

Eosinophils and Eosinophil-derived Substances

Eosinophils are important cells in allergic inflammation. Eosinophilic cationic protein (ECP) is a basic protein that can be detected in the granules of the eosinophil in different forms, with molecular weights ranging from 18.5 kDa to 22 kDa. The number of eosinophils in body fluids correlates highly with the diagnosis of allergic rhinitis, allergic asthma and eosinophilic bronchitis. Sputum eosinophils may also be useful in the diagnosis of asthma and eosinophilic bronchitis and in the follow up to therapy. Elevated levels of ECP have been detected in the serum, sputum and nasal secretions of individuals undergoing a late-phase allergic reaction (usually 6–24 hours after exposure), when an eosinophil influx is predominant at the reactive site. Presently, ECP measurements have shown limited clinical utility as an analyte for monitoring patients with extrinsic asthma and other allergic diseases in which eosinophils may play a role in tissue damage. Several eosinophil chemoattractants (e.g. IL-5, eotaxin) are elevated in nasal and bronchoalveolar lavage fluid from patients with active allergic inflammatory disease associated with recent or concurrent exposure to aerosolized allergens.

MOLECULAR-BASED ALLERGY

Many of the most common allergenic molecules have been cloned and purified for use in serological assays. Their nomenclature which involves the first three letters of their genus, the first letter of their species and a sequence number in order of identification has been established by the World Health Organization and International Union of Immunological Societies (WHO/IUIS) Allergen Nomenclature Subcommittee. For instance, timothy grass allergens are listed as Phl p from *Phleum pratense*. Allergenic molecules have been further classified into protein families, according to their structure and biological function. Many allergenic molecules share common epitopes which mean that the same IgE antibody may bind or cross-react and thus induce an immune response when the individual is exposed to allergenic molecules with similar structures from different allergen sources. Other molecules may serve as unique indicators for specific allergen sources which permit the identification of a primary sensitizing allergen specificity. In some parts of the world where they are reimbursed, molecular allergy diagnostics is used in the diagnosis of allergic patients. This is especially important in the diagnostic evaluation of patients with suspected allergic reactions to foods.

Method

Immunoglobulin E antibodies specific for allergenic molecules may be detected using both singleplex autoanalyzers that detect one specificity per analysis, or multiplex chip, based methods that detect IgE to many allergen specificities in a single analysis. Singleplex assay analysis permits the clinician to individually select those allergenic specificities that may be most useful for the accurate diagnosis of a patient based on their clinical history. The multiplex approach allows for the screening of IgE responses specific for a broad array of preselected allergens, independent of the patient's clinical history. The immunosolid phase allergen chip (ISAC) is one currently available multiplex assay system that measures IgE antibody to 112 individual allergenic components from 51 different allergen sources using 30 microliters of serum. Results are interpolated from a calibration curve in ISAC Standardized Units for specific IgE (ISU-E), which provides a semiquantitative measure of allergen-specific IgE antibody levels. The ISAC which uses small amounts of allergen in a dotted matrix contrasts with the singleplex assays that measures IgE binding under conditions of excess of immobilized allergen. This has consequences for the extent of isotype competition (allergen-specific IgG antibody) and the relative affinities of antibody detected.

Clinical Use

Measurement of IgE antibody to 112 individual allergenic molecules can provide a sensitization profile that is especially well suited for use in patients with complex allergen sensitization patterns. It is more useful than extract-based IgE antibody analyses in distinguishing specific IgE responses which cross-react with structurally similar allergenic molecules. In the field of pollen-related food allergy, molecular allergy testing has demonstrated a unique ability to distinguish primary from cross-reactive sensitization. For instance, in peanut allergic patients, sensitization to Ara h 2 is considered an important marker for identifying a patient who is at risk of a systemic reaction following exposure to peanut allergen. This contrasts with IgE antibody responses to Ara h 8 where cross-reactivity among food allergens and Fagales tree pollen may occur and this immune response is typically associated with mild, oral reactions. Another important application is the ability of molecular allergy diagnostics to aid in distinguishing between pollen and wheat-induced baker's asthma. Table 4.4 illustrates a number of the molecular allergen specificities that identify a low versus high risk for reactions following challenge testing. Another indication for molecular allergen testing comes from the need to accurately identify the allergen specificities to which the patient is sensitized for planning specific immunotherapy. Because subcutaneous immunotherapy is both expensive and long lasting (3–5 years), a correct identification of the primary sensitizing allergen(s) is important for identifying eligible patients.

Molecular allergy diagnostics is most valuable in identifying IgE antibody responses that stem from allergen cross-reactivity. Select allergenic proteins such as the profilins, polcalcins, lipid transfer proteins, pathogenesis-related protein family-10 (PR10) and tropomyosins are highly conserved among a wide variety of allergen specificities. A patient, for instance, who is primarily sensitized to grasses may also test positive for birch pollen. This may be due to cross-reactivity among IgE antibodies that bind to profilin Bet v 2 in birch pollen and Phl p 12 in the grasses. Use of profilin allergens molecules from both birch and grass sources allows for the discrimination between genuine sensitizations and this type of cross-reactivity. Another area where molecular allergy diagnostics improve diagnosis is in the selection of patients for Hymenoptera venom immunotherapy. Sensitization to the major allergens Api m 1 of honeybee and Ves v 1 and 5 from yellow jacket venom can be helpful in discriminating between true double honeybee and yellow jacket sensitization and cross reactivity due to cross-reactivity carbohydrate determinants. Flowchart 4.1 provides an algorithm for how molecular allergen-based testing can guide the planning of an immunotherapy regimen in a polysensitized patient.

Table 4.4: High-versus low-risk molecules from foods giving rise to anaphylaxis.

Source	*High risk*	*Low risk*
Peanut	Ara h 1, 2, 3, 9	Ara h 8, profilin, CCD
Hazelnut	Cor a 8, 9, 14	Profilin, CCD
Walnut	Jug r 1, 2, 3	Profilin, CCD
Soy	Gly m 5, 6, (4)	Profilin, CCD
Rosaceae fruits	Pru p 3, Mal d 3	Pru p 1, Mal d 1, profilin, CCD
Wheat	Tri a 14, Tri a 19	Profilin, CCD

Source: Reused with permission from Canonica GW, Ansotegui IJ, Pawankar R, Schmid-Grendelmeier P, van Hage M, Baena-Cagnani CE, et al. A WAO - ARIA - GA2LEN consensus document on molecular-based allergy diagnostics. World Allergy Organ J. 2013;6:17. (CCD: Cross-reactive carbohydrate determinant).

DEFINITIONS

Allergen Source

A tissue, particle, food or organism inducing allergy (e.g. cat dander, *Dermatophagoides pteronyssinus*, milk, *Aspergillus fumigatus*, *Phleum pratense* pollen, etc.).

Allergen Extract

A crude, unfractionated mixture of allergenic and nonallergenic proteins, polysaccharides, and lipids obtained by extraction from an allergen source (e.g. pollen grains).

Allergenic Molecule (Allergen Component)

A molecule (i.e. protein or glycoprotein) derived from a given allergen source that is identified by allergen-specific IgE antibodies (hereafter referred to as allergen). Allergens can be isolated from natural allergen sources (native, purified allergen) or can be produced by using recombinant DNA technology (recombinant allergen).

A genuine allergen causes specific sensitization to its corresponding allergen source. *Major allergens* are defined as those that bind to IgE in 50% or more of patients with the same allergy; in other words, the majority of patients (≥ 50%) with the same allergy are sensitized to the allergen in question. A *primary allergen* is the original sensitizing molecule (i.e. the driving trigger; in contrast to secondary

Flowchart 4.1: Evaluation of ISAC test results.

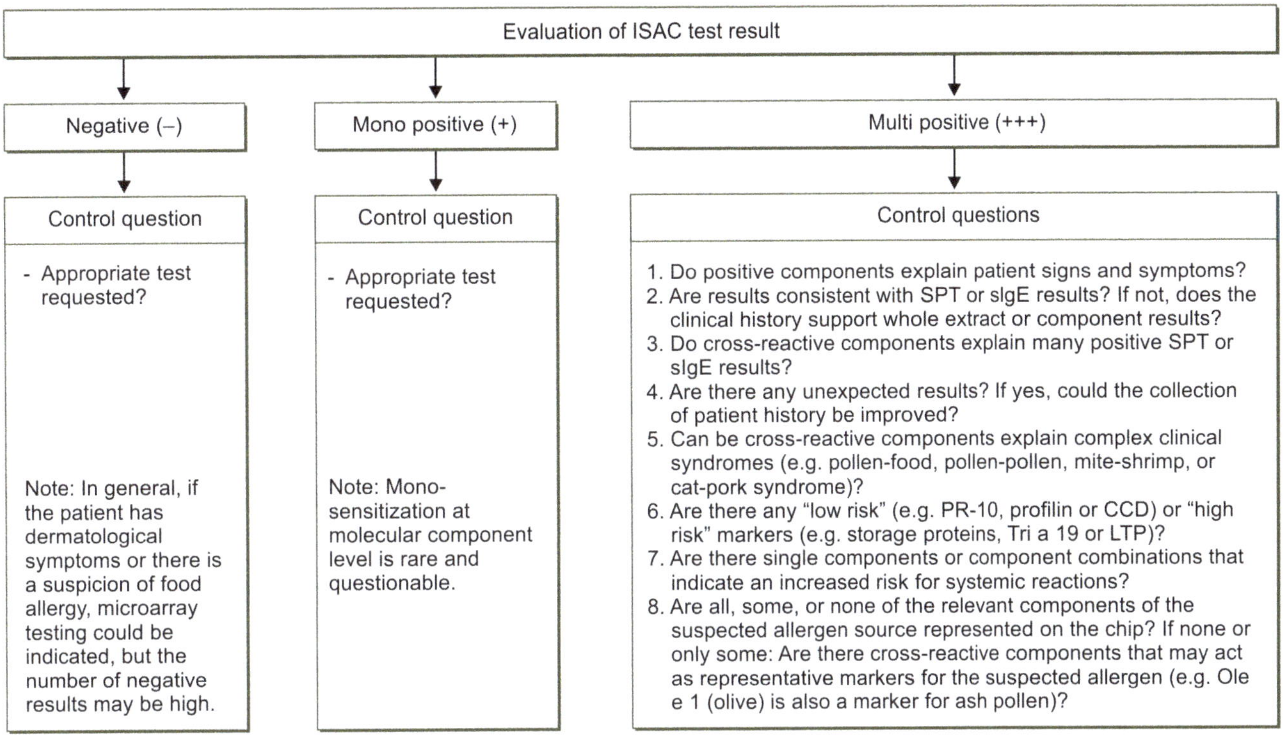

Source: Reused with permission from Canonica GW, Ansotegui IJ, Pawankar R, Schmid-Grendelmeier P, van Hage M, Baena-Cagnani CE, et al. A WAO - ARIA - GA2LEN consensus document on molecular-based allergy diagnostics. World Allergy Organ J. 2013;6:17)
(ISAC: Immunosolid phase allergen chip; SPT: Skin prick testing; sIgE: Allergen-specific IgE; CCD: Cross-reactive carbohydrate determinant; LTP: Lipid transfer protein).

sensitization due to cross-reactivity). In general, major allergens are also genuine and primary. Finally, the abundance of a molecule present in the allergen source is also a parameter to take into consideration.

Cross-Reactivity

The phenomenon of an IgE antibody recognizing, binding and inducing an immune response to similar allergenic molecules (homologs) present in different species; for example, an IgE antibody that binds and reacts to both Bet v 1 in birch pollen and Cor a 1 in hazelnut due to their structural similarity (generally characterized by > 50–70% sequence homology between the primary structures of the proteins). IgE cross-reactivity often occurs between the following:

1. Allergenic molecules in closely related species (e.g. between grass or between mite allergens);
2. Well preserved molecules with similar function present in widely different species that belong to the same protein family (e.g. members of the tropomyosin protein family, such as Der p 10 in house dust mite and Pen m 1 in black tiger shrimp).

Cosensitization

Genuine sensitization to more than one allergen source (e.g. timothy grass and birch), where the sensitization is not due to cross-reactivity.

Stability of Allergens

Allergens that are susceptible to acid pH in context with peptic digestion (relevant at the gastric level) are not able to cross the gastric barrier (except possibly in patients treated with antacid drugs. Temperature (cooking or boiling) susceptibility indicates that the allergen does not maintain its allergenicity after cooking/heating procedures. Heating may occur in the industrial processing of food for production and in domestic cooking. The structure of allergens susceptible to protease digestion is affected by gastric and pancreatic enzymes. Accordingly, allergens sensitive to these factors are considered labile, while those that are not considered to be stable.

Allergen-specific IgE Concentration/Level

1. *High level*: represents a high concentration of allergen-specific IgE antibodies specific for an allergenic extract or molecule. Generally, the higher the allergen-specific IgE level the higher the probability of clinical reactions. Some allergens also have a high probability of inducing severe reactions at low allergen-specific IgE concentrations (e.g. storage proteins and lipid transfer proteins), while others typically do not result in any clinical reactions despite high allergen-specific IgE concentrations [e.g. cross-reactive carbohydrate determinants (CCDs)].
2. *Low level*: represents a low concentration of allergen-specific IgE antibodies specific for an allergen extract or molecule.

Allergen-specific IgE Sensitization

Presence of allergen-specific IgE antibodies in the blood that may occur in the presence or absence of clinical symptoms.

1. *Monosensitization*: Sensitization to one allergen source (*Dermatophagoides pteronyssinus*) or to a closely related taxonomical family or group of allergen sources (i.e. mites).
2. *Poly- or multisensitization*: Sensitization to three or more allergen sources (e.g. mite, birch and grass pollen).

Allergen-specific IgE Detection Based on Allergen Extracts

Singleplex or multiplex platforms for in vitro measurement of allergen-specific IgE reactivity to allergen extracts. Terms such as CAP, radioallergosorbent test (RAST), allergen-specific IgE and in vitro test are often used interchangeably for this technique. However, the performance of different measurement platforms differs and this should be taken into consideration when reporting and comparing results. This approach cannot identify cross-reacting molecules.

Allergen-specific IgE Detection Based on Allergenic Molecules

Singleplex or multiplex platforms for in vitro measurement of allergen-specific IgE reactivity to allergenic molecules.

Cross-reactive Carbohydrate Determinant

The CCDs are carbohydrate moieties of glycoproteins. The most commonly described is MUXF3.

Epitope

The region of the protein recognized and bound by an antibody (i.e. the antibody binding site).

Molecular-based Allergy Diagnostics

A diagnostic approach to define the allergen sensitization of a patient at the molecular level using purified natural or recombinant allergen on singleplex or multiplex measurement platforms.

Panallergen

A cross-reactive allergen, belonging to a protein family well preserved throughout many widely different species, able to trigger IgE antibody binding (e.g. profilins or serum albumins). *See* also definition of cross-reactivity (2).

Recombinant Allergen

An allergenic molecule produced using DNA cloning and protein purification techniques. Recombinant allergens can be produced with consistency in terms of quality and amounts, and without CCD structures. Allergen extracts cannot be produced by recombinant techniques.

BIBLIOGRAPHY AND FURTHER READING

1. Bernstein IL, Li JT, Bernstein DI, Hamilton R, Spector SL, Tan R, et al. Allergy diagnostic testing: an updated practice parameter. Ann Allergy Asthma Immunol. 2008;100:S1-148.
2. Borres MP, Ebisawa M, Eigenmann PA. Use of allergen components begins a new era in pediatric allergology. Pediatr Allergy Immunol. 2011;22:454-61.
3. Bousquet J, Khaltaev N, Cruz AA, Denburg J, Fokkens WJ, Togias A, et al. Allergic Rhinitis and its Impact on Asthma (ARIA) 2008 update (in collaboration with the World Health Organization, GA(2)LEN and AllerGen). Allergy. 2008;63 (Suppl 86):8-160.
4. Bousquet PJ, Brozek J, Bachert C, Bieber T, Bonini S, Burney P, et al. The CONSORT statement checklist in allergen-specific immunotherapy: a GA2LEN paper. Allergy. 2009;64:1737-45.
5. Canonica GW, Ansotegui IJ, Pawankar R, Schmid-Grendelmeier P, van Hage M, Baena-Cagnani CE, et al. A WAO - ARIA - GA2LEN consensus document on molecular-based allergy diagnostics. World Allergy Organ J. 2013;6:17.

6. Ciprandi G, Alesina R, Ariano R, Aurnia P, Borrelli P, Cadario G, et al. Characteristics of patients with allergic polysensitization: the POLISMAIL study. Eur Ann Allergy Clin Immunol. 2008;40:77-83.
7. Ciprandi G, Vizzaccaro A, Cirillo I, Tosca M, Massolo A, Passalacqua G. Nasal eosinophils display the best correlation with symptoms, pulmonary function and inflammation in allergic rhinitis. Int Arch Allergy Immunol. 2005;136:266-72.
8. College of American Pathologist SE Diagnostic Allergy Proficiency Survey. Participant Summary Cycle A, 2004. Diagnostic Immunology Resource Committee. [online] Available from www.cap.org. [Accessed December, 2015].
9. Cox L, Jacobsen L. Comparison of allergen immunotherapy practice patterns in the United States and Europe. Ann Allergy Asthma Immunol. 2009;103:451-9; quiz 459-61, 495.
10. Cox L, Nelson H, Lockey R, Calabria C, Chacko T, Finegold I, et al. Allergen immunotherapy: a practice parameter third update. J Allergy Clin Immunol. 2011;127:S1-55.
11. Dang TD, Tang M, Choo S, Licciardi PV, Koplin JJ, Martin PE, et al. Increasing the accuracy of peanut allergy diagnosis by using Ara h 2. J Allergy Clin Immunol. 2012;129:1056-63.
12. Eden E, Hammel J, Rouhani FN, Brantly ML, Barker AF, Buist AS, et al. Asthma features in severe alpha1-antitrypsin deficiency: experience of the National Heart, Lung, and Blood Institute Registry. Chest. 2003;123(3):765-71.
13. Focke M, Marth K, Flicker S, Valenta R. Heterogeneity of commercial timothy grass pollen extracts. Clin Exp Allergy. 2008;38:1400-8.
14. Focke M, Marth K, Valenta R. Molecular composition and biological activity of commercial birch pollen allergen extracts. Eur J Clin Invest. 2009;39:429-36.
15. Foster B, Schwartz LB, Devouassoux G, Metcalfe DD, Prussin C. Characterization of mast-cell tryptase-expressing peripheral blood cells as basophils. J Allergy Clin Immunol. 2002;109(2):287-93.
16. Hamilton RG, Adkinson NF Jr. Measurement of total serum immunoglobulin E and allergen-specific immunoglobulin E antibody. In: Rose NR, de Macario EC, Fahey JL, Friedman H, Penn GM (Eds). Manual of clinical laboratory immunology, 4th edition. Washington, DC: American Society for Microbiology; 1992. pp. 689-701.
17. Hamilton RG, Marcotte GV, Saini SS. Immunological methods for quantifying free and total serum IgE levels in allergy patients receiving omalizumab (Xolair) therapy. J Immunol Methods. 2005;303(1-2):81-91.
18. Hamilton RG. Accuracy of US Food and Drug Administration-cleared IgE antibody assays in the presence of anti-IgE (omalizumab). J Allergy Clin Immunol. 2006;-117(4):759-66.
19. Heinzerling L, Mari A, Bergmann KC, Bresciani M, Burbach G, Darsow U, et al. The skin prick test—European standards. Clin Transl Allergy. 2013;3:3.
20. Homburger HA. Allergic diseases. In: McPherson RA, Pincus MR (Eds). Henry's clinical diagnosis and management by laboratory methods, 21st edition. New York: WB Saunders Company; 2007. pp 961-71.
21. Jogie-Brahim S, Min HK, Fukuoka Y, Xia HZ, Schwartz LB. Expression of alpha-tryptase and beta-tryptase by human basophils. J Allergy Clin Immunol. 2004;113(6):1086-92.
22. Join Task Force on Practice Parameters. Allergen immunotherapy: a practice parameter. American Academy of Allergy, Asthma and Immunology. American College of Allergy, Asthma and Immunology. Ann Allergy Asthma Immunol. 2003;90(1 Suppl 1):1-40.
23. Klemans RJ, Otte D, Knol M, Knol EF, Meijer Y, Gmelig-Meyling FH, et al. The diagnostic value of specific IgE to Ara h 2 to predict peanut allergy in children is comparable to a validated and updated diagnostic prediction model. J Allergy Clin Immunol. 2013;131:157-63.
24. Lizaso MT, Garcia BE, Tabar AI, Lasa E, Echechipía S, Alvarez MJ, et al. Comparison of conventional and component-resolved diagnostics by two different methods (Advia-Centaur/Microarray-ISAC) in pollen allergy. Ann Allergy Asthma Immunol. 2011;107:35-41.
25. Marogna M, Massolo A, Berra D, Zanon P, Chiodini E, Canonica GW, et al. The type of sensitizing allergen can affect the evolution of respiratory allergy. Allergy. 2006;61:1209-15.
26. McCoy KD, Harris NL, Diener P, Hatak S, Odermatt B, Hangartner L, et al. Natural IgE production in the absence of MHC class II cognate help. Immunity. 2006;24:329-39.
27. Melioli G, Bonifazi F, Bonini S, Maggi E, Mussap M, Passalacqua G, et al. The ImmunoCAP ISAC molecular allergology approach in adult multi-sensitized Italian patients with respiratory symptoms. Clin Biochem. 2011;44:1005-11.
28. Melioli G, Compalati E, Bonini S, Canonica GW. The added value of allergen microarray technique to the management of polysensitized allergic patients. Curr Opin Allergy Clin Immunol. 2012;12:434-9.
29. Mertens M, Brehler R. Suitability of different glycoproteins and test systems for detecting cross-reactive carbohydrate determinant-specific IgE in Hymenoptera venom-allergic patients. Int Arch Allergy Immunol. 2011;156:43-50.
30. Mittermann I, Zidarn M, Silar M, Markovic-Housley Z, Aberer W, Korosec P, et al. Recombinant allergen-based IgE testing to distinguish bee and wasp allergy. J Allergy Clin Immunol. 2010;125:1300-7.e3.
31. Muller U, Schmid-Grendelmeier P, Hausmann O, Helbling A. IgE to recombinant allergens Api m 1, Ves v 1, and Ves v 5 distinguish double sensitization from cross-reaction in venom allergy. Allergy. 2012;67:1069-73.
32. Nelson HS. Specific immunotherapy with allergen mixes: what is the evidence? Curr Opin Allergy Clin Immunol. 2009;9:549-53.
33. Nicolaou N, Custovic A. Molecular diagnosis of peanut and legume allergy. Curr Opin Allergy Clin Immunol. 2011;11:222-8.
34. Noah TL, Tudor GE, Ivins SS, Murphy PC, Peden DB, Henderson FW. Repeated measurement of nasal lavage fluid chemokines in school-age children with asthma. Ann Allergy Asthma Immunol. 2006;96(2):304-10.

35. Nopp A, Johansson SG, Ankerst J, Bylin G, Cardell LO, Grönneberg R, et al. Basophil allergen threshold sensitivity: a useful approach to anti-IgE treatment efficacy evaluation. Allergy. 2006;61:298-302.
36. Pali-Scholl I, Jensen-Jarolim E. Anti-acid medication as a risk factor for food allergy. Allergy. 2011;66:469-77.
37. Radauer C, Bublin M, Wagner S, Mari A, Breiteneder H. Allergens are distributed into few protein families and possess a restricted number of biochemical functions. J Allergy Clin Immunol. 2008;121:847-52.e7.
38. Salib RJ, Lau LC, Howarth PH. Nasal lavage fluid concentrations of eotaxin-1 (CCL11) in naturally occurring allergic rhinitis: relationship to disease activity, nasal luminal eosinophil influx, and plasma protein exudation. Clin Exp Allergy. 2005;35(8):995-1002.
39. Santos A, Van Ree R. Profilins: mimickers of allergy or relevant allergens? Int Arch Allergy Immunol. 2011;155:191-204.
40. Sastre J, Landivar ME, Ruiz-Garcia M, et al. How molecular diagnosis can change allergen-specific immunotherapy prescription in a complex pollen area. Allergy. 2012;67:709-11.
41. Sastre J. Molecular diagnosis in allergy. Clin Exp Allergy. 2010;40:1442-60.
42. Shreffler WG. Microarrayed recombinant allergens for diagnostic testing. J Allergy Clin Immunol. 2011;127:843-9; quiz 850-1.
43. Tripodi S, Frediani T, Lucarelli S, Macrì F, Pingitore G, Di Rienzo Businco A, et al. Molecular profiles of IgE to Phleum pratense in children with grass pollen allergy: implications for specific immunotherapy. J Allergy Clin Immunol. 2012;129:834-9.e8.
44. US Department of Health and Human Services; Radioallergosorbent Test (RAST) Methods for Allergen-Specific Immunoglobulin E (IgE) 510(k)s; Final Guidance for Industry and FDA. Washington, DC; 2001. pp. 1-15.
45. Valenta R, Ferreira F, Focke-Tejkl M, Linhart B, Niederberger V, Swoboda I, et al. From allergen genes to allergy vaccines. Annu Rev Immunol. 2010;28:211-41.
46. Valenta R, Kraft D. Recombinant allergen molecules: tools to study effector cell activation. Immunol Rev. 2001;179:119-27.
47. Valenta R, Twaroch T, Swoboda I. Component-resolved diagnosis to optimize allergen-specific immunotherapy in the Mediterranean area. J Investig Allergol Clin Immunol. 2007;17 (Suppl 1):36-40.
48. Vereda A, van Hage M, Ahlstedt S, Ibañez MD, Cuesta-Herranz J, van Odijk J, et al. Peanut allergy: clinical and immunologic differences among patients from 3 different geographic regions. J Allergy Clin Immunol. 2011;127:603-7.
49. Weber RW. Cross-reactivity of pollen allergens: impact on allergen immunotherapy. Ann Allergy Asthma Immunol. 2007;99:203-11.
50. Williams PB, Barnes JH, Szeinbach SL, Sullivan TJ. Analytic precision and accuracy of commercial immunoassays for specific IgE: establishing a standard. J Allergy Clin Immunol. 2000;105(6 Pt 1):1221-30.
51. Wood RA, Segall N, Ahlstedt S, Williams PB. Accuracy of IgE antibody laboratory results. Ann Allergy Asthma Immunol. 2007;99:34-41.
52. Yu J, Yoo Y, Kim DK, Kang H, Koh YY. Bronchial responsiveness and serum eosinophil cationic protein levels in preschool children with recurrent wheezing. Ann Allergy Asthma Immunol. 2005;94(6):686-92.
53. Zijlstra WT, Flinterman AE, Soeters L, Knulst AC, Sinnema G, L'Hoir MP, et al. Parental anxiety before and after food challenges in children with suspected peanut and hazelnut allergy. Pediatr Allergy Immunol. 2010;21:e439-45.

Chapter 5

Tuberculosis Diagnostics: *In Vivo* and *In Vitro* Techniques

Claudio Sorino, Tiziana Cappelletti

BACKGROUND

The infection by *Mycobacterium tuberculosis* (MTB) affects near one-third of the world population, and kills almost 2 million people each year. The most desirable characteristics of a diagnostic tool for tuberculosis are affordability, rapidity and accuracy. In the last years, old diagnostic options have been improved and several new diagnostic options have been added and are commercially available.

However, the ideal diagnostic paths are often not applied to most of the people who need them, due to multiple social and economic circumstances, and factors related to the host and the pathogen.

Clinical screening and optimizing sample collection are key steps in the diagnostic process.

This requires that the physician has great knowledge about the epidemiology of tuberculosis (TB) in the different populations, as well as of risk factors, clinical manifestations, and way of transmission of the disease.

Tuberculosis is acquired through the inhalation of airborne droplets containing the responsible organism, i.e. MTB (also known as Koch's bacillus or BK). The lungs are the primary site of infection.

The risk of infection is related to:

- Degree of infectiousness of the person with TB (the most infectious patients are those with cavitary disease, since this creates a local environment favoring bacterial growth and an easy way out of mycobacteria from the lungs). Often these patients have the direct examination of sputum positive for BK.
- Adequacy of antimicrobial defense of the exposed subject (individuals with the highest risk are those with immunodeficiency; this can be due to human immunodeficiency virus [HIV] infection, which has the greatest influence and impact on the course of TB worldwide, or to immunosuppressive therapy, organ transplantation, malignancy and advanced age).
- Frequency of contact.
- Environment where contact occurs (high-risk environments includes poorly ventilated and crowded places, such as prisons, hotels, refugee camps, poor neighborhoods of large metropolitan centers).
- Virulence of the infecting organism.

The majority of exposed individuals is able to contain the infection and remains asymptomatic; although at risk of reactivation later in life, especially in cases of immunosuppression.

DIAGNOSIS OF LATENT TUBERCULOSIS INFECTION

Until recently, the only test for detecting latent tuberculosis infection (LTBI) was an in vivo technique, the *tuberculin skin test (TST).* A significant progress in the diagnosis of LTBI has been obtained through the creation of in vitro blood tests based on specific cell-mediated immune response. They are *interferon-gamma release assays (IGRAs)*, and measure T cell release of interferon (IFN)-gamma following stimulation by antigens unique to MTB.

Tuberculin Skin Test

The *Mantoux test* is the recommended TST worldwide. The standard Mantoux test consists in the intradermal injection of 5 *tuberculin units* (TU) of *purified protein derivative (PPD)* solution (usually corresponding to 0.1 mL). It becomes positive within 3-8 weeks after the acquisition of the infection.

A 27-gauge needle and a tuberculin syringe are typically used, and the volar surface of the forearm is the usual site for the test (Figs. 5.1A to C). Areas of skin with veins, rashes or excess hair should be avoided. Before the injection, the area should be cleansed with alcohol swab, and wait for it to dry. If the operator correctly injects all the antigen just below the surface of the skin, he creates a 6-10 mm wheal (a pale, raised area with distinct edges, which does not disappear immediately). If no wheal forms, or if a wheal forms that is less than 6 mm of induration, the test should be repeated immediately, on the other arm or at about 5 cm from original site. If minor bleeding occurs, the injection site can be dabbed with a cotton swab. Coverage of the area with a bandage or application of pressure should be avoided. At the same time, the patient should be instructed not to scratch the site, but to use cool compress to relieve any itching or swelling. The date, time and location of TST administration should be record and the reading done after 48-72 hours. It is good practice to provide written information on TST; in many countries, it is necessary to obtain a written consent of the patient before performing the test. If available, the knowledge of the results of previous TST is very useful.

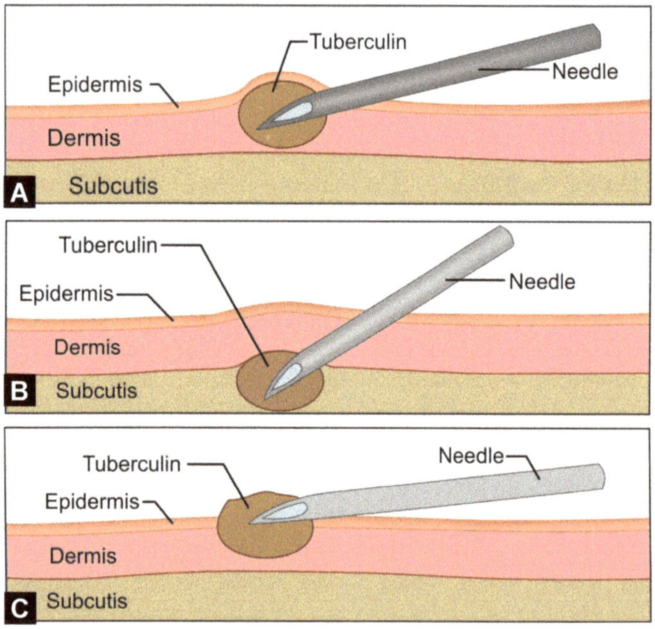

Figs. 5.1A to C: Tuberculin skin test. (A) Proper intradermal injection: a clear characteristic skin wheal is formed; (B) The needle angle is too deep: a diffuse shallow swelling on skin surface occurs; (C) The needle angle is too shallow: tuberculin is leaked on skin surface.

Reading of TST is made by measuring the induration (hard bump) and not erythema. The reader should palpate the area with fingertips, and measure the diameter of induration perpendicular to the long axis of the arm. A ballpoint pen can be used to mark edges of induration, and a tuberculin skin testing ruler or ruler with millimeters to measure such a diameter. It is preferable to record results in millimeters of induration (0 mm, if there is no induration) rather than as positive or negative. PPD solution should be stored and transported in the dark as much as possible; it must be kept refrigerated at 36°- 46°F and fluctuations in temperature should be avoided. Syringes must be filled immediately prior to administration.

The sensitivity of the skin test is reduced in patients with HIV infection, other causes of immune deficiency, advanced age or other comorbidities, which may be anergic.

Tuberculin skin test is considered both safe and reliable throughout the course of pregnancy, but it should be reserved only in the presence of a true real risk for acquiring LTBI or for progression from LTBI to TB disease.

Interpretation of Tuberculin Skin Test

Classification of TST reactions is based on the measurement of the reaction in millimeters. The result is considered positive for different increments of induration diameter (5 mm, 10 mm, or 15 mm) according to the person's risk of acquiring TB infection or the risk of progression to disease in infected subjects. As shown in Table 5.1, in subjects without risk factors, the positivity is given by an induration greater than or equal to 15 mm, while in individuals at risk the threshold can be 10 mm (e.g. in immigrants, resident or employed in prisons, hospitals) or even 5 mm (e.g. in HIV-positive subjects).

Some people infected with *M. tuberculosis* may have a negative reaction to the TST if many years have passed from infection. A positive reaction can result to a subsequent TST because the initial test stimulates the ability to react to the test. This is commonly referred to as the *booster phenomenon* and should not be considered erroneously as a skin test conversion (from negative to positive). The booster phenomenon may occur at any age, but is more frequent in older individuals. A double procedure or "two-step method" is recommended in health care workers that may be tested periodically. If the first test result is negative and the second (performed after 1-3 weeks) becomes positive the person should be considered infected and treat accordingly. If the subject has had a documented TST within the last 12 months, that TST can be counted as the first step in two-step testing.

Table 5.1: Classification of tuberculin skin test reactions according to the individual's risk factors.

A TST reaction of ≥5 mm of induration is considered positive in:
• HIV-infected persons
• Subjects with recent contacts with an infectious TB patient
• Persons with nodular or fibrotic changes on chest X-ray consistent with prior TB
• Patients with organ transplants and other immunosuppressed patients (including patients taking the equivalent of ≥15 mg/day of prednisone for 1 month or more or those taking TNF-α antagonists)
A TST reaction of ≥10 mm of induration is considered positive in:
• Subjects arrived within last 5 years from high-prevalence areas
• Injection drug users
• Residents or employees of high-risk congregate settings (e.g. prisons, correctional facilities, long-term care facilities, hospitals and other health care facilities, residential facilities for patients with HIV infection/AIDS, and homeless shelters)
• Mycobacteriology laboratory personnel
• Persons with clinical conditions that increase the risk for progression to TB disease
• Children younger than 5 years of age
• Infants, children, and adolescents exposed to adults in high risk categories
A TST reaction of ≥15 mm of induration is considered positive in:
• People with no known risk factors for TB (such cases skin testing are usually conducted for employment or school attendance regardless of risk)

(AIDS: Acquired immune deficiency syndrome; HIV: Human immunodeficiency virus; TB: Tuberculosis; TNF: Tumor necrosis factor; TST: Tuberculin skin test).

Interferon-Gamma Release Assays

Interferon-gamma release assays are in vitro techniques, designed for the diagnosis of LTBI. Two IGRAs are today commercially licensed for this purpose: *QuantiFERON®-TB test* (QFT-G; Cellestis, Victoria, Australia), and *T-SPOT® TB test* (Oxford Immunotec, Oxford, United Kingdom). Such tests are performed on peripheral blood samples and are based on the release of interferon gamma by T lymphocytes in response to simulation with exclusive *Mycobacterium tuberculosis* antigens.

Specifically, the first (QuantiFERON) is an enzyme-linked immunosorbent assay (ELISA)-based whole blood test, while the second (T-SPOT) is an enzyme-linked immunospot (ELISPOT) performed on separated peripheral blood mononuclear cells (sensitivity for T-SPOT appears to be higher than for QFT-GIT).

They have a sensitivity of 70-90% for the diagnosis of LTBI, and a specificity of 95-99% (thus greater than TST). Moreover, they are not affected by previous *Bacillus Calmette-Guérin (BCG)* vaccination (so do not cause false positive reactions in BCG recipients). For this reason IGRAs are preferred in endemic countries where BCG is given at an early age (or repeated) to protect infants and young children from serious, life-threatening disease such as miliary TB and TB meningitis.

Furthermore, since the IGRA antigens are not present in most of *environmental mycobacteria or nontuberculous mycobacteria (NTM)*, false positive tests due to NTM exposure or infection are less likely to occur with IGRAs than with TST.

Another advantage of IGRAs is the absence of the above described booster phenomenon, so that using IGRAs for serial testing, a second test is not necessary. Moreover, IGRAs require only one patient visit, there are no health care workers involvements or bias, and results are availability within 24 hours. As for TST, IGRAs cannot distinguish between latent infection and active TB disease. At this time, there are limited data on use in children younger than 5 years of age, individuals with recent exposition to TB, immunocompromised patient. As for TST, IGRAs also are safe to use during pregnancy, but have not been evaluated for diagnosing TB infection in pregnant women.

Sample testing must be performed within 8-30 hours after collection. Laboratories should provide both the

Table 5.2: Expected results of TST and IGRAs in different conditions.

Clinical condition	*TST*	*IGRA*
Non-infected subjects	Negative	Negative
Active tuberculosis	Positive	Positive
Latent tuberculosis infection	Positive	Positive
Recent exposition to *M. tuberculosis*	Positive	Positive
Exposition to environmental mycobacteria	Positive	Negative
BCG vaccination	Positive	Negative

(BCG: Bacille Calmette-Guérin; IGRA: Interferon-gamma release assay; TST: Tuberculin skin test).

Table 5.3: Comparison of the main characteristic of tuberculin skin tests and interferon-gamma release assays.

	TST	*QuantiFERON*	*T-SPOT*
Result format	mm of induration	Concentration of interferon gamma (IU/mL)	Number of spots on a plate
Cross-reacts with BCG and NTM	Yes	No	No
Time frame to get blood to laboratory	NA	<14 hours	<8 hours
Cost to the health system	Low	Moderate	Moderate
Number of visits required	2	1	1
Operator influence	Yes	No	No
Adverse reactions	Rare but possible (skin blistering and ulceration)	Absent	Absent

(BCG: Bacille Calmette-Guérin; NTM: Nontuberculous mycobacteria; TST: Tuberculin skin test).

qualitative (positive, negative, borderline) and quantitative results. Since the results of IGRAs should be interpreted with other relevant clinical information, some TST/IGRA algorithm have been developed to facility the interpretation. Table 5.2 schematizes the conditions when TST and IGRAs are positive or negative. Table 5.3 makes a short comparison of TST and the two IGRAs.

Special considerations in testing for TB infection should be reserved to particular conditions as *HIV infection*. In patient with both LTBI and untreated HIV infection the risk of progression from LTBI to TB disease is 7–10% each year, whereas persons with LTBI but without HIV infection have a 10% risk over their lifetime. Antiretroviral therapy (ART) for HIV infection reduces this risk but this remains much higher than in HIV-negative individuals with LTBI. So HIV infected should be tested for LTBI as soon as their HIV status becomes known. Sensitivity of IGRA in subjects with HIV infection is reduced to 60–80%, thus a negative IGRA result is far from exclude LTBI and annual testing would be appropriate in HIV-infected patients with a risk for exposure to *M. tuberculosis*. Additional control for LTBI in HIV-infected persons with negative result is also recommended after starting ART because the immune response may be restored by ART.

DIAGNOSIS OF ACTIVE PULMONARY TUBERCULOSIS

The gold standard for the diagnosis of active pulmonary TB is the culture isolation of the organism on sputum, bronchial or gastric aspirates. The main disadvantage of the culture is that the mycobacterium can take from 4 to 6 weeks for the growth, resulting in delay in diagnosis.

In individuals with positive tests for TB infection, *chest X-ray* may help differentiate between LTBI and pulmonary TB disease. Useful recommendations include:

- To perform chest X-ray as part of a medical evaluation for subjects with positive TST or IGRA results
- To perform chest X-ray and start treatment for LTBI (e.g. "window prophylaxis" in a young child or

immunocompromised person) in individuals who are in close contact with an infectious TB patient, even without a positive test result for TB infection
- To consider a treatment for LTBI, after TB disease is excluded, in subjects with nodular or fibrotic lesions consistent with old TB at chest X-ray; on the contrary, fully calcified, discrete granulomas do not represent an increased risk for progression to TB disease.

Smear Microscopy

Sputum smear examination is indicated for persons with positive test results for TB infection and either an abnormal chest radiograph or the presence of respiratory symptoms (even when the chest radiograph is normal).

The isolation of MTB from smear required an adequate sample preparation. Because most of sputum samples are rich in mucin, it is necessary a preliminary homogenization with mucolytic agents as N-acetyl-L-cysteine (NAC).

Sputum often contain a great deal of nonmycobacterial microorganisms, thus the specimen must be mixed and treated with decontamination agents (such as solutions of sodium hydroxide 1–2%, sulfuric acid 8%, oxalic acid 5%). So the procedure is less aggressive, but enough to ensure the monitoring of contaminants, than the diagnostic results are best.

The direct microscopic detection of alcohol-acid resistant bacilli (acid-fast bacilli, AFB) in smears is the most rapid bacteriological testing for the presence of mycobacteria in the sample (with a semi-quantitative estimation) and provides preliminary confirmation of the suspected diagnosis. The data are used in the estimation of the infectivity of the patient in question with great importance in clinical and epidemiological prescription of insulation measures and research and identification of contacts at risk.

Two procedures are commonly used for staining: methods to carbol fuchsin (which include Ziehl-Neelsen stain) and methods based on using fluorochrome auramine-O.

Several studies have shown that there must be 5,000–10,000 bacilli × milliliter of sample to allow detection of bacteria in stained smears.

From 50 to 80% of patients with pulmonary TB infection presented a sputum examination positive for AFB. Test sensibility can be significantly increased until 90% with some clinical (repetition of sample on 3 consecutive days) and laboratory precautions (concentration procedures). The percentage of samples AFB positive that result negative in culture is less than 1% (great specificity). Most of the positive samples by microscopic examination, with negative bacterial culture, were observed in patients receiving antibiotic therapy, although not intentionally antimycobacterial (such as fluorochinolons).

The presence of acid alcohol resistant bacilli identified on smear can be both diagnostic of active infection by MTB from NTM. On clinical front is important to remember that the positivity of a microscopic examination for AFB must achieve isolation of the patient and the establishment of infection control measures in the contacts: family, social and working.

All clinical specimens suspected of containing mycobacteria should be cultured because:
- Culture is much more sensitive than microscopic examination
- Growth of the organisms is required for the identification of species
- Tests for drug sensitivity require the isolation of bacteria
- Genotyping of cultured organisms may be useful.

Culture and Drug-Susceptibility Testing

Sputum culture is the gold standard for laboratory confirmation of active TB, and growing bacteria are required to perform drug-susceptibility testing and genotyping.

While there should be 5,000–10,000 bacilli/mm of specimen to allow the detection of bacteria in stained smears, 10–100 bacilli are enough for a positive culture.

The diagnostic sensitivity of culture is about 80-85% with a specificity of 98%. Three different culture media are available for the isolation and identification of MTB: lots based on egg protein (*lowenstein-jensen*), lots agar enriched and liquid media (*broths*). Growth occurs in 3–8 weeks.

Although the diagnosis of active TB is mainly bacteriological, it remains based on clinical-epidemiologic data in 20% of cases in adults, and until 50% in pediatric or in immunocompromised patients. The commercially available broth culture systems (e.g. BACTEC™, MGIT™, VersaTREK, MBBACT) allow detection of most mycobacterial growth in 4–14 days compared to 3–6 weeks for solid media. Laboratories should report initial positive *M. tuberculosis* cultures as soon as possible to the primary health care provider.

All individuals suspected of having TB disease should have sputum specimens collected for microscopy examination and culture, even if respiratory symptoms are absent. At least three consecutive sputum specimens are required, each collected in 8- to 24-hour intervals, with at least one being an early morning specimen. If possible, specimens should be obtained in an airborne infection isolation room or other isolated, well-ventilated area (e.g. outdoors)

Gastric aspiration is a procedure sometimes used to obtain a specimen for culture when a patient cannot cough up adequate sputum (e.g. children). A tube is inserted through the mouth or nose and into the stomach to recover sputum that was coughed into the throat and then swallowed. Gastric aspiration usually requires hospitalization and should be done in the morning before the patient gets out of bed or eats, as it is the optimal time to collect swallowed respiratory secretions from the stomach. Specimens obtained by gastric aspiration should be transported to the lab immediately for neutralization or neutralized immediately at the site of collection.

Since TB disease may involve almost any anatomical site, several clinical specimens other than sputum may be collected for examination when *extrapulmonary* TB disease is suspected. These include urine, cerebrospinal fluid, pleural fluid, pus and biopsy specimens. It should be highlighted that specimens placed in formalin for histologic examination cannot be used for culture.

Drug-susceptibility testing is aimed at finding out which drugs the TB bacteria are sensitive to, and to identify drug-resistant TB. Whenever *M. tuberculosis* is isolated, it should be tested for resistance to the first-line anti-TB drugs: isoniazid, rifampin, ethambutol and pyrazinamide. The results of drug-susceptibility tests help the clinicians to choose the appropriate drugs for treating each patient.

The laboratory should promptly forward the drug-susceptibility results to the physician. Drug-susceptibility tests should be repeated for patients who do not respond as expected or who have positive culture results despite 3 months of adequate treatment.

The Xpert (GeneXpert) MTB/RIF test is a new molecular test which enables simultaneous the diagnoses of TB through the detection of *M. tuberculosis*, and rifampicin (RIF) resistance. The Xpert MTB/RIF a ssay was endorsed by WHO in December, 2010. This assay was specifically recommended for use as the initial diagnostic test for suspected drug-resistant or HIV-associated pulmonary tuberculosis. By June, 2012, two-thirds of countries with a high TB burden and half of countries with a high multidrug-resistant TB burden had incorporated the assay into their national TB program guidelines.

DNA Technology and Nucleic Acid Amplification

The development of DNA technology has allowed to generate fast, highly sensitive and specific procedures such as the hybridization of nucleic acids and the high-performance liquid chromatography (HPLC).

The first uses molecular probes extracted from mycobacteria of the TB complex or the *M. avium* complex, capable to specifically bind the mycobacterial DNA.

HPLC is based on the observation that the synthesis of mycolic acids, structural components of the cell wall, is different for each species of mycobacterium and therefore allows the identification of the species.

The nucleic acid amplification (NAA) tests are used to amplify DNA and RNA segments to rapidly identify the microorganisms in a specimen. Due to their capability to detect even a low number of pairs of DNA, they represent the major new strategy in TB diagnosis.

CDC recommends that NAA testing be performed on at least one respiratory specimen from each patient with signs and symptoms of pulmonary TB for whom a diagnosis of TB is being considered but has not yet been established, and for whom the test result would alter case management or TB control activities, such as contact investigations.

The main utility of NAA tests include:

- To quickly diagnose TB by identifying DNA or RNA of MTB in biological samples reducing the time from weeks to 24–48 hours
- To rapidly confirm whether the AFB microorganisms identified by microscopic examination are MTB or NTM
- To identify drug-resistant strains of MTB through the highlighting of genetic modifications associated with antimycobacterial agents resistance.

However, it is believed that the NAA tests are not yet reliable enough to replace the traditional diagnostic methods. The most common mistake in the use of NAA tests is the false negative result due to the low local density of mycobacteria in the sample. Furthermore polymerase inhibitors present in respiratory secretions interfere with test of amplification. It should be highlighted that the sensitivity of NAA tests for smear negative specimens is as low as 66%.

According to the current recommendations of the Centers for Disease Control and Prevention (CDC) for the use of NAA tests, they should be interpreted within the context of the patient's signs and symptoms, and should always be performed in conjunction with AFB smear and

Table 5.4: Combined interpretation of AFB smear and NAA test and relative suggested approach. In all cases, confirmation by respiratory specimen culture result is required.

AFB smear microscopy	*NAA test (respiratory specimens)*	*Considerations*
+	+	*Presume TB disease.* Start contact investigation, TB medications and keep isolated until determined no longer contagious.
+	–	*Suspect nontuberculous mycobacteria in the specimen.* This does not rule out the possibility of TB. It may be appropriate to remove the patient from isolation, and to delay starting TB medications and contact evaluations until a diagnosis is made. If the patient is highly suspected of having TB and lives in a congregate setting or with high-risk individuals, requesting a NAA test on a second specimen may be justified to assist with treatment and isolation decisions.
–	+	*Likely TB disease* Consider submitting another specimen for NAA testing to verify. A patient can be presumed to have TB if two or more specimens are NAA positive. Use clinical judgment to decide if appropriate to begin TB treatment, start contact investigation and place on isolation.
–	–	*A diagnosis of TB cannot be excluded.* Rely on clinical judgment to determine whether or not to pursue further diagnostic work up or start the patient on treatment while waiting for culture results. Requesting a NAAT on a second specimen may be justified to assist with treatment decisions. A contact investigation may be delayed and the patient presumed non-infectious if three sputum smear results and all NAAT results are negative.

(AFB: Acid fast bacilli; NAA: Nucleic acid amplification; TB: Tuberculosis).

culture (Table 5.4). A single positive NAA test, NAA is considered diagnostic for pulmonary TB in patients with positivity of microscopic examination for AFB. In AFB negative patient, two consecutive positive NAA test are required for diagnosis.

BIBLIOGRAPHY AND FURTHER READING

1. Bodmer T, Ströhle A. Diagnosing pulmonary tuberculosis with the Xpert MTB/RIF test. J Vis Exp. 2012;(62):e3547.
2. Cattamanchi A, Smith R, Steingart KR, Metcalfe JZ, Date A, Coleman C, et al. Interferon-gamma release assays for the diagnosis of latent tuberculosis infection in HIV-infected individuals: a systematic review and meta-analysis. J Acquir Immune Defic Syndr. 2011;56(3):230-8.
3. Center for Disease Control and Prevention. Updated Guidelines for the Use of Nucleic Acid Amplification Tests in the Diagnosis of Tuberculosis. 2009. [online] Available from www.cdc.gov/mmwr/preview/mmwrhtml/mm5801a3.htm?s_cid=mm5801a3_e [Accessed December, 2015].
4. Chang KC, Leung CC. Systematic review of interferon-gamma release assays in tuberculosis: focus on likelihood ratios. Thorax. 2010;65(3):271-6.
5. Lawn SD, Mwaba P, Bates M, Piatek A, Alexander H, Marais BJ, et al. Advances in tuberculosis diagnostics: the Xpert MTB/RIF assay and future prospects for a point-of-care test. Lancet Infect Dis. 2013;13(4):349-61.
6. Mazurek GH, Jereb J, Vernon A, LoBue P, Goldberg S, Castro K, et al. Updated guidelines for using Interferon Gamma Release Assays to detect Mycobacterium tuberculosis infection - United States, 2010. MMWR Recomm Rep. 2010; 59:1-25.
7. Mazurek GH, Jereb J, Vernon A, LoBue P, Goldberg S, Castro K, IGRA Expert Committee, Centers for Disease Control and Prevention (CDC). Updated guidelines for using Interferon Gamma Release Assays to detect Mycobacterium tuberculosis infection - United States, 2010. MMWR Recomm Rep. 2010;59(RR-5):1-25.
8. Menzies D, Pai M, Comstock G. Meta-analysis: new tests for the diagnosis of latent tuberculosis infection: areas of uncertainty and recommendations for research. Ann Intern Med. 2007;146(5):340-54.
9. Metcalfe JZ, Everett CK, Steingart KR, Cattamanchi A, Huang L, Hopewell PC, et al. Interferon-g release assays for active pulmonary tuberculosis diagnosis in adults in low- and middle-income countries: systematic review and meta-analysis. J Infect Dis. 2011;204 (Suppl 4):S1120-9.
10. Pai M, Kunimoto D, Jamieson F, Menzies D. Diagnosis of latent tuberculosis infection. Canadian TB Standards, 7th Edition. Can Respir J. 2013;20 (Suppl A):23A.
11. Pai M, Zwerling A, Menzies D. Systematic review: T-cell-based assays for the diagnosis of latent tuberculosis infection: an update. Ann Intern Med. 2008;149(3):177-84.
12. van Zyl-Smit RN, Zwerling A, Dheda K, Pai M. Within-subject variability of interferon-g assay results for tuberculosis and boosting effect of tuberculin skin testing: a systematic review. PLoS One. 2009;4(12):e8517.
13. Wallis RS, Kim P, Cole S, Hanna D, Andrade BB, Maeurer M, et al. Tuberculosis biomarkers discovery: developments, needs, and challenges. Lancet Infect Dis. 2013;13(4):362-72.
14. Zwerling A, van den Hof S, Scholten J, Cobelens F, Menzies D, Pai M. Interferon-gamma release assays for tuberculosis screening of healthcare workers: a systematic review. Thorax. 2012;67(1):62-70.

Section 2

Evaluation of Respiratory Function

Chapter

6

Overview of the Pulmonary Function Tests

Claudio Sorino, Theodore G Liou, Riccardo Pistelli

MEANING OF LUNG FUNCTION

The term *lung function* refers to the efficiency of the respiratory system in carrying out its functions. It can be evaluated through different noninvasive or minimally invasive procedures indicated just as *lung function tests* or *pulmonary function tests (PFT)*. These explore different aspects of lung function, such as the lung volumes and flows (spirometry, body plethysmography), the diffusing capacity of the lungs for gases, the bronchial responsiveness (bronchoprovocation challenge testing), the elasticity of the lungs and the homogeneity of lung ventilation. Other measurements, such as the pulse oximetry, arterial blood gas analysis and exercise testing, are part of the overall assessment of respiratory efficiency, although they are generally not included in the definition of PFT.

Lung volumes are usually divided into *static* and *dynamic* (moving). The former are instantly measured under specific conditions, the latter are measured at certain time intervals and reflect the diameter and the integrity of the airways. A further classification divides lung volumes in *displaceable* (i.e. which can be inhaled or exhaled) and *not displaceable* (which remain within the lungs even at the end of a maximal exhalation).

Some respiratory volumes can be calculated as the sum of different volumes (static and/or dynamic) and are referred to as capacities (Fig. 6.1).

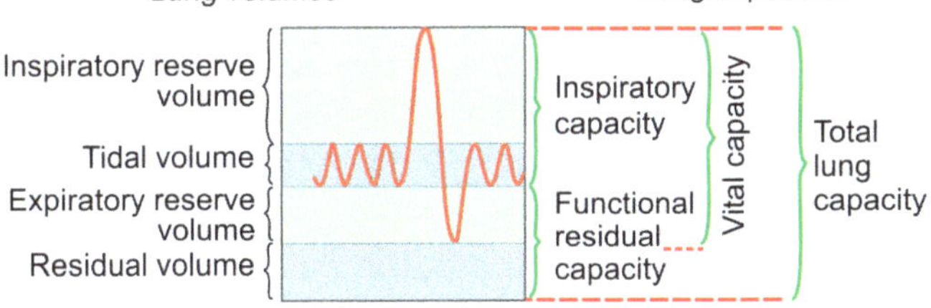

Fig. 6.1: Lung volumes and capacities.

SPIROGRAM AND DISPLACEABLE VOLUMES

The execution of spirometry allow to generate a *spirogram*, consisting of a *volume-time curve* (Fig. 6.2A), often associated with a *flow-volume curve*, in which the signals of flow and volume are reproduced respectively on the y and x axis (Fig. 6.2B).

Although, the two ways of representing the respiratory function today are simultaneously shown in a single report, they were conceived a century one after the other. The spirogram was firstly proposed in 1846 by John Hutchinson, the inventor of the spirometer. He recognized that the volume of air that a subject can exhale after completely inflated the lungs was a great indicator of the capacity for survival. Consequently, he coined the term "vital capacity" (VC) to indicate such a volume, corresponding to the slow expiratory vital capacity (EVC) according to today's terminology. Clinical applications of the "John Hutchinson's mysterious machine" came only after many years. In 1947, the French investigators Tiffeneau and Pinelli changed spirometric measurements to the current form. For the first time they described the forced expiratory maneuver, and proposed measurement of the maximal volume expelled in one second after a deep inspiration, which they called *pulmonary capacity usable on exercise* (capacité pulmonaire utilisable à l'effort) (CPUE). It was intended to substitute the measurement of the "maximum breathing

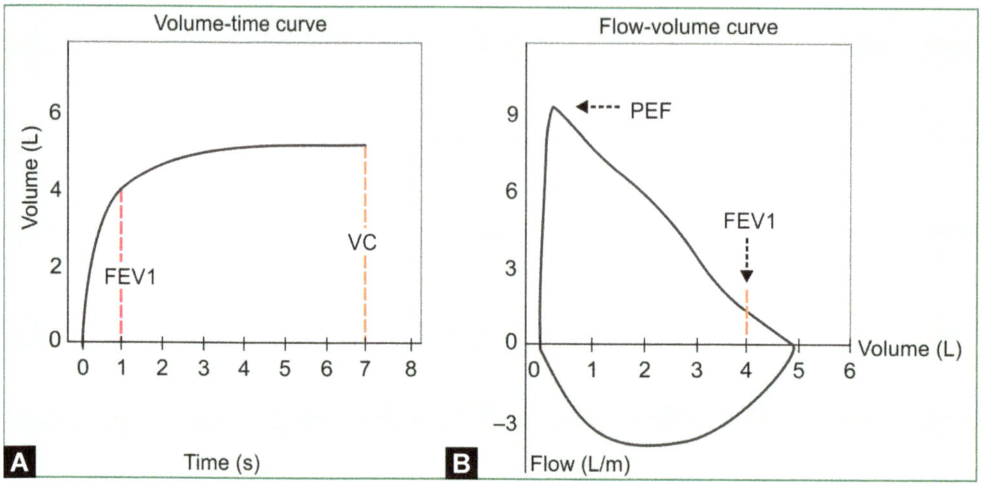

Figs. 6.2A and B: Normal spirogram. (A) Volume-time curve and (B) Flow-volume curve. More than 70% of the air is expelled in the first second of a complete forced expiration.

capacity", which required a laborious and exhausting maneuvre. Such a parameter, subsequently defined *forced expiratory volume in 1 second*, became a key diagnostic index together with the *forced EVC.*

The main parameters that can be determined using simple spirometry are the following:

Forced Expiratory Volume in 1 Second (FEV1)

It is the maximal volume of air expired in the first second of a forced expiration starting from a full inhalation. It depends on the expiratory effort and reflects mainly the diameter of the proximal airways. It is expressed in liters. It depends on the expiratory effort and reflects mainly the diameter of the proximal airways. It is the most reproducible spirometric parameter and can be considered an overall index of airway function, being reduced in both obstructive and restrictive pulmonary diseases. The value of FEV1 is influenced by age, sex, height, and race, and is more accurately expressed as a percentage of the normal predicted value. An FEV can be recorded at any time during the forced expiration. For example, FEV3 is the volume expired in the first 3 seconds, and FEV6 is the volume expired in the first 6 seconds.

Vital Capacity

It is the maximal volume of air that can be inhaled starting after the maximal lung emptying (in this case also called *inspiratory vital capacity* [*IVC*] or vice versa the maximum volume that can be exhaled starting from the maximum filling of the lungs (in this case also called *expiratory vital capacity* [*EVC*]. It is expressed in liters.

Forced Vital Capacity (FVC)

It corresponds to the VC measured during a maximally forced expiration.

FEV1/VC Ratio

It is a clinically useful index of airflow limitation: its reduction is a characteristic of obstructive lung disease, while it remains unchanged in restrictive ventilatory defects due to the reduction of both numerator and denominator. It is calculated as FEV1/VC × 100 expressed as percent value. When VC is recorded only during the forced expiration, the derived FEV1/FVC ratio is also called *Tiffeneau index.*

Forced Expiratory Volume by Time t Seconds (FEVt)

It is the volume of air exhaled at the second t of a forced expiration performed starting from full inspiration (e.g. FEV3 is recorded at the 3rd second, FEV6 at the 6th second).

In patients unable to complete the exhalation, FEV6 can be used as an approximate surrogate of VC in the diagnosis of obstruction, where it is used to normalize the FEV1 (i.e. by calculating the FEV1/FEV6%). The recourse to FEV6 for the evaluation of possible restrictive ventilatory defect can result in a lower sensitivity due to the early interruption of expiration and the consequent underestimation of the exhaled volume of air.

Forced expiratory volume in 3 seconds is usually quite close to the FVC since normal subjects expel most of the air contained in the lungs in three seconds. The ratio FEV3/FVC% indicates the percentage of FVC expelled during the first three seconds of forced exhalation. Its reduction has been suggested as an indicator of mild lung injury when other spirometric parameters are normal.

Tidal Volume

It is the amount of air that is inhaled or exhaled with each breath under resting conditions.

Inspiratory Reserve Volume (IRV)

It is the maximal volume of air that can be further inhaled after a quite inspiration.

Inspiratory Capacity (IC)

It is the amount of air that can be drawn into the lungs after normal expiration. It corresponds to the sum of IRV and TV. It decreases with increasing of the air trapped in the lungs, thus it is increasingly used as a measure of the degree of dynamic hyperinflation in patient with *chronic obstructive pulmonary disease (COPD)*.

NONDISPLACEABLE LUNG VOLUMES

Residual Volume (RV)

It is the volume of air remaining in the lungs after a maximal exhalation.

Total Lung Capacity (TLC)

It is the volume of air contained in the lungs at the end of a maximal inspiration. It can be measured as the sum of VC and RV or the sum of IC and FRC.

Residual volume and TLC can be measured trough different methods including closed circuit dilution (such as the *helium dilution technique* and *nitrogen washout*), *body plethysmography* and, in the research setting, by CT scan. The values obtained by different techniques may significantly differ in the same subject. Indeed, dilutional methods are not able to measure the volume of air contained in spaces closed by severe bronchial obstruction, *body plethysmography* may overestimates lung volume in patients with airflow obstruction if they are panting at greater than or equal to 2 Hz, and CT scan may underestimate lung volumes due to submaximal inspiration in the supine position.

For the above-mentioned reasons, the technique used to measure RV and TLC should always be specified, for example distinguishing TLC-He (Helium), TLC-pleth (plethysmography), and TLC-n (nitrogen washout).

Functional Residual Capacity (FRC)

It corresponds to the volume of air contained in the lungs at the end of expiration at rest. It is the sum of ERV + RV.

Thoracic Gas Volume (TGV)

It is defined as the volume of intrathoracic gas at the time the airway is occluded for the plethysmographic measurement; this is usually at FRC, so that it can be considered synonymous with FRCpleth, but in special circumstances it may not be.

PARAMETERS OF RESPIRATORY FLOW

Peak Expiratory Flow (PEF)

It is the largest flow generated with a maximal forced expiration, started without hesitation after a full inspiration. It is an effort-dependent variable and reflects the diameter of central airways. PEF is usually recorded during the flow-volume maneuver and it is expressed in liters/second. There are portable peak flow meters, used by the patient at home, which often express the PEF in liters/minute.

Peak Inspiratory Flow (PIF)

It is the fastest flow rate recorded during the inspiratory cycle.

Forced Expiratory Flow at 25% of FVC (FEF 25%)

It occurs when 25% of the total volume (FVC) has been exhaled. If maximal patient effort in exhalation is being maintained, then this flow rate would be the reflection of flow through medium-size to large bronchi.

Forced Expiratory Flow at 75% of FVC (FEF 75%)

It is the flow rate measured when 75% of the total volume (FVC) has been exhaled. This point reflects small airway status and is used in the FEF 25-75% calculation. Decreased values in FEF 75% would be expected in the early stages of chronic obstructive pulmonary diseases or in mild asthma, often when the patient is still asymptomatic.

Forced Expiratory Flow between 25% and 75% of FVC (FEF 25–75%)

It is an index of peripheral airways resistance, also known as the *maximum mid-expiratory flow (MMEF)*. It corresponds to the average expired flow over the middle half of the FVC maneuver and is calculated in the test with the largest sum of FEV1 and FVC. The index is highly dependent on the validity of the FVC measure and only in part on the degree of expiratory effort, being measured over the first 25% of FVC. FEF 25-75% is regarded as a more sensitive measure of small airways narrowing than FEV1, but it has a wide range of normality and is less reproducible than FEV1. A considerable reduction in FEF 25-75% (at lower values than 65% of predicted according to some authors) may be considered abnormal and may be the only sign of ventilatory dysfunction in the early stages or very mild broncho-obstructive diseases. This result is expected because most chronic pulmonary diseases are manifest initially in the smallest airways, which contribute significantly toward the end of the expiratory part of the flow volume loop. However, the use of forced flows at low lung volumes as indicative of peripheral airways disease is controversial, because normal values in healthy reference populations are limited and highly variable, so that the confidence limits are very broad.

PARAMETERS OF AIRWAYS RESISTANCE

There are several important determinants of *airway resistance (Raw)*, including the diameter of the airways, and the type of airflow (laminar or turbulent). Usually, the pressure or volume changes of the plethysmograph corresponding to alveolar pressure are plotted versus airflow. Raw is then calculated from the slope of the resulting S-shaped curve (Fig. 6.3). Due to the elastic nature of the tissue that supports the small airways, Raw changes with lung volume. It is not practically possible to measure Raw at a set absolute lung volume, therefore *specific airway resistance (sRaw)* attempts to correct for differences in lung volume at which different measurements of airway resistance were made.

Raw can be measured at a certain flow rate on the linear part of the curve during panting. After the problem of maintaining BTPS conditions in the breathing air was solved, many investigators turned to measuring Raw during quiet breathing instead of panting. It was then proposed to measure Raw over the total range of alveolar pressure *(total Raw)* or over the points of maximum inspiratory and expiratory air flow. For the latter way of interpretation, the term *terminal Raw (Raw t)* has been suggested, because the terminal points of the curve are used.

Raw during panting may be smaller or higher than Raw during quiet breathing depending on frequency, flow rate and normal or abnormal status of the lungs. Therefore, if the equipment of the plethysmograph allows, Raw should be measured during quiet breathing.

Total airway resistance (Raw tot) is defined as the ratio of alveolar pressure to air flow.

Total specific resistance (sRaw, tot) is Raw corrected for lung volume. Specific airway resistance is often measured at FRC, in which case: sRaw = Raw × FRC

Inspiratory airway resistance (Raw, insp) and *expiratory airway resistance (Raw, exp)* respectively refers to the inspiratory and expiratory component of Raw.

Specific Raw is a measure of airway caliber-comprising effects of lung size. sRaw reflects the overall dimensions of the airway, including the effect of lung expansion on the caliber of the airway. Since sRaw is the product of Raw and TGV, it cannot distinguish if improvements are due to either of its two components. Breathing at different levels of lung volume might give the same sRaw, although the

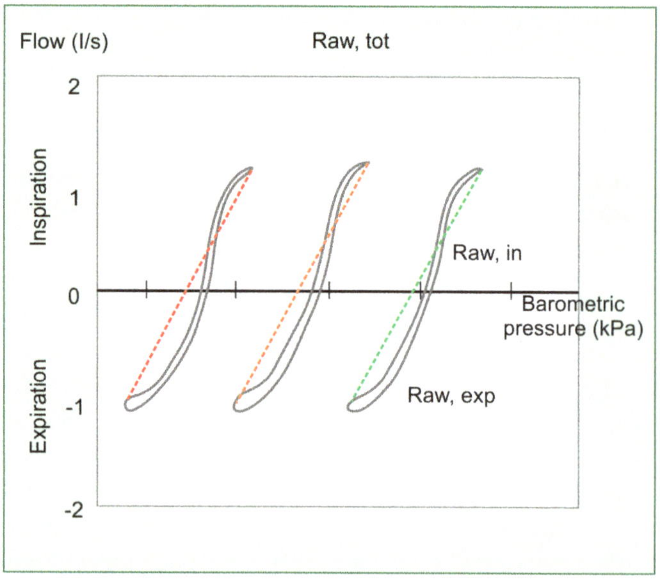

Fig. 6.3: Example of airway resistance loops determined by whole body plethysmography.

relationship between Raw and TGV differs. Likewise, other principles of lung function measurements do not distinguish the effect of lung volume on the flow or resistance.

Any increase, however, of Raw or increase of TGV or both results in an elevated sRaw. Similarly, sRaw will decrease if either Raw or TGV or both are minimized, and a normal sRaw would indicate that both Raw and TGV must be in a normal range. That is why sRaw is the most dynamic parameter, as supported by empiric data comparing sRaw and Raw in asthmatics and healthy subjects. In summary, sRaw is always reflecting the complete respiratory tract, consisting of both resistive and volume properties.

PARAMETERS OF LUNG DIFFUSING CAPACITY

Carbon monoxide diffusing capacity (DL_{CO}): It expresses the lung's ability to transfer a nonreactive test gas, such as carbon monoxide (CO), from inhaled air to the red blood cells in pulmonary capillaries. It is also known as *transfer factor of the lung for carbon monoxide (TL_{CO})*.

Carbon monoxide transfer coefficient (K_{CO}): It is lung diffusion standardized for alveolar volume (VA), and is calculated as DL_{CO}/VA. It had been proposed following the observation that DL_{CO} varies with the depth of inspiration, and hence with the alveolar volume during breath holding. However, the usefulness of K_{CO} as a means for standardizing DL_{CO} has been questioned, since between functional residual capacity and total lung capacity, K_{CO} is not constant, being negatively correlated with alveolar volume.

Methods for measuring lung diffusion capacity are described in detail in a separate chapter.

Tools Used for the Measurement of Lung Function

Spirometry

Spirometry is a simple and noninvasive examination that allows a quantitative assessment of lung displaceable volumes (i.e. those which can be inhaled or exhaled) in function of time. The results provided by spirometry are fundamental for the diagnosis and monitoring of many diseases of the respiratory system.

The tools used for this purpose are the spirometers, which exist in several types based on the use of different technologies. Some spirometers measure as primary signal the volume of mobilized air (bell spirometer, Fig. 6.4); in others spirometers the primary signal recorded is the airflow (pneumotachograph, turbine spirometer, Figs. 6.5A and B). In both cases the spirometer is connected to a computer that converts the signal into numerical values and graphic images.

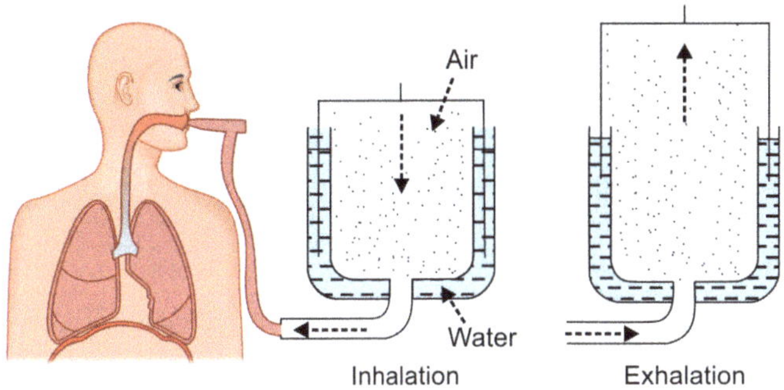

Fig. 6.4: Schematization of a bell spirometer functioning.

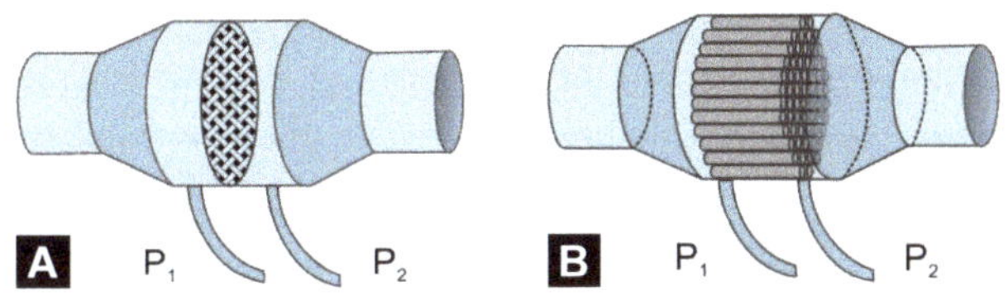

Figs. 6.5A and B: Representation of the two main types of pneumotachographs. (A) Fleisch type; (B) Lilly type.

The *bell spirometer* consists essentially of two bells: the first bell has a double wall and a hollow space filled with water, the second inverted bell is located inside this space; the presence of water ensures the perfect sealing of air or any other gas which is inside of the bells.

The variations of the gas volume present therein induce the sliding of a bell on the other upward and downward. The patient can breathe into the spirometer through a tube equipped with a mouthpiece. This tube is divided into two routes, inspiratory and expiratory, provided of one-way valve; along the tube that leads the exhaled air, there is a container of soda lime which is required to retain the exhaled carbon dioxide (CO_2). All volume-measuring devices, such as the bell spirometer, are subject to Boyles Law describing the effect of atmospheric pressure, temperature and humidity on gas volume. Thus, corrections to body temperature and ambient pressure saturated with water vapor (BTPS) are required and calibration procedures need to be regularly carried out on these types of spirometers as barometric pressure, temperature and humidity frequently change.

The *pneumotachograph* bases its functioning on the Poiseuille's Law, according to which the flow of a gas through a cylindrical duct with rigid walls is proportional to the pressure drop per length unit of the tube. It follows that, by measuring the drop in pressure between two points, the distance of which is known, the flow (liters of air per second) and then the volume can be calculated. There are two main types of pneumotachographs: *Fleisch* and *Lilly*. The Fleisch types are the most used pneumotachographs. They measure the difference in pressure before and after a set of capillaries arranged in parallel with the direction of flow. In the Lilly types the resistance to flow is created by a membrane, but they are usually less reliable than the Fleisch ones.

The main inconvenience of pneumotachographs is that they are very sensitive to temperature, humidity and atmospheric pressure of surrounding air. As a consequence, they must be calibrated very often, at least daily and after each displacement.

Turbine spirometers calculate airflow through a turbine whose rotation is usually measured by infrared. The harder the patient blows, the faster the turbine rotates. The volume of air passed through the tube is calculated from the number of turbine revolutions, while the flow is calculated from the number of turbine revolutions per unit of time. There are two types of turbine: unidirectional, which measure flow only one way (expiratory), and bidirectional, which allow to measure both expiratory and inspiratory flow. The spirometry results are rather reliable and reproducible and not influenced by pressure or humidity.

Spirometers that use ultrasonic waves and the Doppler effect (*ultrasonic spirometers*) are the latest development in this field (Fig. 6.6). Two diagonally opposing piezo-elements send and receive alternatively ultrasonic waves. When there is not gas flow inside the breathing tube, the transit time of the ultrasound waves identical in both directions. An airflow inside the tube accelerates the waves in one direction and slows them down in the other. The higher the flow, the higher the difference between go and return. The results are reliable and precise, the devices are often portable and require no calibration and do not need a thermostat.

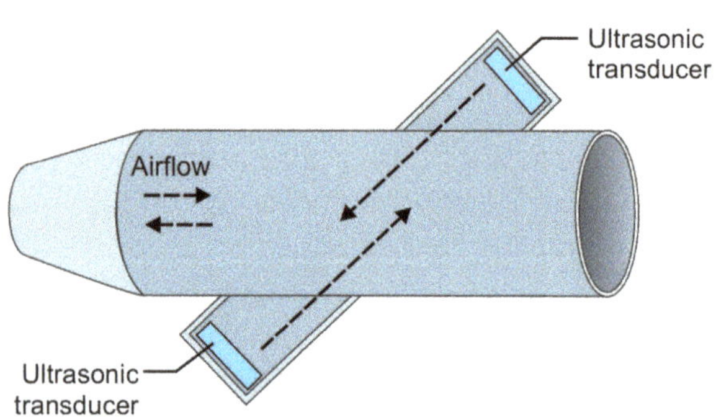

Fig. 6.6: Representation of an ultrasonic spirometer. Two diagonally opposing piezo-elements send and receive alternatively ultrasonic waves. Air flow inside the tube accelerates the waves in one direction and slows them down in the other.

BIBLIOGRAPHY AND FURTHER READING

1. Hutchinson J. On the capacity of the lungs, and on the respiratory functions, with a view of establishing a precise and easy method of detecting disease by the spirometer. Med Chir Trans (London). 1846;29:137-252.
2. Kaminsky DA. What does airway resistance tell us about lung function? Respiratory Care. 2012;57(1):85-96.
3. Macintyre N, Crapo RO, Viegi G, Johnson DC, van der Grinten CP, Brusasco V, et al. ATS/ERS Task Force. Standardisation of the single-breath determination of carbon monoxide uptake in the lung. Eur Respir J. 2005;26:720-35.
4. MacIntyre NR. The future of pulmonary function testing. Respiratory care. 2012;57(1):154-64.
5. Miller MR, Crapo R, Hankinson J, Brusasco V, Burgos F, Casaburi R, et al. General considerations for lung function testing. Eur Respir J. 2005;26:153-61.
6. Miller MR, Hankinson J, Brusasco V, Burgos F, Casaburi R, Coates A, et al. ATS/ERS Task Force. Standardisation of spirometry. Eur Respir J. 2005;26:319-38.
7. Miller MR, Quanjer PH, Swanney MP, Enright PL. Interpreting lung function data using 80% predicted and fixed thresholds misclassifies more than 20% of patients. Chest. 2011;139:52-9.
8. Pellegrino R, Viegi G, Brusasco V, Crapo RO, Burgos F, Casaburi R, et al. Interpretative strategies for lung function tests. Eur Respir J. 2005:26:948-68.
9. Ruppel GL, Enright PL. Pulmonary function testing. Respir Care. 2012;57(1):165-75.
10. Ruppel GL. What is the clinical value of lung volumes? Respir Care. 2012;57(1):26-35.
11. Sorino C, Battaglia S, Scichilone N, Pedone C, Antonelli-Incalzi R, Sherrill D, et al. Diagnosis of airway obstruction in the elderly: contribution of the SARA study. Int J Chron Obstruct Pulmon Dis. 2012:7;1-7.
12. Tiffeneau R, Pinelli A. Air circulant et air captif dans l'exploration de la fonction ventilatrice pulmonaire. Paris Méd. 1947;37:624-8.
13. Wanger J, Clausen JL, Coates A, Pedersen OF, Brusasco V, Burgos F, et al. ATS/ERS Task Force. Standardisation of the measurement of lung volumes. Eur Respir J. 2005;26:511-22.
14. Yernault JC. The birth and development of the forced expiratory manoeuvre: a tribute to Robert Tiffeneau (1910-1961). Eur Respir J. 1997;10:2704-10.

Chapter

7 Displaceable Lung Volumes: Simple Spirometry

Claudio Sorino, Salvatore Battaglia

OVERVIEW OF SIMPLE SPIROMETRY

The mechanical properties of the respiratory system may be affected by several respiratory or systemic diseases. Most of them have consequences upon airway resistance and lung compliance. Simple spirometry is a basic tool for the evaluation of airway function and is commonly the first test performed when a chronic respiratory disease is suspected. By measuring dynamic volumes and flows during forced expiratory and inspiratory maneuvers, it provides a valuable contribute in identifying respiratory diseases associated with some ventilatory defects. It can be used for diagnosing and monitoring respiratory disease, for preoperative risk stratification, and as a tool in epidemiologic and other research studies. The main indications for spirometry are listed in Table 7.1.

Most patients can easily perform spirometry when coached by an appropriately trained technician or other health care provider. The test can be performed in the ambulatory setting, physician's office, emergency department, or inpatient setting. Since several steps should be followed from the preparation to the running of the test, the use of a checklist may be useful to ensure not to overlook some important factors (Table 7.2).

Table 7.1: Main indications for running simple spirometry.

Unexplained, recurrent or persistent respiratory symptoms: dyspnea, cough, or wheezing
Suspected obstructive disease: asthma or chronic obstructive pulmonary disease (COPD)
Presence of risk factors for respiratory diseases (congenital or acquired)
Suspected restrictive disease: suspected interstitial lung disease; chest wall disorders
Assessment of therapy response
Disease follow-up (lung function decline)
Preoperative evaluation of lung function, if indicated

Table 7.2: Example of checklist usable when a spirometry is performed.

- Check the accuracy of the spirometer (daily calibration)
- Record subject's key anthropometric data (gender, date of birth or age, race, standing height, weight).
- Assess if there are contraindications to performing the test (Table 7.3)
- Assess if there are contraindications to administering bronchodilators (Table 7.4)
- Assess which drugs are being used at the present and when they were last taken
- Assess for active smoking (avoid to perform spirometry within 2 hours from the last smoked cigarette).
- Ask the patient to sit for the test
- Ask the patient to loosen restrictive clothing
- Explain the procedure carefully and demonstrate the maneuvers
- Attach nose clip
- Place mouthpiece in mouth and ask the patient to close lips around the mouthpiece
- Ask the patient to inhale quickly and completely (to total lung capacity), then to exhale forcefully without hesitation until no more air can be expelled
- Repeat for a minimum of three valid maneuvers
- Assess the attainment of FEV1 and FVC repeatability, otherwise perform additional maneuvers (up to eight in total)

PREPARATION OF THE EQUIPMENT

Properly calibrated and accurate spirometers are a key element for the correct measurement of respiratory function.

One disadvantage of the new generation of spirometers is that flow sensors can lose accuracy over time, so that calibration checks are needed each day the spirometer is to be used. A 3-liter calibration syringe should be used for this verification. It should be stored near the spirometer so that the two devices remain at the same temperature.

The syringe should be periodically checked for leaks. This can be done by filling the syringe with air, holding the palm against the outlet snout and trying to empty the syringe.

In order to minimize the risk of cross-contamination, the disposable mouthpiece must always be replaced between patients. Moreover, routine hand washing, and proper cleaning of permanent flow sensors are recommended.

PREPARATION OF THE PATIENT AND PRECAUTIONS BEFORE TESTING

Before performing spirometry, the physician should verify that it is safe for the patient. There are absolute and relative contraindications to the spirometry. As shown in Table 7.3, some of these are pathological conditions which are potentially worsened by a forced expiratory maneuver and that may require the postponement of the test until they are resolved (e.g. recent myocardial infarction, pulmonary embolism, pneumothorax, stroke, thoracic, abdominal or eye surgery, uncontrolled hypertension). Other relative

Table 7.3: Absolute and relative contraindications to perform simple spirometry and reasons for this.

Conditions	
Absolute	*Reason: Unsafe for the patient*
Hemoptysis of unknown origin	Risk of exacerbation of the underlying condition with major hemorrhage Possible active pulmonary tuberculosis and consequent risk of cross-infection due to contamination of equipment
Unresolved pneumothorax	Forced expiration may aggravate the problem
Unstable angina or recent myocardial infarction or pulmonary embolism (in the last month)	Risk of precipitating acute coronary syndrome or massive pulmonary embolism, mainly as a consequence of blood pressure changes
Recent thoracic or abdominal surgery (in the last 3 months)	Forced expiration raise intracranial, intrathoracic and intra-abdominal pressures, can cause pain, incisional hernias
Recent eye surgery, e.g. cataract (in the last 3 months)	Forced expiration may cause undesirable raised intraocular pressure
Recent stroke (in the last 3 months)	Risk of recurrence
Uncontrolled arterial hypertension	Risk of dangerous further increase in blood pressure
History of hemorrhagic cerebrovascular events	Precipitation of cerebral bleed
Fractured ribs	Risk of pneumothorax, painful maneuver
Thoracic, abdominal, or cerebral aneurysms	Danger of aneurysm rupture due to increased thoracic pressure
Relative	*Reason: Unsafe for others*
Known or suspected respiratory infection and hemoptysis of unknown origin	Risk of cross-infection due to contamination of equipment Potentially impaired meaning of the results
Relative	*Reason: Suboptimal results*
Nausea, vomiting, or pain	They can affect the patient's ability to perform the test
Confusion, cognitive impairment	Inability to comply with instruction
Oral or facial pain exacerbated by a mouthpiece	The test can be uncomfortable
Stress incontinence	The test can be uncomfortable
Extreme shortness of breath	The test can be uncomfortable
Presence of cough during the test	The test can be unreliable

contraindications are just conditions that may affect the reliability of spirometry measurements (e.g. cognitive impairment, extreme shortness of breath or cough, oral or facial pain, nausea, vomiting).

Moreover, the patients should not have eaten a hearty meal within 2 hours prior to the test (since a full stomach may restrict movement of the diaphragm and cause an underestimation of lung volumes), smoked in the last 2 hours prior to the test or consumed alcohol 4 hours prior to the test (above all if gas transfer or static lung volume measurement are required), undertaken vigorous exercise within 30 minutes prior to the test (since this may affect the quality of spirometry mainly for the measurement of effort-dependent parameters), taken a short-acting bronchodilator within 4 hours prior to the test or long-acting bronchodilator within 12 hours prior to the test (in order to allow the correct measurement of pre- and postbronchodilator values).

Anthropometric data of the patient (race, age, height and weight) are needed for the calculation of predicted values. Height should be accurately measured without shoes, with the feet together, standing as tall as possible with the eyes level looking straight ahead (Fig. 7.1).

Any systemic or inhaled drug able to alter lung function should be recorded, together with its dosage and last intake.

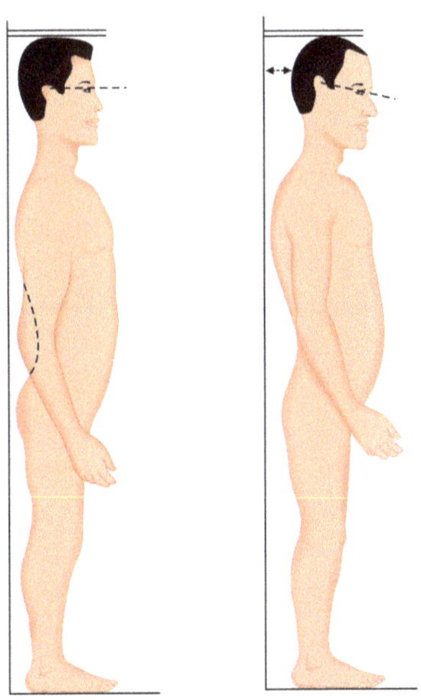

Fig. 7.1: Correct position for the measurement of the height.

TEST EXECUTION

The technician should explain and demonstrate the appropriate technique. Instruction should be detailed but simple and age-appropriate. It is preferable that the patient is sitting, using a chair with arms and without wheels for safety reasons in order to avoid falling due to syncope. When you believe that the patient has understood the instructions, the breathing tube is inserted into his/her mouth, making sure the lips are sealed around the mouthpiece and that the tongue does not occlude it. The use of a nose clip or manual occlusion of the nostril is recommended.

The three key step of a forced expiratory maneuver are the following:

1. Maximal inspiration: the subject should inhale rapidly and completely from functional residual capacity (FRC) to total lung capacity (TLC).
2. Strong exhalation: it is important to prompt the subject to "blast," not just "blow," the air from the lungs.
3. Continued complete exhalation: the subject should be encouraged to fully exhale until the complete emptying of the lung, or at least until the amount of air which exits from the lungs is negligible (*see* end of test criteria).

Reductions in PEF and FEV1 have been observed when inspiration is slow and/or there is a pause higher than 4 seconds at TLC before beginning exhalation. Consequently, it is important that the preceding inspiration is fast and any pause at full inspiration be minimal (ideally only for 1–2 seconds).

The patient's trunk and neck should remain erect during the maneuver, the patient looking straight forward during the entire test without bending over (the latter not only affects the way the trachea is stretched, but may also lead to saliva dripping into the filter mouthpiece and equipment).

In order to more accurately assess the vital capacity (VC), the forced maneuvers can be preceded by two or more slow maneuvers. This can be done in two different ways: (1) starting from end-tidal volume, the subject expires maximally and then makes a full inspiration [inspiratory vital capacity (IVC)] or (2) the subjects make a full inspiration and then exhales maximally [expiratory vital capacity (EVC)].

QUALITY ASSESSMENT OF SPIROMETRY

Before interpreting any spirometry maneuver, it is necessary to evaluate its quality. The reading of the numerical

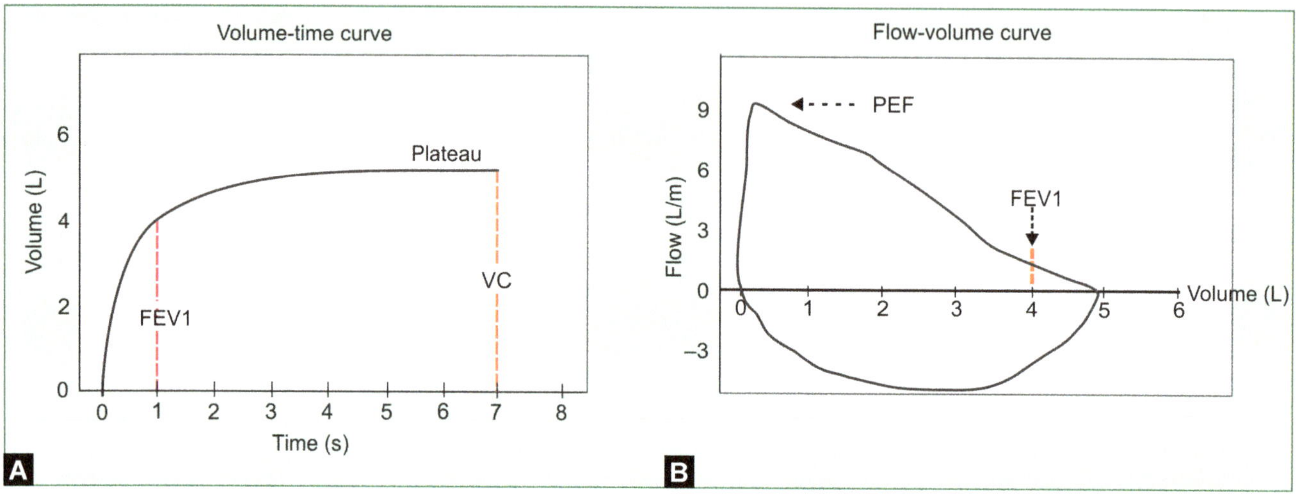

Figs. 7.2A and B: (A) Volume-time curve and (B) Flow-volume curve recorded during a well-performed spirometry in a healthy subject.

data without a review of the quality of the test, as well as the automatic interpretation by the computer, is common sources of interpretation mistakes.

The American Thoracic Society (ATS) criteria, which are the most widely used, suggest to achieve three acceptable maneuvers and verify the repeatability of the main parameters (FEV1 and FVC). They consider the acceptability of the start and the end of each forced spirometric maneuver and repeatability criteria, as discussed below in details.

Evaluation of the Technique and Graphs

Several errors in the patient's execution technique may compromise the interpretation of a spirometry. A careful observation of the patient during the test is essential to assess the adequacy of the technique, in particular of the patient's forced expiratory effort. A correctly performed maneuver should appear to be delivered with maximal effort, starting from the level of maximum inspiration. Forced expiration should start instantaneously and the effort should be sustained at least for one-third of VC. Exhalation should continue until reaching the residual volume, without cough or other interruptions, without evidence for leaks at the mouthpiece, obstruction at the mouth opening due to the tongue or biting the mouthpiece, or to bad-fitting dentures.

The inspection of the volume-time and flow-volume curves is another key element for the quality assessment of a spirometry test. The *volume-time curve* plots volume (in liters) on the vertical axis and time (in seconds) on the horizontal (Fig. 7.2A). The trace must curve upward, be smooth, free of irregularities, and must plateau for at least one second. The *flow-volume curve* plots flow rate (in liters per second or minute) on the vertical axis and volume (in liters) on the horizontal (Fig. 7.2B). The trace should rise almost vertically to a peak flow, then it should go down and merge smoothly with the horizontal axis at FVC at the end of the blow.

A slow start to the forced maneuver often results in a reduced FEV1. In such a case, the volume-time curve has an "S" shape at the start (Fig. 7.3A), whereas the flow-volume curve does not rise steeply (Fig. 7.3B).

When a forced maneuver is performed without enough effort during the initial phase of exhalation, a reduced peak flow can be observed. Moreover, this may result in slightly larger flow rates at middle lung volumes and a higher FEV1, usually due to a reduced gas compression and a lack of sensitivity to lung volume changes when flow is measured at the mouth.

If a maneuver has an obviously hesitant start, the technician may terminate the trial early to avoid an unnecessary prolonged effort. A sudden drop of flow to zero usually suggests a glottis closure or other early interruption of the exhalation, resulting in inaccurate measurement of VC.

Some events that may affect the proper performance and interpretation of spirometry can be easily recognized by observing the graphs (Figs. 7.4A to F).

Even a nonoptimal test can provide useful information. For example, the early interruption of exhalation

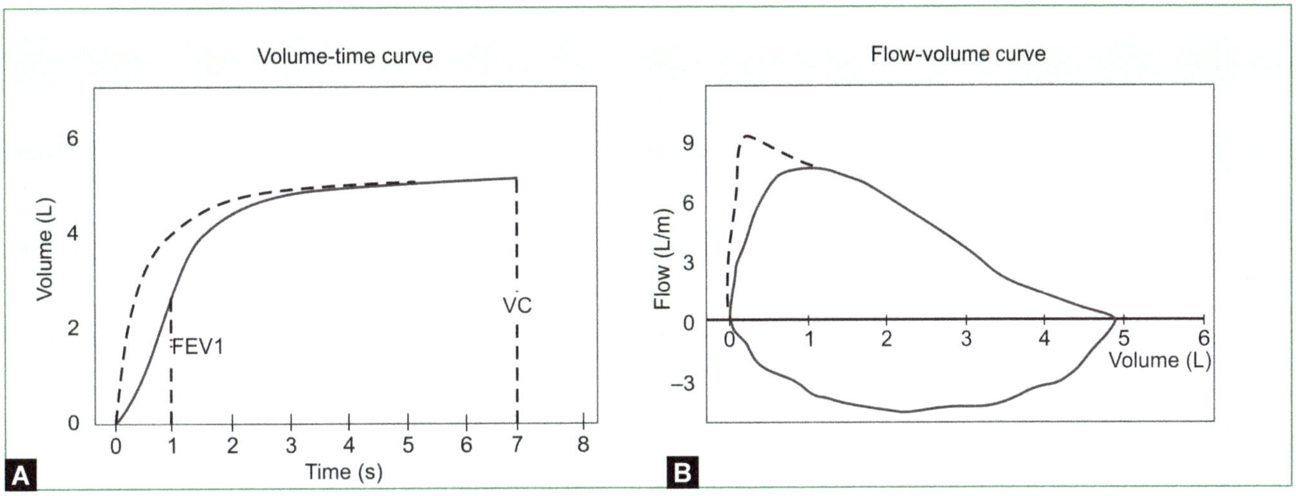

Figs. 7.3A and B: Slow start of forced expiration on the (A) Volume-time and (B) Flow-volume curve. The dashed line indicates the predicted path of the curve without artifacts.

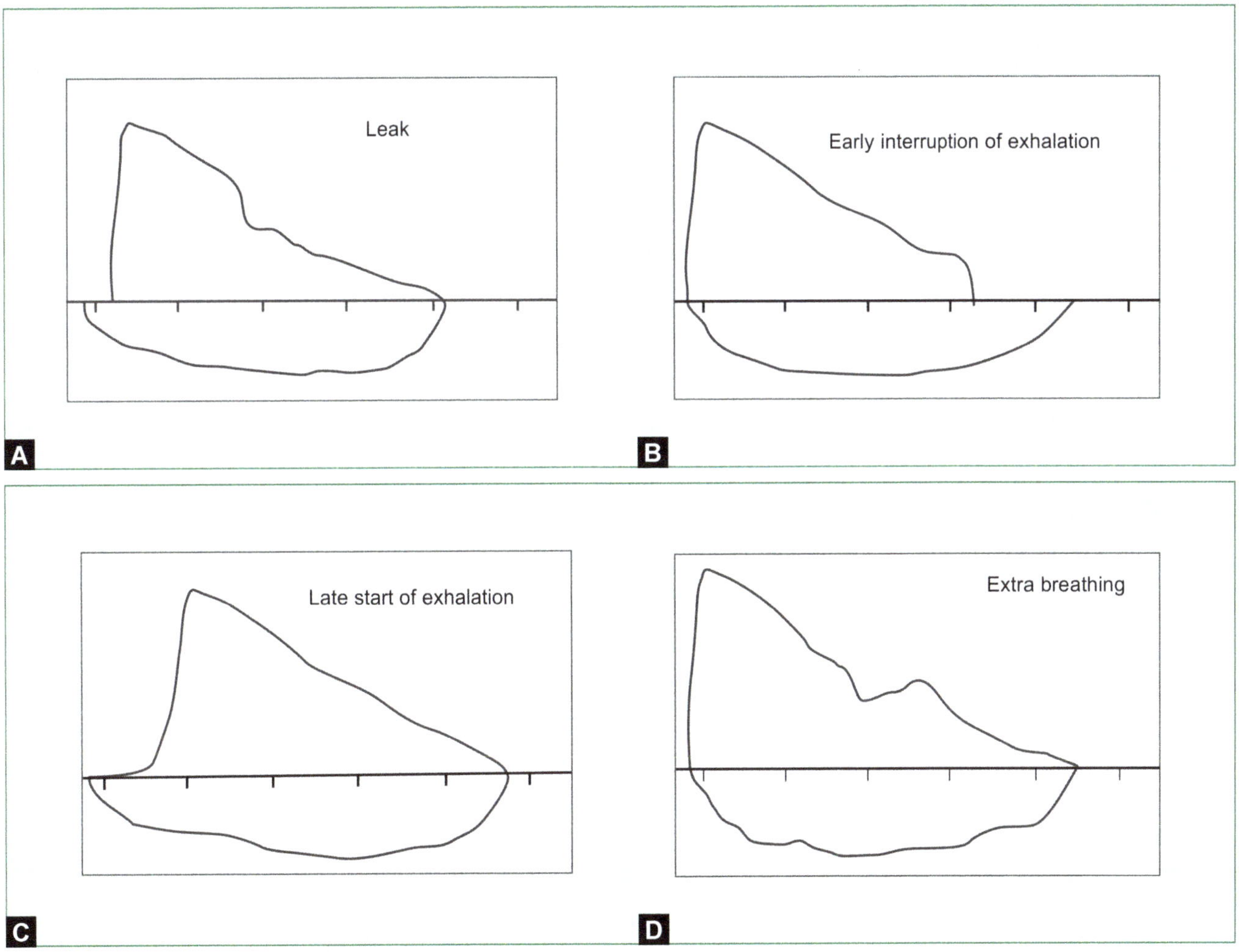

Figs. 7.4A to D

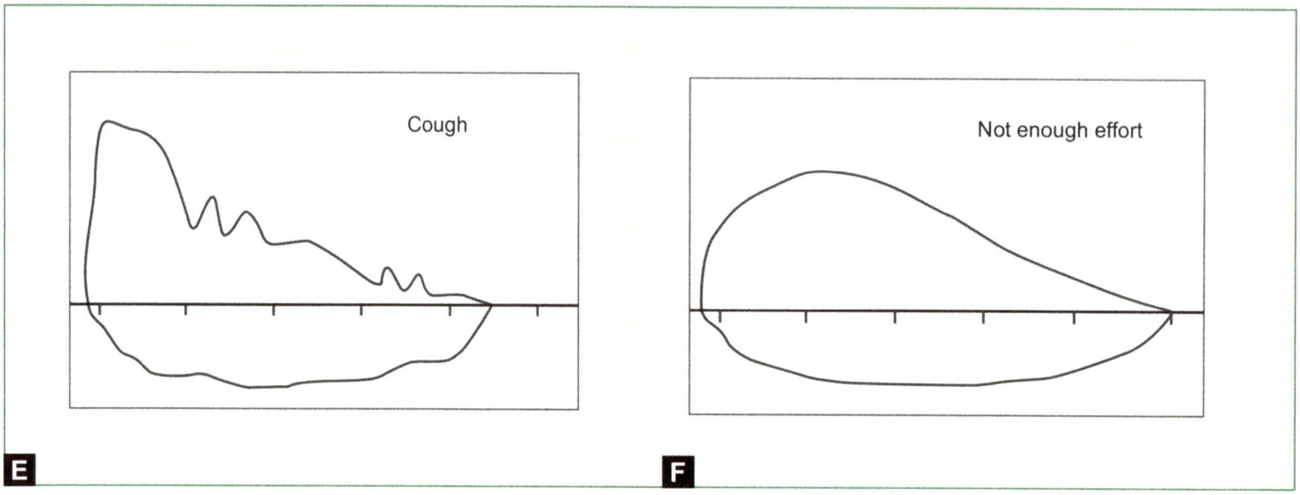

Figs. 7.4A to F: Examples of incorrect maneuvers that can be identified by looking at the graphs.

makes the measurement of FVC unreliable, but it does not affect the measurement of FEV1. In contrast, a weak start of exhalation may prevent a correct calculation of FEV1, but VC can still be measured if the patient completed the lungs emptying.

To ensure a reliability of the spirometry results, the maneuvers must be acceptable and reproducible (*see* below). If all the criteria for acceptability and repeatability are not fully met, the interpreter should comment on the test, pointing out the problems, the direction and magnitude of potential errors.

Within-Maneuver Evaluation (Acceptability)

The acceptability criteria should be applied before reproducibility is checked (Flowchart 7.1). The acceptability is established through "start of test" and "end of test" criteria, which are summarized, together with the repeatability criteria in Table 7.4.

The "start of test" refers to the beginning of forced expiration that should be carried out with the maximal effort and without hesitation. The effective start of timed measurements is determined by the *back extrapolation* method, which provides a new "time zero", and is essential for the accurate calculation of many parameters. In order to achieve an accurate time zero and assure that the FEV1 comes from a maximal effort curve, the EV (back extrapolated volume) must be less than 5% of the FVC or less than 150 mL, whichever is greater. A time to peak expiratory flow (time-to-PEF) less than 120 seconds is an additional start of test criterion. A rapid computerized feedback to the technician is usually given when these criteria are not met.

Flowchart 7.1: Suggested steps for the performance and interpretation of spirometry to obtain a satisfactory quality of the test and accuracy of results.

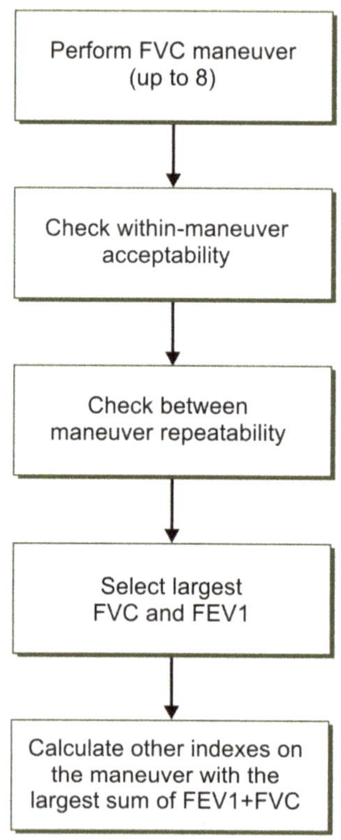

The main end of test criterion is the achievement of a minimum exhalation time of 6 seconds, unless the volume time curve shows a previous clear plateau (i.e. no volume change or <25 mL) of reasonable duration (at least

Table 7.4: Summary of the acceptability and repeatability criteria.

Acceptability
Start of Test
Extrapolated volume <5% of the FVC or <150 mL No hesitation or false start Rapid start to rise time No cough during the first second of the maneuver
End of Test
No early termination of exhalation Exhalation time ≥6 seconds or plateau ≥1 second
Repeatability
Difference of FEV1 from the largest FEV1 <150 mL* Difference of FVC from the largest FVC <150 mL*
* 100 mL if the FVC is <1.0 L

Table 7.5: Stratification of the degree of acceptability and repeatability.

Characteristic	*Grade*	*Criterion*
Acceptability	A	≥3 acceptable maneuvers
	B	2 acceptable maneuvers
	C	Only 1 acceptable maneuver
	D	No acceptable maneuvers
FEV1 repeatability	A	Two largest values match within 100 mL
	B	Two largest values match between 101 mL and 150 mL
	C	Two largest values match between 151 mL and 200 mL
	D	Two largest values do not match (difference >200 mL)
FVC repeatability	A	Two largest values match within 100 mL
	B	Two largest values match between 101 mL and 150 mL
	C	Two largest values match between 151 mL and 200 mL
	D	Two largest values do not match (difference >200 mL)
PEF repeatability	A	Two largest agree within 5%
	B	Two largest agree between 6% and 10%
	C	Two largest agree between 11% and 15%
	D	Two largest do not agree (difference >15%)

1 second). Indeed, some young and healthy people (especially females) complete exhalation and reach a plateau before 6 seconds.

An early interruption of expiration causes an underestimation of FVC (and overestimation of the parameters in which the FVC is the denominator, e.g. FEV1/FVC). However, no maneuver should be eliminated solely because of early termination, since the FEV1 from such maneuvers may be valid.

In addition to the above criteria, no cough (usually revealed by a 50% drop in flow) should be noticed, especially during the first second of the exhalation, and there should not be artifacts, glottis closure, leak at the mouth or obstruction of the mouthpiece by the tongue or teeth.

A minimum of three technically acceptable forced maneuvers are required. If a subject is unable to perform a single acceptable maneuver after eight attempts, testing may be discontinued.

Between-Maneuver Evaluation

After obtaining a minimum of three acceptable FVC maneuvers, *repeatability* (sometimes indicated as reproducibility) should be assessed.

A good repeatability is achieved when the difference between the largest and the next largest FVC is smaller than or equal to 150 mL and the difference between the largest and next largest FEV1 is less than or equal to150 mL. If the FVC is 1.0 L or less, both these values are 100 mL. If these criteria are not met in three maneuvers, additional trials should be attempted, up to, but usually no more than eight maneuvers. Large variability among tests is often due to incomplete inhalations. Some patients may require a brief rest period between maneuvers. Some individual may show a progressive reduction in FEV1 or FVC with each subsequent blow as an expression of high bronchial reactivity. If the cumulative drop exceeds 20% of start value, the test procedure should be terminated in the interest of patient safety.

An overall assessment of the quality of spirometry may be done by assigning a value of acceptability and repeatability, as shown in Table 7.5.

INTERPRETATION OF TEST

The interpretation of spirometry requires the comparison of the parameters measured in the patient with those

Flowchart 7.2: Algorithm for the interpretation of the simple spirometry.

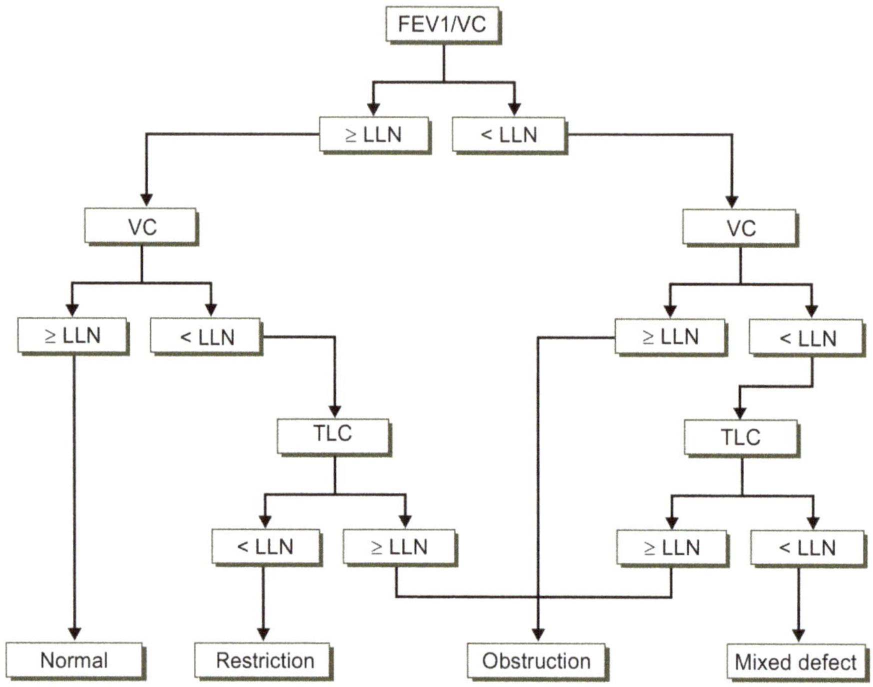

obtained by adequate reference equations. These equations are derived from large cohorts of healthy subjects and allow to calculate the "theoretical" value (or "predicted") for each parameter, as well as the normal ranges with the limits beyond which a result can be considered as pathological. The predicted values are specific for each subject, and vary primarily with gender, age, ethnicity and height of the individual.

On the basis of spirometric parameters, it is possible to identify two large groups of pulmonary disease: obstructive airway diseases, in which there is an expiratory airflow limitation due to a narrowing of the airways [asthma, chronic obstructive pulmonary disease (COPD), etc.] and restrictive lung diseases, characterized by a decrease in lung volumes or in the patient's ability to expand the lungs (obesity, interstitial lung diseases, myopathy, etc.).

The diagnosis of bronchial obstruction require a reduction of FEV1 and of its relationship with the VC or forced vital capacity (FVC) (Tiffeneau Index) at values lower than their respective lower limits of normal (LLN). Lung restriction may be only suspected though a simple spirometry if VC is lower than LLN; its confirmation require the measurement of nondisplaceable lung volumes, showing a reduction of the TLC. Flowchart 7.2 shows a diagnostic algorithm useful for the evaluation of lung function; Figures 7.5A to G show the morphology of the flow-volume curves in normal and pathological conditions.

Forced vital capacity is often used in place of VC because obtained in the same forced expiratory maneuver. However, most recommend to use the largest VC available, which can be obtained either during inspiration (IVC), slow expiration (SVC), or forced expiration (FVC). FVC is usually reduced more than IVC and SVC in airway obstruction. The forced expiratory volume at 6 seconds (FEV6) may be used as a surrogate of VC in subject who cannot complete the exhalation; this requires the use of appropriate LLN for FEV1/FEV6.

The advantages of the use of flow-volume loops include the possibility to identify the probable anatomical location of airway obstruction. An obstructing lesion located in the extrathoracic upper airway (larynx, trachea) can limit airflow in a fixed way and may be identified during the inhalation component on the flow-volume loop.

BRONCHODILATOR REVERSIBILITY TEST

A bronchial reversibility test is always indicated when spirometry reveals airway obstruction (both FEV1 and FEV1/FVC <LLN). After performing a simple spirometry, the patient is asked to inhale a bronchodilator with rapid onset of action (usually 400 mcg of Salbutamol by metered dose inhaler, preferably with a spacer). The forced expiratory maneuver is then repeated about 20 minutes after such an inhalation.

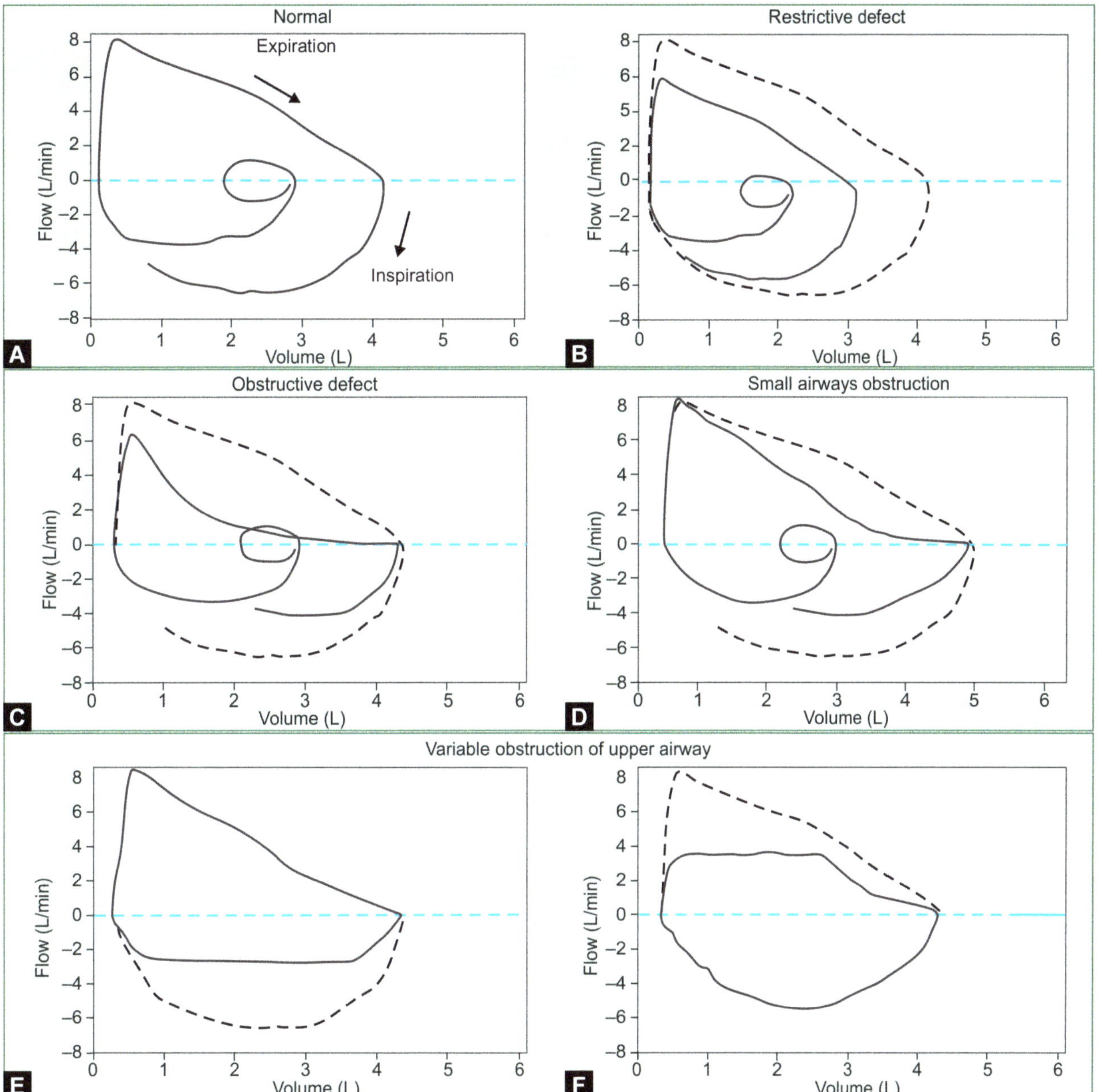

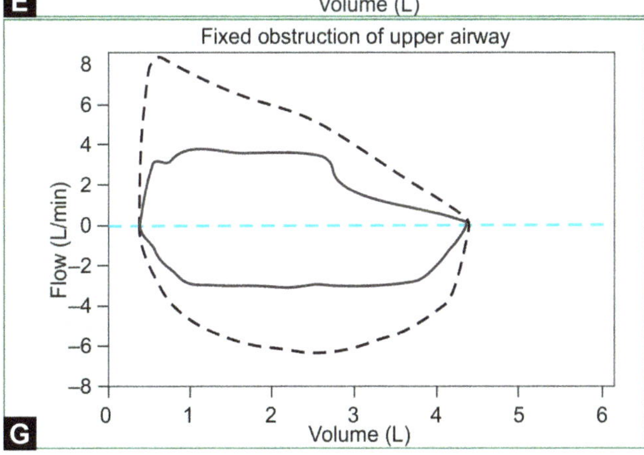

Figs. 7.5A to G: Examples of flow-volume curves in individuals with (A) normal results, (B) reduced lung volumes, and (C) airways obstruction. The loops of subjects with restrictive defect have usually the same shape as normal but are smaller; the loops of subjects with obstructive defect are concave upward. A slight concave shape in the last part of the exhalation curve may be consistent with an early airflow obstruction (small airways), although FEV1 and FVC values are within the normal range (D). Variable and fixed obstruction of upper airway are also shown (E, F, G). The dashed lines indicate the predictive values taking into account parameters, such as patient age, height, weight and ethnicity.

The single administration of inhaled bronchodilators for the reversibility test is generally safe. Hypersensitivity to atropine-like substances is the only rare contraindication to the use of anticholinergics. In some situations, the use of an anticholinergic instead of a β2-sympathomimetic may be a prudent choice. These include thyrotoxicosis, heart failure, hypertension, and diabetes mellitus with poor glycemic control.

Potentially serious hypokalemia and consequent cardiac arrhythmia may result from b2-agonist administration, but the risk concerns mainly patients receiving high doses for therapeutic purposes, especially if endovenous. Caution is advised in patients with hypoxia, concomitant use of heart glycosides (e.g. digoxin, digitalis), xanthine derivatives (e.g. theophylline aminophylline), steroids, diuretics.

β2-sympathomimetic may increase blood sugar levels, and if a diabetic patient is unable to compensate for this, ketoacidosis may occur.

Before undertaking bronchodilator testing, the patient should stop short-acting bronchodilators for 6 hours, long-acting bronchodilators for 12 hours and theophylline for 24 hours.

Test performance is affected by the day of testing, the severity of baseline lung-function impairment. The test is considered positive when it shows an increase in FEV1 and/or FVC or VC of at least 12%, with a simultaneous change in their absolute values of more than 200 mL.

In the past, bronchodilator reversibility has been widely used to differentiate COPD from asthma, since airflow obstruction was thought to be little or no reversible in patients with COPD, and fully reversible in patients with asthma. In effect, no clear cut-off exists between asthmatic and COPD patients. Furthermore, the test is scarcely reproducible over time in the same patient.

Despite this, bronchoreversibility testing is largely used in clinical practice to guide the clinician through the diagnostic and follow-up process. Large increments in the FEV1 from baseline (>400 mL) after the administration of salbutamol support the diagnosis of asthma in patients with a history compatible with the disease.

The presence of chronic airway inflammation may mask the acute reversibility, especially in the elderly; in such cases, if there is a strong clinical suspicion of bronchial asthma, to run a "chronic reversibility test" (or "steroid reversibility test") can be useful. This method, still not well standardized, requires a few weeks period of therapy with oral corticosteroids (e.g. 25 mg of prednisone daily or equivalent for 2 weeks) and/or inhaled corticosteroids (e.g. 200 mcg of beclometasone daily or equivalent inhaled corticosteroid for 6–8 weeks). After this trial, the spirometry is repeated, using criteria for the evaluation response identical to those of acute reversibility.

BIBLIOGRAPHY AND FURTHER READING

1. Bellia V, Sorino C, Catalano F, et al. Validation of FEV6 in the elderly: correlates of performance and repeatability. Thorax. 2008;63:60.
2. Pedone C, Bellia V, Sorino C, et al. Prognostic significance of surrogate measures for forced vital capacity in an elderly population. J Am Med Dir Assoc. 2010;11(8):598-604.
3. Sorino C, Battaglia S, Scichilone N, et al. Diagnosis of airway obstruction in the elderly: contribution of the SARA study. Int J Chron Obstruct Pulmon Dis. 2012;7:389-95.
4. Sorino C, D'Amato M, Steinhilber G, et al. Spirometric criteria to diagnose airway obstgruction in the elderly: fixed ratio vs. lower limit of normal. Minerva Med. 2015; Jan 14. [Epub ahead of print]
5. Sorino C, Sherrill D, Guerra S, et al. Prognostic value of FEV1/FEV6 in elderly people. Clin Physiol Funct Imaging. 2011;31(2):101-7

Chapter

8 Lung Volumes and Further Assessment: Beyond Spirometry

Ann M Granchelli, Theodore G Liou, Richard Kanner, Claudio Sorino

Lung function testing is designed to help answer the question: "Why is this patient short of breath?" In addition to diagnosing disease, lung function testing can help evaluate disease progression, evaluate the effects of treatment designed to improve lung function or monitor the administration of medications that pose a risk to lung function like some chemotherapy agents.

Spirometry is the gold standard for measuring lung function, and is often the most useful and easily available test to diagnose and monitor respiratory disease. While spirometry is commonly used, it does have limitations. Spirometry measures the volume of air that can be inhaled and forcefully exhaled from the lungs, allowing for active measurement of inspiratory and expiratory vital capacities. It cannot, however, measure the residual volume (RV) of gas that remains in the lungs after forceful exhalation.

Because spirometry does not measure RV, the forced vital capacity (FVC) assessed with spirometry is only an approximation of total lung capacity (TLC). How closely the FVC approximates the TLC depends on the subject's age, and ability to participate in active breathing maneuvers. For example, the vital capacity (VC) measurement of a healthy young adult accounts for roughly 75% of the TLC, while this percentage decreases to roughly 60% in old age.

The presence of lung disease can affect the ability of spirometry to estimate TLC. In patients with chronic obstructive lung disease (COPD), a forced exhalation can cause the airways to collapse. The result is an FVC that appears to be reduced because the airway collapsed before a full exhalation could be made. With simple spirometry measurements, such a patient may appear to have mixed ventilator defect (restriction with obstruction) when the patient may in fact have normal or hyperinflated TLC. Thus, spirometry alone is unable to establish the diagnosis of a mixed disorder.

HISTORY OF LUNG VOLUME MEASUREMENT

People have tried to measure lung volumes since the beginning of medicine. Over time these attempts have come closer and closer to measuring a subjects true TLC. Testing methods have progressed from simple anatomical and biomechanical observations to complex clinical analyses of lung physiology.

In 1680, Giovanni Alfonso Borelli, often named the father of biomechanics, first attempted to measure the total amount of air present in the lungs. He was also the first person to advance the idea that lungs do not completely empty with full exhalation, but maintain a RV of air.

Residual lung volume was first measured, in vivo, in 1800 by H Davy who measured the volume of his own lungs by forced breathing of a hydrogen mixture. By inhaling hydrogen, a nonabsorbable gas, he could compare the volume of hydrogen gas withdrawn from a container during forced inhalation with the volume forcibly exhaled and reasoned that the difference was the RV of air left in the lungs.

Ultimately helium replaced hydrogen for gas dilution measurements of lung volumes. Not only was helium easier to get in a pure form (hydrogen was sometimes mixed with arsenic, creating a toxic poison), but it was also less volatile. Meneely and Kaltreider in 1941 created a *closed circuit helium dilution technique* with a spirometer similar

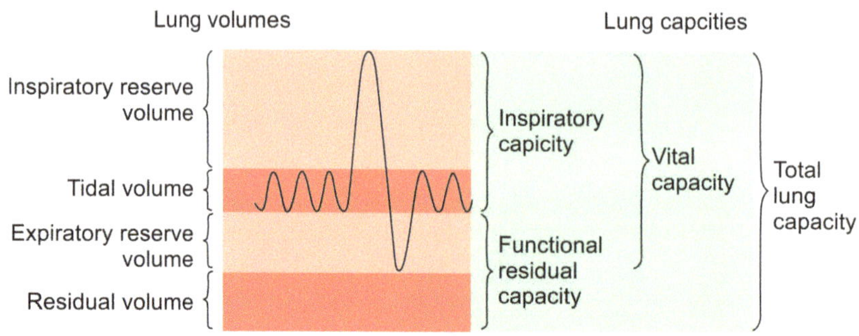

Fig. 8.1: Lung volumes and capacities.

to what is used today. Allowing the subject to breathe a nonabsorbable gas for a set amount of time allowed for equilibrium to occur. In a closed system, the volume, pressure and temperature of each chamber of the spirometer and the quantity of each gas are also known. With this information Meneely and Kaltreider determined a method for calculating the unknown volume of ventilated lung of the subject.

An alternative method, using an *open circuit nitrogen washout technique* was created in 1940 by Darling et al., which measured the progressive washout of alveolar nitrogen by pure oxygen in order to calculate lung volumes including RV. Both helium dilution and nitrogen washout continue to be used to measure lung volumes and will be discussed further later in the chapter.

By the 1950s, body plethysmography was established as another method for measuring lung volumes, and is now generally considered the gold standard. While it had been described as far back as 1878, it was AB DuBois in 1956 who first demonstrated the practical application of Boyle's law, using an airtight chamber designed to detect changes in pressure similar to the modern body plethysmograph.

DEFINITIONS

Before discussing in more detail about the tests used to measure lung volumes, it's helpful to define some common terms.

Lung volume generally refers to the amount of gas present within the lungs as measured by body plethysmography, gas dilution or washout. The volume and location of gas being measured differs slightly based on the method being used, but the same terms are used regardless of method. Lung volumes measured by imaging such as chest radiographs or CT scans are based on the volumes within the outline of the chest and will include both normal and abnormal lung tissue in addition to all intrapulmonary and extrapulmonary gas in the thoracic cavity.

Static lung volumes are measured when the patient is at rest. *Capacities* contain two or more lung volumes.

Definitions involved in measuring the total amount of air in the lungs (Fig. 8.1):

Tidal volume (TV): The volume of air inhaled or exhaled with each breath at rest

Inspiratory reserve volume (IRV): The amount of air that can be additionally inspired when breathing to maximal inhalation from inspired tidal volume.

Expiratory residual volume (ERV): The amount of air that can be additional exhaled from exhaled tidal volume.

Residual volume (RV): The volume of air remaining in the lungs after maximum voluntary exhalation. This cannot be measured by spirometry, and is essential in determining absolute lung volumes.

Vital capacity: The amount of volume change between the positions of full exhalation to full inhalation.

Inspiratory capacity (IC): The amount of air that can be maximally inhaled after tidal volume exhalation includes TV + IC.

Total lung capacity: The volume of air present in the lungs at maximal inspiration. This includes VC + RV.

Functional residual capacity (FRC): The volume of air left in the lungs at the end of exhalation during tidal breathing includes ERV + RV. In healthy young adults, this is the point at which the chest wall is relaxed, and the elastic recoil forces of the lungs and chest wall muscles are equal and opposite.

Intrathoracic gas volume (ITGV) is the absolute volume of gas in the lung at the time of airflow occlusion. It is usually measured at the end of a normal exhalation or at FRC.

Table 8.1: Clinical utility of lung volume measurements.

Clinical value of lung volume measurement	*Examples of usefulness*	*Reference(s)*
Restriction	40–60% of patients with classic restriction by spirometry shown to have normal lung volumes by plethysmography.	Wanger 2005; Miller et al. 2005
ILD	Measurement of VC has a decreased (69.3%) sensitivity for identifying restrictive disease vs plethysmography.	Boros et al. 2004
Asthma	Plethysmography is more sensitive than spirometry at predicting bronchodilator response in mild asthma.	Houghton et al. 2004
Obesity	VC and TLC generally remain within normal limits, but FRC decreases and airway resistance increases.	Jones and Nzekwu 2006, Pelosi et al. 1998, Ferretti et al. 2001
COPD	IC/TLC ratio independently predicts mortality in patients with COPD.	Casanova et al. 2005
Cancer therapy	TLC measurement identifies increasing restriction when chemotherapy is added to radiotherapy for lung cancer	Gopal et al. 2003
Mixed obstruction/restriction	Only 9.5% of patients listed as having mixed obstruction and restrictive disorder by spirometry truly found to have restriction by plethysmography.	Diaz-Guzman et al. 2010

(COPD: Chronic obstructive lung disease; FRC: Functional residual capacity; VC: Vital capacity; IC: Inspiratory capacity; TLC: Total lung capacity; ILD: Interstitial lung disease).

CLINICAL VALUE OF LUNG VOLUME MEASUREMENTS

While it is often easy to see how spirometry measurements will be helpful in diagnosing and managing disease, the clinical value of lung volume measurements is often less clear. Spirometry is often the first test in evaluating a patient with a respiratory complaint. The main reason to move on to lung volume measurements is usually to answer a question that cannot be answered with spirometry. Absolute lung volume measurements can help uncover underlying physiology, such as lung restriction, or hyperinflation. Examples of when lung volume measurements are helpful in a clinical context can be seen in Table 8.1.

Restrictive Lung Disease

Perhaps the most common use of lung volume testing is to evaluate the diagnosis of lung restriction. Spirometry is very good at ruling out restriction in the general population when the VC is normal. The probability of a restrictive defect is less than 3% with a normal VC by spirometry.

Spirometry is far less helpful in correctly diagnosing restriction. Poorly performed spirometry has a tendency to underestimate lung volumes. Even patients with classic patterns of restriction by spirometry have been found to have normal lung volumes in 40-60% of the time with total lung volume measurements. When spirometry shows a decreased VC, The American Thoracic Society (ATS)/ European Respiratory Society (ERS) recommends obtaining lung volume measurements with plethysmography, gas dilution or imaging to correctly diagnose a restrictive ventilatory defect.

Although, generally reliable in ruling out restriction in the general population, in patients with interstitial lung disease, spirometry may have a decreased ability to identify the level of restriction. In one study of patients with an established or probable diagnosis of ILD, the loss of TLC as measured by plethysmography was found to be greater than that of relative loss of VC by spirometry.

Obstruction and Hyperinflation

Hyperinflation refers to the elevation of absolute lung volumes such as RV, FRC, and TLC. The increase in RV in patients with hyperinflation may come from a loss of recoil in emphysema or bullous disease as well as from airway obstruction. Patients with mild emphysema may have loss of recoil without obstruction. Those with asthma generally have obstruction without loss of recoil. Patients with moderate to severe emphysema or COPD may have both loss of recoil and obstructive lung disease. Evaluating patients with lung volume measurements in addition to spirometry can be helpful at determining the underlying disease.

Measuring lung volumes can identify early disease. Patients with early or mild emphysema have been reported to have an increase in RV before obstruction can be clinically apparent on spirometry. Plethysmography is more sensitive than spirometry at predicting bronchodilator response in mild asthma.

While obstructive lung diseases such as COPD are generally diagnosed and monitored with spirometry, there are benefits to further testing and lung volume measurements.

Table 8.2: Comparing physiological methods of lung volumes measurement.

Body plethysmography	*Helium dilution*	*Nitrogen washout*
Accurate measurement even in case of lung obstruction	May underestimate FRC and RV in moderate to severe airflow obstruction.	May underestimate FRC and RV in obstructive lung disease
Requires additional maneuvers beyond tidal breathing	Only tidal breathing required	Only tidal breathing required
Older kids and adults	May be used in all ages — infant to adult	May be used in all ages — infant to adult
Expensive specialized equipment	Less expensive	Less expensive
Requires compliant patient	May be used in patients on ventilator	May be used in patients on ventilator

(RV: Residual volume; FRC: Functional residual capacity).

As previously described, patients with COPD will often appear to have restriction due to airway collapse with forced exhalation. TLC measurement with plethysmography (preferred over gas dilution) will give you a subjects' true lung volume, which is most commonly normal or hyperinflated.

Lung hyperinflation in COPD can decrease with bronchodilator therapy. Neither the baseline hyperinflation nor its improvement with therapy is well captured by spirometry. Plethysmography measurements of FRC and RV are helpful in identifying a response to therapy that may not be captured with spirometry.

Asthma is also classically thought of as causing hyperinflation due to intermittent or persistent airflow obstruction. Patients generally have a TLC within normal limits, but the air trapping caused by premature airway closure during exhalation may result in an increased RV.

Residual Volume Matters

The first task in measuring TLC involves measuring RV or the volume of air remaining in the lungs after a full exhalation. The RV helps show air trapping in obstruction, or lung volume reduction with obesity. It can only be measured with special measurement techniques including *body plethysmography, helium gas dilution,* and *nitrogen washout.*

Each of these techniques produces comparable results for healthy adults, although they measure slightly different volumes. The measurement technique used determines whether you will measure only the amount of gas communicating between the lungs and the environment, or the total amount of gas present in the thorax. Plethysmography measures all compressible gas in the thorax, communicating and noncommunicating, as well as any gas present in the abdomen. Noncommunicating gas includes gas within the esophagus, and any trapped gas within the lungs. Alternatively, gas dilution and washout techniques measure only communicating gas volumes in the lungs. The residual volume will be higher with plethysmography than with helium dilution and nitrogen washout. Plethysmography may therefore be better able to evaluate patients with hyperinflation and obstruction. Table 8.2 shows a comparison of these methods of lung volume measurement including limitations and where they are used.

Imaging techniques (chest X-ray, computed tomography, and magnetic resonance) can also help to estimate the absolute lung volumes and have a role mainly in subjects with limited ability to cooperate.

BODY PLETHYSMOGRAPHY

Body plethysmography is generally considered the gold standard of lung volume measurements. As previously stated, it measures the total volume of gas within the thoracic cavity (and abdominal cavity), including trapped gas that does not communicate with the outside environment. First demonstrated by DuBois in 1955, body plethysmography involves using Boyle's Law and measurements of pressure to determine lung volume. Boyle's law is a simple equation that states that the volume of gas varies in inverse proportion to the pressure to which it is subjected.

In plethysmography, a patient inhales and exhales through a mouthpiece while sitting in a closed airtight glass box. During breathing exercises, the amount of gas present in the lungs can be determined by measuring the changing pressures at the mouthpiece during airway occlusion and panting maneuvers. The two main measurements of lung volume obtained are the FRC and the total intrathoracic gas volume (ITGV or V_{TG}). Plethysmography also allows measurement of airway resistance (Raw).

Equipment

Measurement of lung volume with plethysmography requires a patient to sit in an enclosed body plethysmograph while completing breathing maneuvers. The plethysmograph looks similar to a glass phone booth (Fig. 8.2) and will either measure changes in pressure, volume or airflow depending on the type of device being used. If the chamber is a constant-volume chamber, then the variable measured is the change in pressure (variable-pressure plethysmograph). A constant-pressure setting can either measure volume displacement (volume-displacement plethysmograph), or airflow in and out (flow plethysmograph).

Measurement Technique

Before the test begins, the patient will need to sit in the plethysmograph with the door shut for 1 minute to allow for temperature equilibration. A nose clip is used to occlude the nasal airway, and the patient is asked to form an air-tight seal around the spirometer mouthpiece. The patient then starts the test with normal tidal breathing (breathing at rest).

The spirometer has a shutter valve near the mouth which is initially kept open as the patient takes several comfortable tidal breaths. A short period of time is allowed to let the subject become comfortable breathing through the mouthpiece. This allows a "relaxed" FRC to be measured. A real-time display of the specific resistance curves and the spirogram appears on the screen (Figs. 8.3 and 8.4).

The temperature and humidity of a plethysmograph chamber increases rapidly after the door is closed. Compensation for temperature effects can be done while viewing specific airway resistance (s*Raw*) loops. These plot mouth airflow and shift volume during relaxed tidal breathing (shift volume is the very small change in volume

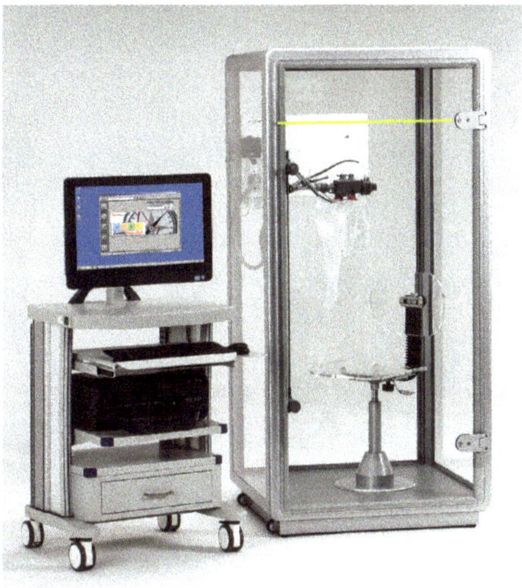

Fig. 8.2: Body plethysmograph.
Source: http://www.morgansci.com/.

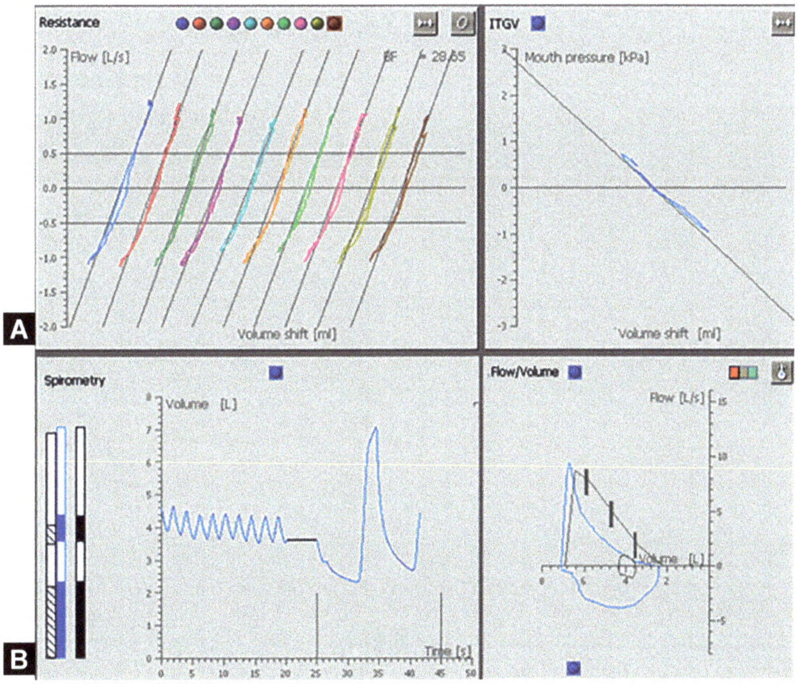

Figs. 8.3A and B: Example of screen display during the (A) resistance measurement and (B) ITGV measurement.

exclusive of airflow that occurs with alveolar compression or decompression during breathing). Drifting of the resistance loops indicates that temperature compensation has not yet been completed (Fig. 8.5A), and ITGV measurements might be not accurate. In this case, it is recommended to wait until the curves write over each other before proceeding further (Fig. 8.5B). If this takes too long, the temperature drift is too high and the pressure compensation valve will have to be opened for a moment and closed again.

If satisfied with the measurement of resistance, the ITGV measurement can begin. The shutter valve is closed at FRC and the patient is asked to pant gently against the closed valve while holding her hands to her cheeks to support breathing (Fig. 8.6).

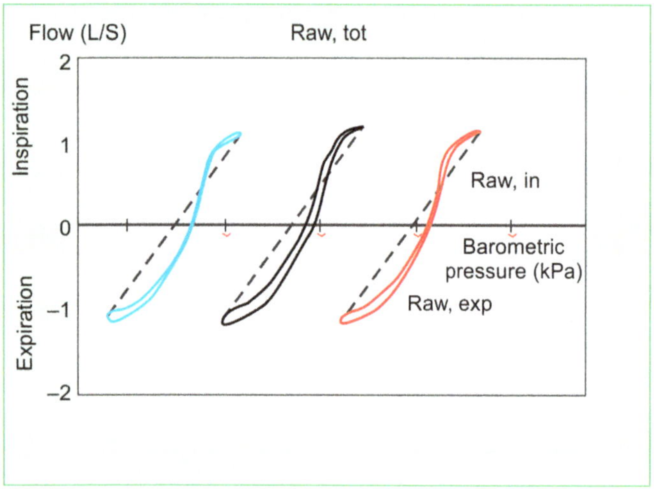

Fig. 8.4: Examples of normal resistance loops.

Panting against a closed shutter valve causes compression and decompression of the air in the lungs.

The change in pressure caused by panting is measured at the mouth by a pressure transducer. This pressure change is compared to the change in volume, which has been measured directly, if using a volume-displacement plethysmograph. If using a variable-pressure plethysmograph, the change in volume is derived mathematically from the measured change in pressure using Boyle's law.

$$P_1 \times V_1 = P_2 \times V_2$$

In the equation above, $P_1 \times V_1$ refers to the initial pressure against the closed valve and initial lung volume before the panting (compression) maneuver is done. $P_2 \times V_2$ refers to the pressure and volume present at the end of the maneuver. Pressure and volume are always inversely related. As the pressure increases, the volume decreases. The volume of the plethysmograph is a fixed constant. The relative change in a patient's lung volume during panting maneuvers can be calculated and is inversely related to the pressure changes measured by the plethysmograph.

The pressure and volume measurements from the panting maneuvers allow for the calculation of the $FRC_{pleth,}$ which is unique for each patient. In order to meet ATS/ERS standards a patient must be able to perform 3–5 panting maneuvers at roughly 1 Hz (this is the speed which reduces errors in measurement). At least two of the calculated FRCpleth values must be within 5% of each other.

Temperature

The relationship of pressure and volume demonstrated by Boyle's law hold true only for a constant temperature,

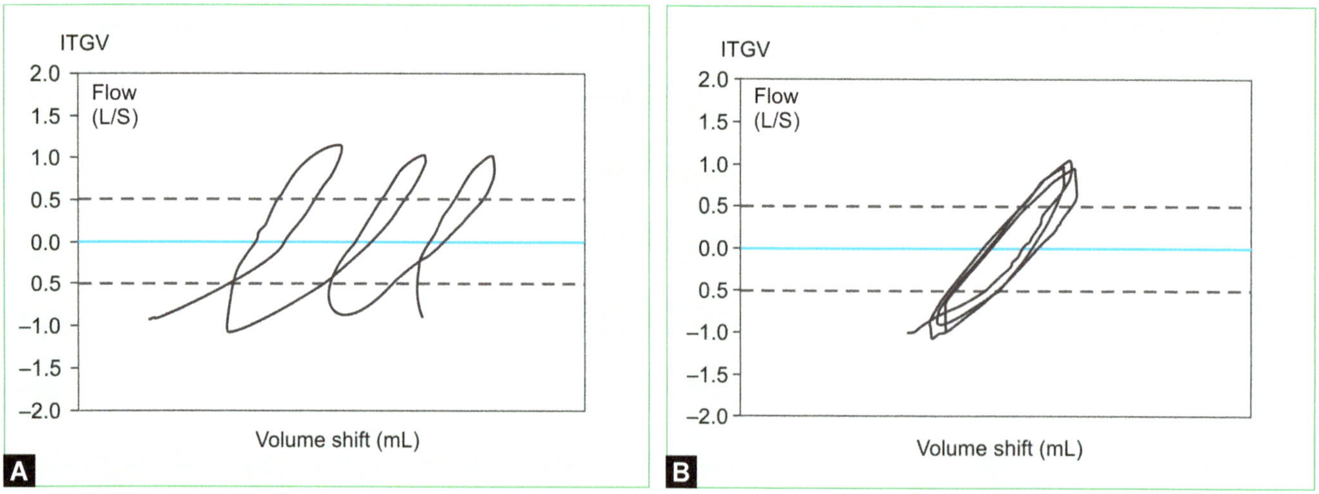

Figs. 8.5A and B: Airway resistance loops (A) before and (B) after compensation for temperature effects.

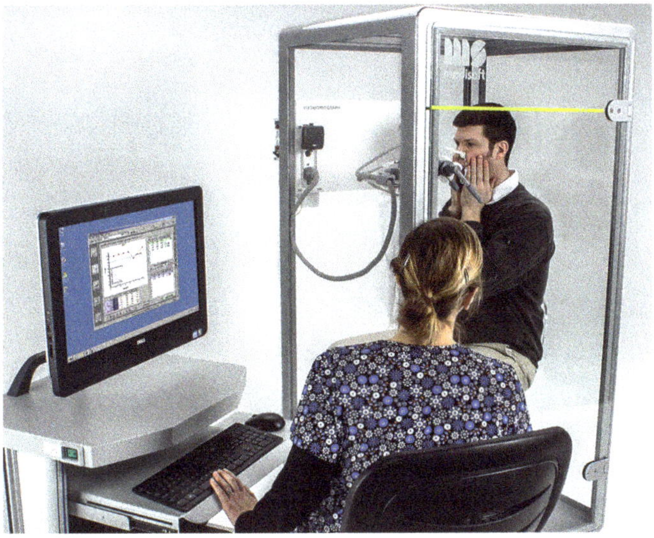

Fig. 8.6: Obtaining FRC (functional residual capacity) in a body plethysmograph.
Source: http://www.morgansci.com/.

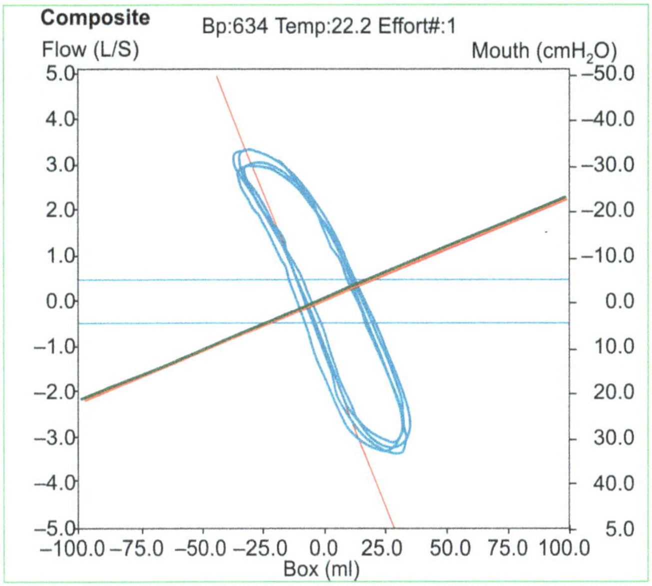

Fig. 8.7: Pressure-volume variation during panting.
Source: http://www.morgansci.com/.

so both the apparatus and mathematical calculations must account for the thermal drift that occurs inside a plethysmograph. Panting 3–4 times against a closed valve provides enough information to plot the relationship of ΔP-ΔV, which varies for each patient, but should look like a series of straight lines and superimposed oval loops on an X-Y plot with some drifting separation due to small changes in temperature during testing (Fig. 8.7).

Other Useful Measurements with Plethysmography

In addition to lung volume measurements, plethysmography can also provide information on airways resistance. This can be useful information for a patient that is being evaluated for airflow obstruction. Airflow obstruction is commonly found in diseases such as COPD and asthma, but patients with obesity can also have significantly increased airflow obstruction. The FRC, which decreases in obesity, has an indirect relationship with airways resistance. Compared to patients with a body mass index (BMI) of 20 kg/m^2, patients with BMI values of 30, 34, and 45 kg/m^2 have an average increase in airway resistance of 33%, 49%, and 62%. This may account for patients' complaints of shortness of breath in the setting of obesity.

The airflow resistance (*Raw*) is the ratio of driving force of airflow to the flow rate of air. This is calculated as the ratio of the pressure difference between the alveoli and the mouth, and the flow rate of air at the mouth. The pressure at the mouth is assumed to be constant during tidal breathing so the calculation only has to account for changing pressure at the alveoli.

$$\text{Raw} = \Delta P_{alv}/V$$

The alveolar pressure is calculated from the pressure-volume curve created by the previously described panting maneuver against a closed shutter. This is the maneuver that also determines the FRC_{pleth}.

Measuring the Total Lung Capacity

After baseline measurements are obtained, the shutter valve is opened again and the patient is told to exhale fully and then take a slow maximal inspiration to TLC (*see* Fig. 8.3B).

When the patient fully exhales after the valve is opened, the expiratory reserve volume is measured. The slow maximal inspiration performed after full exhalation allows the IVC to be determined. The reserve volume can be calculated from FRC_{pleth} -ERV when this preferred method is used.

If it is too difficult for the patient to perform the preferred maneuver after the shutter valve is opened, then an alternate maneuver is used. In the alternate breathing maneuver, the patient maximally inhales from FRC after the valve is opened, and then slowly exhales to RV. This alternative method gives the IC followed by the expired

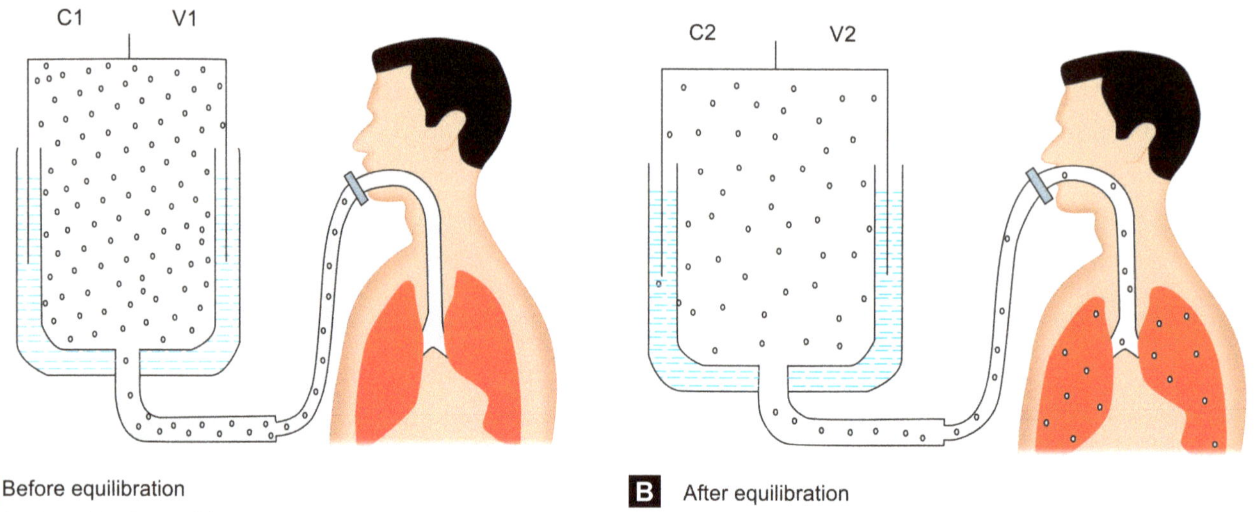

Figs 8.8A and B: Exemplification of the helium dilution technique, before (A) and after (B) equilibration of the helium between the spirometer and the lungs.

vital capacity (EVC). When using this method, the reserve volume will be calculated by subtracting the EVC from the TLC (FRC_{pleth} + IC).

HELIUM DILUTION

Sometimes a patient, who has trouble with spirometry, may also have difficulty with body plethysmography, either because of difficulty following directions, or because of claustrophobia using a plethysmograph. In the case of a child or an adult patient who cannot or has difficulty doing plethysmography, gas dilution can be used to determine FRC and TLC. Helium dilution remains one of the simplest and cheapest ways of measuring lung volumes.

Gas dilution techniques measure the free flowing gas that communicates and equilibrates with the environment. Helium dilution involves a patient breathing a mixed gas through a spirometer in a closed system (Figs. 8.8A and B). The test gas consists of air with added oxygen, usually 25-30%, but higher concentrations are acceptable. The gas in the system apparatus has a known volume (V_{app}) and a known concentration of He (~10%).

Helium is a nonabsorbable gas, so after a period of time the amount of helium within the closed system, including the lungs, will equilibrate. The FRC_{He} of a patient is calculated based on the fraction of helium found in the system at the time of equilibration.

The lung volume is calculated after correcting for the volume of the mouthpiece and valve. The results are corrected for BTPS (body temperature and pressure, saturated) conditions which accounts for the fact that gases have different volumes at different temperatures and pressures.

While helium dilution has the advantage of being cheaper and requires simpler equipment than plethysmography, but like spirometry and plethysmography, achieving accurate results with the helium dilution technique also requires trained operators. This method may not be available at all centers.

Equipment

For measuring lung volumes through the helium dilution technique, systems that utilize a volume-displacement spirometer are usually employed, and the capacity of the spirometer should be more than or equal to 7 liters. The V_{app} with the bell at zero volume, including the circuit tubing to the mouthpiece valve, should be less than or equal to 4.5 liters. Indeed, the smaller the V_{app} is at the time that the patient is switched into the circuit, the larger (and more accurate) the measured changes in helium concentration during the lung volumes measurement will be.

The spirometer should be equipped with a CO_2 absorber, O_2 and helium supply, a gas inlet and outlet, a mixing fan and a water vapor absorber in the line to the helium analyzer. The O_2 concentration is continuously measured and kept relatively constant by adding O_2 to the circuit as necessary. The CO_2 absorber is aimed to maintain the breathing-circuit CO_2 level during testing below 0.5%, thus avoiding patient discomfort and hyperventilation. The activity of the CO_2 and water absorbers should be ensured before each test (either from visual or photocell detection of indicator color changes, or by replacing the absorbent after a specified number of tests or accumulated minutes of equilibration time). The mixing fan should mix the gas throughout the circuit within 8 seconds after the end of exhalation into the circuit.

Measurement Technique

The basic procedure for helium dilution includes the following steps (Fig. 8.9):

- After switching on the instrument, proper warm-up phase should be ensured (variable depending on the equipment)
- The equipment should be calibrated according to manufacturer's instructions
- If the patient has a perforated eardrum, an earplug should be used
- The patient should be seated comfortably. There is no need to remove dentures
- Explain the procedure to the patient, emphasizing the need to avoid leaks around the mouthpiece during the test
- Place the nose clip on the patient
- The patient is asked to breath for 30–60 seconds on the mouthpiece to become accustomed to the apparatus, and to ensure a stable end-tidal expiratory level.
- The patient is connected to the test gas at the end of a normal tidal expiration (usually just by pressing a button)
- The patient is instructed to make regular tidal breaths; while the O_2 flow is adjusted to compensate for O_2 consumption (significant errors in the calculation of FRC can result if O_2 consumption is not adequately accounted for)
- The helium concentration should be observed (it is automatically recorded every 15 seconds): when the change in helium concentration is less than or equal to 0.02% for 30 seconds, helium equilibration is considered to be complete and the patient is disconnected from the test gas of the system.

The test rarely exceeds 10 minutes, even in patients with severe gas-exchange abnormalities. At least one technically satisfactory measurement should be obtained. Due to the extra costs and time in making multiple measurements, and the relatively good inter-day variability in adults, two or more measurements of FRCHe should be performed only for specific clinical or research need or in younger children. If more than one measurement of FRCHe is carried out, the value reported for FRCHe should be the mean of technically acceptable results that agree within 10%.

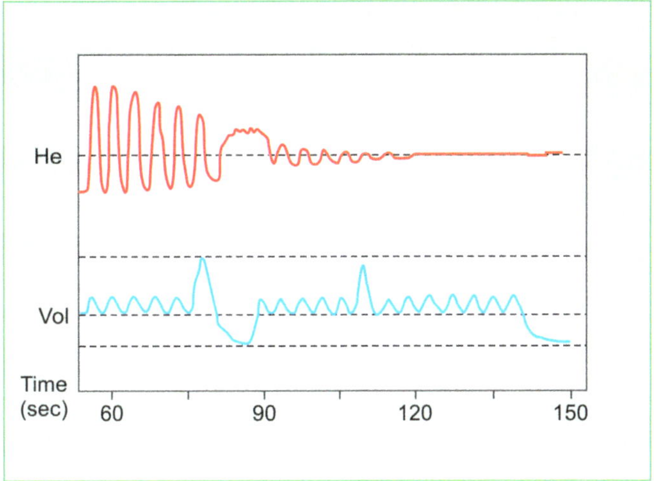

Fig. 8.9: Display of an acceptable profile for a helium dilution test to determine functional residual capacity (FRC).

MULTIPLE-BREATH NITROGEN WASHOUT

First used in 1940, the nitrogen (N_2) washout technique is based on the fact that the alveolar concentration of nitrogen gas is roughly the same as the concentration in the atmosphere: 79%. Nitrogen in the lungs can be washed out and measured from a patient breathing 100% oxygen (Fig. 8.9). This technique is based on the fact that N_2 can be washed out of the lungs of a patient breathing 100% oxygen. The initial concentration of alveolar N_2 and the amount of N_2 that is washed out during the test can be used to calculate the lung volume of the patient. It has most recently been used in measuring the FRV of intubated patients with acute respiratory distress syndrome (ARDS).

Equipment

There are a variety of different systems commercially available that use the nitrogen washout approach and a lack of studies exist comparing different methods. Due to this variation, no single method of measuring FRC by nitrogen washout is currently recommended by the European Respiratory Society. Set up for this test requires a mouthpiece, flow, O_2, and CO_2 sensors, and a reservoir of 100% oxygen. Oxygen should be delivered to mouthpiece through a demand valve, which has low demand valve pressure (<1 kPa or <10 cm H_2O). A one-way valve is also required to prevent rebreathing. The system must be open to allow for the elimination of nitrogen.

Measurement Technique

The technique involves having the patient (wearing a nose clip) take normal breaths through a mouthpiece attached to a 100% oxygen reservoir. The patient needs to breathe 100% oxygen for several minutes starting with the first breath at the end of a normal exhalation or FRC. The percentage of nitrogen expired is measured continually until it reaches 1.5% on three successive breaths (Fig. 8.10). The test is usually run for 7 minutes, but it may take longer for patients with severe obstruction. The total volume exhaled is measured at the end of the test and the initial and final nitrogen concentrations are used to calculate FRC as follows:

$$FRC_{N2} = \frac{(\text{volume } N_2 \text{ washed out}) - (N_2 \text{ tissue excretion})}{\text{Initial} - \text{final lung } N_2 \text{ concentration}}$$

The amount of nitrogen excreted from tissues is small and a set equation is used to estimate the amount for all patients based on body surface area. Like helium dilution, this technique can be used to measure the lung volumes of noncompliant patients, including patients requiring mechanical ventilation. Again the results must be corrected for BTPS conditions and the volume of equipment dead space needs to be subtracted.

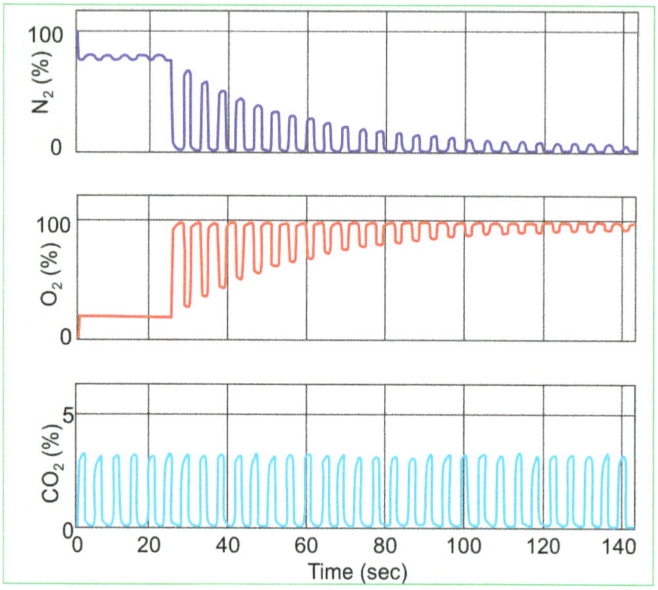

Fig. 8.10: Multiple-breath nitrogen washout test. Gases concentration (nitrogen, oxygen, carbon dioxide) and volume tracings are shown as a function of time.

IMAGING

Chest X-Ray

In addition to breathing tests, lung volume measurements can be made from conventional posterioranterior (PA) chest radiographs, CT scans, and MRIs. The first use of imaging to measure lung volumes involved creating estimations based on the outlines of PA and lateral chest X-rays. There are two major methods of doing this, either by fitting geometrical shapes such as ellipsoids within thoracic outlines or by using planimeters.

In 1960, Barnhard described measuring lung volumes with radiographs using an ellipsoid measurement of thoracic volume. This involved viewing the thorax as a stack of five ellipsoids and calculating the volume using transverse diameters and heights measured from PA and lateral chest radiographs. This method was later modified and computer models were used that could calculate lung volumes using an equation derived from *postmortem* examinations and CT scans.

Planimeters are engineering devices that have been designed to measure the area of irregularly shaped spaces. Subjects have their surface areas converted to TLC through the use of equations derived by physiologic testing and surface area measured by planimetry. Equations are derived from sample studies that seek to create baseline measurements than can then be applied to the population as a whole.

Imaging estimations are dependent on patient effort and ability to breathe hold. The small studies done on the radiographic measurements have differed on the accuracy of both ellipsoid and planimetric calculations compared to plethysmography. One study noted differences between radiographic estimates and plethysmography as high as 1.64 L (20% of the TLC by plethysmography).

One of the reasons for the variation in findings may be that results change depending on patient effort and level of coaching involved during imaging. The patient must be coached to take a maximal inspiration during measurements. This is important during individual testing, but also when creating baseline equations from a sample population. One study published in 1992 to create baseline equations on a sample population stated that the increased accuracy of their results compared to others may be due to population samples with a significant number of chest films with inadequate inspirations. This poses an even greater problem when trying to estimate lung volumes based on routine imaging, as the volume will often differ greatly in size from images required with special coaching.

Lung volume estimations based on imaging involve measuring the area within the thoracic cage, and include not only the amount of gas within the lungs, but also any tissue, both normal and abnormal. While measurements with imaging will likely have similar results to plethysmography for health individuals, patients with airspace occupying disease, such as pneumonia or fibrosis may have overestimated volumes by radiography.

Computerized Tomography Scans

Computerized tomography scans can better distinguish between abnormal and normal lung tissue, and can estimate the amount of abnormal lung tissue as well as the volume of gas present in the lungs. Unfortunately CT lung volume measurements involve algorithms that often involve device-specific proprietary technology that is not available for analysis. Because of the difference in the methodology of different scanners, the same analysis cannot necessarily be applied on different machines. This makes comparisons between images at different facilities difficult. Due to these difficulties ATS/ERS have not recommended any particular method of lung volume measurement by CT scan.

Magnetic Resonance Imaging

Magnetic resonance imaging may also allow for the measurement of lung volume while accounting for both normal and abnormal lung tissue as well as fluid in the lung. Both CT and MRI suffer from two major drawbacks: cost, and positioning of the patient. While lung volumes are physiologically measured with the patient sitting upright, both MRIs and CT scans are done with the patient supine. The difference in position may cause significant changes in results, especially in patients with obesity or neurological disease. MRI technique is discussed further in a separate dedicated chapter of this book.

Interpreting Results

Normal values depend on a person's age, weight, height, ethnicity and gender. Reference values are based on studies of populations meant to representative of different patient populations. Attempts are generally made to match the subject to a reference population with similar characteristics. However, if a patient is from an ethnicity not matching the sample population, the reference values may not apply. This is why many studies have been done, in order to create unique reference values for different ethnic groups so that results can be adjusted for the "normal values" that fit a particular patient. Although there are changes in lung mechanics with age, TLC does not change with aging in healthy adults.

In general, there are three overall patterns of lung volume change in disease: restriction, obstruction and hyperinflation. This becomes somewhat more complicated in patients with more than one disease process. For example, obstruction and hyperinflation often overlap, as in COPD with emphysema. However this is not always the case. In addition to traditional lung diseases, obesity is also becoming a more common contributor to abnormal lung function testing. Understanding how obesity effects lung function and lung volumes will become, unfortunately, more important as the obesity epidemic brings more patients into the pulmonary clinic seeking diagnosis for respiratory complaints.

Table 8.3 depicts general plethysmography results in common lung disorders, ageing and obesity.

Restriction

There are three different categories of disorders that result in restriction; intrinsic, extrinsic, and neuromuscular. Intrinsic causes of restriction include intraparenchymal disease such as pulmonary fibrosis, and alveolitis. Extrinsic restriction includes extrapulmonary disorders

Table 8.3: Plethysmography results in different clinical conditions.

	TLC	*FRC*	*RV*	*VC*
Restriction	Decreased	Decreased	Decreased or normal	Decreased
Obstruction	Normal	Normal or Increased	Normal or Increased	Normal
Hyperinflation	Normal or Increased	Increased	Increased	Normal or Increased
Ageing	No change	Increases	Increases	Decreases
Obesity	Normal or minimally decreased	Decreased	Normal or minimally decreased	Normal or minimally decreased

(FRC: Functional residual capacity; RV: Residual volume; TLC: Total lung capacity; VC: Vital capacity).

such as scoliosis, kyphosis, and congestive heart failure. Neuromuscular restriction results when the patient has diaphragmatic paralysis, or profound muscular weakness such as that seen in ALS.

Restriction is often evaluated with spirometry and measurements of FVC. Although spirometry is clearly easier and cheaper, than other methods, it may fail to correctly identify restrictive disease. Measurement of FVC has been shown in one study to have only 69.3% sensitivity for identifying restrictive changes. It has been suggested that the TLC needs to be measured, in order to identify true restriction.

Hyperinflation

This is most commonly seen in air trapping diseases such as asthma or emphysema. Patients with COPD who also have emphysema will also have evidence of hyperinflation, but not all patients with obstructive lung disease will have hyperinflation. Alternatively, asthma, which is generally a disease of air trapping may present with true restriction. In one study, roughly 8% of patients diagnosed with asthma (by positive bronchodilator response or methacholine challenge test) were found to have a reduced VC without appreciable air trapping and a normal RV.

Combined Obstruction and Restriction

This combination appears to be commonly seen with spirometry. However, when patients are further evaluated with lung volume testing, true combined obstruction and restriction is actually rare. An accurate diagnosis cannot be made with spirometry alone. ATS/ERS guidelines recommend measuring lung volumes when spirometry indicates a decrease FVC.

A retrospective study by the Cleveland clinic showed a mixed disorder present in 2–2.7% of adult patients who underwent spirometry and plethysmography compared with 11% of patients who appeared to have a mixed disorder by spirometry alone. Of the patients initially diagnosed with obstruction and restriction on spirometry, only 9.5% were found to have restriction by plethysmography. True combined restriction and obstruction tends to be a combination of parenchymal and nonparenchymal disease such as COPD with congestive heart failure.

Examples

Patient 1: A 59-year-old Caucasian woman with Alpha-1 antitripsin deficiency. Former smoker, height 177 cm, weight 78.5 kg.

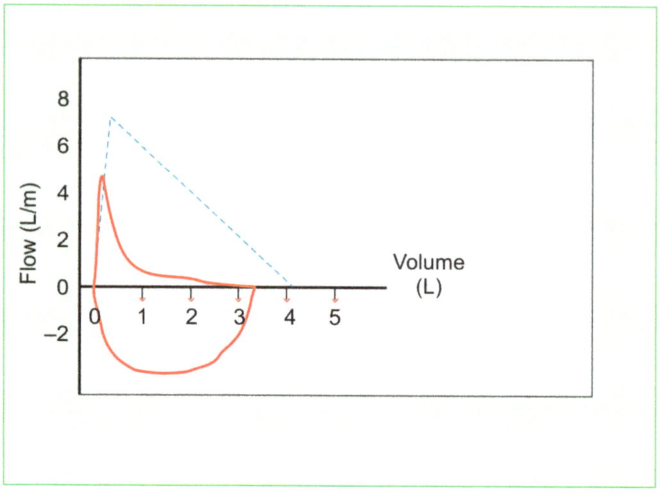

Spirometry

		Predicted	LLN	Measured	% Pred
VCmax	L	4.07	4.07	3.18	78
FEV1	L	3.13	3.13	1.82	58
FEV1/VCmax	%	77	70	57	74
PEF	L/S	6.86	6.86	3.10	45
FEF 25-75	L/S	3.08	1.45	0.86	28
Plethysmography					
TLC	L	5.90	4.90	6.43	108
FRC	L	3.06	2.20	3.83	125
RV	L	2.15	1.57	3.22	149
RAWtot	kPas/L	<0.35	0.30	1.52	434

Interpretation: Simple spirometry confirms the presence of airway obstruction (FEV1/VCmax < LLN) consistent with alph1-antitrypsin deficiency related lung disease. It also suggest a possible associated restrictive lung disease (VC < LLN). Plethysmography allows to exclude this, showing that VC is reduced due to a significant hyperinflation: TLC, FRC, and RV are all increased, with the RV being the most severely increased.

Patient 2: A 66-year-old Caucasian man with pulmonary fibrosis. Former smoker, height 172 cm, weight 72.3 kg.

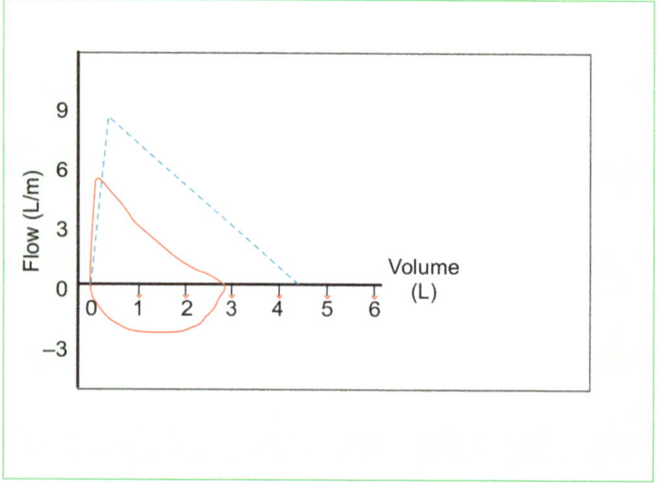

Spirometry					
		Predicted	*LLN*	*Measured*	*% Pred*
VCmax	L	4.17	3.30	2.92	70
FEV1	L	3.10	2.27	2.48	80
FEV1/VCmax	%	74	64.5	85	115
PEF	L/S	7.95	6.02	5.41	68
FEF 25–75	L/S	3.20	1.52	2.05	64
Plethysmography					
TLC	L	6.59	5.51	4.09	62
FRC	L	3.44	2.54	2.27	66
RV	L	2.24	1.80	1.21	54
RAWtot	kPas/L	0.30	0.30		

Interpretation: Simple spirometry suggest mild restriction (FEV1/FVC > LLN, VCmax < LLN). The level of restriction is often different with plethysmography. Plethysmography shows this patient to have moderate restriction with reduction in TLC, FRC and RV. Plethysmography helped to confirm that this patient truly had restriction and that the spirometry was not just decreased due to limited effort.

Patient 3: A 65-year-old Caucasian man with asthma. Former Smoker, height 187.5 cm, weight 103.5 kg.

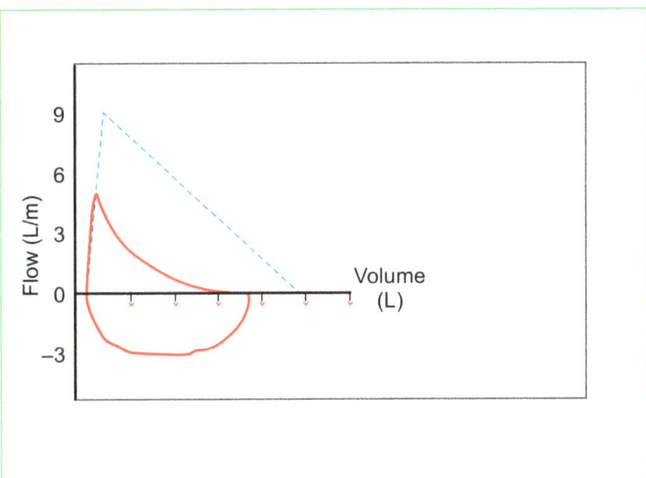

Spirometry					
		Predicted	*LLN*	*Measured*	*% Pred*
VCmax	L	4.97	4.05	3.52	71
FEV1	L	3.69	2.85	2.45	66
FEV1/VCmax	%	75.5	65.7	67	88.7
PEF	L/S	8.87	6.88	5.89	66
FEF 25-75	L/S	3.54	1.84	2.21	62
Plethysmography					
TLC	L	7.90	6.75	6.77	87
FRC	L	3.88	2.90	3.86	93
RV	L	2.66	1.98	2.95	114
RAWtot	kPas/L	0.30	0.30	0.85	283

Interpretation: Simple spirometry testing consistent with restrictive lung disease (FEV1/FVC > LLN, VC < LLN). The plethysmography results show a normal TLC and an increased RV, consistent with air trapping. This is an example of pseudo-restriction, which can occur in patients with obstructive lung disease when the forced exhalation causes collapse of airways with consequent VC result smaller than expected. In such cases, forced VC is usually more reduced than slow VC.

Patient 4: A 57-year-old Caucasian man with dyspnea, morbid obesity. Never smoker, height 178 cm, weight 156.4 kg.

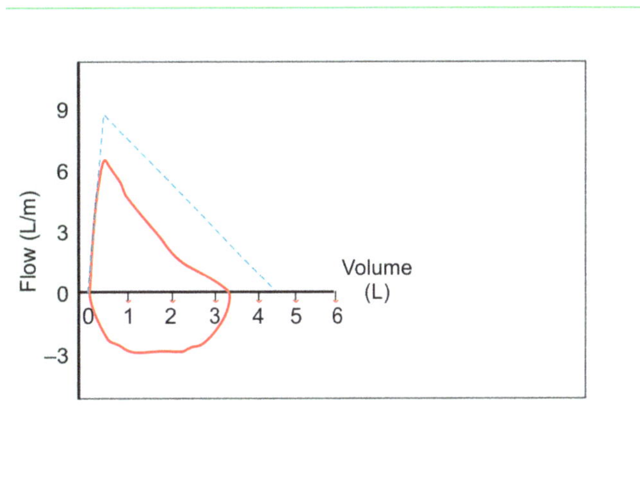

Spirometry					
		Predicted	*LLN*	*Measured*	*% Pred*
VCmax	L	4.42	3.32	3.46	78
FEV1	L	3.45	2.53	2.79	81
FEV1/VCmax	%	78	67	81	104
PEF	L/S	8.50	6.47	6.80	80
FEF 25–75	L/S	2.95	1.29	2.78	94
Plethysmography					
TLC	L	6.79	5.65	5.57	82
FRC	L	3.62	2.54	2.68	74
RV	L	2.37	1.67	1.99	84
RAWtot	kPas/L	0.30	0.30	0.38	126

Interpretation: Simple spirometry shows VC slightly below the lower limit of normal, suggesting a restrictive lung disease. This is commonly seen in obese patients. It has been showed that obesity causes a roughly 0.5% decrease in VC, TLC, and RV with each point increase in BMI. Although decreased, TLC generally remain normal by plethysmography, even in patients with morbid obesity, which have a much larger effect on other lung volumes, specifically the FRC, which decreases rapidly as body weight increases. In such patients, FRC has an indirect relationship with airway resistance.

EVALUATION OF THE RESPIRATORY MUSCLE STRENGTH

The strength of the respiratory muscles can be studied by measuring the pressure generated by inspiratory or expiratory efforts during airway occlusion.

The main parameters used to define an impairment of respiratory muscle strength are the *maximal inspiratory pressure* (MIP or PImax) and the *maximal expiratory pressure* (MEP or PEmax). Other tests to assess inspiratory muscles strength are the *maximal sniff nasal inspiratory pressure* (SNIP), and the *airway occlusion pressure 0.1 second after onset of inspiration* (P 0.1). In addition to the MIP and MEP which are both static measures, the strength of respiratory muscles can be inferred from dynamic maneuvers with the maximal voluntary ventilation (MVV).

Maximal inspiratory pressure (sometimes called *Negative Inspiratory Force: NIF*), corresponds to the highest value of negative pressure a person can generate during a static inspiratory effort (Müller maneuver). It is expressed in centimeters of water (cm H_2O) and can be measured soon after complete emptying of the lungs until the residual volume (MIP_RV) or at functional residual capacity (MIP_FRC).

It is an important and noninvasive measurement of diaphragm and accessory inspiratory muscle strength, useful for diagnosing or monitoring the respiratory involvement in several diseases with neuromuscular dysfunction. The measurement of MIP is also helpful in assessing the inspiratory muscle strength of subjects with alteration of the respiratory mechanics due to lung disease, such as pulmonary emphysema or severe chest deformity. Decreased MIP is common in emphysema and chest wall deformities such as kyphosis.

Maximal inspiratory pressure is useful in assessing patients on mechanical ventilation to determine if they can be extubated. The probability of successfully removing patients from mechanical ventilation increases with the increase of the MIP. Successful extubation occurs in less than 50% of patients with MIP below or equal to 30 cm H_2O.

Maximal expiratory pressure is the greatest positive pressure a person can generate during expiration against a closed valve. The value of MEP is recorded after the patient has inhaled to TLC. It reflects the strength of the abdominal muscles and other expiratory muscles. Figure 8.11

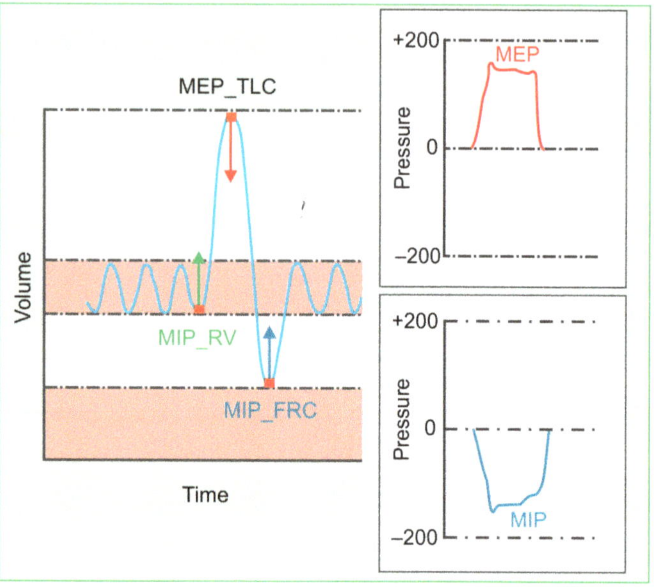

Fig. 8.11: Execution of MIP and MEP maneuvers.
(FRC: Functional residual capacity; MEP: Maximal expiratory pressure; MIP: Maximal inspiratory pressure; RV: Residual volume; TLC: Total lung capacity).

shows when the measurement of MIP and MEP are performed during breathing. Decreased MEP can be seen in patients with neuromuscular disease as well as obstructive lung disease (COPD) and restriction (pulmonary fibrosis).

Maximal inspiratory pressure and MEP measurements are dependent on patient effort. A low value may reflect poor effort rather than a true decrease in respiratory muscle strength.

MIP and MEP maneuvers are performed with the patient in the sitting position with a noseclip in place. The patient breathes through a mouthpiece attached to a tube with a device that prevents glottic closure and recruitment of the orofacial musculature. To record the MIP, the patient is asked to breathe out to residual volume, and then to perform a maximum inspiratory effort for at least 1 second, while a three-way valve or a shutter mechanism is actuated to obstruct the flow and a manometer records mouth pressure. MEP measurement is performed similarly to MIP, by asking the patient to exhale forcefully against a partially occluded airway, beginning from TLC. Subjects can be seated opposite the monitor in order to provide a visual feedback able to improve the quality of test. At least three technically satisfactory and reproducible measurements are required (variation in MIP and MEP <10% or 10 cm H_2O). The patient should be allowed to rest for about one minute before repeating the maneuver. No more than five maneuvers are recommended.

The highest value sustained for 1 second is considered and compared with the predicted value.

When the MIP maneuver is performed at low lung volumes, inspiratory pressures are usually higher. However, measuring PImax at FRC rather than RV is preferable since at this volume the negative recoil pressure of the respiratory system is negligible and only the force of the inspiratory muscles is assessed.

The technique and equipment employed can significantly affect the results of MIP and MEP. Both parameters should be measured using a large-bore circular mouthpiece or a scuba-diving mouthpiece with the cheeks supported. The ranges of normal values are quite large and vary by age and gender.

Maximal volume ventilation (MVV) is the total volume of air exhaled during 12 seconds of rapid, deep breathing. The volume measured after 12 seconds is compared with the predicted MVV which is the FEV1 multiplied by a constant (35 or 40). It correlates well with FEV1 and therefore is not commonly used. Unlike FEV1, which relies largely on expiratory effort, MVV depends on both inspiratory and expiratory strength. For this reason, it has some usefulness as a measurement of neuromuscular weakness and ventilatory reserve during exercise.

MVV can be assessed at the end of spirometry with a subject sitting while wearing a nose clip. The patient needs to make an airtight seal with her lips around the mouthpiece of the spirometer. After at least three resting tidal breaths, the patient is asked to breathe as fast and as deep as possible. The ideal rate is 90–110 breaths per minute. Previous studies suggest encouraging the patient to breathe faster if the rate is not at least 60 breaths per minute, and deeper if the tidal volume is less than 40% of the FVC. The patient should be allowed to rest in between attempts with the greatest of at least two efforts used as the final measurement. The final MVV is reported in L/minute BTPS. A measured MVV that is less than 80% of the predicted MVV suggests either poor effort or disease.

Sniff nasal inspiratory pressure is a simple and reliable means of measuring inspiratory muscle strength. It does not involve the use of a mouthpiece, thus it might be better than VC or mouth pressures for assessing and monitor respiratory function in patients with bulbar disease or motor neuron disease. Measurements are usually made at functional residual capacity, with the patients seated comfortably, using a hand-held meter. Special nasal pillows are inserted into the nostril and the patient is asked to take a series of short sharp sniffs with the mouth closed, each 20 seconds apart. The highest of five results is recorded.

Airway occlusion pressure 0.1 second after onset of inspiration corresponds to the pressure generated at the mouth 0.1 second after the beginning of inspiration against an occluded airway. P 0.1 provides an indirect assessment of the neural drive to the respiratory muscles, as it reflects the neuromuscular component of the output of the central respiratory controller. P 0.1 interpretation requires a great deal of caution. It is most reliable when end-expiratory volume remains constant and there are no important phase lags between flow and pressure.

BIBLIOGRAPHY AND FURTHER READING

1. Aaron SD, Dales RE, Cardinal P. How accurate is spirometry at predicting restrictive pulmonary impairment. Chest. 1999;115:869-73.
2. Bancalari E, Clausen J. Pathophysiology of changes in absolute lung volumes. The Eur Respir J. 1998;12(1):248-58.
3. Barnhard, HJ. Pierce JA, Joyce JW, Bates JH. Roentgenographic determination of total lung capacity. Am J Med. 1960;28:51-60.
4. Borelli DA. De motu animalium. 2 vol. Rome, Bemabo, 1680±1681. 106.
5. Boros PW, Franczuk M, Wesolowski S. Value of Spirometry in Detecting Volume Restriction in Interstitial Lung Disease Patients. Respiration. 2004;71(4):374-79.
6. Brown R, Leith DE, Enright PL. Multiple breath helium dilution measurement of lung volumes in adults. Eur Resp J. 199811(1), 246-55.
7. Brown R, Pearse D, Pyrgos G, Liu M, Togias A, Permutt S. 2006. The structural basis of airways hyperresponsiveness in asthma. Journal of Applied Physiology. 2006;101(1): 30–9.
8. Casanova C, Cote C, de Torres JP, Aguirre-Jaime A, Marin JM, Pinto-Plata V, et al. Inspiratory-to-total lung capacity ratio predicts mortality in patients with chronic obstructive pulmonary disease. Am J Respi Crit Care Medicine. 2005;171(6):591-7.
9. Cazzola M, Rogliani P, Curradi G, Segreti A, Ciaprini C, Pezzuto G, et al. Pulmonary pharmacology & therapeutics. Pulm Pharmacol Therap. 2009;22(6):522-5.
10. Clausen JL, Wanger JS. Consensus statement on measurements of lung volumes in humans. ATS/NHLBI Consensus Document. November 12, 2003.
11. Clausen JL, Zarins LP, Ries AL. Measurements of abnormal increases in pulmonary tissue in restrictive lung disease. Am Rev Respir Dis. 1978;117(Suppl.):322.
12. Clausen JL. Lung volume consensus. ATS. 2010:1-189.
13. Clausen JL. Measurement of absolute lung volumes by imaging techniques. Eur Resp J. 1997;10(10):2427-31.
14. Clayton N. Review series: lung function made easy: assessing lung size. Chron Respir Dis. 2007;4(3):151-7.
15. Coates AL, Peslin R, Rodenstein D, Stocks J. Measurement of lung volumes by plethysmography. Eur Respir J. 1997;10(6):1415-27.
16. Crapo RO, Montague T, Armstrong J. Inspiratory lung volume achieved on routine chest films. Invest Radiol. 1979;14:137-40.

17. Crapo RO. Pulmonary Function Testing. In: Crapo JD, Glassroth J, Karlinsky JB, King TE (Eds). Baum's textbook of pulmonary diseases. 7th edition. Philadelphia, PA: Lippincott Williams & Wilkins; 2004. p. 36.
18. Criée CP, Sorichter S, Smith HJ, Kardos P, Merget R, Heise D, et al. Body plethysmography — its principles and clinical use. Respir Med. 2011;105(7):959-71.
19. Darling RC, Cournand A, Richards DW. An open circuit method for measuring residual air. J Clin Invest. 1940;19:609-18.
20. Diaz-Guzman E, McCarthy K, Siu A, Stoller JK. Frequency and causes of combined obstruction and restriction identified in pulmonary function tests in adults. Respir Care. 2010;55(3):310-6.
21. Dillard TA, Hnatiuk OW, McCumber TR. Maximum voluntary ventilation: spirometric determinants in chronic obstructive pulmonary disease patients and normal subjects. Am Rev Respir Dis. 1993;147:870-5.
22. DuBois AB, Botelho SY, Bedell GN, Marshall R, Comroe JH. A rapid plethysmographic method for measuring thoracic gas volume: a comparison with a nitrogen washout method for measuring functional residual capacity in normal subjects. J Clin Invest. 1956;35:322-6.
23. Ferretti A, Giampiccolo P, Cavalli A, Milic-Emili J, Tantucci C. Expiratory flow limitation and orthopnea in massively obese subjects. Chest. 2001;119:1401-8.
24. Fischbach F, Dunning MB. A manual of laboratory and diagnostic tests. 8th edition. Lippincott Williams and Wilkins. 2008.
25. Flesch JD, Dine CJ. Lung volumes. Chest. 2012;142(2):506-10.
26. GOLD Spirometry for Health Care Providers. 2010:1-14. www.goldcopd.org.
27. Gopal R, Starkschall G, Tucker SL, Cox JD, Liao Z, Hanus M, et al. Effects of radiotherapy and chemotherapy on lung function in patients with non-small-cell lung cancer. Int J Radiat Oncol Biol Phys. 2003;56(1):114-20.
28. Hegewald MJ, Crapo RO. Pulmonary function testing. In: Mason RJ, Broaddus VC, Martin TR, et al. (Eds). Murray and Nadel's textbook of respiratory medicine. 5th edition. chap 24. Philadelphia, Pa: Saunders Elsevier; 2010.
29. Houghton CM, Woodcock AA, Singh D. A comparison of lung function methods for assessing dose-response effects of salbutamol. Br J Clin Pharmacol. 2004;58(2):134-41.
30. Jones RL, Nzekwu MM. The effects of body mass index on lung volumes. Chest. 2006;130(3):827-33.
31. Kilburn KH, Warshaw RH, Thornton JC, Thornton K, Miller A. Predictive equations for total lung capacity and residual volume calculated from radiographs in a random sample of the Michigan population. Thorax. 1992;47(7):519-23.
32. Liou T, Kanner R. Spirometry. Clin Rev Allergy Immunol. 2009;37:137-52.
33. Lumb A. Nunn's applied respiratory physiology. 7th edition. Elsevier Health Sciences; 2012.
34. Meneely GR, Kaltreider NL. Use of helium for determination of pulmonary capacity. Proc Soc Exper Biol Med. 1941;-46:266-9.
35. Miller A, Palecki A. Restrictive impairment in patients with asthma. Respir Med. 2007;101(2):272-6.
36. Miller MR, Hankinson J, Brusasco V, Burgos F, Casaburi R, Coates A, et al. Standardisation of spirometry. Eur Respir J. 2005;26(6):319-38.
37. Newth CJ, Enright P, Johnson RL. Multiple-breath nitrogen washout techniques: including measurements with patients on ventilators. Eur Respir J. 1997;10:2174-85.
38. Patroniti N, Bellani G, Manfio A, Maggioni E, Giuffrida A, Foti G, et al. Lung volume in mechanically ventilated patients: measurement by simplified helium dilution compared to quantitative CT scan. Intensive Care Med. 2004;30(2):282-9.
39. Pelosi P, Croci M, Ravagnam I, Tredici S, Pedoto A, Lissoni A, et al. The effects of body mass on lung volumes, respiratory mechanics and gas exchange during general anesthesia. Anesth Analg. 1998;87:654-60.
40. Petty TL, Silvers GW, Stanford RE. Mild emphysema is associated with reduced elastic recoil and increased lung size but not with air-flow limitation. Am Rev Respir Dis. 1987;136:867-71.
41. Pierce RJ, Brown DJ, Holmes M, Cumming G, Denison DM. Estimation of lung volumes from chest radiographs using shape information. Thorax. 1979;34:726-34.
42. Pride NB. Ageing and changes in lung mechanics. Eur Resp J. 2005;26(4):563-5.
43. Rodenstein DO, Sopwith T, Denison DM, Stanescu DC. Reevaluation of the radiographic method for measurement of total lung capacity. Bull Eur Physiopathol Respir. 1985;21:521-5.
44. Rubin AE, Bruderman I. Overdistension of lung due to peripheral airwasy obstruction. Chest. 1973;63:948-51.
45. Ruppel GL. What is the clinical value of lung volumes? Respiratory Care. 2012;57(1):26-38.
46. Teklu B, Gray WM, Mills RJ, Moran F. A critical appraisal of a rapid radiographic method of determining total lung capacity. Scott Med J. 1986;31:99-102.
47. Vulterini S, Bianco MR, Pellicciotti L, Sidoti AM. Lung mechanics in subjects showing increased residual volume without bronchial obstruction. Thorax. 1980;35:461-6.
48. Wanger, J. Standardisation of the measurement of lung volumes. Eur Resp J. 2005;26(3):511-22.
49. Yernault J-C, Pride N, Laszlo G. How the measurement of residual volume developed after Davy (1800). Eur Respir J. 2000;16:561-4

Chapter 9

Bronchoprovocation Challenge Test

Claudio Sorino, Diego Bagnasco, Fulvio Braido

OVERVIEW OF BRONCHOPROVOCATION CHALLENGE TEST AND CLINICAL INDICATIONS

A bronchoprovocation challenge test is a tool used to assess bronchial hyperresponsiveness. The test requires the administration of an agent able to irritate airways and cause their narrowing in susceptible subjects.

The main indication for bronchoprovocation challenge test is the confirmation of a diagnosis of asthma in subjects with a clinical suspicion but without functional evidence of airway obstruction (normal spirometry). This mainly occurs in patients with mild asthma, in which the airflow obstruction may be absent at the time of spirometry. Less frequently, the bronchoprovocation test can be used to assess response to therapy in patients already diagnosed with asthma, or to identify the triggers when environmental or occupational asthma are suspected. Finally, a bronchoprovocation challenge test is indicated for subjects such requiring a screening test for asthma, such as scuba divers, military personnel, or other individuals in whom bronchospasm during their activities would be particularly dangerous.

BRONCHIAL HYPERRESPONSIVENESS

Bronchial (or airway) hyperresponsiveness is a condition in which the airways respond more than usual to irritative stimuli. One of the main manifestations of this response is the reduction of the airway size (airway narrowing). This is mainly due to the contraction of bronchial smooth muscle ("bronchoconstriction" or "bronchospasm"), but airway inflammation, remodeling and mucus production may help the process. Airway narrowing causes airflow limitation, makes it harder to expel the irritants, and may occur with breathlessness and cough.

Bronchial hyperresponsiveness is one of the main functional features of bronchial asthma, but may be present with varying intensity in other acute and chronic respiratory diseases.

The same smooth muscle stimulation can provoke a very higher degree of airway narrowing in subjects with airway hyperresponsiveness than in subjects with normal bronchial responsiveness. Moreover, smooth muscle relaxants are very helpful in quickly relieving bronchoconstriction in subjects with airway hyperresponsiveness, but they do not change the underlying bronchial hyperresponsiveness.

SPECIFIC AND NONSPECIFIC AIRWAY RESPONSIVENESS

The bronchoconstrictor stimuli can be classified as specific or nonspecific. *Specific stimuli* include *allergens* like the excreta of house dust mites, which are often found in house dust and bedding, since mites feed on skin which scales off from humans or animals. Other antigenic substances comprise animal dander (e.g. cat, dog, horse), pollen from plants (e.g. grasses and trees) and spores from molds.

If inhaled, these materials induce a type I, immunoglobulin E (IgE)-mediated immunological response in the airways in atopic subjects sensitized to a specific allergen. Specific responsiveness to substances with antigenic features is a hallmark of atopic asthma.

Nonspecific stimuli eliciting airway narrowing are nonallergic agents. Their nature can be physical (e.g. cold air,

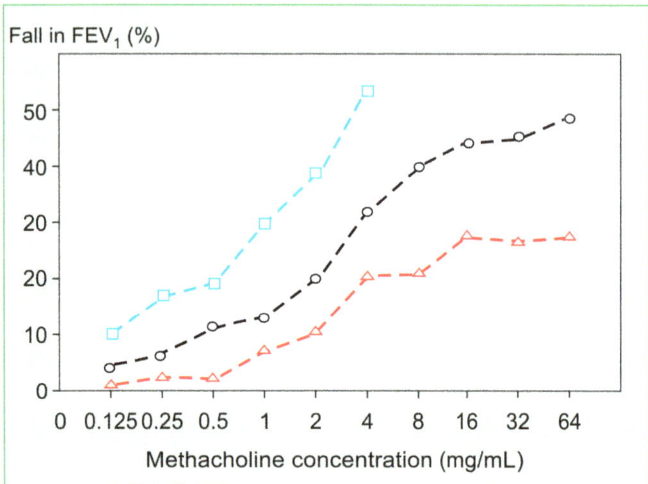

Fig. 9.1: Fall in FEV_1 during a bronchoprovocation challenge test in a healthy subject (triangles), with mild asthma (circles), and moderate asthma (squares).

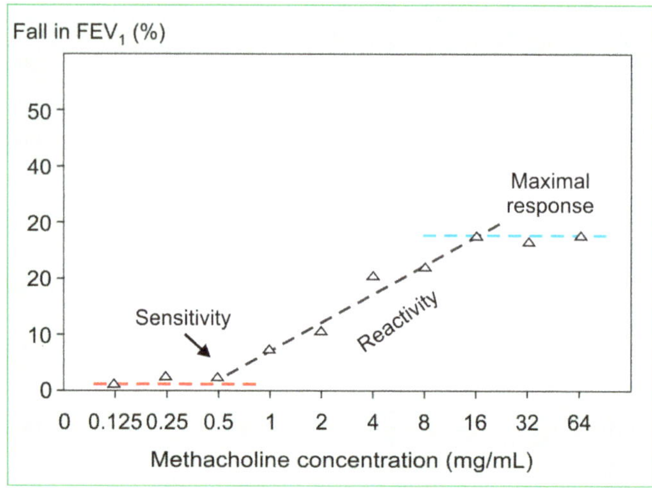

Fig. 9.2: Identification of sensitivity, reactivity, and maximal response in a subject undergoing a bronchoprovocation challenge test.

dry air, hyper- or hypotonic solutions), pharmacological (e.g. histamine, methacholine, adenosine, mannitol), chemical (e.g. sulfur dioxide, ozone), or physiological (e.g. exercise). Nonspecific stimuli generally exert their action through multiple cell types within the airways.

The airways of nonasthmatic subjects do not respond to specific stimuli; they often respond to nonspecific stimuli, but at a greater dosage of irritant and with a lesser extent than the airways of asthmatic subjects (Fig. 9.1).

Airway responsiveness may vary with time and can be measured in laboratory through bronchial challenge tests (dose-response test).

Methacholine and *histamine* are known as *direct bronchoconstrictor* stimuli since they act directly on bronchial smooth muscle; the response to them is reproducible and easy to control.

Eucapnic hyperventilation, ultrasonic mist of *hypertonic or hypotonic solutions* and *exercise* are considered *indirect bronchoconstrictor* stimuli as their action is mediated by the release of inflammatory mediators from bronchial cells. Challenges that use indirect stimuli are poorly standardized.

HOW TO EXPRESS AIRWAY RESPONSIVENESS?

Airway responsiveness to a specific or nonspecific irritant can be assessed by observing the relationship between the dose of irritant which the subject is exposed and the degree of subsequent airway narrowing. This relationship is expressed by a dose-response curve, from which we can deduce the *sensitivity*, *reactivity*, and *maximal response* to the agent (Fig. 9.2).

The airway response to an agent is usually evaluated by measuring the change (reduction) of the maximal volume of air which can be expired in the first second of a forced expiration starting from a full inhalation [forced expiratory volume in one second (FEV_1)]. Less frequently the airway response is assessed by measuring directly the increase of airways resistance through whole body plethysmography.

The main ways to express bronchial responsiveness are the *provocative concentration* (µmol/L or mg/mL) and the *provocative dose* (µmol or mg) able to produce a decrease in FEV_1 by 20% from the initial value or baseline value prior to inhalation of the provocative agent (abbreviated as PC_{20} and PD_{20}, respectively).

Alternatively, the responsiveness can be expressed as the concentration or the dose of agonist which causes airways resistance to double from the initial value, i.e. increase to 200% (PC_{200} and PD_{200}, respectively).

The cumulative dose of provocative agent at the inflection point of dose-response or concentration-response curves reflects the minimum dose required for the airways reaction, and is considered the expression of the bronchial *sensitivity* to the inhaled substance.

In several studies, the concentration of an agent able to produce a decrease in FEV_1 by 6% from the initial value (PC_6) or a decrease in specific airway conductance by 25% has been considered as a sensitivity parameter.

The slope of the dose-response curve corresponds to the variation of the fall in FEV_1 in relation to the increase of the cumulative dose of provocative agent, and expresses the bronchial *reactivity*.

A decrease in PC_{20} may be due to a steeper curve (hyperreactivity) and/or a curve shift to the left (hypersensitivity).

Increased sensitivity (hypersensitivity) and reactivity (hyperreactivity) usually occur together. The nonspecific term "airway (or bronchial) hyperresponsiveness" is often used to designate any difference in the dose-response curve related to sensitivity, reactivity or the maximal response. The *maximal response* expresses the cumulative dose of provocative agent beyond which further bronchoconstriction and fall of FEV1 do not occur. It is often absent or cannot be evaluated in patients with asthma for safety reasons.

HOW TO PERFORM A BRONCHOPROVOCATION CHALLENGE TEST?

Bronchoprovocation challenge testing can be performed with pharmacological, physical and sensitizing stimuli. Airway responsiveness is most frequently assessed by inhalation of histamine or methacholine aerosol. In recent years inhaled mannitol is increasingly used; it increases the osmolarity at the airway surface and thus liberates mediators.

CONTRAINDICATIONS AND PRECAUTIONS

Several conditions can result dangerous for patients or may compromise the quality of a bronchoprovocation challenge test, consequently listed as absolute or relative contraindications.

Absolute contraindications include severe airflow limitation (FEV_1 <50% of predicted or <1 L), known aortic aneurysm, heart attack or stroke in last 3 months, uncontrolled hypertension with systolic blood pressure above 200 mm Hg or diastolic above 100 mm Hg (bronchospasm induction may cause hypoxic vasoconstriction resulting in further increase in blood pressure).

Relative contraindications include moderate airflow limitation at baseline spirometry with FEV_1 under 60% of predicted value or less than 1.5 L in adult people, pregnancy or breastfeeding, therapy with cholinesterase-inhibitor medication due to myasthenia gravis, inability to perform an acceptable-quality spirometry.

PHARMACOLOGIC CHALLENGE TESTS

Several bronchial provocation tests with different pharmacological stimuli can be used in the clinical practice. They include methacholine, mannitol, adenosine, and histamine challenges.

Methacholine Challenge

Methacholine (acetyl-P-methylcholine chloride), is considered the agent of choice for nonspecific bronchoprovocation challenge testing. It is available as a dry crystalline powder and is very hygroscopic. Bulk powder should be stored with a desiccator in a freezer, whereas sealed prepackaged vials do not require desiccation or freezing. Sterile normal saline (0.9% sodium chloride) with or without 0.4% phenol may be used as the diluent. The addition of a preservative such as phenol has the potential to reduce the risk of bacterial contamination, but there is no evidence that this is necessary. Methacholine solutions should be mixed by a well-trained individual using sterile technique. The vials should be labeled as methacholine with the concentration and an expiration date, and stored in a refrigerator at about 4°C. In such a condition, methacholine solutions of 0.125 mg/mL and greater, prepared with saline diluents, can be stable for 3 months. Solutions of methacholine should be warmed to room temperature before testing begins. Any unemployed methacholine solution remaining in a nebulizer should be discarded.

Several different dosing protocols have been proposed for methacholine challenge, each of which has advantages and disadvantages. The American Thoracic Society narrowed the choices to two methods: (1) the two-minute tidal breathing and (2) the five-breath dosimeter (Table 9.1).

Four common methods of aerosol generation and inhalation are used, providing similar results:

1. Dosing during a deep inhalation, using a Y tube occluded by the thumb
2. Five breaths of a fixed duration, using a dosimeter at the beginning of a deep inhalation
3. A hand bulb nebulizer activated during inhalation
4. Continuous nebulization while tidal breathing for 2 minutes.

After instructing the patient on the proper performance of the test, a baseline spirometry should be performed and the absolute value of FEV_1 at which the test will be considered positive should be calculated (baseline FEV_1 in Liters × 0.8).Then the patient is asked to hold the nebulizer upright, with the mouthpiece in his/her mouth, while methacholine is nebulized and delivered.

FEV_1 should be successively measured about 30 and 90 seconds after the nebulization of methacholine is completed. Repeated attempts may be required to obtain a good quality proof. No more than three or four maneuvers should be performed after each dose. It should take no more than 3 minutes to perform these maneuvers. To keep the cumulative effect of methacholine relatively constant,

Table 9.1: American Thoracic Society protocols and dilution schemes for bronchial challenge test with methacholine

Two-minute tidal breathing protocol	*Five-breath dosimeter protocol*
Methacholine concentration	
Solvent	Solvent
0.031 mg/mL	–
0.0625 mg/mL	0.0625 mg/mL
0.125 mg/mL	–
0.250 mg/mL	0.250 mg/mL
0.500 mg/mL	–
1 mg/mL	1 mg/mL
2 mg/mL	–
4 mg/mL	4 mg/mL
8 mg/mL	–
16 mg/mL	16 mg/mL

the time interval between the commencements of two subsequent concentrations should be kept to 5 minutes. If the 20% reduction in FEV_1 in the proof with the best quality has not been reached, and the maximum dose of methacholine has not been administered, the operator can proceed with the next step.

If the 20% reduction in FEV_1 is reached, further methacholine must not be administered, symptoms and signs should be noted, a dose of short-acting beta agonists (SABA) should be administered and spirometry should be repeated after 5–10 minutes.

Table 9.2: Dose steps for mannitol challenge with Aridol™.

Dose steps for osmohale challenge			
Dose#	*Dose (mg)*	*Cumulative dose (mg)*	*Capsules per dose*
1	0	0	1
2	5	5	1
3	10	15	1
4	20	35	1
5	40	75	1
6	80	155	2 × 40 mg
7	160	315	4 × 40 mg
8	160	475	4 × 40 mg
9	160	635	4 × 40 mg

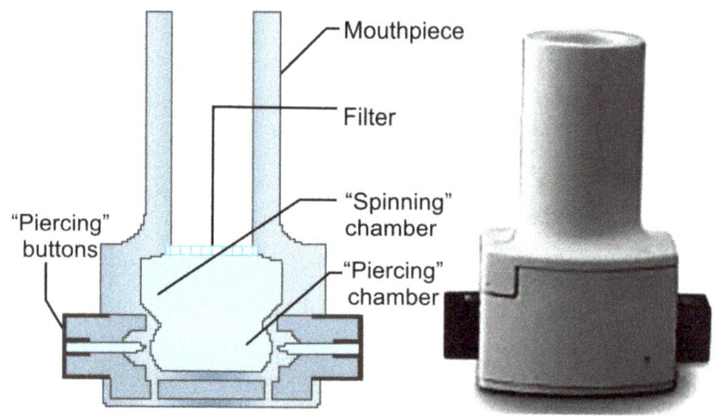

Fig. 9.3: Aridol™ device for inhalation of mannitol.

Mannitol Challenge

Spray-dried mannitol powder, packed in gelatin capsules containing 5 mg, 10 mg, 20 mg, and 40 mg, is inhaled in doubling doses up to 160 mg and repeated three times (Table 9.2), using the *Inhalator Pharmaxis Ltd. (French Forest, Sydney, Australia)*, shown in Figure 9.3.

The test is continued until a fall of FEV_1 by 15% is occurred, or the maximal cumulative dose of 635 mg had been administered. The provocative dose causing a 15% fall in FEV_1 (PD_{15}) is calculated by linear interpolation of the relationship between the percentage decrease in FEV_1 and the cumulative dose of mannitol required to provoke this decrease. The response dose ratio (RDR) is calculated as the percentage fall in FEV_1 after the last dose, divided by the cumulative dose, in milligrams. The test result is considered positive if FEV_1 fell greater than 15% regardless of the dose to provoke this response (or a 10% incremental reduction in FEV_1 between consecutive doses).

Examples of positive challenges include the following:

1. FEV_1 fall following dose step 2: 3%
   FEV_1 fall following dose step 3: 8%
   FEV_1 fall following dose step 4: 16%
   As the total fall is 16% (≥ 15%), the test is positive.
2. FEV_1 fall following dose step 2: 3% FEV_1 fall following dose step 3: 14%

Although the total fall is less than 15%, the incremental fall is 11% (≥ 10%) and the test is positive.

Several computer programs are commercially available to calculate the change in FEV_1 in relation to increasing doses of mannitol administered to the patients during the

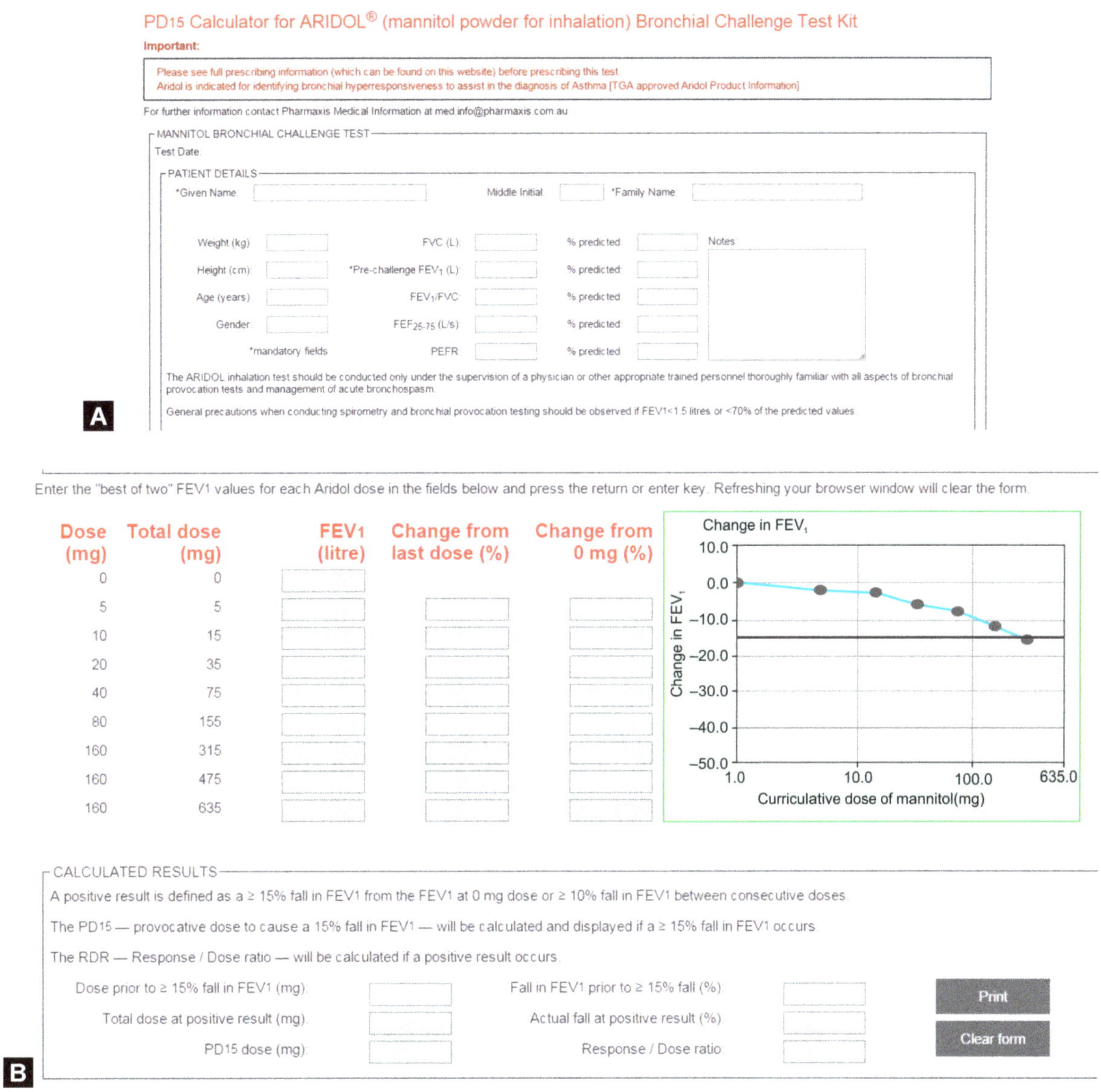

PD15 Calculator for ARIDOL® (mannitol powder for inhalation) Bronchial Challenge Test Kit

Important:

Please see full prescribing information (which can be found on this website) before prescribing this test
Aridol is indicated for identifying bronchial hyperresponsiveness to assist in the diagnosis of Asthma [TGA approved Aridol Product Information]

For further information contact Pharmaxis Medical Information at med.info@pharmaxis.com.au

MANNITOL BRONCHIAL CHALLENGE TEST

Test Date:

PATIENT DETAILS

*Given Name: Middle Initial: *Family Name:

Weight (kg): FVC (L): % predicted: Notes:
Height (cm): *Pre-challenge FEV_1 (L): % predicted:
Age (years): FEV_1/FVC: % predicted:
Gender: FEF_{25-75} (L/s): % predicted:
*mandatory fields PEFR: % predicted:

The ARIDOL inhalation test should be conducted only under the supervision of a physician or other appropriate trained personnel thoroughly familiar with all aspects of bronchial provocation tests and management of acute bronchospasm.

General precautions when conducting spirometry and bronchial provocation testing should be observed if FEV1<1.5 litres or <70% of the predicted values.

A

Enter the "best of two" FEV1 values for each Aridol dose in the fields below and press the return or enter key. Refreshing your browser window will clear the form.

Dose (mg)	Total dose (mg)	FEV1 (litre)	Change from last dose (%)	Change from 0 mg (%)
0	0			
5	5			
10	15			
20	35			
40	75			
80	155			
160	315			
160	475			
160	635			

CALCULATED RESULTS

A positive result is defined as a ≥ 15% fall in FEV1 from the FEV1 at 0 mg dose or ≥ 10% fall in FEV1 between consecutive doses.

The PD15 — provocative dose to cause a 15% fall in FEV1 — will be calculated and displayed if a ≥ 15% fall in FEV1 occurs.

The RDR — Response / Dose ratio — will be calculated if a positive result occurs.

Dose prior to ≥ 15% fall in FEV1 (mg): Fall in FEV1 prior to ≥ 15% fall (%):

Total dose at positive result (mg): Actual fall at positive result (%):

PD15 dose (mg): Response / Dose ratio:

Print

Clear form

B

Figs. 9.4A and B: Example of a report for mannitol challenge.

test and to indicate whether there was a reduction in FEV_1 in accordance with the above criteria (Figs. 9.4A and B).

Adenosine Challenge

Adenosine 5′-monophosphate (AMP) is an indirect stimulus that causes bronchoconstriction, through degranulation of mast cells and release of proinflammatory mediators and by neuronal mechanisms. The adenosine challenge test is an old and desuetude method to assess bronchial hyperreactivity, mainly used for clinical trials, today replaced by the methacholine test.

Histamine Challenge

Histamine is administered using a dosimetric nebulizer. The nebulization time is usually 0.4 s, set to start 100 ms after the beginning of inspiration, with a peak inspiratory flow not exceeding 0.5 L/s, and a nebulization pressure of 2 bars. These settings give a calibrated output of 6.5 μL per inhalation. Histamine diphosphate is inhaled at a starting dose of 25 μg, with fourfold increments until the FEV_1 has fallen 15%, or until the maximal dose of 1,600 μg has been administered. The PD_{15} and RDR values are calculated as above, but using noncumulative doses. The most commonly used cut-off value for a positive response is PD_{15} smaller than or equal to 1.0 mg and PD_{15} smaller than or equal to 0.4 mg.

EXERCISE CHALLENGE TEST

Exercise induces airway narrowing in the majority of patients with asthma. The main stimulus by which exercise causes the airways to narrow is the loss of water in bringing large volumes of air to body conditions in a short time.

As consequences, the main factors that determine severity of such a phenomenon are the pulmonary ventilation reached and sustained during exercise and the water content and temperature of the inspired air.

Exercise challenge test is used to diagnose exercise induced asthma in people who have dyspnea inducted from physical activity with negative methacholine challenge test. Exercise testing is also used to determine the effectiveness and optimal dosages of medications prescribed to prevent exercise-induced bronchoconstriction.

In addition to the contraindication of methacholine challenge, exercise challenge test should not be performed in patient with unstable cardiac ischemia or malignant arrhythmias, as well as in people with orthopedic limitations to exercise. In patients over 60 years old, a recent 12-lead electrocardiogram (within the past year) should be available prior the test. The patient should dress comfortable clothes and running or gym shoes having consumed no more than a light meal and having had bronchodilators withdrawn as suggested for methacholine challenge test. In addition, antihistamines should have been withheld for 48 hours. Vigorous exercise should be avoided for at least 4 hours before testing, since prior exercise has been found to exert a protective effect.

Spirometry should be performed in the seated position before exercise and then serially at the end of the challenge and after the recovery time (at 5-10-15-20-30 minutes) to assess the occurrence of exercise-induced bronchoconstriction and to take the patient to baseline pulmonary function. If the FEV_1 has returned from its nadir to the baseline level or greater, spirometry testing may be terminated at 20 minutes postexercise.

The presence of exercise-induced bronchoconstriction is defined by plotting FEV_1 as a percentage of the pre-exercise baseline FEV_1 at each postexercise interval. A decrease below 90% of the baseline FEV_1 (i.e. a 10% decrease) is a generally accepted abnormal response. Some authors suggest a value of 15% is more diagnostic of exercise-induced bronchoconstriction, particularly if exercise has been performed in the field.

There are two different protocols for this challenge, which use (1) a motor-driven treadmill with adjustable speed and grade and (2) an electromagnetically braked bicycle ergometer.

The use of a pulse oximeter and a three-lead electrocardiographic configuration should be used to monitor oxyhemoglobin saturation and heart rate.

During the whole challenge, the patient needs to inspire dry air at a temperature below 25°C, with a noseclip in place. This can be guaranteed through a conditioner equipped with a thermometer and a hygrometer, and set to maintain air in the room at a temperature comprised between 20 and 25 degrees and a humidity of less than 50%.

Bicycle Ergometer Protocol

The first step is to determine the maximum working load for the patient to be examined. The following equation can be used with this aim: (53.76 × measured FEV_1) - 11.07. The work rate is set to 60% of the target in the first minute, 75% in the second minute, 90% in the third minute and 100% in the fourth minute.

Treadmill Protocol

Treadmill speed and grade are chosen to produce 4–6 minutes of exercise at near-maximum targets with a total duration of exercise of 6–8 minutes.

COLD AIR CHALLENGE TEST

Exercise induced asthma is considered a specific bronchial response to the loss of water vapor from the airway, joined with a thermal (cold) stimulus. It is possible to evaluate such a response by producing a specific stimulus: cold, dry air.

The patients is asked to breath such a frigid air (temperature range –14.6 to –10.2°C) for 4 minutes at a specified minute ventilation calculated as prechallenge FEV_1 × 25. In order to maintain eucapnia, the inflow of carbon dioxide is calculated as target minute ventilation × 0.05. Spirometry is performed in triplicate before the challenge and in duplicate at 3 minute, 5 minute, and 10 minute after the end of the challenge. The greater of the two FEV_1 values at each time point are used for the analysis. The response is calculated as prechallenge FEV_1 minus the lowest value for FEV_1 measured after the challenge, divided by the prechallenge FEV_1, and expressed as percentages. A greater than or equal to 9% fall in FEV_1 may be used as cut-off value for a positive response.

EUCAPNIC VOLUNTARY HYPERPNEA

Eucapnic voluntary hyperpnea (EVH), also known as isocapnic voluntary hyperventilation, is another type of challenge for assessing airway hyperresponsiveness.

Hyperventilation of dry air causes drying of the mucous membrane and hyperosmolarity of the airway surface (similar to the test of exercise-induced broncho), with release of inflammatory mediators from inflammatory cells such as mast cells. EVH is one of the recommended challenge tests for identifying exercise inducted bronchoprovocation in Olympic athletes.

Eucapnic voluntary hyperpnea reproduces exercise-induced asthma by hyperventilation of dry gas containing 5% CO_2, 21% O_2, and balanced N_2. These concentrations are safe for people who do the challenge and stimulate ventilation. The normal end-tidal CO_2 level is held through the test. Inhalation of the gas dries the liquid on the airway surface, resulting in an increased osmolarity. This activates mast cells to release inflammatory mediators, whereby airway narrowing occurs, similar to exercise.

Two different protocols can be used requiring different levels of maximum voluntary ventilation (MVV, calculated as FEV_1 multiplied by 35).

First Protocol

Used for medium and severe exercise-induced asthma. It uses three different steps:

1. 3 minutes at 30% of MVV
2. 3 minutes at 60 % of MVV
3. 3 minutes at 90 % of MVV

After 1, 3, 5, 7 minutes from the end of each step are performed pulmonary function tests.

Second Protocol

Used for mild exercise-induced asthma, is a single step protocol. Subjects for 6 minutes need to ventilate at 85% of MVV ($FEV_1 \times 35$), after 15 minutes from this challenge we need to perform pulmonary function tests.

Both tests can be considered positive if a fall in FEV1 by at least 10% is observed.

ANTIGEN CHALLENGE TEST

Bronchoprovocation challenge with specific agents is performed in specialized centers and under strict medical supervision because patients may have severe response and require immediate hospitalization.

These tests consist of exposing subjects to occupational agents in a hospital laboratory or, occasionally, at work.

When these tests are carried out in a hospital laboratory, low doses of the occupational agent are used to avoid a nonspecific irritant effect. Dose response curves are constructed in which the dose (concentration multiplied by duration) is progressively increased and compared with lung function changes.

BIBLIOGRAPHY AND FURTHER READING

1. Ali Z. How to diagnose exercise induced asthma? Asian J Sports Med. 2011;2(2):63-7.
2. Anderson SD, Brannan JD. Bronchial provocation testing and collection of sputum with inhaled mannitol. Clin Exp Allergy. 2010;40:193-6.
3. Anderson SD, Charlton B, Weiler JM, Nichols S, Spector SL, Pearlman DS, et al. Comparison of mannitol and methacholine to predict exercise-induced bronchoconstriction and a clinical diagnosis of asthma. Respir Res. 2009;10:4.
4. Anderson SD, Kippelen P. Airway injury as a mechanism for exercise-induced bronchoconstriction in elite athletes. J Allergy Clin Immunol. 2008;122:225-35.
5. Anderson SD. Indirect challenge tests. Airway hyperresponsiveness in asthma: its measurement and clinical significance. Chest. 2010;138(2 suppl):25S-30S.
6. Boulet LP, Gauvreau G, Boulay ME, Clinical Investigative Collaboration, Canadian Network of Centers of Excellence AllerGen. The allergen bronchoprovocation model: an important tool for the investigation of new asthma anti-inflammatory therapies. Allergy. 2007;62:1101-10.
7. Brannan JD, Anderson SD, Perry CP, Freed-Martens R, Lassig AR, Charlton B, et al. The safety and efficacy of inhaled dry powder mannitol as a bronchial provocation test for airway hyperresponsiveness: a phase 3 comparison study with hypertonic (4.5%) saline. Respir Res. 2005;6:144.
8. Busse WW. The relationship of airway hyperresponsiveness and airway inflammation: Airway hyperresponsiveness in asthma: its measurement and clinical significance. Chest. 2010;138(2 suppl):4S-10S.
9. Crapo RO, Casaburi R, Coates AL, Enright PL, Hankinson JL, Irvin CG, et al. Guidelines for methacholine and exercise challenge testing-1999. Am J Respir Crit Care Med. 2000;161:309-29.
10. Polosa R, Holgate ST. Adenosine bronchoprovocation: a promising marker of allergic inflammation in asthma? Thorax. 1997;52:919-23.
11. Porsbjerg C, Brannan JD, Anderson SD, Backer V. Relationship between airway responsiveness to mannitol and to methacholine and markers of airway inflammation, peak flow variability and quality of life in asthma patients. Clin Exp Allergy. 2008;38:43-50.
12. Rioux JP, Malo JL, L'Archevêque J, Rabhi K, Labrecque M. Workplace-specific challenges as a contribution to the diagnosis of occupational asthma. Eur Respir J. 2008; 32:997-1003.

13. Rundell KW, Slee JB. Exercise and other indirect challenges to demonstrate asthma or exercise-induced bronchoconstriction in athletes. J Allergy Clin Immunol. 2008;122:238-46.
14. Sterk PJ, Fabbri LM, Quanjer PH, Cockcroft DW, O'Byrne PM, Anderson SD, et al. Airway responsiveness. Standardized challenge testing with pharmacological, physical and sensitizing stimuli in adults. Report Working Party Standardization of Lung Function Tests, European Community for Steel and Coal. Official Statement of the European Respiratory Society. Eur Respir J Suppl. 1993;16:53-83.
15. Vandenplas O, Malo JL. Inhalation challenges with agents causing occupational asthma. Eur Respir J. 1997;10:2612-29.

Chapter

10

Diffusing Capacity or Transfer Factor of the Lung

Riccardo Pistelli, Claudio Sorino

PATHOPHYSIOLOGY OF PULMONARY DIFFUSION

The main function of the respiratory system is to ensure, in cooperation with the cardiovascular system, the supply of oxygen (O_2) to the tissues and the removal of carbon dioxide (CO_2) from them.

This function is carried out through four fundamental processes: *pulmonary ventilation* (inhalation and exhalation), *lung perfusion* (blood supply to the perialveolar vessels), *diffusion of gases* through the alveolar-capillary membrane, *transport of gases,* through the bloodstream from the lungs to the periphery and vice versa.

Lung diffusion consists in the passing of O_2 from the alveolar air to the blood of perialveolar capillaries and of CO_2 in the opposite direction; it is regulated by gradients of partial pressure of these gases. The capacity of the lung to exchange gases across the alveolar-capillary interface is determined by its structural and functional properties. The structural properties include path length for diffusion in the gas phase, thickness and area of the alveolar capillary membrane, any effects of airway closure and the volume of blood in capillaries supplying ventilated alveoli. The functional properties include absolute levels of ventilation and perfusion, the uniformity of their distribution with respect to each other, the composition of the alveolar gas, the diffusion characteristics of the membrane, the concentration and binding properties of hemoglobin (Hb) in the alveolar capillaries and the gas tensions in blood entering the alveolar capillaries in that part of the pulmonary vascular bed which exchanges gas with the alveoli.

ALTERATIONS OF LUNG DIFFUSION CAPACITY

The factors capable to limit the pulmonary diffusing capacity include both alterations of the alveolocapillary membrane, and alterations related to the transportation of blood.

The first can occur in diseases characterized by qualitative modifications in the interstitial tissue interposed between the alveolar cells and the alveolar capillaries (such as in pulmonary fibrosis, where the interstitium is thickened for the accumulation of fibrotic tissue, or in pulmonary edema, where it is filled with water) and in diseases causing destruction of the alveolar-capillary membrane (e.g. in pulmonary emphysema).

In diseases involving the pulmonary interstitium, frequently the lung diffusion capacity is also limited by a restrictive defect, characterized by a reduction in lung volumes and therefore in the surface area available for gas exchange.

In contrast, in pulmonary emphysema the destruction of many alveolar septa is accompanied by an expiratory obstructive defect and the replacement of regular pulmonary alveoli with vast peripherals areas more difficult to reach than normal alveoli by the molecules of the inspired gas. This results in a reduced efficiency of the "alveolar mixing", i.e. the mixture of the inspired air with the air in the alveoli from the preceding inhalation (this process is related to the random motion of gas particles; under normal conditions it occurs so fast as not to be a significant limitation to gas exchange). More importantly, however, this enlargement of alveolar volume (VA) is associated with a reduction of the number of alveoli and a reduction of the surface area available for gas exchange.

It should be noticed that in these conditions the impairment of gas exchange is due mainly to concurrent disorders in the ventilation/perfusion ratio rather than to the reduction in the diffusing capacity of the alveolar-capillary membrane.

A reduction in lung diffusion capacity may be the sole abnormal test hinting to a pulmonary vascular disorder like chronic thromboembolic disease or other causes of pulmonary vascular obliteration, as well as in pulmonary arterial hypertension and vasculitis.

Pulmonary diffusing capacity may vary with variations in the blood levels of hemoglobin and erythrocytes: it is reduced in subjects with anemia, and increased in the case of polycythemia. Moreover, the diffusing capacity of the lung is also amplified in special conditions characterized by high amounts of hemoglobin, such as in the alveolar hemorrhage that may occur in Goodpasture's syndrome.

OVERVIEW OF LUNG DIFFUSION MEASUREMENT

Diffusing capacity of the lung for carbon monoxide (DLCO) provides an objective measurement of lung function and measures the ability of the lungs to transfer gas from inhaled air to the red blood cells in pulmonary capillaries.

The *single-breath* determination of DLCO ($DLCO_{SB}$) involves measuring the uptake of carbon monoxide (CO) from the lung over a breath-holding period. This technique was first described by Marie Krogh. It is based on the assumption that after inspiring a gas mixture containing CO, the alveolar CO fraction, measured by the dilution of a nonsoluble gas included in the inspired mixture, decreases exponentially with time during breath holding as CO diffuses into the blood.

Because the transfer of gas depends only in part on alveolar-capillary diffusion, today the term *transfer factor* of the lung for carbon monoxide (TLCO) is often preferred over DLCO.

Diffusing capacity has been extensively investigated in a wide variety of pulmonary disorders. The lung diseases most frequently associated with a reduction of DLCO are the interstitial or vascular diseases or emphysema. Other lung diseases, as asthma, or abnormalities such as obesity, are usually associated with increased values of DLCO. An increase in the capillary blood volume is the most popular, albeit not definitely demonstrated, explanation for that increase of DLCO.

ADVANTAGES OF USING CARBON MONOXIDE

Carbon monoxide has physical-chemical properties similar to oxygen with regard to diffusion across the alveolar-capillary membrane but the affinity of CO for Hb is about 200 times higher than the affinity of O_2 and this is the reason for choosing CO as a tracer to measure the efficiency of the transfer of gas from the alveolar air to blood in humans. Actually, that transfer is defined as a decrease of the concentration of a gas in a time interval and over a pressure gradient. The direct measurement of the pressure of a gas in alveolar capillaries is impossible and the attempts to derive a pressure estimation by indirect methods in the past gave unreliable results. The unique possibility to assume a null capillary pressure for CO was first used by Maria Krogh in her pioneering study published in 1915. Since that time on that assumption is never been questioned and still is the fundamental basis of the single breath method.

PATIENT PREPARATION

Before performing the test, the operator should carefully explain the procedure to the patient and simulate the maneuver without inhaling any gas. The subject should be seated comfortably throughout the test procedure. The room temperature should be stable, comfortable and within manufacturer's equipment specifications.

The patient should be asked to avoid smoking or other CO exposures on the day of the test. Indeed, COHb causes an acute and reversible reduction in DLCO, mainly due to a diminished Hb-binding sites for CO from the test gas (the so-called "anemia effect"). Since cigarette smoking is the most common source of COHb, the time of the last cigarette smoked should be recorded and noted for the interpretation. Adjustments for CO back pressure are available and recommended for recent or heavy cigarette smoking.

Just before starting the test, the subject may take a sip of water, since dry mouth or throat sometimes makes a subject feel like coughing.

PROCEDURE

The *single-breath diffusing capacity test* ($DLCO_{SB}$) is the most common method to assess the lung diffusion capacity.

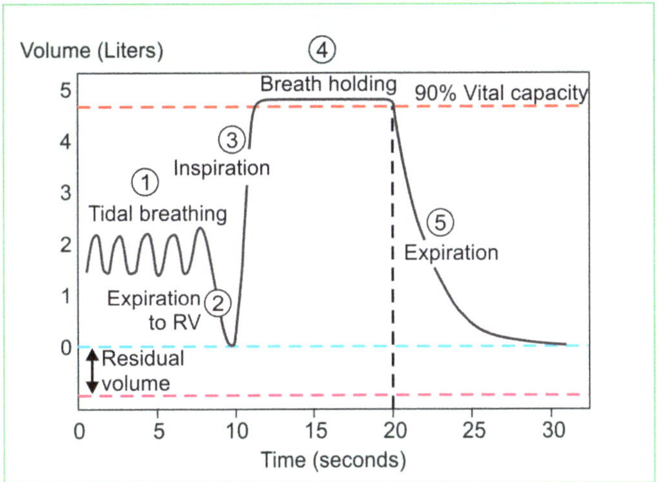

Fig. 10.1: Graphic representation of a single-breath diffusing capacity test.

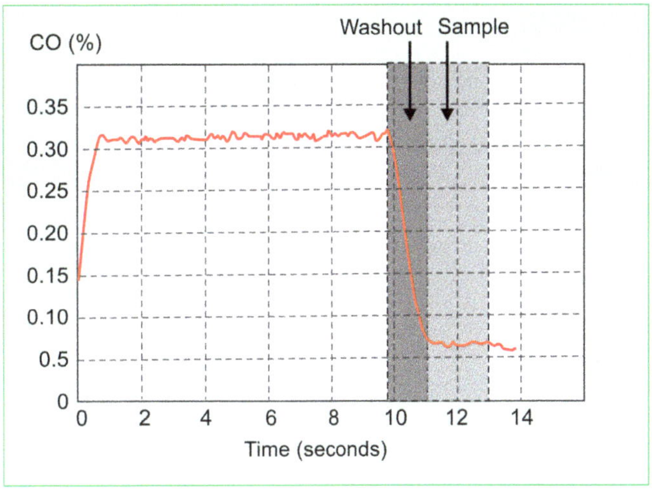

Fig. 10.2: Carbon dioxide (CO_2) variation during a single-breath diffusing capacity test.

The challenge of $DLCO_{SB}$ is to obtain a representative sample of gas from an area of the lungs where diffusion is taking place. When a DLCO test is performed in the Pulmonary Function Laboratory, it takes about 10–20 minutes.

It is imperative that other tests that require breathing special gas mixtures are not performed before any CO diffusion measurements. For example, breathing the 100% oxygen during the Nitrogen (N_2) washout can significantly reduce the calculated DLCO.

Before to perform a DLCO test, the operator must know the value of the SVC of the subject because only tests performed with an inspiratory volume close to the value of SVC can be accepted.

The subject, seating in the upright position and wearing a nose clip, must be tightly connected by a mouthpiece to the respiratory apparatus.

As shown in Figure 10.1, the procedure for such a test can be divided into five steps:

1. The subject is asked to perform a few cycles of *tidal breathing* at room air; tidal breathing should be carried out for a sufficient time to assure that the subject is comfortable with the mouthpiece. Deep inspirations should be avoided during this period as they can increase subsequent CO uptake.
2. The subject *breathes out to residual volume*; this can be noted by the absence of further significant expiratory flow, but the patient may also be asked to indicate with a gesture of his hand when he is unable to exhale additional air.
3. The subject is *connected to the test gas* and invited to *deeply and rapidly inhale up to total lung capacity.* The usual composition of the gas mixture is the following: carbon monoxide 0.3%; helium 10%, an *inert insoluble gas* used to determine the lung volume and by dilution the concentration of CO at the beginning of the breath holding time, oxigen 21%, nitrogen the balance to 100%.
4. The subject *holds his breath at total lung capacity* for 10 seconds. Often a valve mechanism helps to hold the breath for the required time.
5. The subject *slowly breathes out to residual volume* (in a relaxed way). Many machines provide a graphical indication which helps the physician and the patient to understand, if the speed of exhalation is adequate.

Flows are usually measured with a flow transducer and the inspired and expired volumes are obtained by integration of the flow signal in time. At the beginning of expiration, an amount of air corresponding at least to the dead space (usually the first 750 mL exhaled) is discarded and not used for analyzes. A subsequent sample of expired gas (usually 0.5–1.0 L) undergoes gas analysis. This sample is used to determine the alveolar concentration of CO at the end of the breath-holding time (Fig. 10.2).

ACCEPTABILITY AND REPEATABILITY

The current American Thoracic Society (ATS) guidelines recommend to perform at least two acceptable tests. It is suggested to wait for at least 4 minutes before to repeat a DLCO test, and the reported DLCO value is calculated as the mean result of two acceptable and reproducible tests. The following are the suggested criteria for acceptability and reproducibility.

Acceptability

- Inspired volume 85% or greater of the best vital capacity,
- Total lung capacity level achieved within 4 seconds from the beginning of the inspiratory maneuver,
- Breath holding time between 8 and 12 seconds,
- Sampling of expired gas must be completed within 4 seconds from the beginning of the expiratory maneuver.

Repeatability

At least two acceptable measurements of DLCO should agree within 10% or 3 mL/minute/mm Hg of their average value.

INTERPRETATION OF DATA

As mentioned above, the physiological interpretation of the results of a DLCO test are based on the knowledge of the multiple factors that may interfere with the transfer of gas from the alveolar air to the capillary blood and on some modeling of those factors. A useful model for the clinical interpretation of DLCO has been proposed by Roughton and Foster more than 50 years ago. That model assumes that all factors interfering with the transfer of CO can be reduced to only two limiting resistances: the membrane resistance (M) and the capillary blood volume (Vc). Of course both M and Vc include many factors. Shortly, M includes: gas diffusion in the alveolar spaces, area of the membrane, thickness of the membrane, diffusivity of gas across the membrane; Vc includes: the volume of blood in the lung capillary vessels, the amount of Hb in the blood, the plasticity of red cells and the length each CO molecule must travel before to reach a Hb molecule within a capillary Actually, if we take the reciprocal of DLCO, that has the physical dimension of a conductance, we obtain a resistance that can be split in the sum of two resistances in series.

$$\frac{1}{\text{DLCO}} = \frac{1}{\text{DMCO}} + \frac{1}{\Theta\text{CO} \cdot \text{Vc}}$$

This equation, as clearly shown for any x gas in Figure 10.3, represents a straight line whose intercept and slope are represented by the reciprocal of the membrane and capillary diffusing capacities, respectively. By taking different measures of DLCO in different conditions of affinity of CO (ΘCO) for hemoglobin (for example by changing the oxygen concentration in the gas mixture), it is possible to calculate the value of the two resistances, in this way

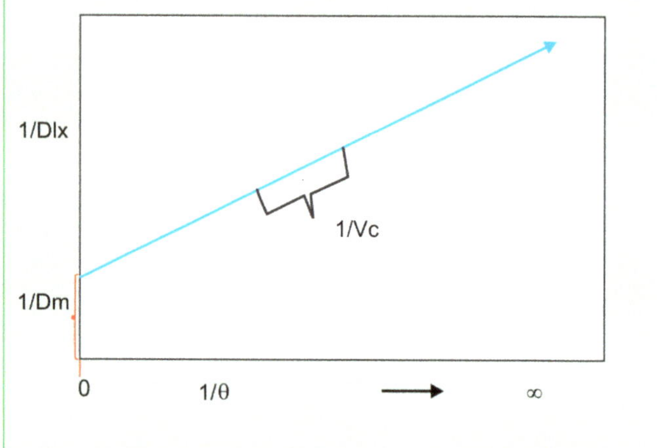

Fig. 10.3: A graphical representation of The Roughton and Foster model (*see* text for explanation).

allowing for an interpretation of DLCO results according to the model proposed by Roughton and Foster.

An example of such interpretation may be easily reproduced in each laboratory by looking at the increase of DLCO in the supine position with reference to the value obtained in the standardized upright position. The interpretation of such an increase obtained by applying the Roughton and Foster's method is fully in agreement with the well know gravity-related filling of lung vessels in the supine position. However, we must say that the interpretation of changes of DLCO by applying that method in many diseases has often given inconsistent results.

It is mandatory to examine a further crucial point in the interpretation of data. DLCO is calculated as the difference of concentration of CO in the alveolar air between the beginning and the end of the breath-holding period times the VA, measured from the volume of the inspired mixture and the dilution of trace gas in the resident alveolar air. It is clear that quite different DLCO values may be obtained from identical CO differences of concentration when those are measured in subjects with quite different VAs. If the ratio of DLCO and VA is taken, the result (KCO) is the difference of concentration adjusted to the selected time and pressure units. Sometimes, this adjustment may lead to some misunderstanding, when an abnormal DLCO is interpreted as uniquely caused by the reduced alveolar exchange area, if KCO is within normal limits. We remind that the relation of VA with the alveolar surface area is not linear and KCO may overestimate the efficiency of gas exchange in smaller alveolar units. Moreover, DLCO is a quite complex parameter including many factors affecting the overall efficiency of gas transfer in the lung. As a consequence of this, the interpretation of a reduction of DLCO as due to a specific factor may be always inaccurate and cautiously proposed when clinically useful.

BIBLIOGRAPHY AND FURTHER READING

1. Blakemore WS, Forster RE, Morton JW, Ogilvie CM. A standardized breath holding technique for the clinical measurement of the diffusing capacity of the lung for carbon monoxide. J Clin Invest. 1957;36:1-17.
2. Forster RE, Cohn JE, Briscoe WA, Blakemore WS, Riley RL. A modification of the Krogh carbon monoxide breath holding technique for estimating the diffusing capacity of the lung; a comparison with three other methods. J Clin Invest. 1955;34:1417-26.
3. Forster RE, Fowler WS, Bates DV, Van Lingen B. The absorption of carbon monoxide by the lungs during breath holding. J Clin Invest. 1954;33:1135-45.
4. Krogh A, Krogh M. On the rate of diffusion of carbonic oxide into the lungs of man. Skandinav. Arch J Physiol. 1909;23:236.
5. Krogh M. Diffusion of gases through the lungs of man. J Physiol. 1915;49:271-300.
6. MacIntyre N, Crapo RO, Viegi G, Johnson DC, van der Grinten CP, Brusasco V, et al. Standardisation of the single-breath determination of carbon monoxide uptake in the lung. Eur Respir J. 2005;26:720-35.
7. Piiper J, Sheid P. Model for capillary-alveolar equilibration with special reference to O2 uptake in hypoxia. Respir Physiol. 1981;46:193-208.
8. Roughton FJ, Forster RE. Relative importance of diffusion and chemical reaction rates in determining rate of exchange of gases in the human lung, with special reference to true diffusing capacity of pulmonary membrane and volume of blood in the lung capillaries. J Appl Physiol. 1957;11: 290-302.
9. Sheid P, Piiper J. Diffusion. In Crystal RG, West JB, Weibel ER, Barnes PJ (Eds). The Lung, Scientific Foundations. Philadelphia, New York: Lippincott-Raven; 1997. pp. 1681-91.
10. Wagner PD. Diffusion and chemical reaction in pulmonary gas exchange. Physiol Rev. 1977;57:257-312.

Chapter 11

Ventilation Homogeneity and Lung Elasticity

Riccardo Pistelli, Claudio Sorino

LUNG VENTILATION

The term *lung ventilation* refers to the process in which a gas mixture continuously cycles between entering and leaving the air spaces of the lung. Traditional subdivisions of the overall lung ventilation are: alveolar space ventilation and dead space ventilation, which refer to the ventilation of air spaces delimited and nondelimited by alveoli, respectively. Ventilation is crucial to the gas exchange process, a phenomenon greatly enhanced by the large surface area available for a close contact between alveolar air and capillary blood. This has been achieved by the subdivision of the lung volume into millions of alveoli delimited by extremely thin walls. Such an arrangement requires a long and quite complex branching conduit from the entrance in the respiratory system to the alveoli so that fresh gas can be transported to, and mixed with, the alveolar gas. Convective flow and molecular diffusion are the principal mechanisms responsible for the transport and mixing of the inspired gas (Fig. 11.1).

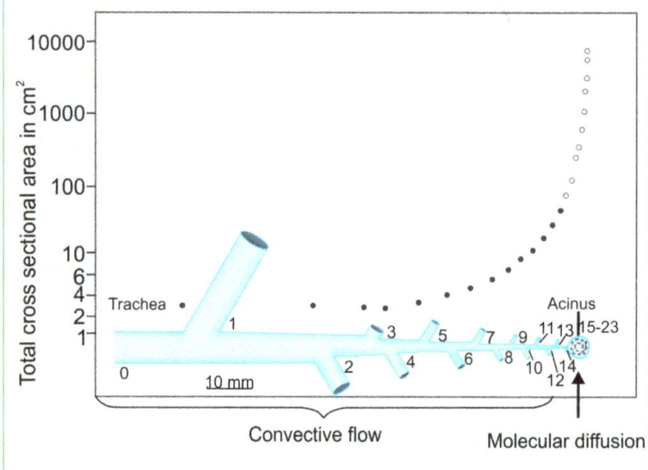

Fig. 11.1: Convective flow and molecular diffusion. Principal mechanisms responsible for the transport and mixing of the inspired gas.

As it can easily be appreciated from Figure 11.1, convective flow driven by a pressure gradient is largely prevalent in more than 95% of the conduit length, being the molecular diffusion mechanism driven by a concentration gradient prevalent in the very last part of the conduit, the acinus, where the airways are mainly delimited by alveolar spaces. Convective or bulk flow refers to the movement of all gas species within a mixture at the mean velocity of the overall airstream. The increase in total cross-sectional area as a function of distance along the conduit determines a fall of the convective velocity and a change of the type of flow, which is predominantly turbulent in the proximal and laminar in distal airways. Turbulence provides a potential mechanism of mixing and homogenization of gas mixture inside the lung, but being confined to the proximal airways its contribution to ventilation homogeneity is minimal.

Molecular diffusion is the principal mechanism of gas mixing in the lung. It is due to the random movement of gas molecules and results in a net transfer of given gas species from regions of high concentration to regions of low concentration. In steady state condition, the diffusive flow of gas across an ideal area A is represented, according to the Fick's first law of diffusion, by the following equation:

$$dQ/dt = -AD^*dc/dx$$

where Q is the quantity of gas, t is time, c is the concentration of the gas, x is the linear distance, and D is the diffusion coefficient of each gas species.

A further contribution to gas mixing is given by dispersion processes that include cardiogenic gas mixing and

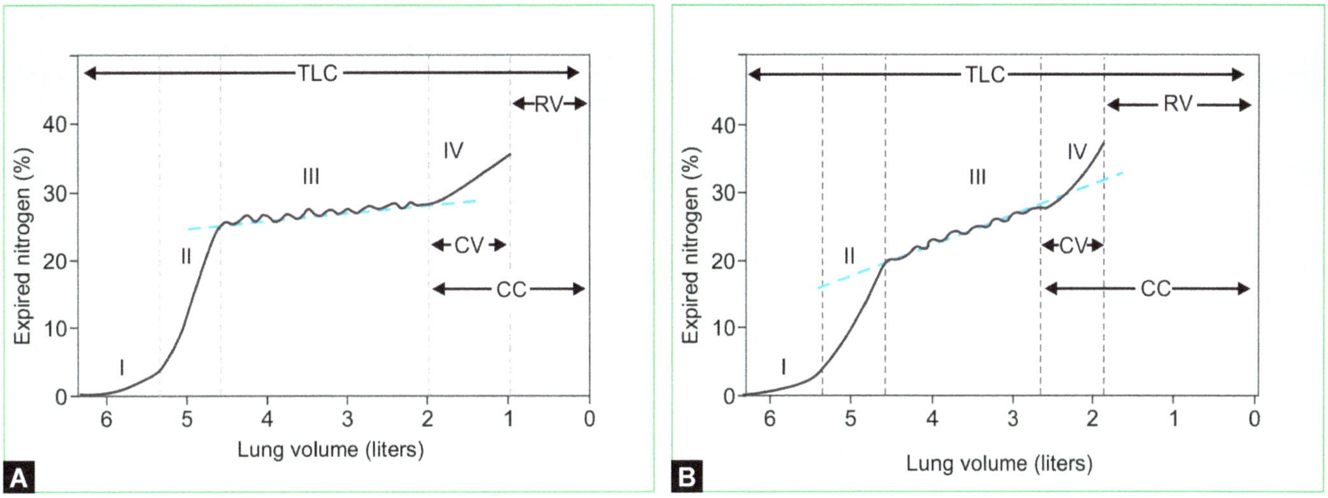

Figs. 11.2A and B: Single-breath nitrogen washout maneuver. (A) Normal lung; (B) Abnormal lung (emphysema). Closing volume (CV) is the quantity of air remaining in the lungs when the small airways begin to close during a maximum exhalation. Closing capacity (CC) equals total lung capacity (TLC) – [CV + residual volume (RV)].

Taylor-type phenomena. The first phenomenon can be easily appreciated in the Figures 11.2A and B, which refers to a maneuver of slow exhalation after a deep inhalation of oxygen and a short breath-holding time. The contribution of the mechanical action of the heart to the mixing of alveolar and dead space air can be seen as small waves in the concentration of nitrogen during the phase III (alveolar plateau) of the exhalation.

In zones where the laminar flow dominates, Taylor dispersion on the border of the parabolic profile of the advancing inhaled gas can enhance its mixing with the resident gas during inhalation. However, theoretical and experimental evidence suggest that both cardiogenic mixing and Taylor dispersion contribute only a minor effect to the overall gas mixing and ventilation homogeneity.

In the above-reported graph, representing the plot of N_2 concentrations during the slow exhalation from TLC down to RV, it is customary to distinguish four phases: Phase I, representing the gas coming from the anatomic dead space; Phase II, representing the crossing of the border between the gas coming from the dead space and the alveolar spaces; Phase III, representing gas coming from the alveolar spaces; Phase IV, representing gas coming from alveolar spaces still open after the closure of some distal bronchiole. It is interesting to pay attention to the sharp increase of the N_2 concentration during the Phase II, in this way suggesting the presence of a stationary diffusion front separating the zones in which predominate convective and diffusive mechanisms of gas transport. Some theoretical models of gas transportation applied to the Weibel's model of the lung showed the substantial independence of the position of this front from the speed of inspiratory flow and breath-holding time. Moreover, it is quite easy to get the empirical confirmation of that theory, in a clinical physiology setting, by repeating the slow exhalation manoeuver while varying the velocity of the inspirations of pure O_2 and the breath-holding time.

There is now a general agreement about the achievement of homogeneous gas concentrations within each acinus, at least during quiet breathing and in not extremely enlarged, or ventilating in series, alveolar spaces. Actually, the difference of N_2 concentrations in the alveolar plateau of the slow exhalation, clearly evidenced by the straight line connecting the data points in Figures 11.2A and B, are interpreted as dependent from nonhomogeneity between acini and not within each acinus of the lung, as it was suggested for the first time by Rauwerda in his dissertation at the Groningen university in 1946. Actually, we may say that nonhomogeneity of ventilation and gas mixing in the lung is convection and convection-diffusion dependent. The mechanical properties of the lung and their distribution are the determinants of ventilation nonhomogeneity in normal and diseased humans.

LUNG ELASTICITY: STATICS

The thoracic respiratory system includes two major elastic organs: the rib cage and the lung. Those organs have their specific elastic characteristics, the interaction of which determines the elastic behavior of the overall respiratory system (Fig. 11.3). The respiratory muscles activity

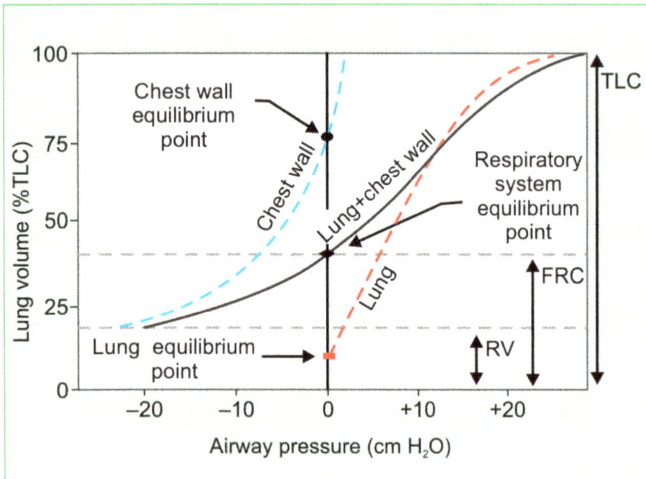

Fig. 11.3: Pressure-volume curves of the lung, chest wall, and the combined respiratory system.
(TLC: Total lung capacity; FRC: Functional residual capacity; RV: Residual volume).

allows for increasing or decreasing the lung volume above or under the FRC level, identified as the lung volume at which the rib cage elastic forces are perfectly balanced with the lung elastic forces (respiratory system equilibrium point). In Figure 11.3 the elasticity of lung and chest cage are represented by considering both elastic organs as homogeneously developing elastic forces and homogeneously changing their volume. This simplified approach may be useful for measuring and interpreting the elastic component of the work of breathing but it is too simplistic when analyzing the nonhomogeneous and variably time-dependent filling and emptying of thousands of respiratory units during each respiratory cycle.

Actually, it has been demonstrated that the intrapleural pressure is less negative (~7 cm H_2O) near the dependent area of the lung. This situation is caused by the weight of the lung, being close to the diaphragm in the upright position or close to the back in the supine position. The consequence of this difference of pressure is the different volume of alveoli, as percentage of their volume at TLC, in the upper and lower zones of the lung. During inspiration, respiratory muscles determine a decrease of the overall intrapleural pressure and the filling of each alveolar unit, which is dependent on the volume of the same unit at the beginning of the inspiration. At that time, the volume of alveoli, as percentage of their volume at TLC, is much higher in the upper than in the lower zones of the lung and the relative increase of volume during inspiration

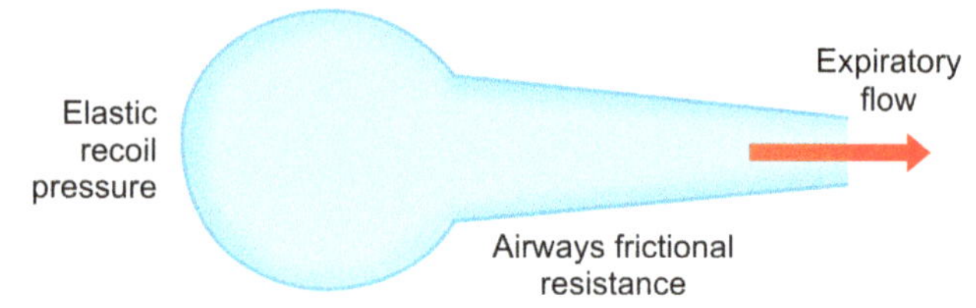

Fig. 11.4: Exemplification of expiratory flow in a respiratory unit.

is much higher in the lower zone than in the upper zone of the lung. As a consequence of this, the convective dilution of the resident gas in the lower zone of the lung is much higher than in the upper zone, also while admitting that the elastic properties of the respiratory units are identical across the entire lung. Of course, in the reality, many and many thousands of respiratory units do have different elastic properties inside each zone of the lung. This is true in the normal humans and must be amplified in lung diseases. We can summarize the static contribution of elasticity to lung ventilation by saying that the intrapleural gradient of pressure determines a between regions nonhomogeneity of ventilation while the different elastic properties of the lung units determine a within regions nonhomogeneity of lung ventilation.

LUNG ELASTICITY: DYNAMICS

The flow speed that can be achieved during the inspiratory and expiratory phases is the limiting factor of ventilation. Ventilation is an alternating process in which the limitation of one phase necessarily limits the other. Each respiratory unit is characterized by a variable, usually referred as time constant, that derives from the combination of its elastic and frictional resistive properties (Fig. 11.4).

Shortly, the speed of the expiratory flow (ExpFlow) is determined by the propulsion due to the elastic recoil pressure (ERP) of a respiratory unit and by the airways frictional resistance (AWR) according to the following relation:

$$\text{ExpFlow} = \text{ERP/AWR}$$

A transformation to the physical units gives:

$$V/T = P/V*1/P*V/T = I/T$$

which obviously represents the negative relation between flow and time. By taking the reciprocal of the above equation, it is easy to demonstrate that the filling or emptying time of a respiratory unit is dependent on the product of the AWR and on the reciprocal of the ERP, or compliance, of the respiratory unit. Any combination of those two variables determines the emptying or filling time of a specific respiratory unit. The many thousands respiratory units of the lung can be in this way grouped according to their ventilation speed and it is necessary to look at the implications of this situation for the ventilation homogeneity. Figures 11.5A to E show an extremely simplified model with only two respiratory units, representing different situations of ventilation nonhomogeneity due to the mechanical characteristics of the respiratory units. In panels A and B are represented situations in which the respiratory units have equal time constants. However, in panel A both resistance and compliance are identical between units while in panel B one unit has half the compliance and twice the resistance of the other. The consequence of this situation is that, at any time during inspiration, the dilution of the resident gas will be quite different between units while the pressure of units will be identical. In panel C and D the respiratory units do have different time constants. However, in panel C there is only a resistance twice the resistance of the other unit and in panel D there is only a compliance half the compliance of the other unit. In panel C, if the filling inspiratory pressure is sustained for a very long time, the dilution of resident gas and the recoil pressure are identical in the two units, but, for a shorter time of inspiration, the dilution of gas and the recoil pressure are different in the units and some gas may be redistributed, following the gradient of pressure, between units. In panel D, also with a long time of inspiration the dilution of gas is different between units. For a shorter time of inspiration, some gas can be transferred to the slow unit in force of

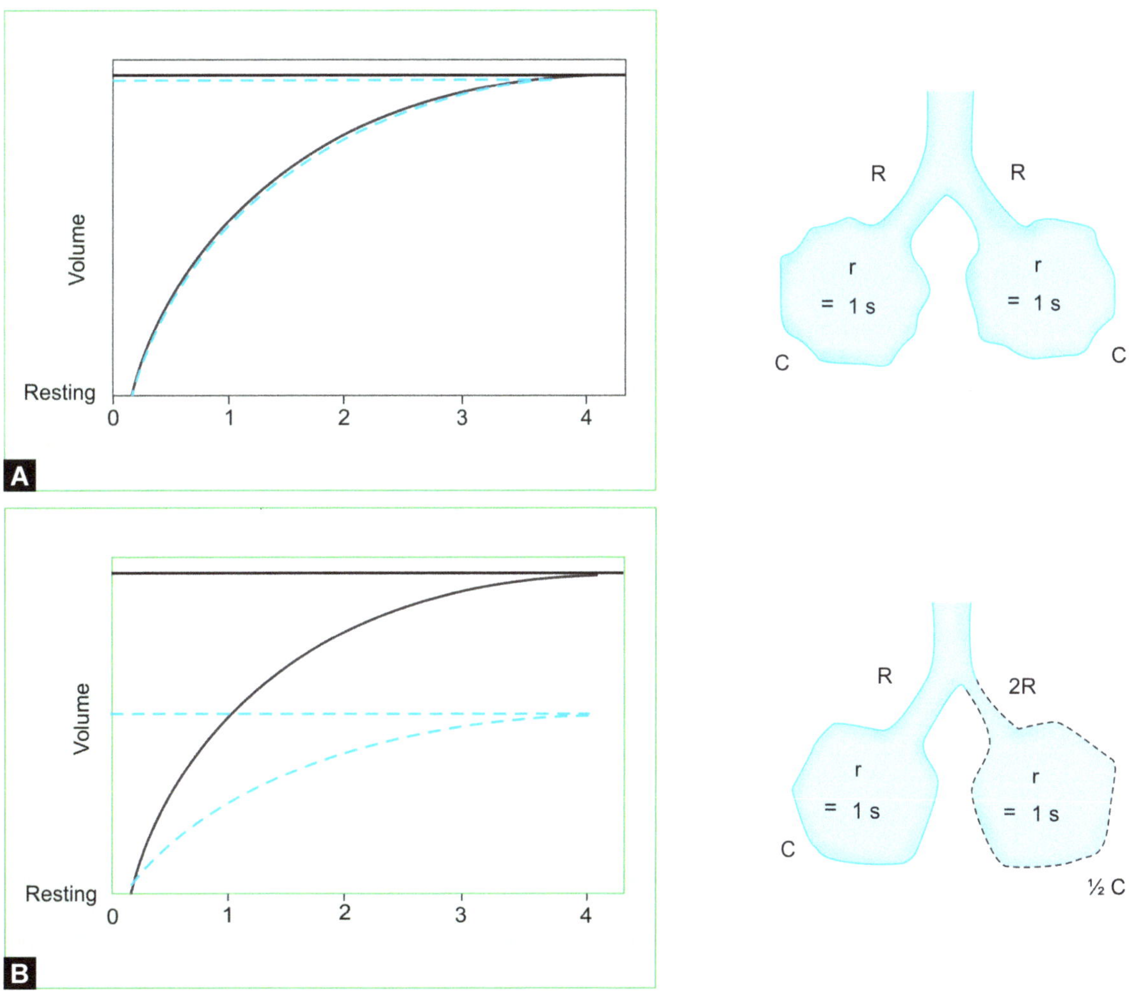

Figs. 11.5A and B

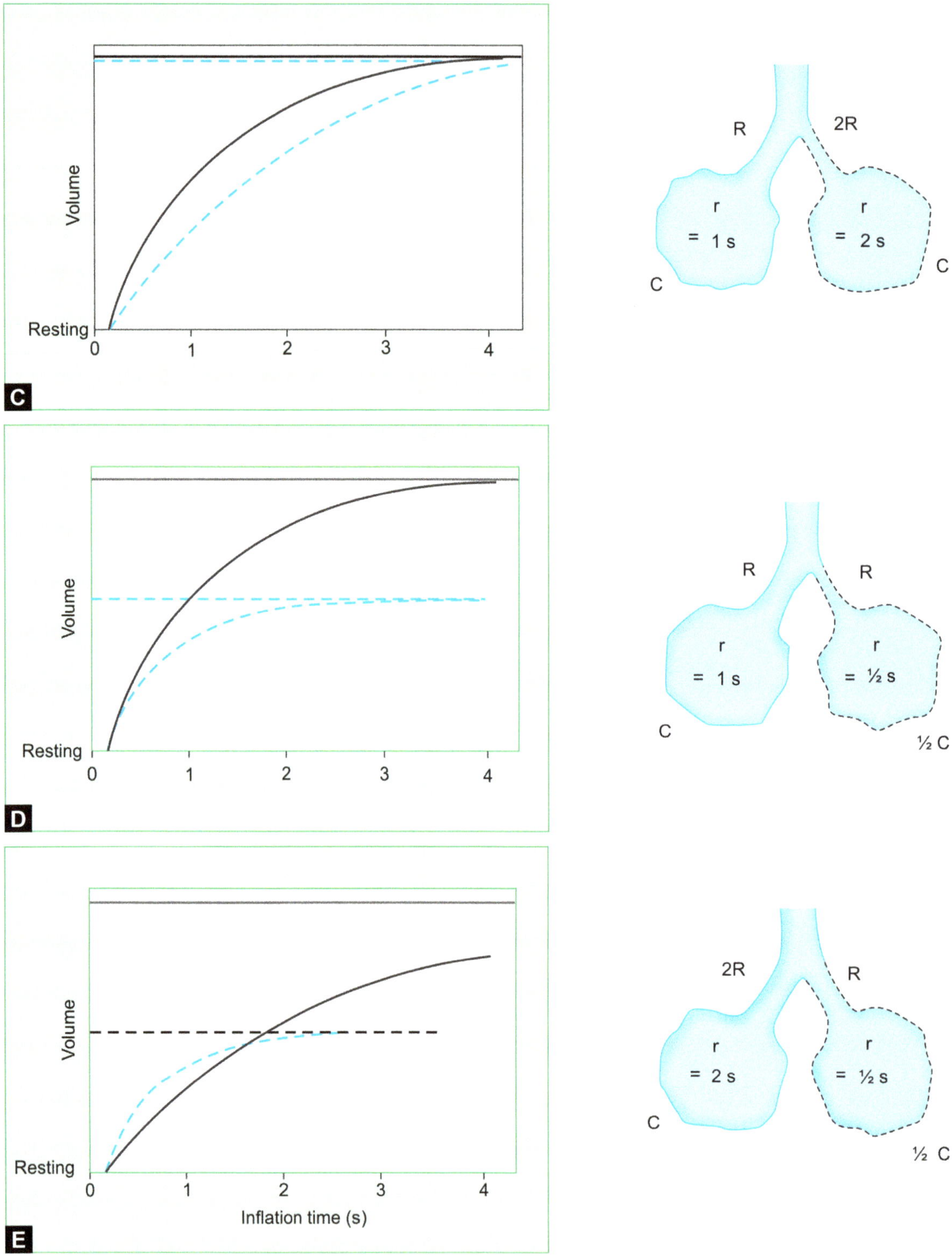

Figs. 11.5A to E: Simplified model representing different situations of ventilation nonhomogeneity.

the quick increase of pressure in the rapid unit. The panel E shows a more complex situation, in which both resistance and compliance are different between units and the gas dilution and pressure are always different between units. In this case, the direction of the redistribution of gas between units may change at different time during inspiration.

This oversimplified approach to the description of the interaction between mechanical properties of the respiratory units and the time limited process of ventilation can give to the reader an idea of the main determinants of ventilation nonhomogeneity inside each region of the lung. Imaging techniques can be useful to investigate the nonhomogeneous distribution of ventilation between regions, however only physiological techniques can be applied to describe the intraregional distribution of ventilation. The next paragraph will shortly describe those techniques.

PHYSIOLOGICAL METHODS TO STUDY THE DISTRIBUTION OF VENTILATION

The experimental studies of gas mixing in humans are mainly performed by the analysis of the expired gas at the mouth. The inert gases, either inspired or resident, are only minimally affected by gas exchange and hence are more useful for specifically examining unequal ventilation and gas mixing.

Resident N_2 can be analyzed after an inspiration of O_2 either with a tidal breath from the FRC level or with a vital capacity breath from RV up to the TLC level. The first method is only seldom used, and gives only partial scarcely reproducible results. The second method is routinely used with inspiratory and expiratory flows standardized at 0.5 l/second. The results of this test are quite reproducible and supply information on both interregional and intraregional inhomogeneities of ventilation. Figures 11.2A and B represent the N_2 concentration in the expired gas at the mouth plotted versus the expiratory volume from TLC down to RV. The increase of N_2 concentration during the expiration of alveolar air is caused by different dilutions of the resident gas due to the inhalation of pure O_2 in different respiratory units. Those differences are certainly attributable to differences in elasticity and possibly to differences in time constants of the respiratory units. However, only the time constants differences between the respiratory units are responsible for that increase of N_2 concentration (slope of the phase III), because the differences of mixing and resident gas concentration between areas with the same time constants would be hidden by the of alveolar air mixing in large bronchi and trachea well before the sampling point at the mouth. The phase IV in the same figure mainly represents the interregional differences in gas mixing. Actually, when O_2 is inspired from RV up to TLC, the respiratory units in the dependent areas of the lung begin to inflate from a smaller volume than volume of respiratory units in the upper areas of the lung and the dilution of the resident gas in the dependent areas will be higher and the concentration of resident N_2 lower than in the upper areas. When the conducting airways in the dependent areas begin to close during the expiration, the contribution of the upper areas to the gas mixture at the mouth increases, as it is demonstrated by the sharp increase of the N_2 concentration. The inflection point between phase III and IV may be used to measure what is known as closing volume—that is the volume expired from the inflection point down to RV. The slope of the phase IV is always higher than the slope of the phase III, in this way demonstrating that the sequential exclusion of some areas greatly improves our capability to detect differences of ventilation and gas mixing between areas.

A quite similar plot can be obtained also by inhaling a bolus of a tracer gas at the beginning the inhalation of air from RV up to TLC. In this case the dilution of the bolus will be higher in the dependent zones than in the upper zones and the plot of the concentration of the tracer gas will be quite similar to the plot obtained during the single breath N_2 washout.

Ventilation inhomogeneity can be also studied by analyzing the washout of a resident inert gas in a multiple-breath maneuver. When the mixing between inspired and resident gas is uniform, consecutive tidal breath of O_2 will make the alveolar concentration of N_2 (F_AN_2) decrease by a constant fraction. This means that F_AN_2 decreases exponentially and the plot of the logarithm of F_AN_2 versus the breath number should be linear. We may approximate F_AN_2 in that plot by using the end tidal N_2 concentration or we may plot the end tidal N_2 concentrations versus the cumulative ventilation corresponding to each breath. In any case, those semi-logarithmic plots should be linear. However, also in young normal subjects, it is rarely possible to obtain quite linear plots because some ventilation inhomogeneity is always present in humans.

Some methods have been developed to describe or to get information from the alinearity of the multiple-breath N_2 washout curve. The first approach was introduced many years ago by fitting two or more exponential function to the N_2 curve, in this way identifying different compartments characterized by some different efficiency of gas mixing. The second approach was developed more recently and it was based on the possibility of a computer of repeatedly check by numerical analysis how well the experimental data fit the data of a model of lung composed by a fixed number of compartments, each one with its own ventilation efficiency.

Finally, it is important to emphasize that physiological methods may be used to detect also a small inhomogeneity of ventilation. However, we do not have information about the amount of inhomogeneity attributable to a lung disease with a measured sensitivity and specificity for each test. This is the major obstacle to a widespread use of these tests in the clinical physiology setting.

BIBLIOGRAPHY AND FURTHER READING

1. Crawford AB, Cotton DJ, Paiva M, Engel LA. Effect of airway closure on ventilation distribution. J Appl Physiol. 1989;66:2511-5.
2. Engel LA. Intra-regional gas mixing and distribution. In: Engel LA, Paiva M (Eds). Gas mixing and distribution in the lung. Lung biology in health and disease. New York: Marcel Dekker; 1985. pp. 287-358.
3. Leblanc P, Raff F, Milic Emili J. Effects if age and body position on airway closure in man. J Appl Physiol. 1970;28:448-51.
4. Lewis S, Evans JW, Jalowayski AA. Continuous distribution of specific ventilation recovered from inert gas washout. J Appl Physiol. 1978;44:416-23.
5. Milic-Emili J. Topographical inequality of ventilation. In: Crystal RG, West JB, Weibel ER, Barnes PJ (Eds). Topographical inequalitiy of ventilation. The Lung, Scientific Foundations. Philidelphia, New York: Lippincott-Raven; 1997. pp. 1415-23.
6. Paiva M, Engel LA. The anatomical basis for the sloping N_2 plateau. Respir Physiol. 1981;44:325-37.
7. Piiper J, Sheid P. Diffusion and convection in intrapulmonary gas mixing. In Handbook of physiology. Vol 4, Gas exchange, section 3: The respiratory system, Bethesda, MD: American Physiological Society; 1987. pp. 51-69.
8. Verbanck S, PaivaM. Model simulations of gas mixing and ventilation in human lung. J Appl Physiol. 1990;69:2269-79.
9. Weibel ER. Morphometryof the human lung. Heidelberg: Springer Verlag; 1963.
10. West JB, Hugh-Jones P. Pulsatile gas flow in bronchi caused by the heart beat. J Appl Physiol. 1961;16:697-802.

Chapter 12

Lung Function Testing in Preschool Children

Stefania La Grutta, Giuliana Ferrante, Enrico Lombardi, Claudia Calogero, Giorgio Piacentini, Giancarlo Tancredi, Caterina Lambiase, Claudio Sorino, Giovanni Viegi

OVERVIEW OF LUNG FUNCTION TESTING IN PRESCHOOL CHILDREN

Measuring lung function in preschool (2–5-year-old) children is extremely important due to the high frequency of respiratory infections in this age group and the fast growth and development of the respiratory system in the first years of life. However, children in this age range also have a short attention span and are physiologically different from older children, with the consequence of being often unable to perform the voluntary forced expiratory maneuvers required for spirometry. For these reasons and for the fact that sedation is not an option in preschool children to try to perform the same techniques used in infants, lung function testing in preschool children has been neglected for long.

In recent years the availability of new techniques that can be performed during tidal breathing without sedation has made it possible to measure lung function in preschoolers. Also, the international community has agreed on new criteria for spirometry in preschool children. For most of these techniques standard operating procedures, repeatability and cut-offs for bronchodilator response (BDR), and international reference values are now available, making these techniques suitable tools for the evaluation of lung function in preschool children. Their clinical applications in young children with recurrent wheezing, cystic fibrosis (CF) or bronchopulmonary dysplasia (BPD) have also been recently reviewed.

The measurement of diffusing capacity of the lung is extensively addressed in Chapter 10 of this book.

INTERRUPTER TECHNIQUE

The interrupter technique was firstly published in 1927, but it only reached popularity toward the end of the last century, when its physiological aspects became clear and its capability of informing about lung function in awake preschool children breathing quietly was largely appreciated.

The main physiological assumption of the interrupter technique is that, during a sudden interruption of the air flow, alveolar pressure will rapidly equilibrate with mouth pressure allowing for an estimate of alveolar pressure at the mouth. Corollary assumptions are that compliance of the upper airways is negligible and valve closure is instantaneous. Hence, dividing mouth pressure during the interruption by air flow at the mouth right before the interruption, resistance of the respiratory system can be measured (classical interrupter technique). An alternative method in which airflow is measured right after the interruption (opening interrupter technique) has been proposed. The two methods cannot be used interchangeably. The American Thoracic Society/European Respiratory Society (ATS/ERS) recommendations have focused on the classical interrupter technique.

The interruption should be short (100 ms), to prevent the subject from breathing against it. The interrupter resistance (R_{int}) should be interpreted as resistance of the respiratory system. When mouth pressure is back-extrapolated to the start of the interruption (as in the classical interrupter technique), R_{int} approaches airway resistance, but still contains some amount of lung tissue resistance and chest wall resistance; when, vice versa, mouth pressure is measured at the end of the interruption (as in the opening interrupter technique) R_{int} tends toward an estimate of the actual resistance of the respiratory system. Since R_{int} is not pure airway resistance, it is not surprising that the comparisons between R_{int} and plethysmographic airway resistance (R_{aw}) show a significant difference between the two techniques.

As always when dealing with young children, special caution should be used in approaching the child, since the success of the measurement depends on the capability of the operator to initiate a good relationship with him/her. Measurements should be performed during quiet tidal breathing, with the child seated and breathing through a bacterial filter with a mouthpiece (Fig. 12.1). Head should be slightly extended and cheeks should be supported to avoid upper airway compliance. According to the ATS/ERS recommendations, occlusions should be triggered by peak flow during tidal expiration, ten interruptions should be performed with the aim of retaining a minimum of five acceptable interruptions, and the median of all technically acceptable interruptions should be reported.

Feasibility of the interrupter technique is more than 80% in preschool children. Several reference values have been published for R_{int} in preschoolers and schoolchildren and have been recently collated to create international reference equations for 3–13-year-old children. Information on between-measurement repeatability (both short-term and long-term) and BDR in normal is also available, contributing to make this technique a suitable tool for measuring lung function in preschool children.

A recent ATS document has assessed the clinical applications of the interrupter technique in preschool children. R_{int} has mainly been used in children with recurrent wheezing and BDR was found to better distinguish between health and disease than baseline values, with specificity between 70% and 92% and sensitivity between 24% and 76%. R_{int} was also used to assess response in pharmacological intervention studies.

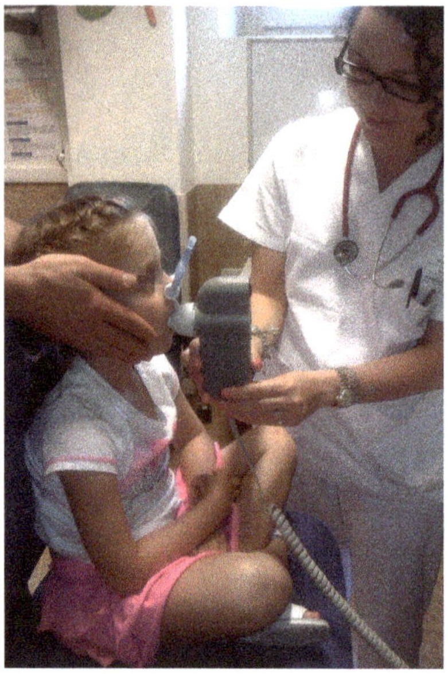

Fig. 12.1: Interrupter technique in preschool children: Measurement conditions.

FORCED OSCILLATION TECHNIQUE

The forced oscillation technique (FOT) also allows lung function measurements during tidal breathing and is hence very appealing in preschool children. Its principle is that, while pressure oscillations generated by a low frequency loudspeaker are transmitted to the respiratory system through the mouthpiece, flow and pressure changes can be measured at the mouth to calculate the impedance of the respiratory system (Z_{rs}) with its two components, resistance (R_{rs}) and reactance (X_{rs}). Hence, with respect to the interrupter technique, FOT has the advantage of also measuring X_{rs}, which can be interpreted as compliance of the respiratory system.

Single-frequency or multiple-frequency signals have been used, both as sinusoidal waves or impulses, with frequencies between 5 Hz and 10 Hz being considered as those that best reflect total airways.

Forced oscillation technique measurement conditions are very similar to those of the interrupter technique (Fig. 12.2). The child is seated and breathes quietly through a bacterial filter and mouthpiece, with the nose clipped and cheeks supported to avoid upper airway compliance. The mean of 3–5 measurements, each lasting 8–16 s, is reported. The coefficient of variation of the 3–5 measurements should also be reported as a quality indicator.

The feasibility of FOT in preschool children is also greater than 80%. Reference values for the 2–13 age range have been reported, as well as short-term repeatability and BDR, making FOT an appealing tool at the disposal of researchers and clinicians with an interest in lung function in preschool children.

Regarding the clinical applications of FOT, significantly higher R_{rs} values and lower X_{rs} values have been shown in preschool wheezers than in healthy subjects, and R_{rs} BDR was reported to have sensitivity between 76%

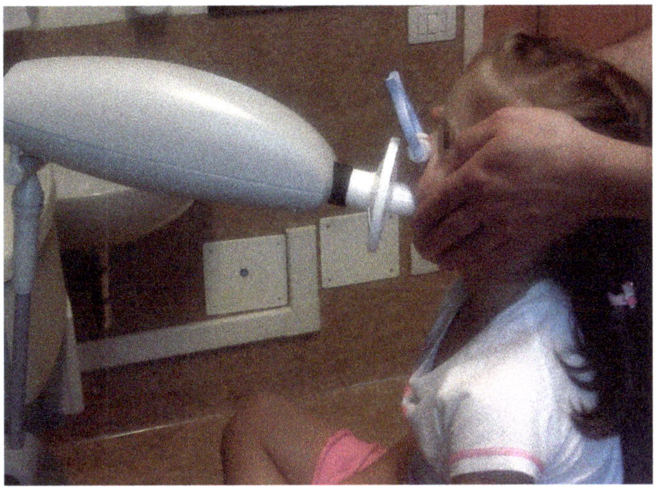

Fig. 12.2: Forced oscillation technique in preschool children: Measurement conditions.

and 90% and specificity between 55% and 65% in detecting preschool children with recurrent wheezing from normal. FOT indices were also shown to be able to detect the effects of anti-inflammatory treatment in preschool children with asthma.

SPIROMETRY IN COOPERATING CHILDREN

Spirometry represents a cornerstone of assessment in respiratory health, both in adults and in children. This test measures how an individual inhales and exhales air as a function of time; the primary signal measured may be volume or flow. Whilst in the past the standard instrument was a water-bell spirometer or a dry rolling seal spirometer, currently the required equipment is an electronic device that usually incorporates a pneumotachograph or an ultrasonic flow-meter to measure flow, whereas volume is subsequently obtained by differentiation.

The most important values in assessing lung function are:

- *Forced vital capacity (FVC)*: The volume delivered at the end of full and forced expiration, after a full inspiration
- *Forced expiratory volume (FEV_1) in one second*: The volume delivered in 1 second, which is the first second of an FVC maneuver
- *FEV_1/FVC*: Relationship between the volume exhaled in one second and the forced vital capacity
- *FEF_{25-75}*: The mean forced expiratory flow between 25% and 75% of FVC
- *PEF*: The highest flow achieved from a maximum forced expiratory maneuver after a maximal lung inflation.

There are three phases in a FVC maneuver:

1. Maximal inspiration
2. Fast and forced exhalation
3. Continued and complete exhalation until the end of the test.

The breathing tube should be inserted into the subject's mouth, making sure that the lips are sealed around the mouthpiece and that the tongue does not occlude it. Then, the subject should inhale rapidly and completely, without any hesitation, from the level of functional residual capacity (FRC). After a minimal pause (only 1-2 seconds) at fully inspiration, the subject should exhale with maximal force until no more air can be expelled (≥3 s in children aged <10 years; ≥6 s in subjects aged >10 years). During this maneuver, enthusiastic coaching, with appropriate body language and phrases, is required. A prior demonstration of the appropriate technique by the technician or the doctor is also advised. The test operator should visually inspect the performance of each maneuver: the flow-volume curve shows the magnitude of the effort during the initial part of the maneuver; the volume-time graph gives more details about the latter part of the maneuver.

Children as young as 5 years are often able to perform acceptable spirometry. Technicians and doctors involved in the lung function testing of children should be specifically trained. Encouragement, lack of intimidation, detailed but simple instructions and visual feedback are advised. The use of a nose clip is recommended. For safety reason, testing should be done in the sitting position, using a chair with arms and without wheels; other positions must be documented on the report.

Individual spirograms are acceptable if:

- They are free from artefacts (i.e. cough during the first second of exhalation, glottis closure, early termination, lack of maximal effort, leak, obstructed mouthpiece)
- They have good starts (extrapoled volume <5% of FVC or 0.150 L)
- They show satisfactory exhalation.

After those three acceptable maneuvers have been obtained, it should be checked that:

- The two largest values of FVC must be within 0.150 L of each other
- The two largest values of FEV_1 must be within 0.150 L of each other

If both of these criteria are not met the test should be continued until they are both met or until a total of eight tests have been performed or the subject cannot continue to perform the test. After examining the data from

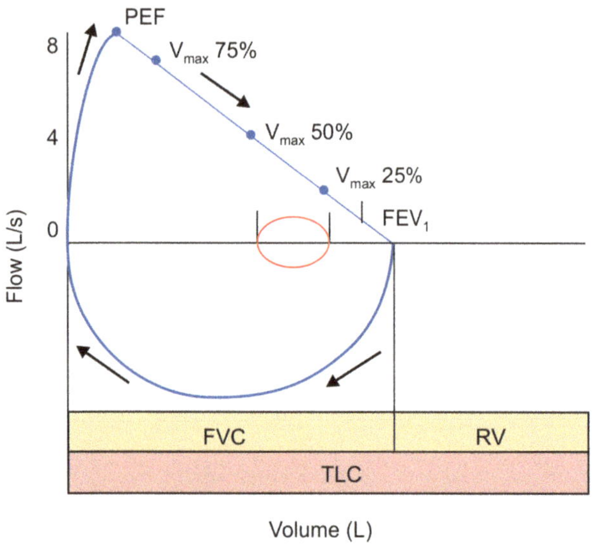

Fig. 12.3: Flow–volume curve.
Source: Modified from La Grutta S. Spirometry in cooperating children. Pneumologia Pediatrica. 2006;22:33-41.

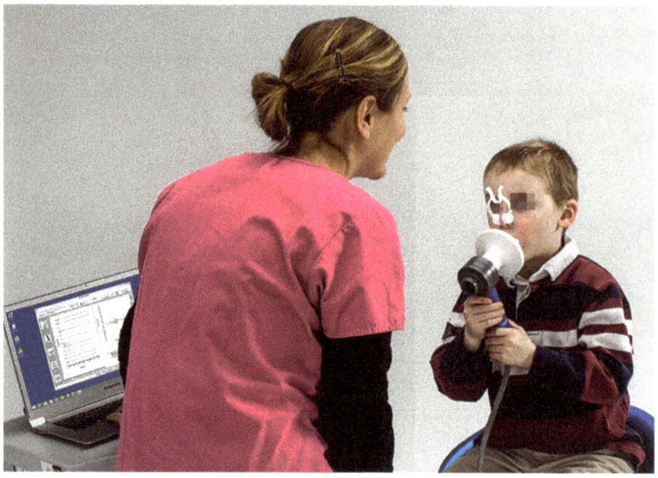

Fig. 12.4: Spirometry in a preschool child.
Source: http://www.morgansci.com/

all the usable curves, the largest FVC and FEV_1 should be recorded, even if they do not come from the same curve. Other indices such as FEV_1/FVC, $FEF_{25-75\%}$ and PEF should be taken from the curve with the largest sum of FEV_1 and FVC. A flow-volume curve is shown in Figure 12.3.

PRESCHOOL SPIROMETRY

Preschool children (2–5 years) are physiologically different from schoolchildren. It is important that the operator gains the trust of the child and that he/she is able to obtain measurements without causing distress (Fig. 12.4). It is also recommended the laboratory environment to be friendly, with games, videos and space for play. During a forced expiratory maneuver their lungs tend to empty in less than 1 s and using the forced expiratory volume in one second (FEV_1) as the main index (as for spirometry in schoolchildren and adults) is often unrealistic. For the same reason, adult spirometry criteria as the requirement to expire for at least 6 s can obviously not be reached. Also, due to the poor attention span of preschool children, reproducibility criteria are often impossible to meet.

The ATS/ERS Working Group for Lung Function Testing in Preschool Children has modified the acceptability criteria for spirometry, making them suitable for preschool children. First of all, preschool children need time to get acquainted with the machine and the maneuver. Computerized incentives may be used, although not mandatory, and in this case a volume-driven or a flow- and volume-driven incentive should be preferred. Regarding the start of test criterion, the volume of back extrapolation (V_{BE}) should be less than 80 mL or 12.5% of forced vital capacity (FVC), but maneuvers that do not meet this criterion should not be necessarily rejected. The use of FEV in 0.5 s ($FEV_{0.5}$) or 0.75 s ($FEV_{0.75}$) instead of FEV_1 is recommended. If the maneuver stops at a flow higher than 10% of peak flow, premature termination is evident and FVC should not be reported, but it may still be possible to report $FEV_{0.5}$ or $FEV_{0.75}$. At least two acceptable curves should be obtained (with the two FVC and $FEV_{0.5}$ or $FEV_{0.75}$ within 0.1 L or 10%), but a single acceptable curve should not be rejected because of poor repeatability.

The principles of spirometry quality control in preschool children are the same as in adults. Visibly inadequate maneuvers have to be excluded. Since preschoolers are likely to become bored or tired if the session is too prolonged, the operator should visualize the curves on the screen, or at least before the next effort in order to encourage the child to improve his/her technique, if necessary.

The feasibility of spirometry is reported to be not far from that of the interrupter technique and FOT in 5-6-year-old children, but is much lower at age below 5 years. Also, due to the complexity of spirometry in preschool children, a circumspect approach to its interpretation should be undertaken in this age group. The recent availability of international multiethnic reference values from 3 to 95 years of age (Global Lung Function Initiative 2012) has made it easier to interpret spirometry in preschool children.

Types of Ventilatory Defects

- *Obstructive abnormalities*: An obstructive ventilatory defect, such as in asthma, is a disproportionate reduction of maximal airflow in relation to the maximal volume that can be displaced from the lung. It implies airway narrowing during exhalation and is defined by a reduced FEV_1/FVC ratio. The slowing of expiratory flow is reflected in a concave shape of the flow–volume curve. A determination of the airflow-limitation reversibility with drug administration is commonly considered as part of lung function testing. The subject should undergo the baseline test without taking any drugs before (i.e. short acting agonists such salbutamol should not be assumed within 4 hours of testing; long acting agonists such salmeterol or formoterol should not be used for the 12 hours prior to the test). After that FEV_1 and FVC have been recorded as described previously, the drug is administered at a standardized dose (for example, 400 µg of salbutamol) and three additional acceptable curves are recorded after 10–15 minute. Values greater than 12% and 200 mL compared with baseline during a single-testing session suggest a "significant" bronchodilatation. However, the lack of a response to bronchodilator testing in a laboratory does not preclude a clinical response to bronchodilator therapy (Table 12.1).
- *Restrictive abnormalities*: A restrictive ventilatory defect, as occurs in CF, may be suspected when FVC is reduced, the FEV_1/FVC is increased and the flow–volume curve shows a convex pattern.
- *Mixed abnormalities*: A mixed ventilatory defect is characterized by the coexistence of obstruction and restriction and is defined physiologically when both FEV_1/FVC and TLC are reduced.

Examples of flow–volume curves in subjects with different ventilatory defects are shown in Figures 12.5A to C.

Clinicians are used to express lung function results as percent predicted (100*[observed/predicted]), where the predicted value comes from a reference equation incorporating sex, age and height. In childhood height is the preferred predictor of pulmonary function test, since predicted values based on age may overestimate expected values if the child suffers from any significant degree of growth retardation associated with the respiratory disease. Several spirometry equations have been available throughout these years. However, the use of different equations has been shown to lead to different interpretation, depending on the way patients were assessed with. For this reason, in 2012, a European Respiratory Society Task Force (GLI-Global Lung Function Initiative) published a new equation that collects the 3–95-year age range and covers five ethnic groups. This equation produces z-scores. A z-score is the deviation of an individual's value from the median value of a reference population, divided by the standard deviation of the reference population; it indicates how many SDs an individual is below or above the predicted mean for any given parameter. The use of z-scores, that account for the interindividual variability of the normal distribution, let the clinician interpret test results independently from age, height, sex and ethnic group, unlike the use of percent of predicted that is associated with significant biases. Hence, the GLI 2012 reference equation offers the opportunity to standardize the interpretation of spirometry world-wide and its increasing use is envisaged in clinical and research settings.

Table 12.1: Main types of ventilatory defects.

Obstructive abnormalities	*Restrictive abnormalities*
FEV_1/FVC ↓	FEV_1/FVC ↑
FEV_1 ↓	VC ↓
FEF_{25-75} ↓	TLC ↓

(FVC: Forced vital capacity; FEV_1: Forced expiratory volume in one second; FEF: Forced expiratory volume; TLC: total lung capacity; VC: Vital capacity)

EXHALED NITRIC OXIDE

Exhaled NO (eNO) is currently considered a marker of airway inflammation and it may be particularly useful in allergic asthmatic patients. The safety of the procedure and the technical improvements in measurement devices has widened the measurement of eNO in the clinical practice both in adults and in children.

Official European Respiratory Society (ERS) and American Thoracic Society (ATS) guidelines have been produced in order to standardize the measurement procedure. The method of single-breath online measurement, assessing the fractional exhaled NO (FeNO), is currently considered the standard procedure for the measurement of nitric oxide for the assessment of lower airway inflammation both in children and in adults.

The maneuver is relatively easy and can be performed adequately even in preschoolers. The patient is requested to inhale to near total lung capacity from a mouthpiece connected to source containing less than 5 ppb of nitric oxide and to immediately exhale at a flow of 50 ml/s against a resistance between 5 and 20 cm H_2O, aimed to

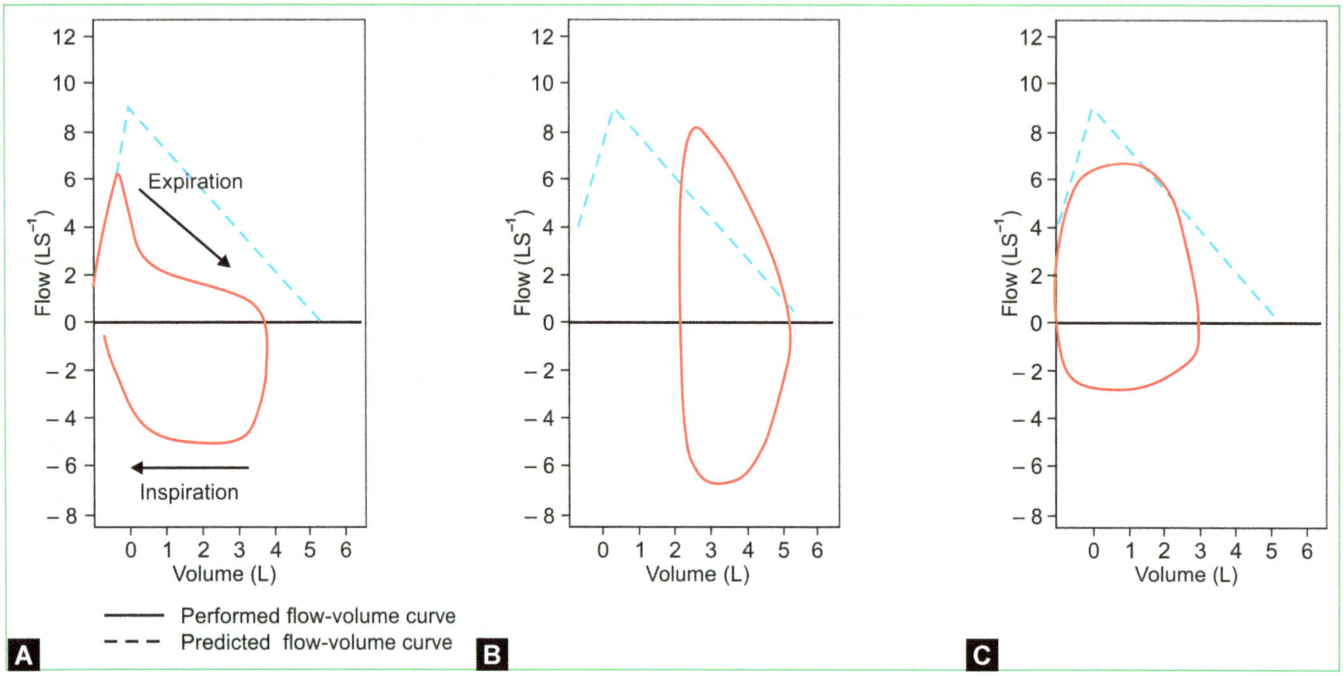

Figs. 12.5A to C: Examples of flow-volume curves. (A) Moderate obstructive deficit in asthmatic patients; (B) Restrictive deficit; (C) Extrathoracic obstruction of the upper airways.
Source: Modified from La Grutta S. Spirometry in cooperating chldren. Pneumologia Pediatrica. 2006;22:33-41.

keep velum closed during the exhalation. Three measurements agreeing within 10% or two within 5% are recommended.

While the first generation of chemiluminescence devices were poorly adequate in order to fulfil the requirements of standardized measurements, in few years a number of devices have been designed to obtain FeNO measurements according to ATS/ERS guidelines. Manual or automatic flow controllers were introduced in order to ensure constant controlled expiratory flow at the required pressure during the measurement maneuvre. Visual feedback aids were also introduced to this purpose.

More recently, FeNO analyzers operating by electrochemical sensors have been introduced in place of chemiluminescence analyzer. Some of these electrochemical analyzers are portable and they have been proposed for ambulatory setting. Factors such as environmental pollution, physical activity, recent meals or beverage or other functional test immediately before FeNO measurement should be considered.

Since FeNO level is well related with the degree of eosinophil airway inflammation, it has been proposed as a noninvasive marker to be used in selected asthmatic patients. A practical role for FeNo measurement in asthma has been proposed for diagnosis, selection of responders to inhaled corticosteroids (ICS), disease control monitoring and treatment tailoring. FeNO levels have been reported to be predictive of asthma with a sensitivity of 88% and specificity of 79% in a population with symptoms of asthma ranging in age 8–75 years. The same study group observed that the combination of increased FeNO levels (>33 ppb) and low FEV_1 (< 80% predicted) can provide the valuable combination of parameters for the diagnosis of asthma with 94% sensitivity and 93% specificity (93%).

During the first years of life, in particular, the determination of asthma phenotype may significantly influence the treatment strategy in the single patient. Since FeNO is well correlated to the level of eosinophil of airway inflammation in asthmatic patients, it has been proposed a possible role of FeNO in distinguishing among the different wheezing phenotypes in children in the preschool age. In fact, though wheezing is very common during the first years of life, only a minority of the children who wheeze at that age will develop asthma in the future. A number of studies has evaluated whether the measurement of FeNO in these subjects may contribute in phenotyping. Taken together these results show that the measurement of FeNO in preschoolers, along with dedicated questionnaires, clinical evaluation and lung function measurements can significantly contribute to early identify the children who will be at higher risk of developing asthma in the future and to address an early appropriate treatment.

Controller therapy for asthma is mainly based upon a regular use of ICS, or in selected patients, leukotriene receptor antagonists (LTRAs). FeNO has been demonstrated to be the only clinical marker capable of predicting a positive response of treatment with ICS in a pediatric population and, therefore it can be proposed as a tool to address treatment choice in daily practice. FeNO has been shown to decrease promptly when ICS treatment is started and to be reduced during prolonged treatment. From a practical viewpoint, therefore, FeNO can be regarded as a tool to assess the optimization of treatment and the level of compliance with the anti-inflammatory therapy.

An additional challenge in the real-life management of asthmatic patient is the assessment of disease control, mainly based upon symptoms, bronchodilator consumption and level of lung function. Nevertheless, though asthma is an inflammatory disease which requires a regular anti-inflammatory treatment, none of these parameters is capable of reflecting the degree of airway inflammation in asthmatic patients and the role of airway inflammation in the clinical outcomes of asthma is still debated. Therefore, a number of studies has been performed aimed to evaluate whether the assessment of FeNO may contribute in assessing the level of asthma control. In the real life, a degree of agreement between the results from validated questionnaires, such as Asthma Control Test (ACT), and FeNO levels has been demonstrated in particular in newly diagnosed children but not in followed-up patients, thus suggesting that the evaluation of disease control is not easy to achieve by a single method but that a combination of evaluation parameters is advisable.

In selected populations of allergic asthmatics, FeNO has been demonstrated to be capable to reflect the level of allergen exposure. FeNO was evaluated in children with mild asthma sensitized to birch pollen while tracking the increasing natural birch pollen exposure. It has been shown an increase in FeNO, paralleling the pollen count, which persisted in the week after the pollen peak, suggesting a prolonged effect of airway inflammation after acute pollen exposure. During the study period no significant change was observed in PEFR or FEV_1, thus suggesting that FeNO may be considered a more sensitive measure of asthma activity than lung function. Similarly, FeNO has been proposed as a marker of disease reactivition in house dust mite sensitized children re-exposed to mite after a period of avoidance, with an interesting evidence of an increase in FeNO 2–3 days before symptom report.

The evidence of a relationship between asthma symptoms and FeNO levels has raised the hypothesis that asthma treatment could be personalized upon the basis of FeNO level rather than on symptoms. A number of studies has been performed to verify this hypothesis with rather discordant results. Though some of these studies showed some advantage in the management of asthmatic patients on the basis of their FeNO levels, some others failed on this hypothesis. Overall, the body of the data from these studies failed to demonstrate a significant benefit of treatment tailoring on the basis of FeNO measurement. Nevertheless, some criticisms were raised to these studies, in particular in consideration that they were designed in a way that individual treatment were modified according to fixed FeNO values without taking into consideration the need to consider individual best FeNO levels rather than population reference values. An approach based upon individual best values is more easily achieved with the most recent portable devices, which can be easily used in office settings and not only in specialized centers.

In the most recent ATS guidelines it has been proposed a practical approach to FeNO measurement in asthma, based on the results of the studies performed so far, suggesting how to interpret FeNO values. The interpretation of FeNO considers the reason for which the test is performed distinguishing between patients with nonspecific symptoms, still undiagnosed, and those with a confirmed diagnosis of asthma. A distinction of patients with eNO values less than 25 ppb (in children <20 ppb) and those who have eNO values greater than 50 ppb (for children >35 ppb) is performed but FeNO values have to be interpreted along with patients' symptoms.

In conclusion, for practical purposes, FeNO can help clinicians in early identifying preschoolers with asthmatic phenotype, diagnosing allergic asthma, predicting the response to ICS in asthmatic patients and, if properly considered, in monitoring treatment compliance and disease control.

EXHALED BREATH CONDENSATE

An impressive number of scientific reports on exhaled breath condensate (EBC) studies and official ATS/ERS guidelines were produced. The rationale of EBC method is based upon the condensation of exhaled breath water vapor, which contains a number of aerosol particles from the respiratory tree, onto a cold surface.

The method requires poor cooperation by the patient and it has been demonstrated to be safe and feasible even in very young children. Nevertheless, a number of factors need to be considered both in sample collection, assaying and data interpretation in order to have reproducible results.

In terms of collection procedure, published studies may differ for a wide number of factors, including collection devices, temperature of condensation, duration of collection, environmental temperature and humidity patients characteristics, respiratory pattern, food or beverages in the hours immediately before collection, circadian variations. For example, it has been demonstrated that both the temperature and the material of the condenser surface may influence the sample content and, therefore, such factors need to be clearly considered in data interpretation if different collection conditions were used. Similarly, the respiratory pattern of the patient may drive the concentration of the collected biomarkers as well as other factors, such as wearing or not a nasal clip.

In practice, the patients is request to sit in a comfortable position, wearing a noseclip and breath tidally for a period of time which is generally between 10 and 30 minutes into a condensing system made of inert surface through a mouthpiece. A salivary trap, but no filters, should be in place. Duration and temperature of collection may be variable and decided according to the purpose of each study but they need to be kept constant for the participating subject and considered when comparing the results with other studies. When the collection is completed, samples need to be immediately processed or stored frozen until processed.

A main advantage of EBC is that it is possible to assay a wide number of biomarkers in the collected samples, including pH, cytokines, arachidonic acid derivatives, nitroxidative compounds, hydrogen peroxidative compounds, aldehydes and others. Furthermore, the samples are suitable for proteomic and metabolomic assays. Nevertheless, it has to be carefully considered that, for most of the investigated biomarkers, internal protocols have been validated only within research groups while standardization of procedures to be used universally with reproducible results is definitely needed.

In the field of asthma, EBC has been proposed for early diagnosis of asthma in children, to discriminate among inflammatory phenotypes, to assess severity of airway inflammation to monitor disease control. It has also been used for research purposes in a number of other broncho-pulmonary diseases, including pneumonia, interstitial lung disease, pulmonary fibrosis, CF, in children and adult, as well as for occupational medicine investigations.

The availability of dedicated analyzers for selected biomarker, such as H_2O_2, opens a perspective for the use of EBC at bedside for clinical purposes, and not only for research.

In summary, EBC represents a relatively simple method for sampling biomarkers from the airways with the purpose of allowing the collection of a variety of biomarkers from the airways in a wide range of respiratory diseases. To the present, it has been mostly used for research purposes but possible clinical applications are expected, after adequate standardization procedure.

STATIC LUNG VOLUMES

Static lung volumes represent the gas within the lungs that is not influenced by air flow. Lung volume measurements are valuable in the assessment of disease severity, functional disability, and response to treatment in infants as well as in children. All static volumes are age-dependent and increase during childhood. Static lung volumes consist in specific volumes and capacity (sum of two or more volumes) (Tables 12.2 and 12.3). The static lung volumes and lung capacities are assessed with the methods of the body plethysmograhy and gas dilution technique.

The body plethysmograph measures the volume of gas in the thorax and it is considered the most accurate method of calculating FRC (Fig. 12.6). This method is more expensive, technically not easy, and requires more subject cooperation than gas dilution-washout methods. Conversely, the multiple breath washout (MBW) with gas dilution methods are relatively simple to perform and require little collaboration from the children. It is necessary to underline that in children with obstructive lung disease the MBW methods can underestimate (undervalue) the FRC because they measure only those parts of the lungs in communication with the mouth (the areas of the lungs that contain trapped gas are excluded). In this way an obstructive lung disease can be incorrectly classified as mixed obstructive-restrictive lung disease patterns.

Multiple breath washout with gas dilution methods are widely utilized in pulmonary function laboratories because are measured during tidal breathing. These methods are easy to perform in the children and require minimal learning and cooperation. The multiple-breath closed circuit He dilution involves diluting He, an inert gas, in the lungs by rebreathing the gas in a closed system over a short time. In a different way the multiple-breath open-circuit N_2 washout requires removing or washing out

Table 12.2: Static lung volumes.

- *Tidal volume (V_T)*: The volume of gas inhaled or exhaled during the respiratory cycle
- *Inspiratory reserve volume (IRV)*: The maximum volume of gas that can be inhaled from the end-inspiratory level during tidal breathing
- *Expiratory reserve volume (ERV)*: The volume of gas that can be maximally exhaled from the end-expiratory level during tidal breathing
- *Residual volume (RV)*: The volume of gas remaining in the lung after maximal exhalation. RV includes the volume of gas contained in the alveoli and anatomical dead space
- *Thoracic gas volume (TGV or V_{TG})*: The absolute volume of gas in the thorax at any point in time and any level of alveolar pressure. Usually it is measured at functional residual capacity.

Table 12.3: Lung capacities

- *Inspiratory capacity (IC)*: The maximum volume of gas that can be inspired after normal expiration. IC is the sum of tidal volume and inspiratory reserve volume: IC = VT + IRV
- *Expiratory capacity (EC)*: The amount of gas expelled from the lungs with a slow exhalation at the end of a normal inspiration. It is also given by the sum of tidal volume and expiratory reserve volume: EC = TV + ERV
- *Vital capacity (VC)*: Slow vital capacity (SVC) is the maximum volume of air that can be slowly exhaled from a maximum inspiration to a full expiration (expiratory vital capacity: EVC) or inhaled from a position of full expiration to full inspiration (inspiratory vital capacity: IVC). Forced vital capacity (FVC) is the volume of gas that is exhaled during a forced expiration, starting from a position of full inspiration and ending at complete expiration.
- *Functional residual capacity (FRC)*: The volume of gas present in the lung at end expiration during tidal breathing
- *Total lung capacity (TLC)*: The volume of gas in the lungs after maximal inspiration, or the sum of VC+RV.

the N_2 gas in the child's lungs while the patient breathes 100% O_2. A third method utilizes the multiple-breath washin/washout technique with the sulphur hexafluoride (SF_6) a nonresident, inert, non toxic marker gas. The FRC of washout is obtained by dividing the measured expired SF_6 volume by the end tidal SF_6 concentration before washout and by subtracting the volume of the apparatus dead space including the face mask.

Furthermore, it is possible to measure the lung clearance index (LCI), a sensitive index of ventilation inhomogeneity. It is calculated as cumulative expired volume needed to reduce the end tidal SF_6 to a value below 1/40th of its starting concentration, divided by FRC. The obtained value corresponds to the number of lung volume turnovers needed to clear the lung from the tracer gas. Ventilation inhomogeneity is supposed

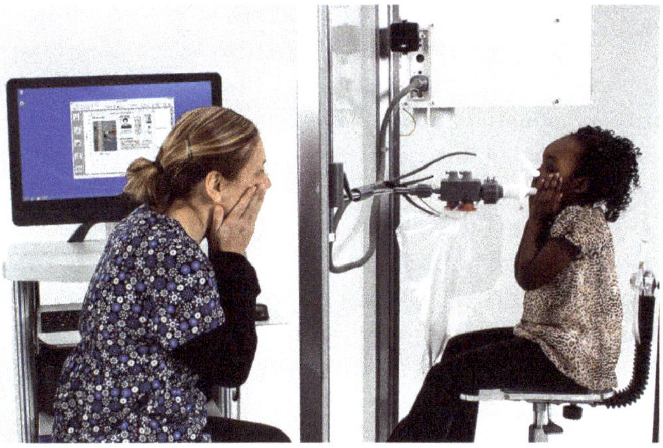

Fig. 12.6: Obtaining functional residual capacity (FRC) by plethysmography in a preschool child.
Source: http://www.morgansci.com/

to reflect changes in peripheral airways which are not apparent with spirometry because FEV_1, in health and early disease, mostly reflects proximal airways. Moreover, LCI is increased in the presence of airway narrowing caused by inflammation and it is largely independent of age. LCI has been shown in CF patients to be more sensitive than spirometry for detecting changes in small airways, and to be the earliest indicator of disease progression during longitudinal follow-up.

BRONCHOPROVOCATION CHALLENGE TEST

Bronchial hyperresponsiveness (BHR) is defined as an increase of airflow limitation in response to bronchoconstrictor stimuli and reflects the variability of bronchial tone in asthmatic children. BHR can be measured by pharmacological agents such as methacholine or histamine producing directly contraction upon the bronchial airways.

Other indirect methods of measurement of nonspecific BHR are the response to dry cold air inhalation, hyperventilation or inhalation of other substances such as adenosine monophosphate (AMP) or the hyperosmolar agent mannitol.

Mannitol challenge is included in the category of osmotic aerosols, whose main reference is hypertonic saline. It is easy to perform, and induces the increase of airways osmolarity and the delivery of histamine from mast cells. It also shows a good correlation with the level of bronchial inflammation.

Respiratory virus infection (rhinovirus) and air pollution (including second hand smoke) increase bronchial responsiveness.

Exercise test is an indirect method to measure exercise-induced bronchoconstriction (EIB). It is more specific and can differentiate asthma from other chronic lung diseases, but it is less sensitive than bronchial provocation with methacholine or histamine in diagnosing asthma. Some authors observed that bronchial provocation challenge by exercise and methacholine or histamine does not always identify the same individuals. Moreover, sensitivity of the exercise test on a treadmill can be significantly amplified adding another stimulus such as the inhalation of cold and/or dry air.

The prevalence of bronchial asthma in children is around 10% and 40–90% of these patients have EIB, a manifestation that is frequently undiagnosed. EIB is defined as a condition in which physical activity triggers acute airway narrowing in children with heightened airway reactivity. Increased ventilation during physical activity leading to augmented water loss and heat loss through respiration. Consequently, these modifications determine smooth muscle contraction and mucosal edema in predisposed children through reflex parasympathetic nerve stimulation. The diagnosis of EIB is suggested by the clinical history (cough, wheezing, tightness in the chest, shortness of breath or dyspnea) and demonstrated by a decrease of 10–12% in forced expiratory volume in one second (FEV_1). The challenge consists in performing an exercise test on a treadmill. The slope and speed of the treadmill is administered according to a standardized protocol for 6–8 minutes, to induce a heart rate at a level of 80-90% of the maximum predicted (220-age in years) during the last 4 minutes of the test. In overweight and unfit children it may be difficult to maintain the target heart rate for 4 minutes. Before the test, the children should not take bronchodilators nor inhaled corticosteroids. The nose clips is applied to ensure mouth breathing. During exercise an electrocardiogram can be utilized to determine heart rate and to detect possible arrhythmias. Arterial oxygen saturation (SpO_2) is monitored with a pulse oximeter through a probe attached to the index finger. FEV_1 is measured at 1, 5, 10, 15, 20, and 30 minutes after exercise and the lowest FEV_1 recorded over this period is used to calculate the maximal percentage fall from baseline by the following equation: Percent fall in FEV_1 = (pre-exercise FEV_1 – lowest FEV_1 post-exercise)/pre-exercise $FEV_1 \times 100$.

Figure 12.7 shows the trend of FEV_1, as percentage of predicted values, assessed at the time points (5, 10, 15, 20, and 30 minute) after two different exercise test (treadmill vs 3-minutes step test).

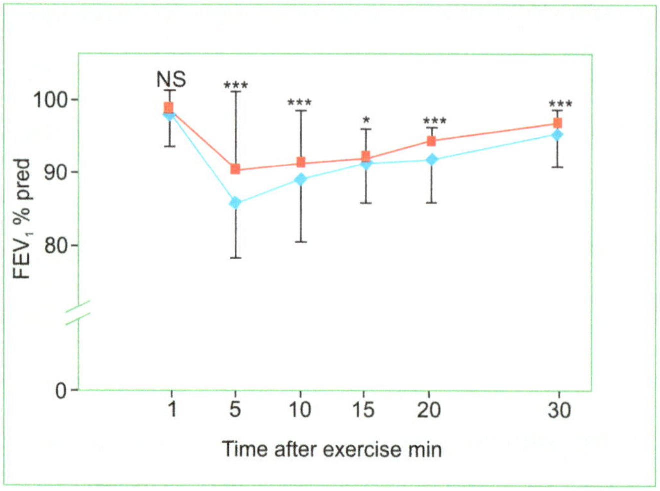

Fig. 12.7: Forced expiratory volume in one second (FEV1) (% predicted) after the treadmill test (♦) and the 3-minute step test (•). ns: nonsignificant; *: $p < 0.05$; ***: $p < 0.001$.
Source: Tancredi G, Quattrucci S, Scalercio F, De Castro G, Zicari AM, Bonci E, et al. 3-Min step test and treadmill exercise for evaluating exercise-induced asthma. Eur Respir J. 2004;23:569-74.

It is necessary to underline that the reasons to perform an exercise test are numerous. An exercise test gives information about physical skill, fitness and motor development. It is possible to study the response to exercise of cardiovascular and respiratory system and skeletal muscles. Furthermore exercise test is a useful screening tool to evaluate children with respiratory disease, as well as diagnostic and prognostic tool for lung and heart transplantation, physical fitness, and rehabilitation programs.

Exercise testing is essential because pulmonary and cardiac function testing at rest cannot reliably predict exercise performance or functional capacity and the overall health status will correlate more closely with exercise tolerance than with measurements taken at rest.

In conclusion, BHR tests are a valuable tools in assessing the severity of childhood asthma, but they cannot replace a comprehensive medical evaluation including history and physical examination.

BIBLIOGRAPHY AND FURTHER READING

1. Aurora P, Stocks J, Oliver C, Saunders C, Castle R, Chazip-arasidis G, et al. Quality control for spirometry in preschool children with and without lung disease. Am J Respir Crit Care Med. 2004;169:1152-9.
2. Baraldi E, de Jongste JC. European Respiratory Society/American Thoracic Society (ERS/ATS) Task Force Measurement of exhaled nitric oxide in children ERS/ATS statement. Eur Respir J. 2002;20: 223-37.

3. Beydon N, Davis SD, Lombardi E, Allen JL, Arets HGM, Aurora P, et al. on behalf of the American Thoracic Society/ European Respiratory Society Working Group on Infant and Young Children Pulmonary Function Testing. An Official American Thoracic Society/European Respiratory Society Statement: Pulmonary Function Testing in Preschool Children. Am J Respir Crit Care Med 2007;175:1304-145.
4. Calogero C, Simpson SJ, Lombardi E, Parri N, Cuomo B, Palumbo M, et al. Respiratory impedance and bronchodilator responsiveness in healthy children aged 2 to 13 years. Pediatr Pulmonol. 2013;48:707-15.
5. Dweik RA, Boggs PB, Erzurum SC, Irvin CG, Leigh MW, Lundberg JO, et al. An official ATS clinical practice guideline: interpretation of exhaled nitric oxide levels (FeNO) for clinical applications. Am J Respir Crit Care Med. 2011;184: 602-15.
6. Fuchs SI, Gappa M. Lung clearance index: clinical and research applications in children. Paed Respir Rev. 2011;12:264-70.
7. Gajdocsi R, Bikov A, Antus B, Horvath I, Barnes PJ, Kharitonov SA. Assessment of reproducibility of exhaled hydrogen peroxide concentration and the effect of breathing pattern in healthy subjects. J Aerosol Med Pulm Drug Deliv. 2011;24:271-5.
8. Horváth I, Hunt J, Barnes PJ, Alving K, Antczak A, Baraldi E, et al. Exhaled breath condensate: methodological recommendations and unresolved questions. Eur Respir J. 2005;26:523-48.
9. Krogh M. The diffusion gases through the lungs of man. J Physiol. 1915;49:271-300.
10. Latzin P, Roth S, Thamrin C, Hutten GJ, Pramana I, Kuehni CE, et al. Lung volume, breathing pattern and ventilation inhomogeneity in preterm and term Infants. PLoS ONE. 2009;4:e4635.
11. Latzin P, Thamrin C, Kraemer R. Ventilation inhomogeneities assessed by the multibreath washout (MBW) technique. Thorax. 2008;63:98-9.
12. Macintyre N, Crapo RO, Viegi G, Johnson DC, van der Grinten CP, Brusasco V, et al. Standardisation of the single-breath determination of carbon monoxide uptake in the lung. Eur Respir J. 2005;26:720-35.
13. Mele L, Sly PD, Calogero C, Bernardini R, Novembre E, Azzari C, et al. Assessment and validation of bronchodilation using the interrupter technique in preschool children. Pediatr Pulmonol. 2010;45:633-8.
14. Merkus PJ, Stocks J, Beydon N, Lombardi E, Jones M, McKenzie SA, et al. Reference ranges for interrupter resistance technique: the Asthma UK Initiative. Eur Respir J. 2010;36:157-63.
15. Miller MR, Hankinson J, Brusasco V, Burgos F, Casaburi R, Coates A, et al. ATS/ERS Task Force. Standardization of spirometry. Eur Respir J. 2005;26:319-38.
16. Pellegrino R, Viegi G, Brusasco V, Crapo RO, Burgos F, Casaburi R, et al. Interpretative strategies for lung function tests. Eur Respir J. 2005;26:948-68.
17. Piacentini GL, Peroni DG, Bodini A, Bonafiglia E, Rigotti E, Baraldi E, et al. B Childhood Asthma Control Test and airway inflammation evaluation in asthmatic children. Allergy. 2009;64:1753-7.
18. Quanjer PH, Stanojevic S, Cole TJ, Baur X, Hall GL, Culver BH, et al. ERS Global Lung Function Initiative. Multiethnic reference values for spirometry for the 3–95 years age range: the global lung function 2012 equations. Eur Respir J. 2012;40:1324-43.
19. Quanjer PH, Weiner DJ. Interpretative consequences of adopting the Global Lungs 2012 reference equations for spirometry for children and adolescents. Pediatr Pulmonol. 2014;49:118-25.
20. Rosenfeld M, Allen J, Arets BH, Aurora P, Beydon N, Calogero C, et al. American Thoracic Society Assembly on Pediatrics Working Group on Infant and Preschool Lung Function Testing. An official American Thoracic Society workshop report: optimal lung function tests for monitoring cystic fibrosis, bronchopulmonary dysplasia, and recurrent wheezing in children less than 6 years of age. Ann Am Thorac Soc 2013;10:S1-S11.
21. Smith AD, Cowan JO, Taylor DR. Exhaled nitric oxide levels in asthma: personal best versus reference values. J Allergy Clin Immunol. 2009;124:714-8.
22. Stanojevic S, Wade A, Stocks J, Hankinson J, Coates AL, Pan H, et al. Reference ranges for spirometry across all ages: a new approach. Am J Respir Crit Care Med. 2008;177:253-60.
23. Wanger J, Clausen JL, Coates A, Pedersen OF, Brusasco V, Burgos F, et al. Standardisation of the measurement of lung volumes. Eur Respir J. 2005;26:511-22.

Chapter 13

Arterial Blood Gas Analysis and other Tools for the Evaluation of Gas Exchange Efficiency

Claudio Sorino, Angelo Corsico

OVERVIEW OF THE MEASUREMENT OF GAS EXCHANGE EFFICIENCY

Arterial blood gas analysis (ABGA) allows to assessing the efficiency of the respiratory system and the acid-base equilibrium by evaluating several parameters. These include blood pH (logarithmic measure of hydrogen ion concentration), partial pressure of oxygen (pO_2) and carbon dioxide (pCO_2) in systemic arterial blood, bicarbonate ion (HCO_3^-), base excess and oxygen saturation (SpO_2). ABGA is a relatively easy investigation, widely performed in emergency departments and intensive care units (ICU). It gives precious information to guide the management and monitor patients with acute respiratory failure as well as other several acute and chronic diseases involving an acid-base disorder. ABGA also has some applications in general practice, such as to evaluate the need for long-term domiciliary oxygen therapy in patients with chronic pulmonary disease. Interpretation of an arterial blood gas result should not be done without considering the clinical findings. Factors relating to sampling technique, specimen processing and environment may influence the results.

Pulse oximetry is a simple and noninvasive tool which estimates SpO_2 of peripheral capillary blood, defined as the ratio of oxyhemoglobin (HbO_2) to the total concentration of hemoglobin (Hb) present in the blood. Pulse oximetry functioning is based on the absorption of light from light-emitting diodes positioned in a finger clip or adhesive strip probe (spectrophotometry). *Transcutaneous oxygen (StO_2) evaluation* is possible through electrodes which incorporated a thermostatically controlled heating element to maximize local blood flow. StO_2 differs from the SpO_2 measured by pulse oximetry, since StO_2 is a local measure of oxygen saturation in the microcirculation where oxygen is exchanged with tissue, while pulse oximetry assesses the systemic oxygen saturation of arterial blood.

Transcutaneous carbon dioxide analysis is a noninvasive technique able to provide a continuous estimate of pCO_2. It is particularly useful in ventilated patients, when blood CO_2 values may rapidly change. In such conditions, getting a continuous monitoring of the pCO_2 values may be preferable than observing them intermittently by ABGA.

End-tidal CO_2 ($ET\text{-}CO_2$) measurement, also known as *capnography*, provides continuous values of the expired CO_2 tension at the airway. It is part of the routine monitoring during anesthesia in the operating rooms and is increasingly used in the ICU; however, several patient-related issues such as ventilation-perfusion mismatch may influence the correlation of the $ET\text{-}CO_2$ with arterial pCO_2 measured by ABGA.

The *diffusing capacity of lungs for carbon monoxide (DLCO)* provides complementary information to ABGA on gas exchange efficiency. The test can be performed only in clinically stable and cooperative patients, and does not provide information on the transport of gases and consequently on the effective amount of O_2 that reaches the peripheral tissues, and the effectiveness of CO_2 removal. DLCO measurement technique has been extensively addressed in a dedicated chapter.

Arterial Puncture

Arterial blood gas analysis is usually performed on blood withdrawn from the radial artery since its superficial

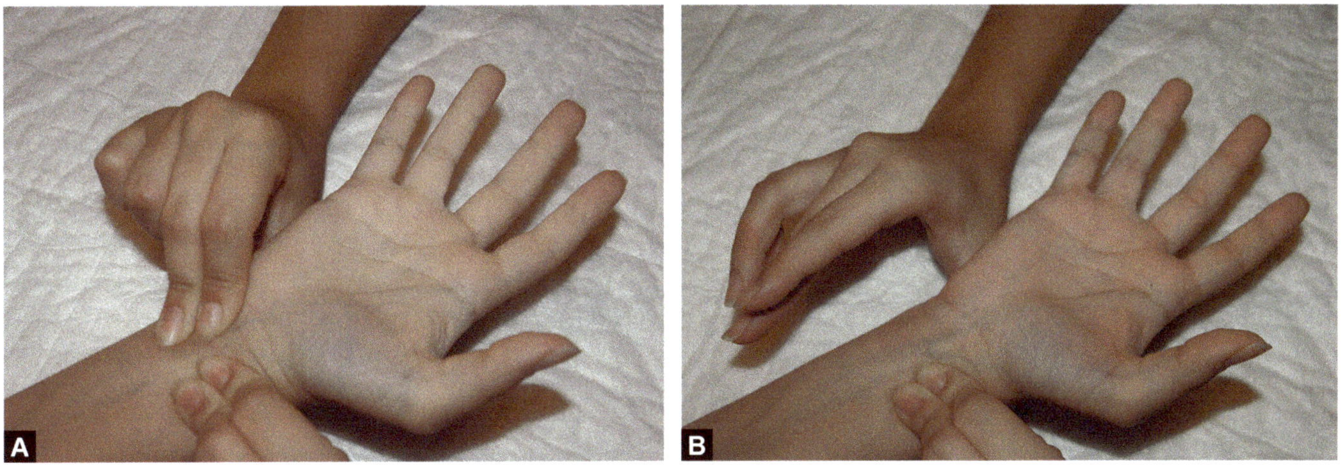

Figs. 13.1A and B: Allen's test. (A) Pressure is applied over the ulnar and the radial arteries so as to occlude both of them; the hand should appear blanched; (B) Ulnar pressure is released and the color should return in a few seconds.

anatomic presentation makes it easily palpable and accessible. Collateral blood supply to the hand is usually good, but this should be verified before performing a radial arterial puncture.

Allen's test (Figs. 13.1A and B) is the most widely performed test with this purpose: both the radial and ulnar arteries are compressed at the same time until the hand becomes white; then the ulnar artery is released and the color should return to the hand in a few seconds. This ensures an adequate blood supply to the hand if the ABGA cause a blockage in the radial artery.

The radial artery arises from the bifurcation of the brachial artery and runs distally along the lateral (radial) side of the forearm to the wrist. If the radial pulse is diminished or distal perfusion is compromised, femoral or brachial artery puncture can be performed instead. The use of ultrasonography allows more precise identification, delineation and targeting of the chosen vascular structure.

To perform a radial arterial puncture, the patient's arm is supinated and the wrist extended (Fig. 13.2). A towel can be placed under the wrist to facilitate this position. The puncture site should be cleaned with alcohol, iodine or an antiseptic swab. A local anesthetic (such as 2% Lidocaine) can be infiltrated to make arterial puncture less painful but it is not routinely done. The syringe that is used is heparinized and has a 23 or 25 gauge needle. The needle should be inserted at 30–45 degrees to the skin at the point of maximum pulsation of the radial artery (Fig. 13.3). The needle is advanced until arterial blood flushes into the syringe, then it should be kept as motionless as possible, while the arterial pressure allows the blood to fill the syringe. A small quantity of blood (about 2 mL) is usually sufficient. Bright red and pulsating blood is usually a visual confirmation that the arterial sample has been correctly collected. These features may be less noticeable or absent if the patient has severe respiratory failure or low blood pressure.

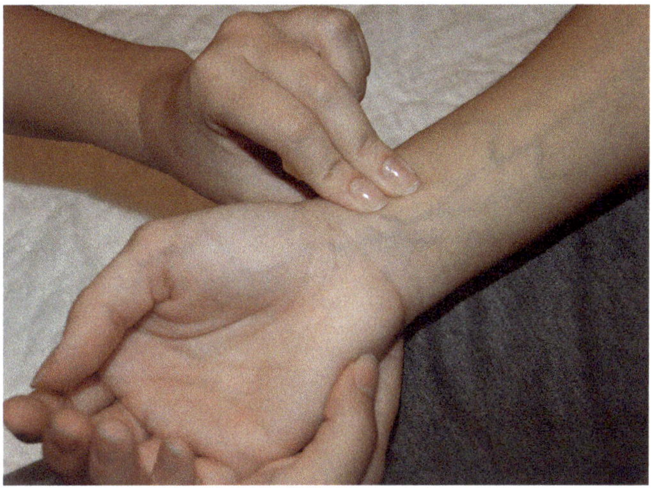

Fig. 13.2: Detection of the radial artery. Index and middle fingers are placed half way between the tendons that run down the center of the forearm and the edge of the thumb side of the arm, down at the wrist, pressing lightly.

While removing the needle from the artery, you should put a sterile gauze over the puncture site and apply a pressure. It is preferable to apply a medical tape to keep the pressure on the gauze for several minutes to obtain hemostasis.

A different site (e.g. the contralateral radial artery) should be used if ABGA needs to be repeated. The insertion

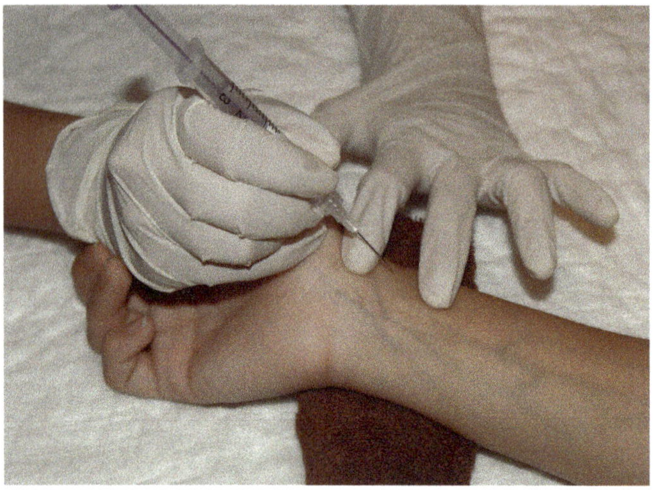

Fig. 13.3: Radial artery puncture for ABGA. The needle is inserted at 30–45 degrees angle at a point just below the index and middle fingers of the operator's nondominant hand.
(ABGA: Arterial blood gas analysis).

of an arterial line can be useful if you expect to perform ABGA repeatedly. Table 13.1 reassumes the main advantages and disadvantages of arterial puncture and arterial line use.

Complications of arterial puncture are not common and include arteriospasm, artery damage, prolonged bleeding, infection, thrombosis, hematoma and vasovagal response.

Pain, numbness or paresthesia from inadvertent puncture of radial nerve may occur mainly when multiple punctures are performed.

Preanalytical Phase

The preanalytical phase, that is the phase which precedes the transfer of the blood sample in the analyzer, is crucial since it is mainly responsible for errors in the measurement of arterial blood gases.

An arterial blood sample provides information about the status of the patient at the time of sampling. Many of the measured parameters can vary significantly even within a few seconds. It is therefore recommended to correlate the values of arterial blood gas analysis with respiratory and circulatory parameters recorded at time of arterial blood sampling.

The syringe for arterial blood sampling is usually prepacked and contains heparin in an amount sufficient to prevent coagulation. If the syringe is not properly heparinized, clot can form inside it, block the analyzer or cause inaccurate measurement of pCO_2, pH, and hemoglobin.

It is recommended to use pre-heparinized syringes with anhydrous (dry) heparin. The heparin in solution (liquid) dilutes the sample and causes an underestimation of the actual values.

Moreover, if electrolytes are measured, balanced heparin for the electrolytes should be used to avoid errors in the results, since unbalanced heparin interferes with the measurement of electrolytes by binding with cations, for example with calcium or potassium.

Immediately after sampling, any air bubbles inadvertently introduced during sampling must be promptly evacuated. To do so, the syringe held vertically and taped,

Table 13.1: Advantages and disadvantages of samples collected by arterial puncture or by aspiration from an indwelling arterial catheter.

Arterial puncture	*Arterial line*
Advantages	
• Less risk of bias than arterial-line and capillaries if performed correctly	• Easy to obtain samples because of indwelling line
• Can be carried out in an emergency situation	• Not painful to the patient
• No catheter needed	• Elimination of risk associated with multiple punctures
• Requires less blood volume than catheter sampling	
Disadvantages	
• Painful to the patient, hyperventilation can potentially change blood gas values	• Risk of infection with invasive catheter
• It can be difficult to locate arteries	• Risk of clotting leading to thromboses or emboli
• Risk of complications for the patient, not always advisable to perform arterial puncture	• Risk of anemia because too much blood is removed (typically 5–6 mL per sample including waste)
• User safety—risk of needle stick accidents	• Risk of locally diminished or blocked blood flow leading to necrosis
• Requires trained/authorized personnel	• Risk of air contamination from catheter connections, etc.
	• Risk of dilution errors if catheter is flushed insufficiently

while its tip is covered with a piece of gauze. When the air bubbles have been expelled, the sample should be closed with a tip cap and mixed thoroughly to dissolve the heparin. In room air at sea level, partial pressure of O_2 (pO_2) is approximately 150 mm Hg and partial pressure of CO_2 (pO_2) is 0 mm Hg. Consequently, air bubbles that mix and equilibrate with arterial blood sample tend to increase its values of pO_2 and to reduce those of pCO_2.

A label identifying the patient should be placed on the syringe together with other information which can affect the interpretation of the ABGA, such as patient temperature and *fraction of inspired oxygen* (FiO_2).

Generally, by entering the patient temperature into the blood gas instrument when analyzing the sample, the analyzer will be able to display temperature corrected results. FiO_2 allows to calculate the *shunt fraction (Fshunt)* that in normal subjects is less than 0.05 (<5%). In pathological conditions the shunt fraction is significantly greater and even breathing 100% oxygen does not fully oxygenate the blood. Thus, giving pure oxygen at 100% for 20 minutes does not raise the arterial pressure of O_2; this is because although the PO_2 of alveolar gas (PAO_2) has been changed by giving pure supplemental O_2, the PaO_2 will not increase that much because the V/Q mismatch still exists and it will still add some de-oxygenated blood to the arterial system via the shunt. Because shunt represents areas where gas exchange does not occur, 100% inspired oxygen is unable to overcome the hypoxia caused by shunting.

$$\frac{Q_S}{Q_T} = \frac{(P_AO_2 - P_3O_2)\times(0.003)}{4+(P_4O_2 - P_aO_2)\times(0.003)}$$

Where the constant 4 is the assumed arteriovenous difference in volume%, and 0.003 is the solubility coefficient of oxygen in plasma at 37°.

Less than 10%	=	normal lungs
10–20%	=	minimal effect
20–30%	=	significant pulmonary disease
Greater than 30%	=	life-threatening

In general, samples should be analyzed as quickly as possible to minimize the effects of continued metabolism, diffusion of oxygen through the plastic sampler and potassium leakage from red blood cells. If it is not possible to analyze the sample immediately, it must be analyzed within 30 minutes after collection. The recommended storage temperature is room temperature.

The practice of placing the syringe in a container with ice after collection, which was historically performed to prevent metabolic consumption of oxygen, is no longer recommended for plastic syringes.

Just before analysis, it is important to mix the sample thoroughly by repeatedly, to ensure that the part of the sample that is transferred to the analyzer is homogeneous and representative of the whole sample. If not, significant errors can occur, particularly on the hemoglobin parameters.

Parameter Description

Minor differences may exist in the reference ranges for blood gases parameters according to different analysers and laboratories. The most commonly used normal ranges are reported in Table 13.2.

Arterial Blood Gases

Arterial oxygen tension express the partial pressure of oxygen in a gas phase in equilibrium with the blood. It is usually indicated as pO_2, but depending on the sample, the symbol used may be $pO_2(a)$ for arterial blood or $pO_2(v)$ for mixed venous blood.

The arterial oxygen tension is an indicator of the oxygen uptake in the lungs. High and low pO_2 values of arterial blood indicate hyperoxemia and hypoxemia, respectively. The classification of hypoxemia severity is arbitrary: the cut-off point or normality at sea level is about 80 mm Hg, while there is respiratory failure when PaO_2 is below 60 mm Hg. This value of PaO_2 has been chosen because of physiology: it is the critical point in which the sigmoidal (S-shaped) HbO_2 saturation curve becomes steeper and when PaO_2 is below 60 mm Hg small changes in PaO_2 are associated with large changes in hemoglobin saturation, thus in arterial oxygen content. When the value of pO_2 is between 60 mm Hg and 79 mm Hg, generally the patient is considered to have mild hypoxemia; a value between 45 mm Hg and 59 mm Hg is indicative of moderate hypoxemia; values less than 45 mm Hg express severe hypoxemia.

The normal range for pO_2 is affected by age and altitude. Due to a worsening of ventilation-perfusion ratio, normal PO_2 declines with advancing age. In order to estimate this decrease, several reference equations have been created based by analyzing healthy lifetime nonsmokers; some disparity in the results exists due to heterogeneous study populations and not uniform study conditions. One of the simplest formula to calculate the normal value of pO_2 expected for age is the following:

$$pO_2 = 109 - 0.43\,(\text{age in years})$$

Unfortunately, many traditional reference studies did not include adequate samples of subjects over age 60, yet

Table 13.2: Reference ranges for the main arterial blood gas parameters.

		Alternative unit of measure
pH	7.35–7.45	
PaO_2*	83–108 mm Hg	11.1–14.4 kPa
$PaCO_2$	35–45 mm Hg	4.7–6.0 kPa
HCO_3^-	22–26 mmol/L	
Base excess	–2 to +2 mmol/L	
ctO_2	7.1–9.9 mmol/L	15.8–22.3 mL/dL
p50	25–29 mm Hg	3.3–3.9 kPa
Anion Gap (K+)	10–20 mmol/L	
Lactate	0.5–1.6 mmol/L	(4.5–14.4 mg/dL)

* Age and altitude dependent (*see* text).
(kPa: Kilopascals: to convert pressures to kPa, divide mm Hg by 7.5).

they were used to extrapolate beyond age 60 the downward trend in PaO_2 seen in those studied from ages 40 to 60. Studies of elderly persons show this assumption of linear decline to be incorrect because a survival effect. Mean PaO_2 remains relatively constant at 83 mm Hg from age 65-90 in healthy elderly persons at sea level. These results suggest that oxygen saturation also does not change over this age range.

At elevations above sea level, the partial pressure of inspired oxygen reduces, and the normal PO_2 decreases concomitantly. For example, the predicted normal pO_2 of a healthy young subject is approximately 95 mm Hg at sea level, whereas it is about 80 mm Hg at 1,500 meters.

The Alveolar-arterial gradient (*A-aO_2* or *A-a gradient*), is the difference between the alveolar and the arterial concentration of oxygen (PAO_2-PaO_2). Its determination helps to determine the efficiency of the lungs in transferring oxygen from the inspired air to the blood. To calculate A-a gradient, the PaO_2 is obtained from the ABG, while the PAO_2 is obtained from the alveolar gas equation: $PAO_2 = (760 - 47) \times FiO_2 - PaCO_2/0.8$ (or 1). Normal A-a gradient is 20 in a health young person.

The ratio of partial pressure arterial oxygen and fraction of inspired oxygen (*PaO_2/FiO_2 ratio or P/F ratio*) is another index useful to assess the integrity of alveolar-capillary unit. It is easier to calculate than A-a gradient, since it does not require the alveolar gas equation. Normal PaO_2/FiO_2 is 300-500. Values lower than 250 indicate a clinically significant gas exchange derangement. According to the major scientific societies, a PaO_2/FiO_2 ratio less than or equal to 300 is necessary for the diagnosis of acute respiratory distress syndrome.

Arterial carbon dioxide tension is defined as the carbon dioxide partial pressure in a gas phase in equilibrium with the blood. High and low values of pCO_2 in the arterial blood indicate blood hypercapnia and hypocapnia, respectively. It is usually indicated as pCO_2, but depending on the sample, the symbol used may be $pCO_2(a)$ for arterial blood or $pCO_2(v)$ for mixed venous blood.

$pCO_2(a)$ reference range for adult is a bit lower in females (32-45 mm Hg than in males (35-48 mm Hg). Normally, carbon dioxide in the inspired air is almost zero, and pCO_2 directly reflects the adequacy of alveolar ventilation in relation to the metabolic rate.

Low pCO_2 (hypocapnia) is due to alveolar hyperventilation and may cause respiratory alkalosis. Possible causes include excessive ventilator treatment, psychogenic hyperventilation, compensation to metabolic acidosis, central nervous system affection, hypoxia. High pCO_2 (hypercapnia) is due to alveolar hypoventilation and may cause respiratory acidosis. Possible causes include various lung diseases, central nervous system depression, either primary, or secondary to sedation or analgesics. It is often part of the therapeutic strategy to accept or aim for values that are lower or higher than the reference range.

Arterial Blood pH

The value of pH is the negative logarithm of the hydrogen ion activity ($pH = -\log[H^+]$). It indicates the acidity or alkalinity of the blood. The normal function of many metabolic processes requires a pH to be within a relatively narrow range, thus its measurement is an essential part of the ABGA.

Depending on the sample, the symbol used may be pH(a) for arterial blood or pH(v) for mixed venous blood.

The reference range for pH(a) in adults is 7.35-7.45. A reduction in the pH(a) to values lower than 7.35 is defined *acidosis*. If this is supported by inadequate ventilation with consequent hypercapnia (increased pCO_2), you can diagnose a *respiratory acidosis*. If such a condition persists for several days, renal bicarbonate excretion will decrease and acidosis will be partly or totally compensated for by increased bicarbonate concentration in the blood. Common causes of acute respiratory acidosis include asthma and chronic obstructive pulmonary disease (COPD) exacerbation, pulmonary edema, depression of the central respiratory center by cerebral disease (e.g. trauma, stroke, hemorrhage, neoplasm) or drugs (e.g. opiates, sedatives, anesthetics), neuromuscular disorders (e.g. Guillain-Barré syndrome, Myasthenia gravis, amyotrophic lateral sclerosis, muscular dystrophy, muscle relaxant drugs, toxins such as organophosphates and snake venom), cervical cord trauma or lesions at or above C4 level, tetanus, over-production of CO_2 due to hypercatabolic disorders (e.g. malignant hyperthermia), increased intake of CO_2 (Rebreathing of CO_2-containing expired gas, insufflation of CO_2 into body cavity for laparoscopic surgery).

Chronic respiratory acidosis may be secondary to many disorders, including COPD, restrictive ventilatory defects (e.g. lung interstitial diseases or thoracic deformities), obesity hypoventilation syndrome (i.e. Pickwickian syndrome) and inadequate mechanical ventilation. Hypoventilation in COPD involves multiple mechanisms, including a decreased responsiveness to hypoxia and hypercapnia, increased ventilation-perfusion mismatch leading to increased dead space ventilation, and decreased diaphragmatic function due to fatigue and hyperinflation.

When pH reduction is sustained by a reduction of plasma concentration of bicarbonates (HCO_3^-) or more in general of the bases, you can diagnose a *metabolic acidosis*. If the patient is spontaneously breathing, this condition is usually partly compensated for by hyperventilation which results in low pCO_2. Common causes of metabolic acidosis include renal failure, ketoacidosis (diabetic, alcoholic starvation), gastrointestinal loss of bicarbonate (longstanding diarrhea), lactic acidosis due to hypoxia and hypoperfusion, drugs (e.g. Metformin, Isoniazid), impaired carbohydrate metabolism.

A pH(a) greater than 7.45 defines a situation of *alkalosis*. A *respiratory alkalosis* is due to the reduction of pCO_2 for alveolar hyperventilation. This can occur as a consequence of head injury, stroke, anxiety, pain, fear, stress, iatrogenic causes (e.g. excessive controlled ventilation).

A metabolic alkalosis is caused by the increase of bicarbonates and bases, and can occur as a consequence of a renal loss of hydrogenions (e.g. patients taking diuretic drugs, hyperaldosteronism) or with gastrointestinal loss of acid (vomiting). Spontaneously breathing patients may decrease their alveolar ventilation slightly to compensate the alkalosis with a slightly increased pCO_2. A metabolic alkalosis can be also observed in patients with chronic hypercapnia and higher bicarbonate levels due to a renal compensation, if CO_2 levels quickly return to baseline after medical therapy or mechanical ventilation.

Both acidosis and alkalosis can be *mixed* when respiratory and metabolic causes are simultaneously present. Moreover, because of the compensatory mechanisms, a pH value in the normal range does not exclude the presence of an acid-base imbalance, whereas the simultaneous evaluation of pCO_2 and $cHCO_3^-$ is required.

Acid-base Status

Actual bicarbonate, indicate as HCO_3^- or $cHCO_3^-$ (P), is the concentration of bicarbonate (hydrogen carbonate) in the plasma of the sample. It is calculated by entering the measured values of pH and pCO_2 in the Henderson-Hasselbalch equation.

$cHCO_3^-$ (P) *reference range for adults is 21-28 mmol/L.* An increased level of HCO_3^- may be due to a metabolic alkalosis or a compensatory response in respiratory acidosis. Decreased levels of HCO_3^- are seen in metabolic acidosis and as a compensatory mechanism in respiratory alkalosis.

Standard bicarbonate, indicated with the symbol *SBC* or *$cHCO_3^-$ (P,st),* is the concentration of hydrogen carbonate in plasma from blood which is equilibrated with a gas mixture with pCO_2= 40 mm Hg (5.3 kPa) and pO_2 100 mm Hg (13.3 kPa) at 37°C. The equilibration of fully oxygenated blood with a pCO_2 of 40 mm Hg (5.3 kPa) is an attempt to eliminate the respiratory component in the acid-base status. In these circumstances, a low standard bicarbonate indicates a metabolic acidosis, and an elevated standard bicarbonate indicates a metabolic alkalosis.

Actual base excess (BE) is the concentration of titratable base when the blood is titrated with a strong base or acid to a plasma pH of 7.40 at a pCO_2 of 40 mm Hg (5.3 kPa) and 37°C at the actual oxygen saturation. Base excess (BE) corresponds to the mmol/L of base that needs to be removed to bring the pH back to normal when pCO_2 is corrected to 40 mm Hg. It is often abbreviated and symbolized as BE. A negative base excess indicates a base deficit or an acid excess in the blood.

Standard base excess is an in vivo expression of base excess. It refers to a model of the extracellular fluid (one part of the blood is diluted by two parts of its own plasma) and is calculated using one third of the *c*tHb for blood in the formula. Alternatively, a standard value for the hemoglobin concentration of the total extracellular fluid (including blood) of 3 mmol/L can be used. SBE is the base excess in the total extracellular fluids, of which blood represents approximately one-third. Buffering capacities differ in the extracellular compartments, which makes the SBE more representative of the in vivo base excess compared to actual BE.

Anion gap is the concentration difference between the cations (sodium and potassium), and the measured anions (chloride and bicarbonate):

Anion Gap $= cNa^+ + cK^+ - cCl^- - cHCO_3^-$.

Normally, anion gap in healthy adults is comprised between 10 mmol/L and 20 mmol/L. Anion gap is a reflection of the unmeasured anions in the plasma, e.g. proteins, organic acids, sulfates and phosphates (although changes in plasma calcium and magnesium also affect the anion gap). Anion Gap may be an aid in the differential diagnosis of metabolic acidosis.

Metabolic acidosis can be classified into two groups:

1. Those with an increase in the anion gap, thus implying the presence of increased amounts of organic acid.
2. Those with normal anion gap, due to loss of bicarbonate.

Decreased anion gap can be caused by:

- Decrease in plasma proteins
- Hyponatremia
- Increase in unmeasured cations.

Increased anion gap can be caused by:

- Ketoacidosis
- Lactoacidosis
- Renal failure
- Intoxication with: salicylate, methanol, and ethylene glycol.

Causes of metabolic acidosis with a normal anion gap include:

- Diarrhea
- Uremic acidosis of recent onset
- Renal tubular acidosis
- Ureterosigmoidostomy

Other Parameters

Arterial concentration of total oxygen (ctO_2), commonly called "O_2 content", is the concentration of the total oxygen in the blood, which comprises of the hemoglobin-bound and physically dissolved oxygen. The hemoglobin-bound oxygen is the large majority of the about 20.5 mL of O_2/100 mL of blood, that is the O_2 content for a normal adult male, while only about 0.3–0.5 mL are in solution. The oxygen content of the blood is an expression of the oxygen transport properties of the blood. It reflects the integrated effects of changes in the arterial pO_2, the effective hemoglobin concentration, and the hemoglobin affinity for oxygen as expressed in the *p*50.

It is calculated by: (O_2 carried by Hb) + (O_2 in solution) = (1.34 × Hb × SpO_2 × 0.01) + (0.023 × PaO_2), where SO_2 = percentage saturation of Hb with oxygen; Hb = hemoglobin concentration in grams per 100 mL blood; PO_2 = partial pressure of oxygen (0.0225 = mL of O_2 dissolved/100 mL plasma/kPa, or 0.003 mL/mm Hg).

Oxygen tension at 50% saturation of blood (p50) is the oxygen tension at half saturation (50%) of blood and is calculated from the measured oxygen tension and oxygen saturation by extrapolation along the oxygen dissociation curve to 50% saturation. The *p*50 reflects the affinity of hemoglobin for oxygen. The position of the oxygen dissociation curve is dependent primarily on the pH, but several physical and chemical changes may affect hemoglobin affinity for oxygen.

Concentration of total hemoglobin (ctHb) is the concentration of total hemoglobin in blood, including all types of hemoglobin, such as Deoxyhemoglobin (HHb), oxyhemoglobin (O_2Hb), carboxy-hemoglobin (COHb), methemoglobin (MetHb). In most analyzers, the very rare and non-oxygen-carrying sulfhemoglobin is not included in the reported *c*tHb.

Thus, *c*tHb = cO_2Hb + *c*HHb + *c*COHb + *c*MetHb

*c*tHb is a measure of the potential oxygen-carrying capacity, whereas the actual oxygen capacity is defined by the effective hemoglobin (*c*tHb minus the dyshemoglobins). High values of *c*tHb (polycythemia) may be primary (polycythemia vera) or secondary to dehydration, chronic hypoxemia, or regular intense aerobic physical activity. These conditions involve a high blood viscosity, which increases the afterload to the heart. Low concentrations of *c*tHb (anemia) may be primary (impaired red cell production) or secondary to hemolysis, bleeding, dilution (overhydration). These conditions imply a risk of tissue hypoxia because of the lowered arterial oxygen content (ctO_2).

Fraction of oxyhemoglobin (FO_2Hb) is the ratio between the concentrations of O_2Hb and all hemoglobins present (tHb) including dyshemoglobins. It is a measure of the utilization of the potential oxygen transport capacity, and is calculated as follows:

FO_2Hb = cO_2Hb/cO_2Hb + *c*HHb + *c*COHb + *c*MetHb

It is normally comprised between *94% and 98%*.

It should be emphasized that not all the blood gas analyzer are provided with the CO-oximeter that allows to detect the COHb. Unfortunately, when the analyzer calculates the patient's oxygen saturation levels from the oxygen partial pressure (PO_2), the arterial SaO_2 may appear normal. Thus CO exposure and CO-poisoned patients may be misdiagnosed delaying treatment and even returning vulnerable patients and their families to potentially lethal environments. Moreover, conventional pulse oximeters

Flowchart 13.1: Example of algorithm for the interpretation of the ABGA.

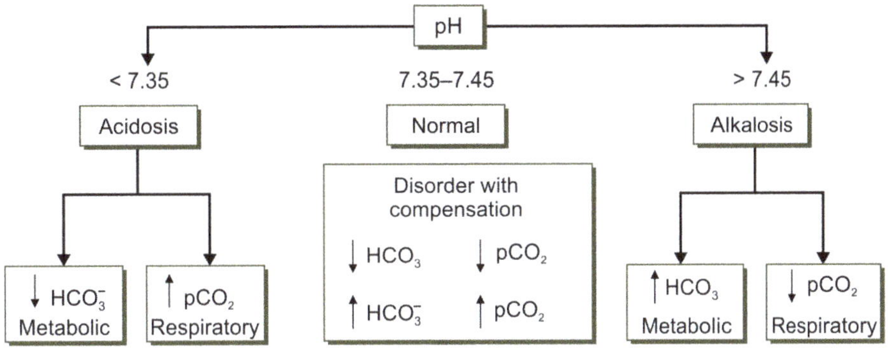

are incapable of isolating the carbon monoxide contaminated Hb from the HbO_2. Thus, pulse oximeters artificially overestimate arterial oxygen saturation in the presence of elevated blood carbon monoxide. Therefore, the readings will be falsely high when carbon monoxide is occupying binding sites on the heme molecule.

Lactate is one of the metabolites commonly assessed by an ABGA, used as a marker of critical imbalance between tissue oxygen demand and oxygen supply. Inadequate oxygen supply, in most cells of the body, cause a shift from normal aerobic to anaerobic metabolism with production of excessive amounts of lactate. In most situations, elevated blood lactate will be caused by hypoperfusion, severely impaired arterial oxygen supply, or a combination of the two. Monitoring of lactate is a way to monitor the adequacy of treatment of the critically ill patient. Decreasing or persistently low levels of blood lactate during critical illness is considered a signal of successful treatment. ABGA often provides arterial concentration of the main electrolytes, such as potassium (K^+), sodium (Na^+), chlorine (Cl^-) and calcium (Ca^{2+}). Table 13.2 shows reference ranges for the main arterial blood gases parameters with alternative unit of measure.

Strategy for Interpretation of Results

Many strategies have been proposed to guide the interpretation of ABGA (Flowchart 13.1). The following five-step process may be used to ensure a complete interpretation ABGA.

1. Assess acid-base status

Look at the pH value: If the pH level is below 7.35, the condition of acidosis is present, if the pH level is above 7.45, the condition of alkalosis is present. A value between 3.5 and 4.5 indicates a normal pH; this may be due to the absence of problems affecting the acid-base balance, or to an abnormal acid-base status with metabolic or respiratory compensation.

2. Determine if the disturbance is respiratory or metabolic

Verify that pCO_2 and plasma HCO_3^- (or BE) values are within their normal range. Abnormal pCO_2 indicates a respiratory involvement, while abnormal amount of HCO_3^- or BE indicates a metabolic involvement. These parameters should be evaluated in light of the arterial pH.

Values of pH lower than 3.5 may be due to an increase of pCO_2 (>45 mm Hg) when a respiratory cause is underlying (respiratory acidosis) or to a reduction of HCO_3^- (< 22 mmol/L) or BE (< –2 mmol/L) when a metabolic cause is underlying (metabolic acidosis). On the other hand, values of pH higher than 4.5 may be due to a reduction of pCO_2 (<35 mm Hg) when a respiratory cause is underlying (respiratory alkalosis) or to an increase of HCO_3^- (>26 mmol/L) or BE (>2 mmol/L) when a metabolic cause is underlying (metabolic alkalosis).

Plotting the values of pH, pCO_2, and HCO_3^- in an acid-base chart like shown in Figure 13.4 may help the identification of acid-base disturbances.

3. Assess for compensation

Once the acid-base disorder is identified as respiratory or metabolic, you should assess if a compensation occurs and its degree. The system that is not primarily responsible for the acid-base abnormality tries to restore the pH to the normal range.

In respiratory acidosis (low pH due to high pCO_2), the compensatory mechanism is a reduction of renal

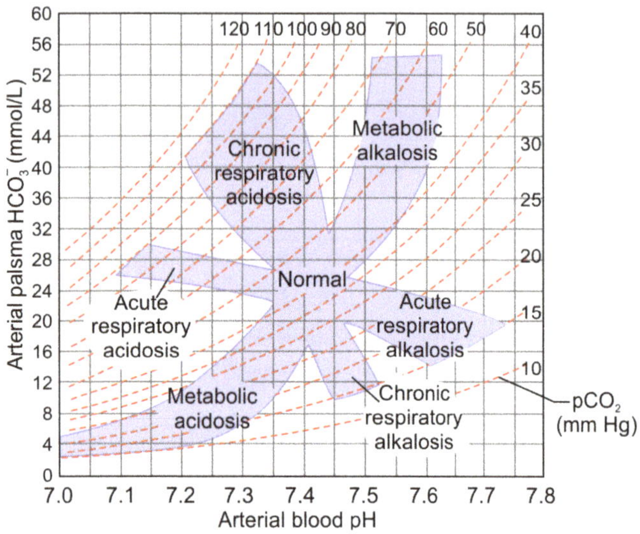

Fig. 13.4: Acid-base diagram.

bicarbonate excretion, with consequent increase of plasma HCO_3^- concentration, while respiratory alkalosis (high pH due to low pCO_2), elicits a compensatory decrease in plasma HCO_3^-.

Since the kidneys respond within hours/days, an acute or acute-on-chronic respiratory failure with increase of pCO_2 initially involve a uncompensated respiratory acidosis.

A metabolic acidosis (low pH due to low HCO_3^-) elicits a respiratory compensation with hyperventilation and consequent decrease in pCO_2, while a metabolic alkalosis (high pH due to high HCO_3^-) causes a compensatory hypoventilation and increase in pCO_2.

We can observe a *complete compensation* when pH is brought into the normal range or a *partial compensation* when pH is still out of the normal range but is in the process of moving toward the normal range.

When interpreting ABGS, it should be noted that the body never overcompensates. Thus, if you observe a pH lower than 7.35, pCO_2 below 35, and HCO_3^- below 22, it is unlikely that the primary disorder is a respiratory alkalosis and that a renal compensation causes a fall of pH to the values of acidosis. On the contrary, this situation usually reflects a metabolic acidosis, due to loss of bicarbonate, with partial respiratory compensation (hyperventilation).

4. Assess the oxygenation status

The PaO_2 does not affect the acid-base balance, but its evaluation is essential, as most of the organs including brain and heart, constantly need oxygen. Hypoxemia in the absence of hypercapnia defines type I respiratory failure, while hypoxemia and hypercapnia define type II respiratory failure.

When assessing the patient's PaO_2 you need to consider it in the context of inspired oxygen.

Indeed, the interpretation of values of pO_2 in the normal range is very different if observed in a patient breathing room air (fraction of inspired oxygen 21%) or 50% oxygen.

Roughly, the difference between the partial pressure of inspired oxygen and PaO_2 should be less than 10 kPa (75 mm Hg) because of the alveolar-arterial (A-a) gradient. Since the fraction of oxygen in room air is 21% (about 21 kPa or 157 mm Hg), we would expect the PaO_2 in the blood to be at least 11 kPa (about 83 mm Hg).

A greater difference is probably due to an impaired efficiency of oxygen transfer from alveoli to blood (e.g. ventilation/perfusion mismatch).

5. If a metabolic acidosis exists, calculate the anion gap

PULSE OXIMETRY

Pulse oximetry is a noninvasive method for determining an oxygen saturation through absorption spectrophotometry. Oxygen delivery to the tissues is a direct function of cardiac output, oxygen capacity (hemoglobin concentration) and the oxygen affinity of the patient's hemoglobin. When both cardiac output and Hb values are normal, measurement of oxygen saturation is a valuable measure of both oxygen exchange and delivery.

The principle of pulse oximetry is based on the different red and infrared light absorption of oxygenated hemoglobin (*oxyhemoglobin*: O_2Hb) and reduced hemoglobin (*Deoxyhemoglobin*: HHb).

Oxyhemoglobin absorbs more infrared light and allows more red light to pass through. Conversely, HHb absorbs more red light and allows more infrared light to pass through.

Pulse oximeters use a light emitter with red and infrared LEDs that shines through a reasonably translucent site with good blood flow. Typical adult/pediatric sites are the finger, toe, pinna (top) or lobe of the ear. Infant sites are the foot or palm of the hand and the big toe or thumb. Opposite the emitter is a photodetector that receives the light that passes through the measuring site.

While noninvasive monitoring of gas exchange efficiency by pulse oximetry is simple, effective and increasingly widely used, it cannot replace ABGA in many circumstances. In fact, pulse oximetry is exclusively an appraise of oxygen saturation and provides no indication about blood pH, CO_2, and HCO_3^- concentrations.

TRANSCUTANEOUS OXYGEN AND CARBON DIOXIDE MEASUREMENT

Transcutaneous oxygen and carbon dioxide (respectively indicated as $tcpO_2$ and $tcpCO_2$) is a local, noninvasive measurement reflecting the amount of O_2 and CO_2 that diffuse from the capillaries, through the epidermis, to an electrode at the measuring site. It provides instant, continuous information about the body's ability to deliver oxygen to the tissue. $tcpO_2$ is dependent on oxygen uptake in the respiratory system, the oxygen transport/capacity of the blood and the general status of the circulatory system. Any impairment of the organism's ability to deliver oxygen to the tissue will be revealed immediately since the skin is ranked very low in the body's system of oxygenation priority.

$tcpO_2$ and $tcpCO_2$ are based on the principle that a heating element in the electrode elevates the temperature of the underlying tissues. This increases the capillary blood flow and the pCO_2, and makes the skin permeable to gas diffusion. It should be remembered that the electrode is measuring the gas tensions of the underlying tissue and not the arterial gas tension. When hemodynamic conditions are stable, the transcutaneous measurements correlate well with arterial values but are not identical.

Technically, the electrode heats the underlying tissue to create a local hyperemia, which intensifies the blood perfusion, increasing the oxygen pressure. In addition, the heat will dissolve the lipid structure of the dead, keratinized cells in the epidermal layer making the skin permeable to gas diffusion. On its way the oxygen may be consumed by the cells if the metabolism is high.

It should be noted that $tcpO_2$ is not the same as the arterial oxygen saturation measured using standard pulse oximeters.

It was initially believed that Ptc, O_2 measurements would not be satisfactory in adults due to their thicker epidermis, but subsequent studies have shown that this technology may work just as well for older children and adults.

In the case of Ptc, CO_2, the elevated temperature at which the transcutaneous electrode operates in order to increase skin permeability will also raise skin metabolism and lead to an increase in CO_2 production. The measured values will, therefore, be significantly higher than arterial values at 37°C. The transcutaneous values can be temperature corrected, thus enabling a readout of values comparable to those at the normal body temperature.

Continuous monitoring of Ptc, CO_2 during sleep may be considered if nocturnal CO_2 retention is to be documented. Transcutaneous monitoring of pCO_2 has been a useful measurement in patients with respiratory failure due to COPD.

The main problem with the use of transcutaneous monitoring is the need to change the site of the electrode to prevent thermal skin trauma if an electrode temperature higher than 43°C is employed. It is possible to obtain effective Ptc, CO_2 at lower temperatures (42°C) giving a site time of up to 8 hours.

The transcutaneous methods of measuring CO_2 require a calibration procedure.

BIBLIOGRAPHY AND FURTHER READING

1. Andrews T, Waterman H. What factors influence arterial blood gas sampling patterns? Nurs Crit Care. 2008;13:132-7.
2. Cinar O, Acar YA, Arziman I, Kilic E, Eyi YE, Ocal R. Can mainstream end-tidal carbon dioxide measurement accurately predict the arterial carbon dioxide level of patients with acute dyspnea in ED. Am J Emerg Med. 2012;30(2):358-61.
3. Geoffrey Baird. Preanalytical considerations in blood gas analysis. Biochemia Medica. 2013;23(1):19-27.
4. Hedberg P, Majava A, Kiviluoma K, Ohtonen P. Potential preanalytical errors in whole-blood analysis: Effect of syringe sample volume on blood gas, electrolyte and lactate values. Scand J Clin Lab Invest. 2009;69:585-91.
5. Howe TA, Jaalam K, Ahmad R, Sheng CK, Nik Ab Rahman NH. The use of end-tidal capnography to monitor non-intubated patients presenting with acute exacerbation of asthma in the emergency department. J Emerg Med. 2011;41(6):581-9.
6. Küme T, Sişman AR, Solak A, Tuğlu B, Cinkooğlu B, Coker C. The effects of different syringe volume, needle size and sample volume on blood gas analysis in syringes washed with heparin. Biochem Med (Zagreb). 2012;22:189-201.
7. May TA, Clancy M, Critchfield J, Ebeling F, Enriquez A, Gallagher C, et al. Reducing unnecessary inpatient laboratory testing in a teaching hospital. Am J Clin Pathol. 2006;126(2):200-6.
8. Restrepo RD, Hirst KR, Wittnebel L, Wettstein R. AARC clinical practice guideline: transcutaneous monitoring of carbon dioxide and oxygen: 2012. Respir Care. 2012;-57(11):1955-62.
9. Rogers KM, McCutcheon K. Understanding arterial blood gases. J Perioper Pract. 2013;23(9):191-7.
10. Scott M, LeGrys V, Klutts J. Eletrolytes and blood gases. In: Burtis C, Ashwood E, Bruns D, (Eds). Tietz textbook of clinical chemistry and molecular diagnostics. St. Louis, MO: Elsevier Saunders; 2006. p. 1008.

Chapter 14

Cardiopulmonary Exercise Testing

Claudio Sorino, Ross Arena, Adriano Di Paco, Daniel Forman

OVERVIEW OF CARDIOPULMONARY EXERCISE TESTING AND MAIN INDICATIONS

The cardiopulmonary exercise test (CPET) is a noninvasive method that facilitates simultaneous assessments of the cardiovascular and respiratory systems at rest and then during exercise with a progressive workload on a cycle ergometer or treadmill. CPET provides an integrated evaluation of ventilation (air inhaled and exhaled), consumption of oxygen and removal of carbon dioxide (through the analysis of exhaled gases), heart rate, electrocardiogram, oxygen saturation and systemic arterial blood pressure, to provide a comprehensive perspective regarding lung, cardiac, vascular and muscle physiology.

Cardiopulmonary exercise test is a valuable tool in several clinical applications including populations that are healthy as well as patients contending with symptoms or known disease. Table 14.1 lists many of the circumstances when CPET is useful. More generally, CPET is a valuable tool for quantifying fitness among healthy adults, stratifying risk among known disease states, and helping with diagnosis when basic clinical data [e.g. history, physical examination, chest X-ray, resting pulmonary function tests and resting electrocardiogram (ECG)] fail to make this clear. Figures 14.1A and B illustrate a CPET being conducted on a cycle ergometer and a treadmill, respectively.

Table 14.1: Main indications for cardiopulmonary exercise test (CPET).

1. Assessment of exercise intolerance of unknown origin
2. Assessment of dyspnea of unknown origin
3. Assessment of cardiorespiratory fitness (for athletic assessment, disability or as a prognostic indicator)
4. Diagnostic, prognostic, and therapeutic efficacy evaluations in patients with cardiovascular disease (e.g. heart failure, coronary heart disease, valvular heart disease)
5. Diagnostic, prognostic, and therapeutic efficacy evaluations in patients with respiratory diseases (e.g. COPD, interstitial fibrosis, pulmonary hypertension)
6. Evaluation of the risk for patients before major surgery (particularly prior to lung resection)
7. Exercise prescription for cardiac and pulmonary rehabilitation and evaluation of post-rehabilitation improvements
8. Evaluation of disability status in patients with specific conditions
9. Evaluation for appropriateness of lung, heart or heart-lung transplantation listing

(COPD: Chronic obstructive pulmonary disease).

EQUIPMENT REQUIRED

Exercise Equipment

The CPET is most commonly carried out through one of two exercise modalities; a *cycle ergometer* or a motor-driven *treadmill*. A cycle ergometer is a stationary bicycle with the capacity to progressively increase pedaling resistance (typically measured as watt) and with an ergometer to measure the work done by the exerciser. A motor-driven treadmill is a device with a moving belt on which a person can walk or run. Work intensity on a treadmill is usually assessed in relation to the incline and speed of the treadmill. While cycle ergometers and treadmills each have proponents, each also has distinctive advantages in relation to specific CPET applications.

A cycle ergometer generates progressive pedaling resistance over time, and thereby increases physical work demands while a subject/patient exercises at a fixed rate. Compared to a treadmill, a cycle ergometer is generally less expensive and requires less space. Furthermore,

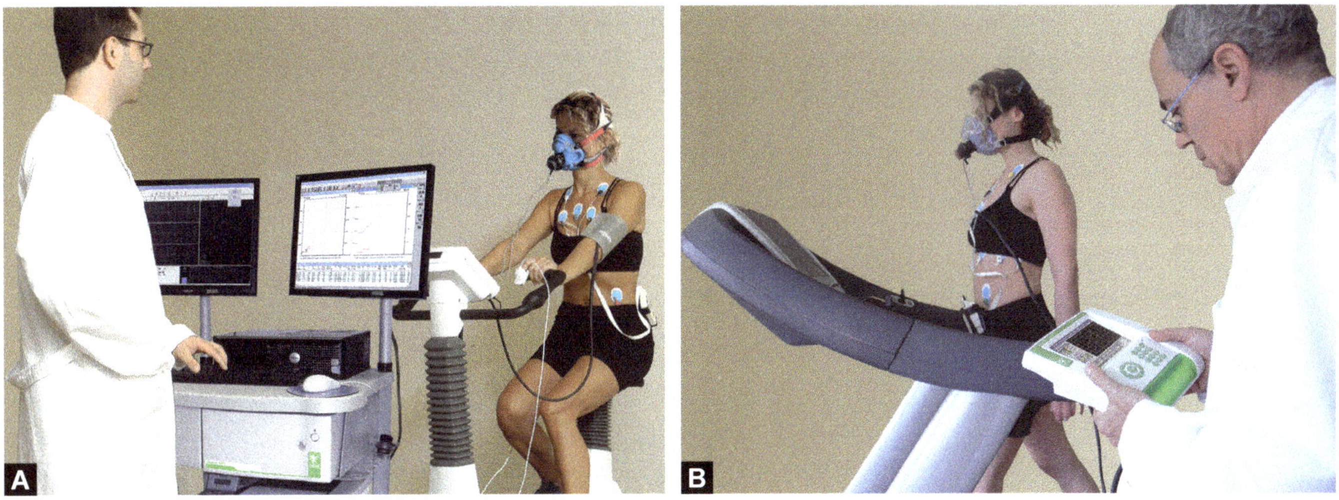

Figs. 14.1A and B: (A) CPET on a cycle ergometer and (B) a treadmill. In both cases, the patient is connected to a mask with a turbine to measure the expired gases, pulse oximeter, blood pressure cuff and ECG electrodes.
Source: COSMED (www.cosmed.com).
(CPET: Cardiopulmonary exercise test; ECG: Electrocardiogram).

performing a CPET on a cycle ergometer is a relatively more stable clinical situation than performing a CPET on a treadmill since the risks of falling are reduced as the subject/patient remains in seated position; this is particularly advantageous for patients prone to exercise-induced arrhythmia or dizziness (such as those with heart failure, valvular heart disease, or known arrhythmic histories). Compared to treadmill exercise, the seated position of a cycle ergometer is also less likely to be associated with movement artifacts that otherwise can distort ECG waveforms and blood pressure auscultation. The influence of body weight on a cycle ergometer is lower than treadmill, as metabolic demands for pedaling in obese subjects only slightly increases in relation to their weight.

Treadmill exercise generates a progressive rise in workload as speed and grade of the treadmill increase. Among the advantages of treadmill exercise testing is that walking/running is often a more familiar activity than cycling for those being assessed. Moreover, walking/running on a treadmill involves the work of a larger muscle mass and more work against gravity, and thereby leading to greater aggregate stress on the organ systems mediating the exercise response. This is valuable in athletes, in whom the determination of cardiorespiratory fitness is critical, but also in heart failure since key decisions in clinical management (e.g. medical treatment vs transplant) may pivot on maximal CPET performance indices, i.e. assessments that may be best discerned using a walking or jogging stimulus vs using a cycle ergometer. Similarly, the relatively higher work demands of treadmill over cycle-based exercise may help better induce abnormalities such as cardiac ischemia or arrhythmia that sometimes occur only at the uppermost metabolic demands. Treadmill exercise also better reflects the workload associated with elevated body weight.

A common criticism of standard treadmill exercise testing (without gas exchange) is the difficulty to precisely estimate the external workload of the subject during treadmill exercise, particularly due to variability of handrail use, as well as to differences in gait efficiency. However, CPET enables workload on a treadmill for each patient to be well-characterized in terms of the metabolic parameters (ventilation indices) that essentially surmount the limitations associated with traditional treadmill-based workload metrics, i.e. ventilation indices determined by CPET can reliably discern each patient's workload irrespective of differences in handrail use, gait efficiency or other individual patient idiosyncrasies.

Airflow or Volume Transducers

Several flow-transducing devices are available for an accurate measurement of ventilation parameters during exercise testing. They include pneumotachographs, mass flow sensors, pitot tube flow meters and turbine volume transducers. The choice of a flow versus a volume transducer is not crucial since one entity can be calculated from knowledge of the other.

Transducers employed for exercise testing should meet established standards by the American Thoracic

Society for flow and volume measurement during spirometry. They should be as lightweight as possible, with low dead space, low resistance to flow (at least in the range of flows occurred during exercise), and not affected by water vapor or pools of saliva that may gather during the test.

Accurate values for ventilation and metabolic parameters obtained from exercise testing are critically dependent on the accuracy of the flow-sensing device. For this reason, accurate calibration is essential and must be verified before each test.

Gas Analyzers

Two types of gas analyzers can be used: a mass spectrometer, which is considered the gold standard and is able to measure all the required respiratory gases [i.e. oxygen (O_2), carbon dioxide (CO_2) and, for some purposes, nitrogen (N_2)], and separate analyzers for O_2 and CO_2. The dynamics of analyzer measurement have two separable components: transport delay (the time needed for gas to go from the sampling site to the analyzer) and analyzer response (i.e. the kinetics of response to a change in the composition of gas conveyed into the analyzer). Computer software allows compensation for gas transport delay, generally on the order of 0.2–0.4 second, depending on the length of the gas-sampling tube and the gas-sampling rate.

Gas Exchange Measurement

Oxygen consumption and carbon dioxide production (VCO_2) each represent the difference between the volume of O_2 and CO_2 inhaled and exhaled per unit of time, respectively. Under steady state conditions, VO_2 and VCO_2 correspond to the rate of O_2 consumption and CO_2 production at the cellular level.

The Douglas Bag collection method is considered the gold standard for determining VO_2 and VCO_2, since it can be performed with simple and basic equipment, requiring only the measurement of large gas volumes and accurate measurement of gas concentrations without the need for rapidly responding gas analyzers. Potential errors in the Douglas bag method may arise from gas concentration analysis, bag residual volume and bag leakage or gas diffusion rates.

A continuous measurement of VO_2 and VCO_2 can also be estimated with a *gas-mixing chamber*: the subject breathes through a two-way valve and expired air is directed through a chamber (usually 5- to 15-L capacity) with baffles that facilitate mixing of the entering gas. The concentrations of CO_2 and O_2 are measured continuously at the distal end of the mixing chamber and averaged every 15–20 seconds. They are correlated with the volume of air exhaled, that is continuously measured by any of the above-mentioned flow devices and also usually averaged every 15–20 seconds. For the final report, the data should be averaged over 10–60 seconds, depending of the time for each stage of the exercise test and the variable being assessed. During steady state exercise, mixing chamber systems are capable of accurate metabolic rate measurements, but inaccurate calculations may occur during a continuously changing workload, due to misaligned volume and gas concentration signals.

However, for incremental protocols commonly used for clinical CPET, ventilation and mixed expired gas concentrations do not change rapidly and, therefore, the accuracy and precision of a well-designed mixing chamber may be comparable to those of the *breath-by-breath* gas analysis technique.

Advancing technology has facilitated the escalation of portable breath-by-breath gas analysis systems that measure gas volumes and concentrations continuously. This has become the most common gas analysis method. With breath-by-breath technique, a signal is measured proportional to expired airflow as well as signals proportional to fractional concentrations of CO_2 and O_2. Gases are sampled 50-100 times per second. In this way, each breath is decomposed into many parts and VO_2 and VCO_2 output are computed for each interval. These measurements are summed over the entire expiration to calculate the total volume of O_2 uptake and CO_2 per breath. The values of each breath are extrapolated to the minute. Such calculations must take into account water vapor, barometric pressure and ambient temperature variations.

Electrocardiographic Monitoring

Continuous display of ECG tracings with 12-lead ECG placement is essential to detect myocardial ischemia and cardiac arrhythmias during exercise. In some exercise tests, a 3-lead ECG may be used to monitor for rhythm disturbances and to screen for ischemia. The R-R interval of the ECG is habitually used to measure heart rate. It is recommended to use electrodes and detection electronics designed for movement artifact rejection. Silver or silver chloride ECG electrodes with circumferential adhesive provide good electrical contact and minimize movement artifacts.

PRETEST RECOMMENDATIONS

Patients performing the CPET should: have a light breakfast but be fasted for at least 2 hours prior to the test, take habitual medications, particularly nodal agents, avoid alcohol 24 hours prior to the test, avoid taking caffeine on the day of the test, abstain from smoking for at least 8 hours prior the test.

Patients should wear comfortable clothing for the test, including trainers/walking shoes, trousers or shorts and a top that avoid them to get too warm during the test.

Preliminary requirements for CPET may include the execution of simple spirometry and the maximal voluntary ventilation (MVV); lung volumes and diffusing capacity can be included if clinically warranted. Resting arterial blood gases should be considered, if feasible, if *pulse oximetry shows low values* oxyhemoglobin saturation (close to or lower than the lower limit of normal). A recent complete blood count and electrolytes are usually evaluated and consultation with a cardiologist is recommended for patients with a history of coronary artery disease.

Before starting CPET, absolute and relative contraindications to exercise testing must be reviewed (Table 14.2).

Table 14.2: Absolute contraindications to exercise testing.

Acute myocardial infarction (3–5 days) or unstable angina
Uncontrolled symptomatic arrhythmias
Active endocarditis
Acute myocarditis or pericarditis
Symptomatic severe aortic stenosis
Acute pulmonary embolism or DVT
Suspected dissecting aneurysm
Uncontrolled asthma
Uncontrolled pulmonary edema
Room air desaturation with SpO_2 <85%
Acute noncardiopulmonary disorder that may affect exercise performance (e.g. infection, orthopedic problem)
Mental impairment leading to inability to cooperate

TEST PROTOCOLS

Cardiopulmonary exercise test is routinely performed as an outpatient test. The time required for the execution of a complete CPET is approximately 1 hour, including time required for subject preparation, equipment calibration and post-CPET monitoring. The effective time in which the patient carries out the exercise is ideally between 8 and 12 minutes if the test is intended to induce maximal physical exertion. Before starting the test, the subject's main anthropometric parameters (i.e. sex, age, height, and weight), medical history and habitual physical activity should be recorded. A recent blood count affords the ability to rule out anemia or to detect polycythemia (sometimes an expression of chronic hypoxemia). Prior to testing, depending on test indication, spirometry for the assessment of lung volumes and flows, mainly forced expiratory volume in 1 second (FEV_1), forced vital capacity (FVC), forced expiratory flow 25-75% ($FEF_{25\text{-}75\%}$) peak expiratory flow (PEF), and inspiratory capacity (IC).

The subject is typically monitored by a 12 lead ECG, blood pressure cuff and pulse oximeter, prior to, during and post-testing. A facemask or snorkel with nose clip is connected to the flow meter and gas analyzer in order to assess VO_2 and VCO_2.

There are a number of protocols that can be used with either a cycle ergometer or a treadmill, which are categorized according the way in which the work rate is applied:

- Progressive incremental exercise, with a constant increase of work rate (every minute or continuous)
- Multistage exercise protocol (increase in work rate every 3 minutes, with relatively stable work at each level)
- Constant work rate (the same work rate, usually for 5-30 minutes)
- Discontinuous protocol, which consists of short periods (3-4 minutes) of constant work rate exercise separated by resting periods and with loads progressively increased (rarely used clinically).

Maximal incremental protocols are typically employed in clinical practice both with cycle ergometry and/or treadmill tests. A progressively increasing work rate protocol enables rapid acquisition of diagnostic data. Since the responses of the major variables [i.e. minute ventilation (VE), VO_2, and VCO_2] lag behind changes in work rate, it may be desirable to use a protocol in which work rate increases at a constant rate. For similar reasons, it may be preferable to begin the incremental phase of exercise from a baseline of unloaded pedaling ("0 W"), rather than rest.

A suggested incremental protocol on a cycle ergometer consists of 5 minutes of rest, 3 minutes of unloaded pedaling and then an incremental phase of exercise. Main ramp protocols involve increments in work rate at intervals of 10-60 seconds, with workload increases from 5 to 25 W/minute, depending on subject fitness level and estimated aerobic capacity. For debilitated patients, it is preferable to select low work rate increments (5–10 W/minute). On the contrary, for the subject who appears to be fit, work rate increments as high as 25–30 W/minute can be chosen. Computer-controlled, magnetically braked, cycle ergometers allow for a continuous increase in work rate, usually every 1–2 seconds in a ramp-like fashion. The protocol should be tailored to the individual to yield a fatigue-limited exercise duration between 8 and 12 minutes. CPET protocols tailored to a subject's baseline activity and/or clinical profile are usually more reliable than a standardized protocol for all. An example of cycle ergometer protocol is shown in Table 14.3. Tables 14.4 and 14.5 show examples of treadmill protocol respectively for people who weigh less than 80 kg or more than 80 kg.

Holding onto the treadmill handrails is often discouraged during exercise testing on a treadmill as handrail support reduces the subject's workload at any given level and alters (usually decreases) the metabolic cost of treadmill exercise. Nonetheless, handrail support may also be a source of stability to patients who are inherently unsteady on a treadmill and/or susceptible to exercise-induced instability. Fortunately, irrespective of differences in handrail use, CPET assessments can discriminate differences in workload, essentially accounting for any variability in treadmill testing that may develop from handrail use, gait efficiency or other methodological variability.

CPET PROCEDURE

Resting Phase of CPET

Pre-exercise systolic and diastolic *blood pressure* should be obtained and recorded. During measurement, the subject should be in a relaxed in a comfortably seated position without clothing in between the cuff and the arm. The correct cuff size for a given subjects arm should be chosen; the bladder width should encircle 40% of the circumference of the arm and there should be at least 2 cm between the bottom of the cuff and the brachial artery.

Heart rate and 12-lead ECG recordings should be started during the rest period and continued during CPET. Interpretation of cardiac rhythms and pattern interpretation on electrocardiograms need to be performed contemporaneously with exercise testing to ensure patient safety. Proper skin preparation is important to ensure a high-fidelity signal, free from motion artefact and electrical

Table 14.3: Example of CPET exercise worksheet for standard subject performing bicycle ergometry. Note that testing is commonly modified relative to baseline fitness.

Elapsed time (minutes)	*Work rate increase at 20 W/ minute*	*RPM (min-1)*	*HR*	*SpO_2 (%)*	*SBP (mm Hg)*	*DBP (mm Hg)*	*Borg dyspnea (1–10)*
–1 (Pre)	Rest	0					
5	Rest	0					
8	0 (unloaded)	60					
9	20	60					
10	40	60					
11	60	60					
12	80	60					
13	100	60					
14	120	60					
15	140	60					
16	160	60					
17	180	60					
18	200	60					
19	220	60					
20	240	60					
>20	+20/minute	60					

(W: Watts; HR: Heart rate; SpO_2: Oxygen saturation; SBP: Systolic blood pressure; DBP: Diastolic blood pressure).

Table 14.4: Example of treadmill protocol for subjects weighing less than 80 kg designed to mirror cycle ergometry with a ≈10 W/minute incremental protocol. Testing is commonly modified relative to baseline fitness.

Elapsed time (minute)	*Work rate (W)*	*Speed (mph)*	*Grade (%)*	*HR (bpm)*	*SpO_2 (%)*	*SBP (mm Hg)*	*DBP (mm Hg)*	*Borg dyspnea (1–10)*
-1 (Pre)	0	Rest	0					
5	5	0.8	2					
8	15	1	5					
9	24	1.1	7					
10	33	1.3	8.5					
11	43	1.5	9.5					
12	51	1.6	10.5					
13	60	1.8	11					
14	70	2	11.5					
15	80	2.2	12					
16	88	2.3	12.5					
17	100	2.5	13					
18	111	2.7	13.5					
19	123	2.9	14					
20	137	3.1	14.5					
21	150	3.3	15					
22	165	3.5	15.5					
>22	150	+0.2/minute	+0.5/minute					

(W: Watts; HR: Heart rate; SpO_2: Oxygen saturation; SBP: Systolic blood pressure; DBP: Diastolic blood pressure).

Table 14.5: Example of treadmill protocol for subjects weighing more than 80 kg designed to mirror cycle ergometry with a ≈10W/minute incremental protocol. Testing is commonly modified relative to baseline fitness.

Elapsed time (min)	*Work rate (W)*	*Speed (mph)*	*Grade (%)*	*HR (bpm)*	*SpO_2 (%)*	*SBP (mm Hg)*	*DBP (mm Hg)*	*Borg dyspnea (1–10)*
-1 (Pre)	0	Rest	0					
5	0	Rest	0					
8	5	0.8	1.5					
9	16	1	4					
10	24	1.1	5.5					
11	36	1.3	7					
12	44	1.5	7.5					
13	50	1.6	8					
14	60	1.8	8.5					
15	70	2	9					
16	82	2.2	9.5					
17	90	2.3	10					
18	98	2.5	10					
19	111	2.7	10.5					
20	125	2.9	11					
21	140	3.1	11.5					
22	155	3.3	12					
>22	164	+0.2/min	+0.5/min					

(W: Watt; HR: Heart rate; SpO_2: Oxygen saturation; SBP: Systolic blood pressure; DBP: Diastolic blood pressure).

interference. This involves removing the hair with a disposable safety razor, cleansing the skin with alcohol or acetone to remove skin oils, followed by light abrasion to remove stratum corneum. Standard limb lead placement on the wrists and ankles is modified for exercise by moving them to the anterior trunk as shown in Figure 14.2.

With subjects sitting on the cycle ergometer or standing on the treadmill, a noseclip is placed and the mouthpiece is inserted. At this time the importance of maintaining a tight seal around the mouthpiece should be emphasized to the patient.

Before starting exercise, a rest period of 3-5 minute is suggested, during which time lab personnel should observe key variables in comparison to reference values to ensure proper calibration and performance of the metabolic measuring system. Table 14.6 provides an example of key resting variables and their expected values.

Warm-up Phase

After the rest period, the patient should receive a verbal command to start pedaling with the cycle unloaded, freewheeling or walking on the treadmill. Depending on the protocol used, this phase lasts between 30 seconds and 3 minutes.

On a cycle ergometer, the patient should be coached to pedal at 60 revolutions per minute (rpm) on the unloaded cycle to become accommodated to this pace. The pedal rate meter should be displayed in clear view of the patient to facilitate compliance with this goal pedaling frequency. An accessory motor should be utilized to rotate the flywheel at a rate of 60 rpm in order to eliminate the inertial force needed to start the flywheel rotating and reach the desired speed.

Incremental Exercise and Criteria for Terminating the Exercise Test

After the warm-up, the work rate is increased according to the chosen protocol. During the CPET, the subject should be verbally encouraged to give a maximal effort with the goal of achieving a physiologic limitation. Subjective perception of effort is obtained by a perceived exertion scale, such as the 10 point modified Borg scale (Table 14.7), where a value greater than 8 may be considered expression of an exhaustive exertion. It can be helpful to print out the Borg scales in large font, so that it is clearly visible to the patient during exercise. The patient should be encouraged to keep eyes open during exercise, and the technician and physician should observe the patient's facial expression.

Heart rate, as measured by ECG, should be recorded every minute. Blood pressure, oxygen saturation, perceived exertion and dyspnea should be recorded every 2 minutes. ECG monitoring is used to ensure electrical stability of the heart during exercise testing as well as determine if signs of myocardial ischemia evolve during or post testing. The physician must be careful to identify and treat conditions that manifest with ECG abnormalities during exercise. These should be then indicated in the final report.

The main criteria for terminating an exercise *test* before symptom limitation are the following:

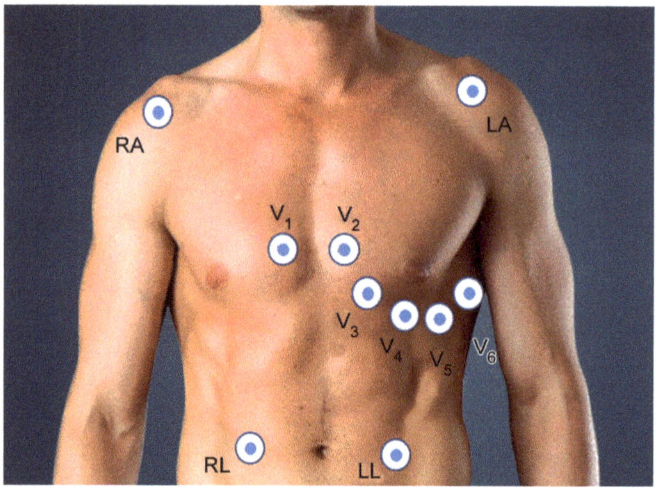

Fig. 14.2: Electrode placement for electrocardiogram recording during exercise.
(RA: Right arm; LA: Left arm; RL: Right leg; LL: Left leg).

Table 14.6: Reference values appropriate for resting conditions.

SBP mm Hg	*DBP mm Hg*	*Heart rate/minute*	*VO_2 ml•kg^{-1}•min^{-1}*	*VO_2 mL/minute*	*VCO_2 mL/minute*
100–140	60–90	60–100	3.5	200–300	140–300
RER	*RR min*	*VE L/min*	*$P_{ET}O_2$ mm Hg*	*$P_{ET}CO_2$ mm Hg*	
0.7–1.0	12–20	6–10	100–105	38–42	

(SBP: Systolic blood pressure; DBP: Diastolic blood pressure; VO_2: Oxygen consumption; VCO_2: Carbon dioxide production; RER: Respiratory exchange ratio; RR: Respiratory rate; VE: Minute ventilation; $P_{ET}O_2$: Partial pressure of end-tidal oxygen; $P_{ET}CO_2$: Partial pressure of end-tidal carbon dioxide).

- Chest pain suggestive of ischemia (angina)
- Ischemic ECG changes (e.g. ST-segment elevation)
- Sustained ventricular tachycardia or other arrhythmias (e.g. complex ectopy, second or third degree atrioventricular block)
- Fall in systolic pressure above 20 mm Hg from the highest value during the test
- Hypertension (> 250 mm Hg systolic; > 120 mm Hg diastolic)
- Severe desaturation: SpO_2 less than 85% when accompanied by symptoms and signs of severe hypoxemia
- Signs of poor perfusion (e.g. sudden pallor or cyanosis)
- Central nervous system symptoms (e.g. mental confusion, loss of coordination, dizziness or faintness)

Table 14.7: Modified 0–10 Borg scale for rating of perceived exertion (RPE). The maximum value is 10. Twice the rating is likely to be twice as hard.

Rating	*Description*	*Level of exertion*
0	Nothing at all	
0.5	Very, very weak	Just perceptible
1	Very weak	
2	Weak (light)	Light
3	Moderate	
4	Somewhat strong	
5	Strong (heavy)	Heavy
6		
7	Very strong	
8		
9		
10	Extreme	Almost maximum

KEY VARIABLES, NORMAL VALUES AND SIGNIFICANCE

While the list of CPET-derived variables is rather long, scientific investigations have allowed for a shorter list of key variables. These variables are presented in Table 14.8. Some variables listed in Table 14.8 have universal applicability, regardless of test indication. Other variables are relevant for specific test indications. Table 14.9 lists recommended equations for calculating predicted peak VO_2 values for sedentary but apparently healthy men and women. Table 14.8 shows the criteria of normality for the main variables measured during the CPET, whereas Table 14.9 describes the patterns of abnormal response to exercise commonly observed in different diseases.

ANAEROBIC, LACTATE, AND VENTILATORY THRESHOLDS

The anaerobic threshold (AT) is a term used to indicate the work beyond which the aerobic metabolism in muscle becomes inefficient and switches to the anaerobic metabolism, with consequent blood lactate overload. AT is used as an indicator of fitness and can be used to diagnose a limitation in exercise. AT usually occurs in about

Table 14.8: Identifying and defining normal responses for key CPET variables.

CPET variable	*Description/Significance*	*Normal value/Response*
Peak VO_2 ($mlO_2 \cdot kg^{-1} \cdot min^{-1}$)	Highest O_2 uptake obtained during exercise. Commonly designated as "peak" value in patient populations described in this document. Expressed as a 10–60 second averaged value depending on ET protocol (i.e. shorter averaging interval for protocols with shorter stages and longer averaging interval for protocols with longer stages). Response influenced by central (CV and/or pulmonary) and peripheral (skeletal muscle) function. Broadly reflects disease severity in a number of patient populations including HF, HCM, PAH secondary PH, COPD, ILD. Universal prognostic marker.	Wide range influenced by age and sex: ≈ 80 to ≈ 15 $mlO_2 \cdot kg^{-1} \cdot min^{-1}$ in young elite athlete and apparently healthy 80-year-old female, respectively; normal age-related decline related to decrease in central and peripheral performance across the lifespan; normal sex-related differences largely influenced my difference in maximal cardiac output. Reporting peak VO_2 as a percent-predicted value using equations provided in Table 14.9 recommended to account for age and sex differences. Percent-predicted values should be ≥100%.
VO_2 at VT ($mlO_2 \cdot kg^{-1} \cdot min^{-1}$)	Submaximal VO_2 where there is a dislinear rise in VE and VCO_2. Generally associated with anaerobic threshold. Represents upper limit of ET workloads that can be sustained for a prolonged period. Valuable in setting inensity for exercise prescription in a highly individualized manner.	≈ 50–65% of peak VO_2. Influenced by genetic predisposition and chronic aerobic training.

Contd...

Contd...

CPET variable	*Description/Significance*	*Normal value/Response*
Peak RER	Defined as the VCO_2/VO_2 ratio. Expressed as a 10–60 second averaged value depending on exercise protocol (i.e. shorter averaging interval for protocols with shorter stages and longer averaging interval for protocols with longer stages). As exercise progresses to higher intensities, VCO_2 outpaces VO_2, increasing the ratio. Currently is the best noninvasive indicator of exercise effort.	Peak value ≥ 1.10 widely accepted as excellent exercise effort.
VE/VCO_2 slope	Relationship between VE, plotted on the y-axis, and VCO_2 plotted on the X-axis; both variables in L/minute. Most commonly calculated using all ET data. Represents matching of ventilation and perfusion within the pulmonary system. Broadly reflects disease severity as well as prognosis in a number of patient populations including HF, HCM, PAH/secondary PH, COPD, ILD.	< 30 considered normal with slight increase with advanced age possible.
EOV	No universally definition currently available. Most commonly defined as an oscillatory pattern at rest that persists for ≥60% of the exercise test at an amplitude of ≥15% of the average resting value. Recommend using 10-second averaged VE data for plotting. Reflects advanced disease severity and poor prognosis in patients with HF.	This is not a normal ventilatory response to exercise under any circumstances.
$P_{ET}CO_2$ (mm Hg) at rest and during exercise	Also represents matching of ventilation and perfusion within the pulmonary system and cardiac function. Broadly reflects disease severity in a number of patient populations including HF, HCM, PAH/secondary PH, COPD, ILD.	Rest: 36–42 mm Hg Increases between 3 and 8 mm Hg by VT. Decrease following VT secondary to increased ventilation response.
VE/VO_2 at Peak Exercise	Expressed as a 10–60 second averaged value depending on exercise protocol (i.e. shorter averaging interval for protocols with shorter stages and longer averaging interval for protocols with longer stages). Reflects ventilatory cost of O_2 uptake at peak ET. Has diagnostic utility in patients with suspected mitochondrial myopathy.	≤ 40 50 = upper limit of normal response
$\Delta Q/\Delta VO_2$ Slope	Relationship between Q, plotted on the y-axis, and VO_2 plotted on the x-axis; both variables in L/minute. Additional equipment needed to measure Q; through foreign gas rebreathing technique. Reflects the relationship between O_2 delivery and utilization in exercising skeletal muscle. Has diagnostic utility in patients with suspected mitochondrial myopathy if anemia is ruled out.	≈ 5
VE/MVV	Ratio between VE at maximal exercise and MVV obtained at rest; both variables in L/minute. Although prediction equations are available (FEV_1 × 40), MVV should be directly measured. Has diagnostic utility in determining if unexplained exertional dyspnea is related to a pulmonary mechanism.	≤ 0.80
FEV_1 (L/minute) and PEF (L/minute)	Components of pulmonary function testing battery. Predicted values automatically generated by CPET unit software packages; influenced by age, sex and body habitus. Has diagnostic utility in determining if unexplained exertional dyspnea is related to a pulmonary mechanism, particularly exercise-induced bronchospasm. When relevant, should be assessed prior to and following CPET for comparative purposes.	< 15% reduction from pre to post CPET for both variables.

Contd...

Contd...

CPET variable	*Description/Significance*	*Normal value/Response*
O_2 Pulse Trajectory (mLO_2/beat)	O_2 pulse defined as the ratio between VO_2 (mlO_2/minute) and HR (beats/minute) Noninvasively reflects stroke volume response to exercise. Has diagnostic utility in patients with suspected myocardial ischemia (i.e. exercise-induced left ventricular dysfunction).	Continual linear rise throughout exercise with possible plateau approaching maximal exertion.
ΔVO_2/DW Trajectory ($mL{\cdot}min^{-1}{\cdot}Watt^{-1}$)*	Plot of the relationship between VO_2 (y-axis in mL/minute) and workload (x-axis in watts). Lower extremity ergometer should be used as exercise mode when assessed. Has diagnostic utility in patients with suspected myocardial ischemia (i.e. exercise-induced left ventricular dysfunction).	Continual linear rise throughout ET. Average slope, calculated with all exercise data, is 10 $mL{\cdot}min^{-1}{\cdot}Watt^{-1}$.
Exercise HR (Beats/minute)	In patients not prescribed a beta-blocking agent; provides insight into chronotropic competence and cardiac response to exercise. Peak HR should not be used as the primary gauge of subject effort given its wide variability.	Increase ~10 beats per 3.5 $mLO_2{\cdot}kg^{-1}{\cdot}min^{-1}$ increase in VO_2, achieve at least 85% of age-predicted maximal HR with good effort.
HRR at 1 minute (beats)	Difference between maximal exercise HR and HR one minute into recovery. Provides insight into speed of parasympathetic reactivation.	> 12 beats is the most commonly used cut point when exercise cool down occurs actively and upright. Other cut points are used when a patient is not active, or if the patient is supine.
Exercise BP (mm Hg)	Provides insight into CV response to exercise and left ventricular afterload.	SBP increase ~10 mm Hg per 3.5 $mLO_2{\cdot}kg^{-1}{\cdot}min^{-1}$ ncrease in VO_2. Upper range of normal maximal SBP is ~210 mm Hg for males and ~190 mm Hg for females. DBP remains the same or slightly decreases.
SpO_2 (%)	Noninvasive estimate of arterial hemoglobin saturation. Has diagnostic utility in determining if unexplained exertional dyspnea is related to a pulmonary mechanism. Desaturation common in patients with COPD, ILD, PAH/secondary PH as disease severity advances.	≥95% at rest and throughout exercise. Should not decrease > 5% (absolute value).
ECG	Insight into stability of cardiac rhythm. Identifies baseline abnormalities and exercise-induced ischemia.	Minimal waveform changes. No significant deviation from normal sinus rhythm.
Subjective symptoms	Used to determine subjects perception of symptoms limiting exercise. Rating of perceived exertion (i.e. Borg scale) as well as dyspnea and angina (using symptom specific scales) should be quantified using separate scales with unique verbal anchors Unusual dyspnea as primary reason for test termination (i.e. 4/4: severely difficult, patient cannot continue) shown to indicate increased adverse event risk in patients assessed for myocardial ischemia and HF.	Limiting factor muscular fatigue with no significant dyspnea or angina.

* $\Delta VO_2/\Delta W$ trajectory is only available for CPET completed with cycle ergometry (since it relies on the assessment of watts).

Source: Adapted and reprinted with permission from EACPR/AHA Scientific Statement: Clinical Recommendations for Cardiopulmonary Exercise Testing Data Assessment in Specific Patient Populations. Circulation. 2012;126:2261-74. ©2012 American Heart Association, Inc.

(CPET: Cardiopulmonary exercise testing; VO_2: Oxygen consumption; ET: Exercise testing; VT: Ventilatory threshold; VE: Minute ventilation; VCO_2: Carbon dioxide production; RER: Respiratory exchange ratio; EOV: Exercise oscillatory ventilation; $P_{ET}CO_2$: Partial pressure of end-tidal carbon dioxide; HF: Heart failure; HCM: Hypertrophic cardiomyopathy; PAH: Pulmonary arterial hypertension; PH: Pulmonary hypertension; COPD: Chronic obstructive pulmonary disease; ILD: Interstitial lung disease; Q: Cardiac output; MVV; Maximal voluntary ventilation; PEF: Peak expiratory flow; FEV_1: Forced expiratory volume in one second; O_2: Oxygen; W: Watt; HR: Heart rate; HRR: Heart rate recovery; BP: Blood pressure; SBP: Systolic blood pressure; DBP: Diastolic blood pressure; SpO_2: Saturation of peripheral oxygen; ECG: Electrocardiogram).

40–50% VO_2max, lower values suggesting impaired release of oxygen or its takeover in muscles and actually reflecting a state of hypoxia in the muscle during exercise. In interpreting a CPET, it is more important to evaluate whether the threshold has been reached, rather than to evaluate the VO_2 value at which it is achieved. AT is a parameter that cannot be voluntarily controlled and not affected by psychological factors.

A direct measurement of serum lactate may allow the determination of the AT, but this invasive method does not have practical applications. Noninvasive methods of AT evaluation are available, by analyzing gas exchange,

Table 14.9: Predicted peak oxygen consumption equations according to *Wasserman and Hansen equations.*

Sedentary male	*Sedentary female*
Step 1: Calculate	*Step 1: Calculate*
Cycle factor = 50.72 – 0.372 (age)	Cycle factor = 22.78 – 0.17 (age)
Predicted weight: = 0.79 (height) – 60.7	Predicted weight: = 0.65 (height) – 42.8
Step 2: Classify weight	*Step 2: Classify weight*
Measured weight </=/> predicted weight	Measured weight </=/> predicted weight
Step 3: Select equation	*Step 3: Select equation*
Measured weight < Predicted weight	Measured weight < Predicted weight
Peak VO_2 (mL/minute) = [(Predicted weight + Actual weight)/2] cycle factor	Peak VO_2 (mL/minute) = [(Predicted weight + Actual weight +86)/2] * cycle factor
Measured weight = Predicted weight	Measured weight = Predicted weight
Peak VO_2 (mL/minute) = Measured weight · cycle factor	Peak VO_2 (mL/minute) = (Measured weight + 43) · cycle factor
Measured weight > Predicted weight	Measured weight > Predicted weight
Peak VO_2 (mL/minute) = (Predicted weight · cycle factor) + 6 · (Measured weight – predicted weight)	Peak VO_2 (mL/minute) = (Predicted weight + 43) · cycle factor + 6 · (Measured weight – predicted weight)
Step 4: Mode of exercise consideration	*Step 4: Mode of exercise consideration*
If treadmill used for test	If treadmill used for test
Multiply predicted VO_2 from step 3 · 1.11	Multiply predicted VO_2 from step 3 · 1.11

Height is expressed in cm; weight is expressed in kg.

Source: Adapted and reprinted with permission from EACPR/AHA Scientific Statement: Clinical Recommendations for Cardiopulmonary Exercise Testing Data Assessment in Specific Patient Populations. Circulation. 2012;126:2261-74. ©2012 American Heart Association, Inc.

(VO_2: Oxygen consumption).

specifically measuring the oxygen consumption and the CO_2 production. After the initiation of the anaerobic metabolism, the resulting lactic acid needs to be buffered by bicarbonate, which produces a disproportionate increase in VCO_2 as compared to oxygen consumption.

The V-slope method is the most used to assess the AT, based on the trend of VCO_2 and its relationship with the VO_2. Before the threshold is reached, VCO_2/VO_2 relationship is linear, the slope corresponding to a parallel line (line of identity) to the hypotenuse of an isosceles angle headpiece which has the acute angles at the level of the abscissa and ordinate of the graph. When the AT is reached, the slope deviates from the line of identity, due to the increase of lactacidemia and the consequent increase of VCO_2. The inflection point of the curve represents the value of the ventilatory anaerobic threshold (Fig. 14.3). This method of detection of the threshold requires a breath by breath analysis of exhaled gases.

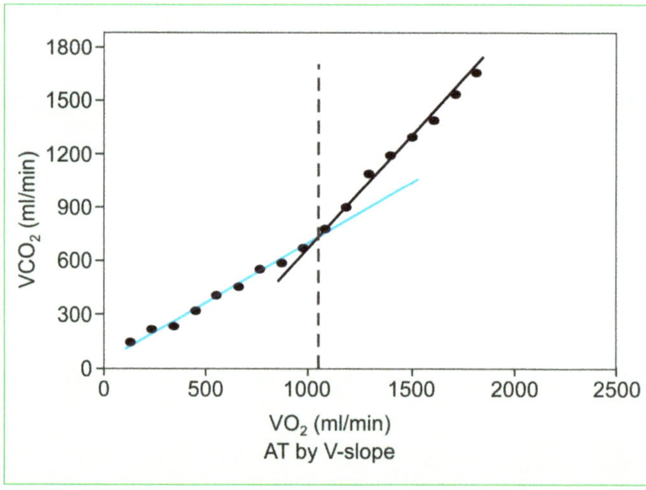

Fig. 14.3: Determination of the anaerobic threshold (AT) through the V-slope method. The AT is the point where the two regression lines explaining VCO_2 as function of VO_2 intersect.

The concept of the anaerobic threshold has been questioned, whereas *lactate threshold (LT)* has been recently considered a more descriptive term for the lactate inflection point described above. Due to the misconception about lactate as the source of fatigue, it was thought that the workload just below lactate accumulation in the blood reflected a maximum sustainable level of performance. Despite the fact that LT is a more descriptive name for the lactate inflection point than AT, current research suggests that it tends to underestimate time trial performance. Moreover, the reliability and accuracy of LT in measuring performance is questionable since there are different methods of measuring and interpreting LT, and each method can produce a different set of results for a given subject. *Ventilatory threshold (VT)* describes the inflection point for ventilation during an incremental exercise test. Ventilation increases at about the same rate as oxygen consumption up to about 50–70% of VO_2max (depending on one's trained level). At this point (just beyond the ventilatory threshold) ventilation increases exponentially.

INTERPRETATION OF RESULTS

Interpretation of CPET results is dependent upon test indication. When CPET is utilized to assess cardiorespiratory fitness in athletes, it provides reliable insight regarding their physical state and training efficacy. When CPET is used in clinical exercise testing laboratories in patients with suspected or known cardiovascular or pulmonary disease, it provides insights regarding prognosis, diagnosis, functional capacity, and therapeutic efficacy. A joint scientific statement was recently published by the European Association for Cardiovascular Prevention and Rehabilitation (EACPR) and the American Heart Association (AHA) which outlined interpretive CPET strategies for common test indications. Tables 14.10 and 14.11 illustrate the criteria of normality for the main variables measured during the CPET and the patterns of abnormal response to exercise in different diseases.

Before interpreting a CPET and drawing up a report, you should verify the appropriateness of the values obtained for the main parameters measured (*see* Table 14.6). In particular, you should review the following parameters:

VO_2 (O_2 uptake) at Rest and during Warm-up Phase

A normal-sized subject should have a VO_2 roughly 250 mL/minute at rest and roughly 400 mL/minute during unloaded pedaling (Fig. 14.4). In obese people, both the resting and unloaded pedaling values are usually higher (around 500 mL/minute and 1,000 mL/minute, respectively).

Respiratory Exchange Ratio: VCO_2/VO_2

Respiratory exchange ratio value should remain between 0.8 and 0.95 for the first 30–40% of the CPET, and should never be below 0.7. Successively, the value of RER increases with the progressively increasing of the effort, raising to between 1.1 and 1.3 at peak exercise, and this is an evidence of good maximal effort. However, for many subjects, especially those who are deconditioned or anxious, this threshold is difficult to achieve. The increase of RER persists for 1–2 minutes after the exercise is terminated, since the muscles eliminate the accumulated CO_2 while O_2 consumption decreases (Fig. 14.5). A decrease of RER as the work load increases, should raise the suspicion that gas sensor does not work well or that a leak in the mask or sampling catheter exists.

VO_2/W Relationship between VO_2 and Workload in Watts

When the subject starts loaded exercise, oxygen consumption (VO_2) and watts expended should increase in a linear and predictable way. VO_2 should raise at around 10-12 mL/watt (Fig. 14.6). Blunted increases suggest disease states (e.g. advanced COPD or HF).

REPORT PREPARATION

The report can be divided into several parts, corresponding to similar steps in the interpretive process.

Table 14.10: Criteria of normality for the main variables measured during the CPET.

Variables	*Criteria of normality*
VO_2max or VO_2peak	> 84% predicted
Anaerobic threshold	40–80% VO_2max predicted
Maximal heart rate	90% age predicted
Heart rate reserve (HRR)	< 15 beats/minute
O_2 pulse (VO_2/HR)	> 80% predicted
Ventilatory reserve	MVV -VEmax:11(L)
Respiratory frequency	< 60 breaths/minute
VE/VCO_2 (at AT)	< 34
VD/VT	< 0.28; < 0.30 for age > 40 years
$P(A–a)O_2$	< 35 mm Hg

Table 14.11: Patterns of abnormal response to exercise in different diseases.

	COPD	*ILD*	*PVD*	*Obesity*	*Deconditioned*	*Chronic heart failure*
VO_2peak	Reduced	Reduced	Reduced	Reduced normal	Reduced	Reduced
Anaerobic threshold	Normal or Low	Normal or low	Low	Low	Normal or low	Low
Ventilatory reserve	Reduced or none	Reduced or normal	Normal	Normal	Normal	Normal
Heart rate recovery	Normal increased	Normal or increased	Normal	Normal	Normal	Reduced or Normal
O_2 Pulse	Reduced	Reduced	Reduced	Normal	Reduced	Reduced
Fall in SpO_2	Present Absent	Present	Present	Absent	Absent	Absent

(COPD: Chronic obstructive pulmonary disease; ILD: Interstitial lung disease; PVD: Pulmonary vascular disease).

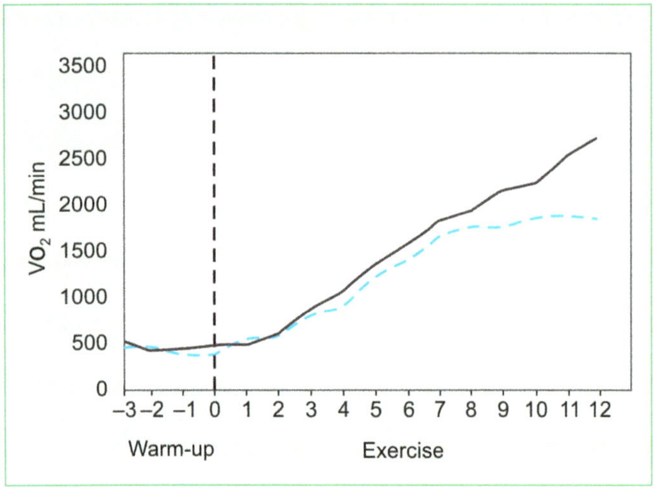

Fig. 14.4: Normal (solid line) and abnormal (dashed line) increase of VO_2 (oxygen consumption) during CPET

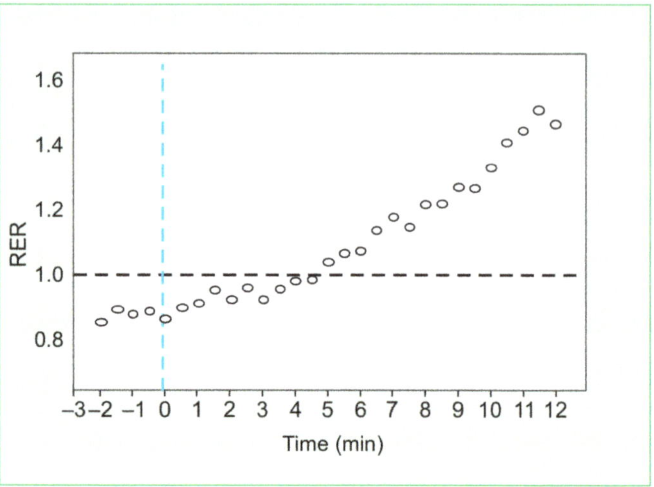

Fig. 14.5: Plot of respiratory exchange ratio (RER) against time in a normal subject.

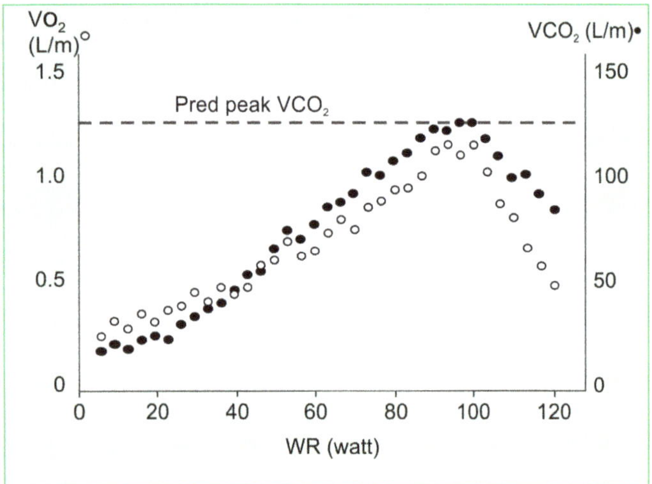

Fig. 14.6: Plot of VO_2 and VCO_2 against work rate (WR) in a normal subject.

Step 1: Quality Control

As preliminary evaluation, the operator should verify the oxygen saturation (SpO_2) data and evaluate whether there are leaks in the system.

SPO_2 Data

A reduction in SpO_2 during the test, it is necessary to assess whether the patient has clinical signs suggestive of a true desaturation. Usually, true desaturation occurs in a steadily and progressively, and the lowest values are observed in the first minute after the load is removed. A fall in SpO_2 due to sensor placement or poor signal is usually characterized by chaotic data, without a clear trend.

Leaks in the System

Even if rarely, gas leaks may occur from the mask or other connections in the system and distort the test data. You can suspect such a problem if you observe a very early VO_2 plateau (i.e. VO_2 fails to rise as work rate continues to rise for more than a 1–2 minute period), inappropriate R-values, and inappropriately high $P_{ET}O_2$ values.

Step 2: Indications for the Test and other Relevant Clinical Data

A typical CPET report should begin with a short review of the primary reasons for performing the test. In this section, you should also note whether the patient takes any relevant cardiac or pulmonary medications (e.g. beta-blockers) that may affect CPET results, and/or whether he/she has undergone any cardiac or thoracic surgical procedures that can affect cardiopulmonary parameters.

Step 3: Factors Limiting Exercise

The report must comprise of the power increment used (e.g. 10 watt/minute ramp), the maximum power attained and the subject's stated reason for interrupt the test (e.g. leg fatigue, dyspnea, chest pain, lightheadedness, etc). You should also describe whether the exercise-limiting symptoms during the test duplicated the exertional symptoms the patient has at home. You should describe if the patient reached the anaerobic threshold and note the point at which it occurred (e.g. at 60% of the VO_2max). In most individuals, AT occurs at about 60% of the VO_2max, while in highly trained endurance athletes, it may occur at 80% of their maximum exercise capacity. Active patients aged over 80 years may show a threshold either very late in exercise or not at all. People with ventilatory limitation usually do not reach the AT.

Step 4: Maximal Exercise Capacity

You should report the VO_2max in absolute value ($mLO_2 \cdot kg^{-1} \cdot min^{-1}$) as well as the weight-normalized values and the percent of the predicted values based on age, height and gender. Be aware that calculated normal values are not appropriate for people under the age of 20, whereas the data for the elderly (especially women) are poor.

Another important point to remember is that a subject's VO_2max may fall within the "normal" range or even exceed the predicted values yet that person may still have exercise limitation. This may occurs in athletes usually able to perform intensive work, who may have a significant reduction of their performance and of their individual VO_2max following a pathological event (e.g. pulmonary embolism), although VO_2max still appears normal if compared to the reference values.

Step 5: Cardiovascular Response

Note the predicted maximum heart rate and the maximal heart rate attained. The difference between these two values, the heart rate reserve, should also be noted. You should also review the ECG report and note whether there were any ST depressions or arrhythmias and when in the progression of the test they were observed. Describe the blood pressure response to exercise. It should rise progressively with exercise, with marked increases beyond the ventilatory threshold. A falling blood pressure may be a sign of significant coronary artery disease and merits further assessment expeditiously. Note the changes in the O_2 pulse, a surrogate marker for stroke volume. This should rise progressively through exercise and plateau once the patient achieves the VO_2max.

Step 6: Ventilatory Response

The aim of this part of the report is to describe if the patient has any signs of ventilatory limitation. After noting the peak respiratory rate and the maximum tidal volume achieved, you should compare the maximum minute ventilation at peak exercise with MVV. In patients with ventilatory limitation, the minute ventilation at peak exercise is over 70% of the MVV, although very fit athletes can raise their minute ventilation up to or above their MVV.

You should also report the ventilatory equivalents for CO_2 and O_2 since these values reflect alveolar ventilation and the extent of ventilation-perfusion matching. Normal VE/VCO_2 values should be about 25–35 at low level exercise below the ventilatory threshold. They will rise to higher levels once a subject passes his/her ventilatory threshold. Values lower than those suggest the patient is hypoventilating while higher values are suggestive of hyperventilation or increased dead space. Many fit athletes get "amped up" when they get on the bicycle and hyperventilate while sitting at rest or during unloaded pedaling. They will demonstrate elevated ventilatory equivalents as a result of this but the values tend to come back down to normal levels once they begin loaded pedaling.

Step 7: Gas Exchange and Blood Gases

The trend of SpO_2 and end-tidal CO_2 should be reported. SpO_2 generally remains constant in normal subjects and in patients with cardiac limitation, whereas it falls in patients with ventilatory limitation and pulmonary vascular or interstitial lung disease. An end-tidal CO_2 falls after the patient reach the ventilatory threshold but increases or remains stable in patients with ventilatory limitation or neuromuscular disease.

If you have arterial blood gas analysis, assessment of the alveolar-arterial oxygen difference may be useful. It usually remains between 10–15 mm Hg until the ventilatory threshold, then it usually increases (although, it may already be maximally widened at baseline in patients with advanced heart failure). Healthy adults usually have an alveolar-arterial oxygen difference of below 20 mm Hg at maximum effort. You should then identify changes in the bicarbonate and the arterial $PaCO_2$. The bicarbonate starts to fall around the ventilatory threshold and the $PaCO_2$ should drop progressively in response to this metabolic acidosis. A stable or increasing $PaCO_2$ is evidence of ventilatory limitation or neuromuscular disease.

Data Analysis

Only a careful and simultaneous evaluation of numerical data and graphs allows us the evaluation and interpretation of a parameter change during the test. The figures are usually compared with reference values for a sedentary population. The American Thoracic Society (ATS) has recommended the use of at least nine graphics for a correct

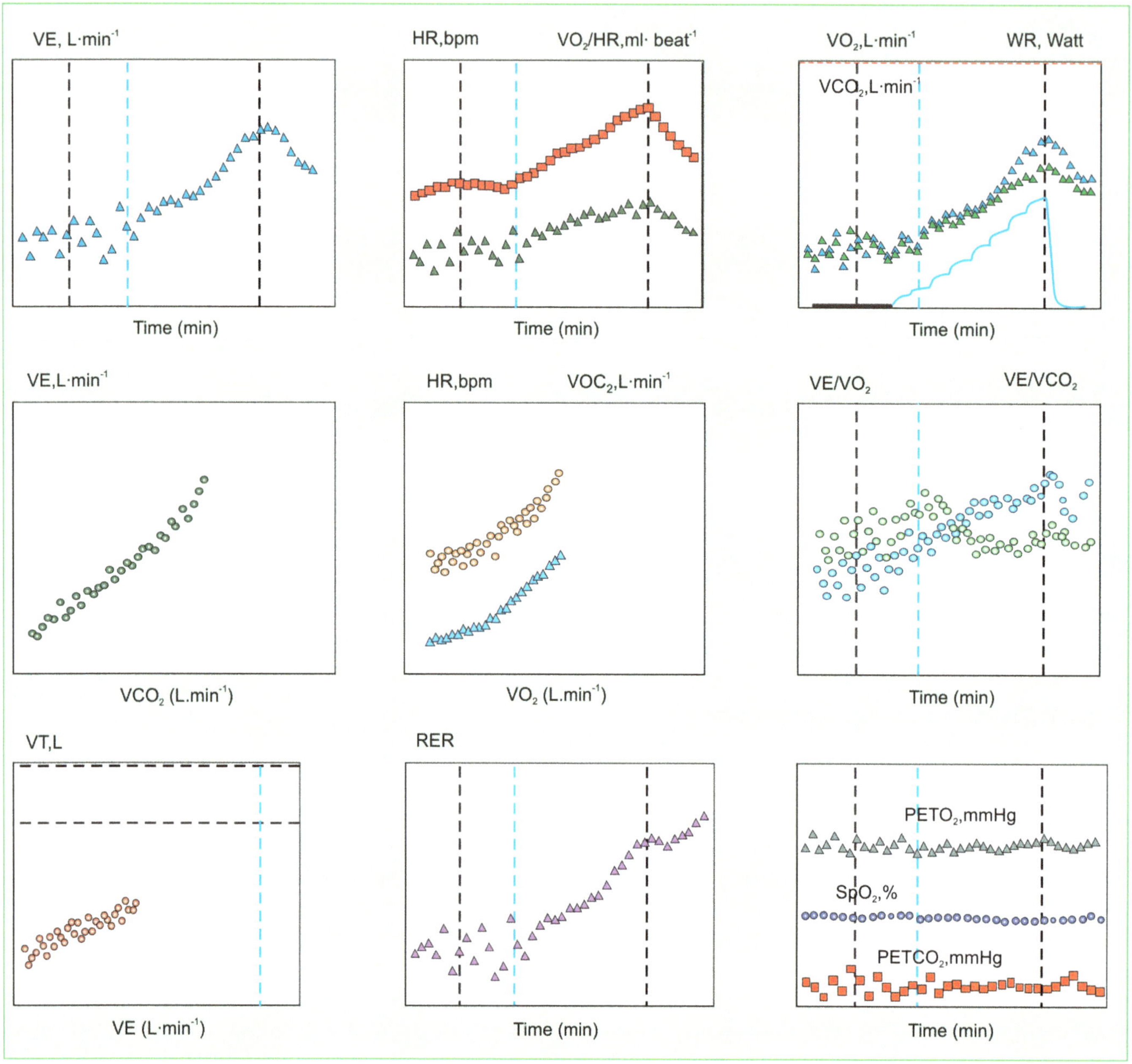

Fig. 14.7: The nine graphics recommended for a complete interpretation of cardiopulmonary exercise test (CPET).

interpretation of CPET parameters (Fig. 14.7). The constellation of differences between a subject an establish norms often reveal distinctive patterns that can be used to differentiate deconditioning, cardiovascular disease, pulmonary disease, or other clinical situations, or relative degrees of stability in patients with known disease. Flowchart 14.1 is a simplified algorithm for the interpretation of CPET.

BIBLIOGRAPHY AND FURTHER READING

1. Abidov A, Rozanski A, Hachamovitch R, Hayes SW, Aboul-Enein F, Cohen I, et al. Prognostic significance of dyspnea in patients referred for cardiac stress testing. N Engl J Med. 2005;353:1889-98.
2. Arena R, Myers J, Guazzi M. The clinical and research applications of aerobic capacity and ventilatory efficiency in heart failure: an evidence-based review. Heart Fail Rev. 2008;13:245-69.

Flowchart 14.1: Simplified algorithm for the evaluation of unexplained dyspnea by cardiopulmonary exercise test (CPET).

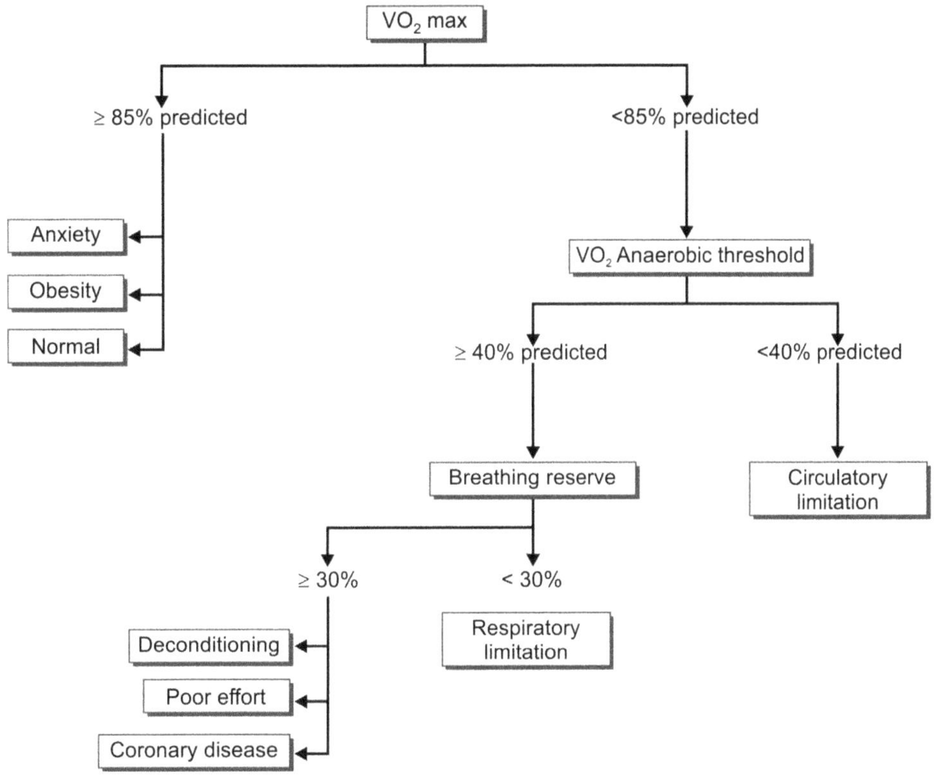

3. Arena R, Myers J, Williams MA, Gulati M, Kligfield P, Balady GJ, et al. Assessment of functional capacity in clinical and research settings: a scientific statement from the American Heart Association Committee on Exercise, Rehabilitation, and Prevention of the Council on Clinical Cardiology and the Council on Cardiovascular Nursing. Circulation. 2007;116:329-43.
4. Arena R, Sietsema KE. Cardiopulmonary exercise testing in the clinical evaluation of patients with heart and lung disease. Circulation. 2011;123:668-80.
5. Armstrong L, Balady G, Berry M, et al. Health-Related Physical Testing and Interpretation. In: Whaley MH, Brubaker PH, Otto R, (Eds]. ACSM's Guidelines for exercise testing and prescription. 7th edition. Philadelphia: Lippincott Williams and Wilkins; 2007. pp. 55-92.
6. Balady GJ, Arena R, Sietsema K, Myers J, Coke L, Fletcher GF, et al. Clinician's guide to cardiopulmonary exercise testing in adults. A Scientific scientific Statement statement From from the American Heart Association. Circulation. 2010;122:191-225.
7. Borg GA. Psychophysical bases of perceived exertion. Med Sci Sports Exerc. 1982;14:377-81.
8. Campbell SC. A comparison of the maximum voluntary ventilation with the forced expiratory volume in one second: an assessment of subject cooperation. J Occup Med. 1982;24:531-3.
9. Chase P, Arena R, Myers J, Abella J, Peberdy MA, Guazzi M, et al. Prognostic usefulness of dyspnea versus fatigue as reason for exercise test termination in patients with heart failure. Am J Cardiol. 2008;102:879-82.
10. Corra U, Giordano A, Bosimini E, Mezzani A, Piepoli M, Coats AJ, et al. Oscillatory ventilation during exercise in patients with chronic heart failure: clinical correlates and prognostic implications. Chest. 2002;121:1572-80.
11. Jain M, Nkonde C, Lin B, Walker A, Wackers FJ. 85% of maximal age-predicted heart rate is not a valid endpoint for exercise treadmill testing. J Nucl Cardiol. 2011;18:1026-35.
12. Myers J, Arena R, Franklin B, Pina I, Kraus WE, McInnis K, et al. Recommendations for clinical exercise laboratories: a scientific statement from the American Heart Association. Circulation. 2009;119(24):3144-61.
13. Myers J, Gujja P, Neelagaru S, Burkhoff D. Cardiac output and cardiopulmonary responses to exercise in heart failure: Application of a new bio-reactance device. J Card Fail. 2007;13:629-36.
14. Myers J, Gullestad L, Vagelos R, Do D, Bellin D, Ross H, et al. Cardiopulmonary exercise testing and prognosis in severe heart failure: 14 mL/kg/min revisited. Am Heart Journal J. 2000;139(1):78-84.

15. Pinkstaff S, Peberdy MA, Kontos MC, Finucane S, Arena R. Quantifying exertion level during exercise stress testing using percentage of age-predicted maximal heart rate, rate pressure product, and perceived exertion. Mayo Clin Proc. 2010;85:1095-100.
16. Taivassalo T, Dysgaard Jensen T, Kennaway N, DiMauro S, Vissing J, Haller RG. The spectrum of exercise tolerance in mitochondrial myopathies: a study of 40 patients. Brain 2003;126:413-23.
17. Wasserman K, Hansen JE, Sue DY, Stringer W, Whipp BJ. Normal Values. In: Weinberg R (Ed.). Principles of Exercise Testing and Interpretation. 4th edition. Philadelphia: Lippincott Williams and Wilkins; 2005. pp. 160-82.

Chapter 15

Diagnostic Tests for Sleep-Related Breathing Disorders

Maria Rosaria Bonsignore, Claudio Sorino, Oreste Marrone

SLEEP VERSUS WAKEFULNESS: WHAT IS DIFFERENT?

Sleep remains a fascinating mystery as its real functions are concerned. Sleep is essential for recovery of all functions of the body, including cerebral activity. It is not a homogeneous state and its structure differs according to age (only adult subjects will be considered in this chapter).

Sleep occurs in cycles of about 90 minutes each, which are repeated during the night for 5 or 6 times, each cycle including stages with and without *rapid eye movements* (REM), (non-REM and REM sleep). Sleep is a continuum, but is analyzed for practical purposes in epochs of 30 s. Non-REM sleep is largely predominant (about 80% of total time), and is characterized by progressive slowing of cerebral activity at the electroencephalogram (EEG). Non-REM *stage 1* is transient, and represents the initial phase of sleep, identified as presence of theta waves for at least half of a 30 s epoch. *Stage 2* is the most represented sleep stage and is characterized at the EEG by two types of activity, *spindles* and *K-complexes*. *Stage 3* is also called *slow-wave sleep*, since EEG activity is highly synchronized with large delta waves. During non-REM sleep, muscle tone progressively decreases, heart rate and respiratory rate slow down, and sympathetic nervous activity declines, with predominance of vagal influences. Respiration remains under control of chemical stimuli (i.e. the level of oxygen and carbon dioxide in arterial blood), but responsiveness is lower compared to wakefulness.

During REM sleep, the brain shows a high degree of activity. REM sleep could represent a phase of "housekeeping" in the brain, necessary for maintenance of normal cerebral functions. A profound muscle hypotonia is typical of REM sleep, and breathing is maintained by the diaphragm, which is the only respiratory muscle that remains active. Control of breathing becomes less dependent on chemical stimuli compared to wakefulness and non-REM sleep. Heart rate and arterial blood pressure are irregular, and the sympathetic nervous system activity is higher than in non-REM sleep and similar to that found in the awake state.

Compared to wakefulness, brain activity and the responsiveness to external stimuli decrease during sleep. This is partially due to the decreased or absent activity of the ascending reticular formation during sleep, which contributes to activation of the central nervous system during wakefulness. With regard to respiration, the equivalent of such activation is the *wakefulness drive*, which stimulates ventilation in the awake state and is absent during sleep.

Although responsiveness is reduced, various stimuli, such as noise, can wake up the subject. Such stimuli often disturb sleep without causing full awakenings, and these events are called *"arousals"* or *"microarousals"* from sleep. *Arousals* are short interruptions of sleep continuity (up to 15 s), characterized by a sudden increase in EEG frequency, often featuring a wake rhythm, for a few seconds. Arousals often occur during sleep-related obstructive respiratory events and contribute to sleep fragmentation and daytime sleepiness. Despite their short duration, arousals are associated with blood pressure and heart rate surges, increased muscle tone, increased ventilation and possibly body movements.

An important consequence of sleep is the tendency of the upper airway to collapse, explaining the pathogenesis of "obstructive" respiratory events during sleep. Several factors contribute to such tendency: (1) the reduction of muscle tone during sleep, leading to inadequate activity of the dilator upper airway muscles, (2) the insufficient downward traction and expansion of the upper airway during inspiration, due to reduced lung volumes in the supine posture, especially in obese subjects, (3) the rostral shift of fluids during recumbency which may cause edema and narrowing of the upper airway in susceptible subjects, i.e. patients with heart failure, renal insufficiency or resistant hypertension. Moreover, the cyclic occurrence of respiratory events during sleep and hyperventilation during arousals from sleep in patients with sleep-related breathing disorders (SRBDs) causes state-dependent fluctuations in neural drive to respiratory and upper airway muscles which may perpetuate sleep disordered breathing of both central and obstructive type.

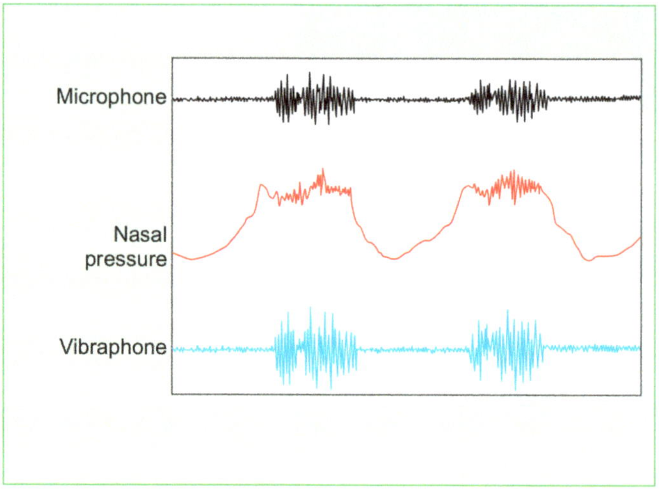

Fig. 15.1: Snoring detection by using microphone, nasal cannula pressure, and vibraphone.

OVERVIEW OF SLEEP-RELATED BREATHING DISORDERS

Sleep-related breathing disorders (SRBDs), previously called *sleep-disordered breathing*, is a term used to encompass different types of abnormal breathing during sleep. These disorders may alter the organization and duration of sleep, with consequential daytime symptoms, i.e. *excessive daytime sleepiness (EDS)* or fatigue, and organ system dysfunction, i.e. cardiovascular or metabolic alterations.

From the point of view of the pulmonologist, SRBDs cause hypoxemia during sleep, either intermittent or continuous. *Intermittent hypoxia* alters cardiorespiratory modulation by the autonomic nervous system, increases the production of inflammatory mediators and oxidative stress, and affects metabolic variables, all these mechanisms likely contributing to the high cardiovascular risk of patients with untreated severe *obstructive sleep apnea syndrome (OSAS)*. On the other hand, *continuous hypoxia* is the consequence of sleep hypoventilation in patients with respiratory impairment, and may affect neurocognitive function during daytime and contribute to the development of polycythemia.

The following paragraphs will briefly summarize the main types of SRBDs encountered in respiratory clinical practice.

Snoring can be defined as a vibratory sound generated during sleep in the upper airways, but its characteristics have been variably described. Snoring is common, but estimated prevalence rates are highly variable in general population studies (between 2% and 85%) and show ethnic-related differences. Risk factors for snoring include male gender, obesity and weight gain, active and passive smoking, and alcohol use, whereas habitual physical activity may exert a protective effect. Snoring has been rarely directly recorded in large studies and criteria of snoring "severity" are lacking. Besides, self-reported snoring might simply reflect the coexistence of OSAS. The impact of snoring, independent of coexisting OSAS, on health outcomes is uncertain.

From a practical point of view, snoring is a very important symptom of obstructive sleep apnea, and as such it deserves attention. Simple snoring can be considered as one end of the spectrum of severity of airway obstruction during sleep with obstructive sleep apnea being the other end. Questions should be asked about the features of snoring in patients referred for suspected obstructive SRBD, i.e. how often a patient snores, whether snoring is loud and disturbing for others, and the occurrence of continuous versus intermittent snoring: in fact, loud intermittent snoring is highly suggestive of OSAS.

Sound measurement by a small microphone placed near the cannula is the most accurate way to detect snoring. Many polysomnography (PSG) studies detect snoring by a sensor which record vibrations (vibraphone), located at the patient's neck. Moreover, also the nasal cannula pressure system is often used to evaluate snoring, since this causes small, fast fluctuations in the airflow signal. Through the use of a specific filter, these fluctuations can be captured and amplified. The morphology of the nasal pressure waveform is very similar to that recorded using snoring microphones and vibraphones (Fig. 15.1).

Table 15.1: Definition of respiratory events in adults.

Event	*Definition*
Obstructive apnea	Reduction of airflow by >90% of pre-event baseline associated with continued or increased thoracoabdominal movements, duration ≥10 s
Central apnea	Reduction of airflow by >90% of pre-event baseline associated with absent thoracoabdominal movements, duration ≥10 s
Mixed apnea	Reduction of airflow by >90% of pre-event baseline with absent thoracoabdominal movements in the initial portion of the event, followed by resumption of respiratory efforts in the second portion of the event, duration ≥10 s
Hypopnea	Reduction of airflow by ≥30% of pre-event baseline, associated with ≥3% oxygen desaturation or arousal, duration ≥10 s *Obstructive hypopnea*: Occurrence of snoring, inspiratory flow limitation or thoracoabdominal paradox during the event *Central hypopnea*: Absence of any criteria listed for obstructive hypopnea
Respiratory effort related arousal (RERA)	Sequence of breaths lasting ≥10 seconds characterized by increasing respiratory effort or by flattening of the inspiratory portion of the nasal pressure waveform leading to arousal from sleep (when the sequence of breaths does not meet criteria for an apnea or hypopnea)
Cheyne-Stokes breathing	Episodes of ≥3 consecutive central apneas and/or central hypopneas separated by a crescendo-decrescendo change in breathing amplitude with a cycle length of ≥40 s, and ≥5 central apneas and/or central hypopneas per hour of sleep associated with the crescendo/decrescendo breathing pattern recorded over ≥2 hours of monitoring
Hypoventilation	Increased $PaCO_2$ or $PtcCO_2$ >55 mm Hg for 10 minutes or increased $PaCO_2$ or $PtcCO_2$ by ≥10 mm Hg compared to wakefulness exceeding 50 mm Hg for ≥10 minutes

Source: Adapted from AASM Manual for the Scoring of Sleep and Associated Events, 2012.

Upper airway resistance syndrome (UARS) has been defined as recurrence of episodes of increased resistance of the upper airway during sleep followed by respiratory arousals in the absence of oxygen desaturation (*"respiratory effort-related arousals"* or *"RERAs"*), and associated with daytime fatigue and/or sleepiness, and possibly systemic hypertension. RERAs represent an intermediate level of airway obstruction between snoring and obstructive hypopneas (Table 15.1 for the complete definition of RERA). Diagnosis requires recording of esophageal pressure during PSG to assess occurrence of respiratory efforts, but this is rarely performed. Instead, the *flow limitation* pattern in the nasal pressure recording is largely used as a reliable marker of incomplete upper airway obstruction (Fig. 15.2). Occurrence of symptoms in a snorer is often labeled as UARS, raising questions on the real existence of this clinical entity. Indeed, differences between PSG recordings of simple snoring and UARS were found to be minor, with the exception of an increased number of arousals in non-REM sleep in the latter.

The obstructive sleep apnea syndrome (OSAS) is the most frequent SRBD in the population. It is characterized by complete or partial collapse of upper airway during sleep, progressive respiratory efforts during airway obstruction, intermittent hypoxia and fragmented sleep. EDS occurs in about 50% of patients with OSAS. Prevalence estimates

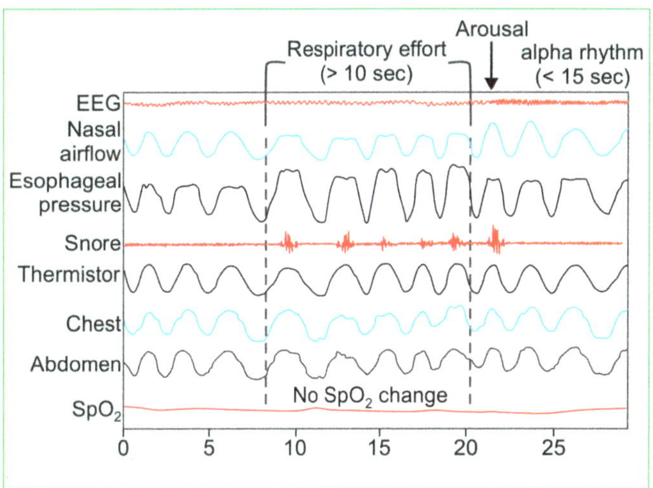

Fig. 15.2: Example of respiratory effort-related arousal (RERA). Even if the definition of a RERA is based on increasing esophageal pressure prior to arousal, the change in shape on the nasal pressure airflow signal is usually present and allows RERAs to be detected non-invasively. During the RERA, changes in phase between chest and abdominal movements may occur. A short interruption of sleep (arousal) follows the respiratory effort. This appears as an abrupt wakefulness (alpha rhythm on the EEG) or change from a deeper stage of non-REM sleep to a lighter stage for a few seconds (if the alpha rhythm last more than 15 seconds, it is considered an awakening).

in the general US population in the early 90s suggested that OSAS, defined as occurrence of more than five respiratory events per hour of sleep associated with EDS, affected 4% of men and 2% of women, but today these figures could be higher due to the increasing prevalence of obesity in the general population. If occurrence of respiratory events was considered irrespective of EDS, prevalence of OSAS was much higher, with estimates of about 24% in men and 9% in women.

Upper airway patency depends on anatomical and functional factors. Reduction of airway lumen can be caused by increased volume of tonsils, uvula or tongue, or by increased collapsibility of pharyngeal wall. Importantly, upper airway muscles counteract increased upper airway resistance by reflex active responses, which decrease or may be lost during sleep, particularly in subjects with OSAS. Upper airways can be modeled as a *Starling resistor*, and the *critical closing pressure of the airways (Pcrit)* is a useful concept. In normal subjects, *Pcrit* is very negative, with progressively less negative values in subjects with snoring, obstructive hypopneas and obstructive apneas. Obesity increases upper airway collapsibility, especially in men.

The typical OSAS patient is a middle aged obese or overweight man, but the disease occurs at all ages and in women as well. Besides the obese phenotype, the other main presentation of the disease is that associated with anatomic abnormalities of upper airways (e.g. micrognathia, enlargement of tonsils). OSAS often occurs in endocrinological disorders, such as hypothyroidism and acromegaly, with obesity explaining at least partly the predisposition for OSAS.

Clinically, OSAS patients report unrefreshing sleep, sometimes morning headaches, tiredness, dyspnea on exertion and nicturia. The bed partner usually refers heavy snoring interrupted by pauses. Untreated severe OSAS carries an increased risk to develop cardiovascular disease, possibly linked to increased sympathetic activation caused by chronic nocturnal intermittent hypoxia with increased risk to develop systemic hypertension. Intermittent hypoxia is also responsible for inflammatory activation in systemic vessels. In addition, OSA may affect metabolic variables, since intermittent hypoxia worsens insulin sensitivity, plasma lipids and liver function with a pattern of proatherogenic dyslipidemia. Severe OSAS is often associated with the metabolic syndrome, but this topic is still under study since obesity is a major confounder. Finally, the mechanical alterations associated with obstructed respiratory efforts may contribute to *autonomic dysregulation* and negatively affect cardiac function by altering transmural cardiac pressures. Patients with OSAS often report concentration difficulties, memory loss and daytime sleepiness, and are at increased risk of car accidents, in part secondary to sleep disruption. An association of OSAS with cancer has been recently reported, with increased mortality in untreated young (age <50 years) patients.

The most effective treatment for OSAS is the application of *continuous positive airway pressure (CPAP)* via nasal or oronasal mask, titrated in each patient to the pressure level which abolishes all respiratory events in all sleep stages and body positions. Effective CPAP (usually at a pressure level ≤15 cm H_2O) maintains upper airway patency and prevents respiratory events and all their consequences. Observational and randomized controlled studies showed that long-term CPAP decreases the risk of car accidents, total and cardiovascular mortality in men, women and elderly patients, systemic blood pressure, and the incidence of hypertension in normotensive patients. Protective effects of CPAP have been recently reported for occurrence of stroke in men and women. All these studies underlined that adherence to CPAP treatment (at least 4 hours of use per night) is needed to achieve positive effects on prognosis. Unfortunately, maintenance of a good compliance to CPAP treatment may be a problem in some subjects.

Other treatments are available. Weight loss decreases OSAS severity and should always be suggested. Weight loss and other lifestyle interventions can improve OSAS, but are generally insufficient to completely normalize respiration during sleep. For mild OSAS, or patients who do not tolerate CPAP, *mandibular advancement devices (MAD)* represent a well-accepted option. The device has to be worn during sleep, is less intrusive than CPAP in the private life of the patient, and has to be titrated with a sleep study, in order to reach a degree of advancement effectively preventing respiratory events. MAD positively affect symptoms and blood pressure.

Obesity hypoventilation syndrome (OHS) was also known as *Pickwickian Syndrome*, from the fatty sleepy boy described by Dickens. It is characterized by chronic daytime hypercapnia in obese subjects in the absence of concurrent lung or neuromuscular disease, and is associated with marked hypoxemia during sleep. Its clinical importance has increased due to the increasing prevalence of obesity worldwide and the high number of patients with morbid obesity [Body mass index (BMI) >40 kg/m^2]. Recently, the *malignant obesity hypoventilation syndrome (MOHS)* has been defined as a severe multisystem disease. Patients with MOHS often require admission to ICU, and their mortality is high.

Obesity places a high demand on the respiratory muscles while causing a restrictive syndrome and this partly explains the susceptibility to develop hypoventilation. Sleep studies are a major part of the diagnostic work-up in OHS patients, since obese patients often show severe OSAS and nocturnal hypoventilation, especially in REM sleep. A recent study compared hypercapnic and normocapnic obese patients referred for suspected OSAS to identify predictors of OHS in this population. Partial pressure arterial oxygen (PaO_2) and serum bicarbonate concentration greater than 27 mmol/L independently predicted daytime hypercapnia. According to other studies, increased CO_2 production, rather than decreased minute ventilation, is the main feature of OHS.

Obesity hypoventilation syndrome patients should be referred for medical or surgical treatment of obesity, and initiated on nocturnal *non invasive ventilation (NIV)*. Due to high morbidity and mortality of the condition, OHS patients need a multidisciplinary approach aimed at correcting not only respiratory, but also metabolic and cardiovascular abnormalities.

Central Sleep Apnea Syndrome and Cheyne-Stokes Respiration

Central sleep apnea (CSA) and Cheyne-Stokes respiration (CSR) are breathing disorders usually caused by instability of the respiratory drive, which becomes evident in non-REM sleep when control of breathing depends only on chemical stimuli.

In the awake state, the wakefulness drive maintains ventilation irrespective of partial pressure of carbon dioxide ($PaCO_2$) values. However, during non-REM sleep respiration ceases when $PaCO_2$ falls below the apnea threshold. If $PaCO_2$ during wakefulness is close to the apnea threshold, the risk to develop central apneas is increased, with hyperventilation at the end of the respiratory event triggering subsequent cessation of breathing. *In normal subjects,* short central apneas can occur while falling asleep, but respiration becomes regular when sleep stabilizes. *At high altitude,* however, the low $PaCO_2$ associated with hypoxia-driven hyperventilation triggers the cyclic occurrence of central apneas in non-REM sleep.

Subjects without heart failure can experience central sleep apnea during sleep, but the "idiopathic central sleep apnea syndrome" (ICSA) is rare compared to OSAS. These patients often show fragmented sleep. Short sudden hyperventilation associated with arousals can lead $PaCO_2$ below the apnea threshold, and central apneas occur. In some subjects, administration of Zolpidem, a hypnotic drug, may effectively stabilize both sleep and ventilation. Treatment with opioids is an additional, recently identified cause of CSA.

Central sleep apneas/hypopneas are highly prevalent in subjects with chronic heart failure, where they show the typical crescendo-decrescendo pattern of CSR. Several factors concur in the pathogenesis of CSA/CSR in heart failure. First, these patients often show increased central chemoresponsiveness, and tend to hyperventilate. Second, pulmonary congestion causes a reflex increase in ventilation, contributing to hypocapnia. Furthermore, altered cerebrovascular responses to CO_2 may amplify central chemoreceptor responses. Interstitial lung edema and decreased lung volume due to cardiomegaly and/or pleural effusion may also play some role. While the duration of central apneas does not correlate with cardiovascular function, the length of the ventilation period between apneas is directly proportional to the circulation time from the lungs to the peripheral chemoreceptors, and inversely proportional to cardiac output. Therefore, heart failure patients typically show quite prolonged ventilatory periods between events. Compared to patients with obstructive events in whom arousals usually precede hyperventilation, patients with CSA/CSR often show arousals during hyperventilation. Therefore, arousals are not necessary for interruption of central event but may significantly contribute to the ventilatory overshoot that triggers the subsequent apneic cycle. Old age (>60 years), male sex, awake $PaCO_2$ below or equal to 38 mm Hg, and presence of atrial fibrillation are risk factors for CSA/CSR.

The symptomatic consequences of CSA/CSR are less dramatic than those of OSAS. Cardiac patients with CSA/CSR rarely complaint of daytime sleepiness, possibly as a result of high sympathetic activation. Hypoxemia caused by central apneas is usually less severe compared to that observed after OSA. Hypertensive peaks, however, occur in the interapneic period after both types of apneas, and contribute to increase cardiac O_2 demand in patients with heart failure.

It is still unclear whether CSA/CSR is a marker of CHF severity or contributes independently to worsen mortality. Randomized controlled trials currently under way will answer this question. Until the effect on survival will be clarified, indications for treatment of CSA/CSR are not well defined. Optimization of treatment for CHF should be the first step, while patients who complain of poor sleep quality or show severe cardiac impairment are candidate to further treatment for CSA/CSR. Nocturnal O_2 administration reduces the number of respiratory events, but rarely normalizes ventilation during sleep. Inhalation of CO_2 is immediately successful in eliminating CSA, but increases sympathetic nervous activity and is not used clinically. CPAP has been used, and in some subjects may exert positive effects through multiple mechanisms, including decreased pulmonary congestion and increased lung volume, but this treatment has been superseded by the development of noninvasive modalities of ventilation specifically designed to correct CSA/CSR. *Adaptive servo-ventilation (ASV)* stabilizes respiration but today its safety in chronic heart failure is under debate.

Hypoventilation during sleep frequently occurs in respiratory disorders, from COPD to neuromuscular diseases. Nocturnal respiratory failure usually precedes the onset of diurnal hypoventilation. Initially in the natural history of chronic respiratory failure, hypoventilation occurs only in REM sleep, and extends to non-REM sleep in the most severe cases. Reduction in intercostal and accessory respiratory muscles activity in REM sleep is one of the main causes of sleep hypoventilation, especially in subjects with altered diaphragm function. Worsening of ventilation/perfusion inequalities may give some contribution to deterioration of blood gases during sleep in some subjects. Hypoventilation limited to, or predominant in, non-REM sleep is typically observed in the rare central hypoventilation syndromes, where absence of the wakefulness drive associated with altered or absent chemoresponsiveness heavily reduce ventilation in that sleep state.

To diagnose hypoventilation, it is necessary to monitor arterial or *transcutaneous PCO_2 ($PtcCO_2$)* during sleep, the latter being preferred because it is noninvasive. $PtcCO_2$ undergoes slow changes compared to $PaCO_2$, and this has to be considered in the analysis of tracings. $PtcCO_2$ monitoring is also useful when nocturnal noninvasive ventilation (NIV) is started, to optimally adjust the ventilator setting.

Daytime arterial blood gases values may imperfectly predict nocturnal desaturations and hypoventilation. They are variably correlated with the nocturnal values, also depending on the disease by which the patient is affected. Pulse oximetry during sleep may provide findings suggestive of hypoventilation, i.e. prolonged desaturation periods, but its sensitivity in detecting hypoventilation is low, especially in patients using supplemental oxygen.

Table 15.2: The Epworth sleepiness scale.

Situation	*Chance of dozing*
Sitting and reading	0 – 1 – 2 – 3
Watching TV	0 – 1 – 2 – 3
Sitting inactive in a public place (e.g. a theater or a meeting)	0 – 1 – 2 – 3
As a passenger in a car for an hour without a break	0 – 1 – 2 – 3
Lying down to rest in the afternoon when circumstances permit	0 – 1 – 2 – 3
Sitting and talking to someone	0 – 1 – 2 – 3
Sitting quietly after a lunch without alcohol	0 – 1 – 2 – 3
In a car, while stopped for a few minutes in traffic	0 – 1 – 2 – 3

TESTS FOR MEASURING EXCESSIVE DAYTIME SLEEPINESS

Excessive daytime sleepiness is a major symptom of SRBDs. It can be evaluated subjectively by questionnaires, and objectively by more complex tests, like the *multiple sleep latency test (MSLT)*. Patients with suspected SRBD should always be asked about their sleeping habits, occurrence of sleepiness during daytime, need for naps and sleepiness while driving.

The *Epworth sleepiness scale (ESS)* is the most widely used questionnaire to assess subjective daytime sleepiness (Table 15.2). It is a very short questionnaire, which asks the subject to rate his/her probability of dozing off in eight different situations that most people experience in their daily lives. Scoring of the answers is 0–3, with 0 being "would never doze" and 3 being "high chance of dozing". A sum of 10 or more from the 8 individual scores reflects above normal daytime sleepiness and need for further evaluation. Despite its limitations, it is simple, cheap and is part of the standard evaluation of patients with suspected OSAS.

Multiple sleep latency test is an objective test performed in the sleep laboratory after PSG, and measures the time necessary to fall asleep at different times of the day, due to the physiologic variability in sleep propensity during daytime. It is highly time-consuming and is not indicated in routine respiratory clinical practice.

HOW TO STUDY SLEEP?

According to the practice parameters published in 1994, diagnostic methods for the diagnosis of respiratory sleep disorders can been classified as shown in Table 15.3.

While this classification underwent no major changes in the last 20 years, the large number of patients requiring

Table 15.3: Diagnostic tests according to practice parameters of American Sleep Disorders Association (ASDA), 1994.

Level 1. Standard polysomnography (PSG)	Minimal requirements include recording of electroencephalogram (EEG), electrooculogram (EOG), chin electromyogram (EMG), electrocardiogram (ECG), airflow, respiratory effort and oxygen saturation. Body position must be documented or objectively measured. Trained personnel must be in constant attendance and able to intervene.
Level 2. Comprehensive portable PSG	Same as for level 1 except heart rate instead of ECG is acceptable, and no personnel attends the recording.
Level 3. Modified portable sleep-apnea testing	Minimum requirements include recording of ventilation (at least two channels of respiratory movement, or respiratory movement and airflow), ECG or heart rate and oxygen saturation. Personnel are needed for preparation, but the ability to intervene is not required for all studies.
Level 4. Continuous (single or dual) bioparameter recording	Only one or two physiologic variables need be recorded. The ability to intervene is not required.

diagnosis and treatment for SRBD, the high cost of full PSG, and the increasing cuts to public health costs, together with improvements in technology, have gradually changed clinical practice with increasing use of portable monitoring devices, and use of traditional PSG in the laboratory in highly selected cases.

The major advancement in clinical research on portable monitoring versus in-lab PSG was provided by some randomized controlled trials reporting no significant difference in outcome between patients undergoing ambulatory management, i.e. diagnosis and treatment, for OSAS and patients undergoing usual diagnosis and CPAP titration in the sleep laboratory. Ambulatory management was by cardiorespiratory polygraphy and automatic positive airway pressure (APAP) ventilation at home for a few days to identify the correct level of fixed CPAP (abolition of respiratory events in all sleep stages and body positions during sleep). Importantly, these data apply only to patients with severe OSAS and no comorbidities. Patients usually accept well the home titration by APAP, since it does not alter sleeping habits compared to the need to sleep in a different environment. Patients have to be carefully instructed to correctly use the ventilator and apply the mask, and need to return to the sleep clinic for a few times during the titration process (*see* below).

Recently, good results have been reported on use of cardiorespiratory polygraphy in the diagnosis of CSR in heart failure patients.

Polysomnography is the gold standard diagnostic tool used to evaluate sleep disorders (Fig. 15.3). It allows identification of sleep and wakefulness, sleep stages and arousals. Respiratory events (apneas and hypopneas, RERA, periodic breathing, and Cheyne-Stokes respiration) can be identified. Alterations in EEG (e.g. in epilepsy) and periodic leg movements can be detected. Other sleep-related

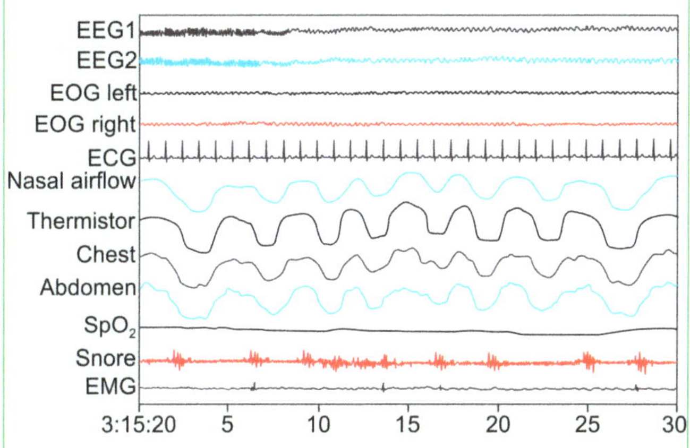

Fig. 15.3: Example of normal polysomnogram during the transition from stage 0 (wakefulness) to stage 1.
(EEG: Electroencephalogram; EOG: Electrooculogram; ECG: Electrocardiogram; EMG: Electromyogram).

abnormalities, such as parasomnias, like REM-related sleep behavior disorders, can be diagnosed by PSG associated with video-recording. When PSG is obtained in the sleep laboratory *(level 1),* a technician insures surveillance of the patient and quality control of the recordings for the whole night. Ambulatory PSG is considered *level 2,* but is quite rarely used in usual clinical practice.

Nocturnal cardiorespiratory polygraphy (PG) (level 3) is the most commonly used test for the diagnosis of SRBD. Eight-channels are available in the majority of devices, including the registration of airflow and thoraco- abdominal movements, ECG, heart rate and arterial oxygen saturation (SpO_2), a sensor for body position, and a microphone to record snoring. Mask pressure during CPAP or NIV can also be recorded. PG allows to identify the respiratory events (reduction or disappearance of airflow) and to differentiate central, obstructive, and mixed apneas in relation to the presence or absence of chest and abdomen respiratory efforts (Fig. 15.4). Ideally, two different sensors should be used for airflow: the *nasal pressure cannula* which provides a signal sensitive to quantitative (like in hypopneas) and qualitative (like with inspiratory flow limitation) variations in airflow, and the *thermistor*, which records flow by changes in air temperature and is more accurate in the identification of apneas. PG does not record sleep, with some implications in the calculation of the apnea-hypopnea index and the scoring of hypopneas (*see* below).

Level 4 devices are available. The *Watch-PAT* recorder uses peripheral arterial tonometry to identify obstructive events, and has been validated against PSG.

Nocturnal oximetry is the simplest and most widespread measurement obtained in clinical practice for investigations on nocturnal respiratory disorders. It can be recorded at home or hospital. It involves the use of a probe similar to a clothespin worn on a finger or earlobe that provides a continuous noninvasive measurement of SpO_2 and heart rate. Software programs usually provide a summary on the number, frequency and degree of desaturation events (usually defined as a SpO_2 reduction ≥ 4% from baseline). Oximetry can be used as a screening tool for sleep disorders. However, by night pulse oximetry alone, it is not possible to identify occurrence of respiratory disorders that do not involve reduction of SpO_2.

Other level 4 devices are also available. *Nasal pressure recording*, alone or in combination with oximetry, has been validated against PSG in patients with high clinical suspicion of OSAS.

Despite some investigations have found some level 4 devices useful for OSAS diagnosis, especially in severe cases, they are not recommended by guidelines for diagnostic purposes. Their use could be more appropriate in follow-up or screening studies.

According to recent recommendations, patients with OSAS should undergo 24-hour monitoring of arterial blood pressure (ABPM). This technique is mandatory to identify isolated nocturnal hypertension associated with OSAS. SRBD is a major cause of "masked hypertension", i.e. normal office blood pressure associated with increased mean 24-hour blood pressure.

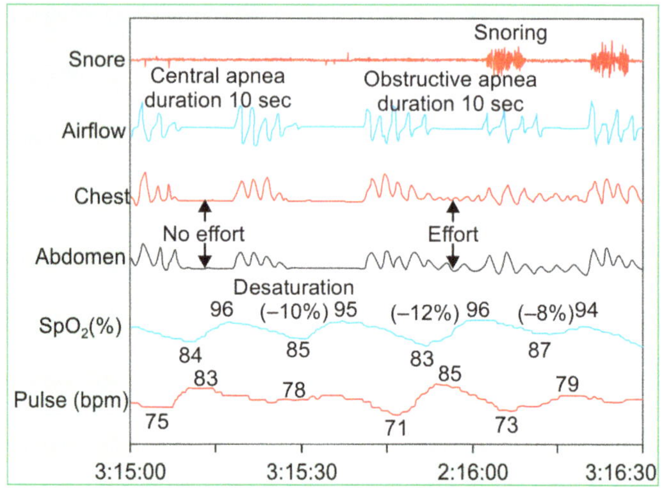

Fig. 15.4: Example of nocturnal cardiorespiratory polygraphy showing central and obstructive apneas. An apnea is defined as an 80–100% reduction in airflow signal for at least 10 seconds. The apnea is considered to be central if no effort is noted on both the thorax and abdominal effort channel. When there is no airflow but there is effort to breathe, the apnea is classified as obstructive. Note that the apneas are often followed by a reduction oxygen saturation and an increase in heart rate. Whereas snoring is commonly associated with obstructive events, it is usually not found with central sleep apnea.

HOW TO SELECT THE MOST APPROPRIATE DIAGNOSTIC PROCEDURE?

All patients with suspected SRBD should undergo full clinical evaluation, including clinical history, assessment of cardiovascular and metabolic comorbidities (i.e. coronary heart disease, hypertension, heart failure, cerebrovascular disease, type 2 diabetes, metabolic syndrome) and current treatment. The bed partner can provide information on snoring and breathing pauses. Weight and height should be measured to calculate the BMI.

In patients with high clinical suspicion of OSAS, current AASM guidelines recommend to use full-night PSG in the laboratory. Alternatively, in patients without comorbidities, ambulatory PG can be used, while Level 4 devices are not recommended. Similarly, for CPAP/NIV titration, attended PSG is the gold standard.

Automatic CPAP (diagnostic mode) is a good alternative to manual CPAP titration in the laboratory, as confirmed by several randomized studies. Different ventilator models are available, and all use detection of obstruction as the signal to regulate the pressure delivered. After a few nights during which the patient uses the auto-CPAP machine at home, the pressure to be delivered in the fixed mode can be identified as the 95th percentile, and the patients is switched to fixed CPAP to complete titration. The automatic CPAP machines, originally developed to improve compliance to treatment, are very useful for ambulatory titration, since they provide data on pressure delivered and leaks, allowing optimization of the interface. In addition, they provide an estimate of central and obstructive residual events. A sleep study (PSG or PG) is, however, necessary at the end of the titration procedure to confirm effectiveness of treatment.

Scoring PG raises some problems. First, in PSG the apnea-hypopnea index (AHI) is calculated as the total number of respiratory events divided by total sleep time (TST). When sleep is not recorded, recording time is used with obvious "dilution" of respiratory events if wakefulness occurs during the night. Therefore, the AHI of PSG is generally higher than the AHI of PG. Second, scoring of hypopneas according to the most recent rules requires a reduction in airflow associated with either 3% oxygen desaturation or an arousal. Since arousals cannot be scored in PG, a lower AHI will result compared to the AHI calculated in a PSG recording, due to lack of identification of hypopneas terminating with arousals. Similarly, respiratory related arousals (RERA), typical of UARS, will also be missed in PG. For all these reasons, it would be appropriate to use specific rules for scoring of events recorded during PG.

Despite these limitations, cardiorespiratory polygraphy is very useful in the management and follow-up of OSAS patients, and possibly of patients with CSR as well. Besides sleep studies at the end of the CPAP titration procedure, we routinely obtain PG in patients on noninvasive bilevel ventilation, in order to identify problems in the setting of the ventilator (i.e. insufficient pressure, asynchronies, trigger problems, backup rate). Some rules have been proposed to scoring these events during PSG or PG, but built-in software of NIV machines already provides some information on residual respiratory events during use.

PREPARATION OF THE PATIENT FOR POLYGRAPHY

Since PSG is currently used much less than PG for diagnosis of sleep disorders in respiratory patients, the interested reader is referred to the AASM Manual for Scoring Events for detailed description of technical requirements for PSG.

Figure 15.5 illustrates how devices for PG should be mounted. Place the bands around the chest and abdomen (outside of a patient's t-shirt) for recording their movements during respiration. Bands of different sizes are usually available, to be chosen according to the characteristics of the patient. Place the sensor underneath the nose for recording airflow. Place the probe (the sensor) for the oxyhemoglobin saturation to a finger of a hand or earlobe). If a snore microphone is available, place it on the face close to the source of snoring. A hypoallergenic medical tape can help to maintain the microphone in the desired position throughout the night.

The device should be programmed to record from the usual bedtime to the usual wake-up time of the patient.

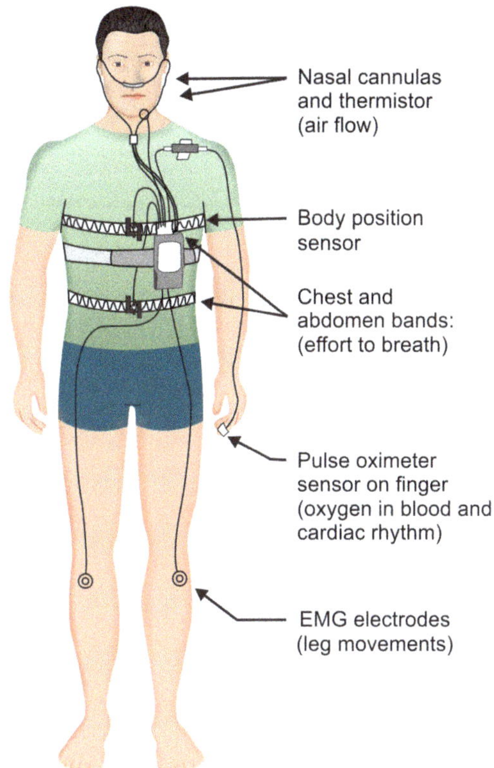

Fig. 15.5: How to use a cardiorespiratory monitoring device.

ANALYSIS AND INTERPRETATIVE STRATEGIES

All nocturnal recordings should be manually revised, since automatic readings are often unreliable. Duration of the recording should be at least 5 hours, and shorter recordings or recordings of bad quality should be repeated. Lack of sleep in supine position is also a reason to repeat the study if PG results negative, since severity of SRBD could be underestimated in the absence of the supine position. A sleep diary is recommended to estimate sleep duration in case of ambulatory PG.

Severity of SRBD is expressed as the apnea hypopnea index (AHI), i.e. the number of apneas and hypopneas per hour of sleep (PSG) or recording (PG). Recently, the new Classification of Sleep Disorders (ICSD-3) introduced the term respiratory event index (REI) as the number of respiratory events per hour of recording, in order to immediately distinguish between PSG- and PG-derived results, and recommended to exclude periods of obvious wake from the analysis of the PG recording. The respiratory disturbance index (RDI) differs from AHI because it also includes respiratory-related arousals (RERA), but is less widely used compared to AHI.

SRBDs are classified as mild for AHI between 5 and 15/hour, moderate for AHI between 15 and 30/hour, and severe for AHI more than 30/hour. Some Centers use a higher cut-off of 10 for the diagnosis of OSAS, especially in elderly patients.

Assessment of OSA severity includes analysis of oxygen desaturation, in particular mean SpO_2, lowest SaO_2, and the percentage of time spent at SaO_2 less than 90%. The oxygen desaturation index (ODI) is the number of oxygen dips per hour of sleep (PSG) or recording (PG). Since ODI can be calculated based on both 3% and 4% desaturation, the degree of oxygen desaturation should be always included in the report (ODI3% or ODI4%). Figures 15.6 to 15.12 show some examples of polygraphic recordings from "real-life" patients with obstructive and central events.

FACTORS TO BE INCLUDED IN A SUMMARY REPORT

An example of summary report is shown in Table 15.4. The main factors to be included in a summary report of cardiorespiratory polygraphy are the following:

1. Setting in which the monitoring was performed:
   - Respiratory conditions (room air, with oxygen support, during noninvasive mechanical ventilation)
   - Environment (at home, in the laboratory)
   - Instrumentation used (portable device, number of channels)
2. Indicators of the duration of sleep (Lights Out, Lights On, Total Recording Time)
3. Indicators of the patient's oxygenation status:
   - Baseline SpO_2 (awake)
   - Mean SpO_2 during sleep
   - Lowest oxygen saturation reached during the night (nadir SpO_2)
   - Mean lowest SpO_2
   - Sleep time with SpO_2 <90% and <80%
   - Oxygen desaturation index (ODI) according to desaturation threshold (3 or 4%).

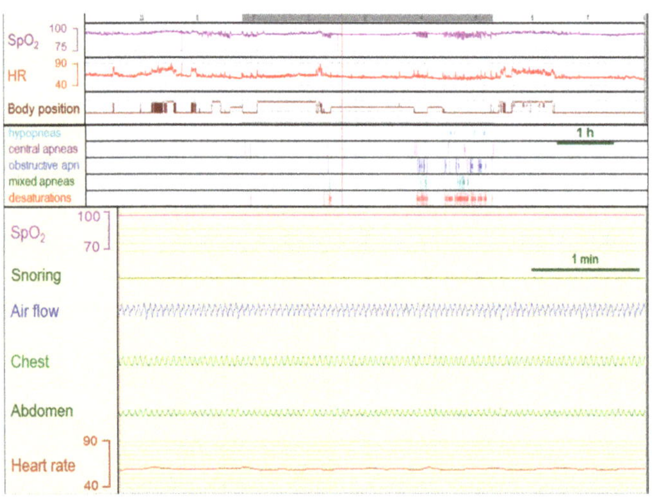

Fig. 15.6: Period of normal breathing in a patients with mild OSAS (cardiorespiratory polygraphy). The upper and middle boxes report data for the entire recording, the lower box shows respiratory signals occurring at the point marked by a vertical red line in upper and middle boxes. Oxygen desaturations and obstructive events occur at some points during the night in right lateral decubitus, and may be associated with REM sleep (PSG would be necessary to define the sleep stage). The lower box corresponds to a period of the night during which respiration is regular without respiratory events or oxygen desaturations.
(PSG: Polysomnography; SpO_2: Oxygen saturation by pulse oximetry; HR: Heart rate).

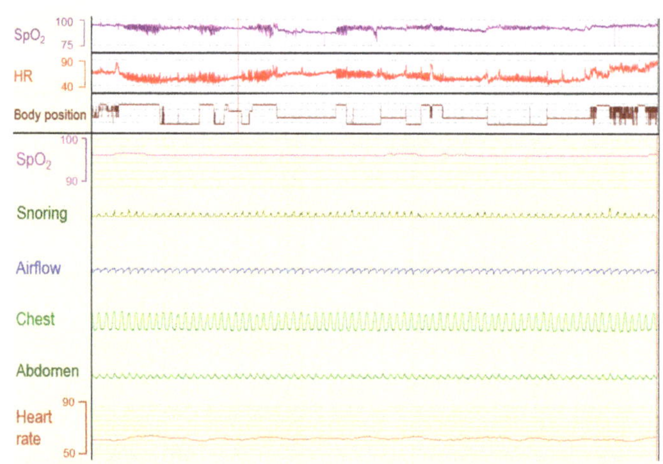

Fig. 15.7: Period of snoring and flow-limitation in a patient with OSAS (cardiorespiratory polygraphy). The upper box reports data for the entire recording, the lower box shows respiratory signals occurring at the point marked by a vertical red line in the upper box. Oxygen desaturations occur intermittently during the night. The lower box corresponds to a period of the night during which snoring occurs. Note the aspect of inspiratory flow limitation in the airflow tracing with inspiratory flattening of the curve instead of the normal rounded appearance (nasal cannula).
(SpO_2: Oxygen saturation by pulse oximetry; HR: Heart rate).

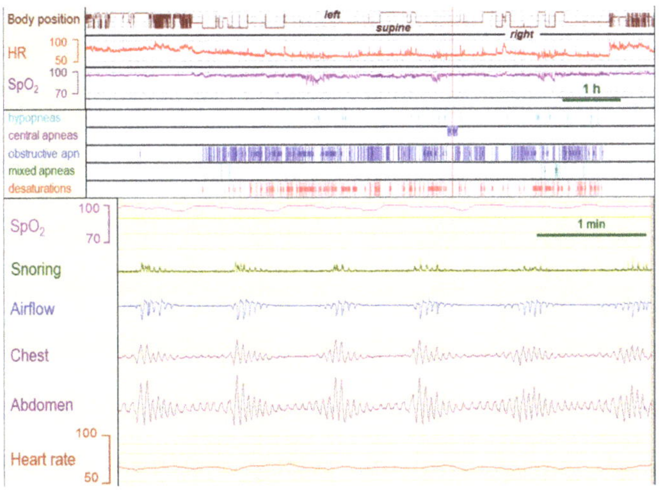

Fig. 15.8: Obstructive apneas (cardiorespiratory polygraphy). The upper and middle boxes report data for the entire recording, the lower box shows respiratory signals occurring at the point marked by a vertical red line in upper and middle boxes. Mild oxygen desaturations occur during the night. The lower box corresponds to a period of the night during which obstructive apneas occur. Note the absence of airflow associated with progressive increase in respiratory movements, and occurrence of intermittent snoring at the time of airway reopening. In this patients, respiration is highly disturbed (note the high frequency of obstructive apneas in all body positions) but apneas cause only a mild degree of oxygen desaturation.
(SpO_2: Oxygen saturation by pulse oximetry; HR: Heart rate).

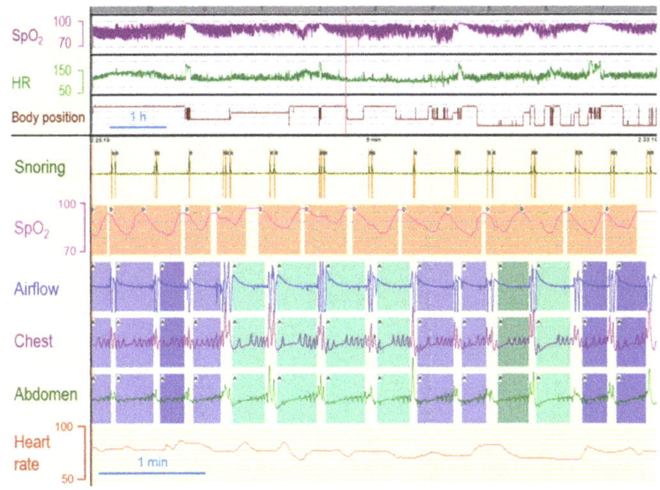

Fig. 15.9: Severe obstructive sleep apnea syndrome (cardiorespiratory polygraphy). The upper box reports data for the entire recording, the lower box shows respiratory signals occurring at the point marked by a vertical red line in upper box. Severe and highly frequent oxygen desaturations occur during the night. The lower box corresponds to a period of the night during which obstructive (marked in blue) and mixed (marked in green) apneas occur. In this patients, respiration is highly disturbed (note the high frequency of obstructive apneas in all body positions). Note absence of respiratory movements in the initial portion of mixed apneas, and the continuous oscillations of oxygen saturation and heart rate.
(SpO_2: Oxygen saturation by pulse oximetry; HR: Heart rate).

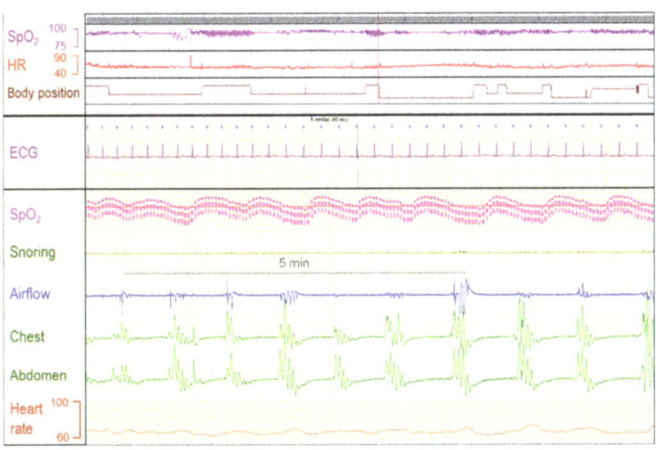

Fig. 15.10: Central sleep apneas (cardiorespiratory polygraphy). The upper box reports data for the entire recording, the middle box shows ECG at 5 mm/s, the lower box shows respiratory signals occurring at the point marked by a vertical red line in upper box. Mild oxygen desaturations occur during the night. The lower box corresponds to a period of the night during which central apneas occur. Note the absence of airflow associated with absence of respiratory movements, and little snoring. The interapneic phase does not show the features of Cheyne-Stokes breathing (no crescendo-decrescendo pattern, *See* Figure 15.11).
(ECG: Electrocardiogram; SpO_2: Oxygen saturation by pulse oximetry; HR: Heart rate).

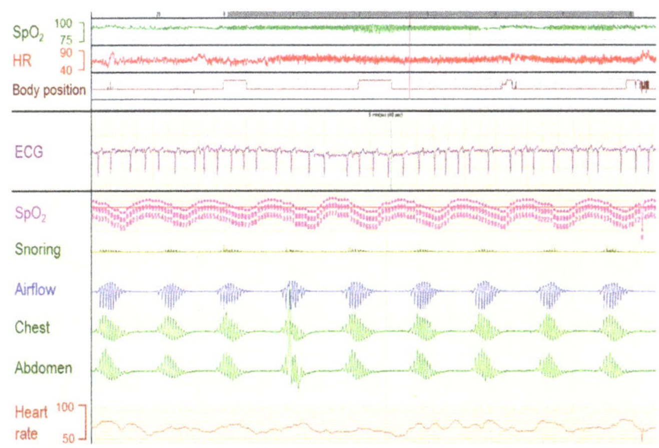

Fig. 15.11: Cheyne-Stokes respiration (cardiorespiratory polygraphy). The upper box reports data for the entire recording, the middle box shows ECG at 5 mm/s (atrial fibrillation), the lower box shows respiratory signals occurring at the point marked by a vertical red line in upper box. The lower box shows central apneas separated by ventilatory periods with a clear crescendo-decrescendo pattern, typically found in patients with chronic heart failure. Note the absence of airflow associated with absence of respiratory movements. Oxygen desaturations associated with central apneas tend to be smoother and more "rounded" compared to those observed during obstructive apneas.
(ECG, Electrocardiogram; SpO_2: Oxygen saturation by pulse oximetry; HR: Heart rate).

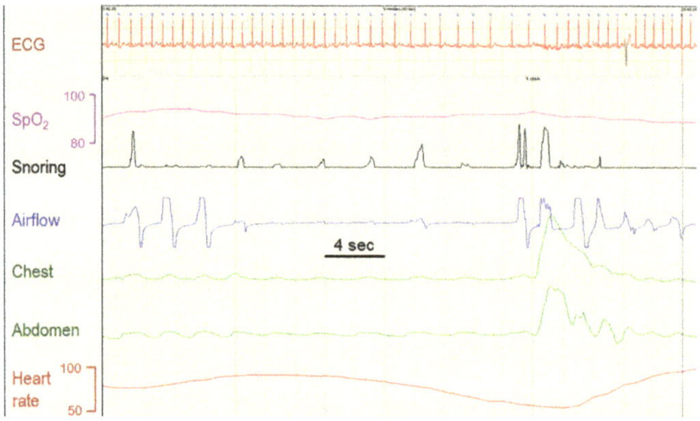

Fig. 15.12: Obstructive hypopnea (cardiorespiratory polygraphy) with marked changes in heart rate. Note occurrence of snoring, and decreased airflow with aspect of inspiratory flow limitation, during the event, associated with significant O2 desaturation. Recording of electrocardiogram (ECG) during polygraphy is highly advisable, since it may show slowing of heart rate during the respiratory event followed by tachycardia at resumption of breathing.

Table 15.4 : Example of polysomnogram summary report.

Patient	Adrian Rossi	Age	60 years, 3 months		
Gender	Male	Height	172		
Date of birth	June 20, 1954	Weight	86		
Type	Adult	BMI	29		
Date of the exam	March 25, 2014	Referring Physician	Dr. Claudio Sorino		
Number PSG	2014_145	Technician	Angelo Longoni		
*Summary of sleep structure**					
Lights off	22:15:30 PM				
Lights on	07:40:45 AM				
Total recording time	9 hours, 25 minute, 15 sec				
Total sleep time	7 hours, 12 minute, 4 s				
Summary of respiratory events					
		Body position		*Sleep state*	
	Total	*Non-Supine*	*Supine*	*NREM*	*REM*
Sleep time (minute)	432	164 (38%)	268 (62%)	346 (80%)	86 (20%)
Obstructive apneas	65	12	53	44	21
Mixed apneas	4	0	4	0	4
Central apneas	5	2	3	0	5
All	74	14	60	44	30
hypopneas	23	8	15	15	8
Apneas + Hypopneas	97	22	75	59	38
RERA	22	2	20	12	10
Apnea Index	10.3	5.2	13.4	7.6	20.9
Hypopnea Index	3.2	2.9	3.4	2.6	5.6
AHI	13.5	8.1	16.8	10.2	26.6
RDI	16.5	8.8	21.2	12.3	33.6
Duration of respiratory events					
	Mean	*Maximum*			
Apneas	34.0 s	50.6 s			
Hypopneas	21.5 s	26.6 s			
RERAs	15.2 s	21.2 s			
*Summary of oxygen saturation***					
Total desaturations	105				
ODI	14.6				
Mean SpO_2	94%				
Minimum SpO_2	83%				
Maximum SpO_2	98%				

Contd...

Contd...

*Summary of oxygen saturation***	
Time < 90%	1 hours 15 minutes, 24 s
Time < 80%	0 hours, 22 minutes, 15 s
Summary snoring	
Total number of snoring episodes	68
Total time with snoring	73 minutes (16.9% of sleep)
Summary of heart rate	
Mean pulse (bpm)	73
Min pulse (bpm)	58
Max pulse (bpm)	96

*Sleep Efficiency Index: Total Sleep Time/Total Recording Time.
**Desaturation Events are defined as a drop in $SpO_2 \geq 4$.

4. Indicators of airflow abnormalities during the sleep:
   - Number of apneic episodes (obstructive, central, and mixed), hypopneas
   - Occurrence of periods with an inspiratory flow limitation pattern (narrative comments)
   - Indexes (number of events per hour of sleep) of the aforementioned episodes. They can be considered separately or in combination, such as in the apnea-hypopnea index (AHI).

It is recommended to express these indexes also by body position.

If PSG is performed, the following indicators of sleep should be included:

- Total sleep time (TST)
- Sleep efficiency (TST/time in bed, percent)
- Sleep onset latency and REM sleep latency
- Cumulative duration of sleep stages throughout the night (hypnogram) and of wakefulness after sleep onset (WASO)
- Arousal index (number of arousals per hour of sleep)

DIAGNOSTIC CRITERIA FOR RESPIRATORY EVENTS

The most widely accepted definitions of the respiratory events during sleep are listed in Table 15.1.

BIBLIOGRAPHY AND FURTHER READING

1. Araghi MH, Chen YF, Jagielski A, Choudhury S, Banerjee D, Hussain S, et al. Effectiveness of lifestyle interventions on obstructive sleep apnea (OSA): systematic review and meta-analysis. Sleep. 2013;36:1553-62.
2. Ayappa I, Norman RG, Suryadevara M, Rapoport DM. Comparison of limited monitoring using a nasal-cannula flow signal to full polysomnography in sleep-disordered breathing. Sleep. 2004;27:1171-79.
3. Ayas NT, Pittman S, MacDonald M, White DP. Assessment of a wrist-worn device in the detection of obstructive sleep apnea. Sleep Med. 2003;4:435-42.
4. Berry RB, Brooks R, Gamaldo CE, Harding SM, Lloyd RM, Marcus CL, et al. The AASM Manual for the Scoring of Sleep and Associated Events: Rules, Terminology and Technical Specifications, Version 2.0.3. [online] Available from www.aasmnet.org, Darien, Illinois: American Academy of Sleep Medicine, 2014. [Accessed December 2015].
5. Bonsignore MR, Marrone O, Insalaco G, Bonsignore G. The cardiovascular effects of obstructive sleep apnoeas: analysis of pathogenetic mechanisms. (Review) Eur Respir J. 1994;7:786-805.
6. Bonsignore MR, Masa JF. Cardio-respiratory monitoring during sleep. ERS Handbook: Respiratory Sleep Medicine. In: Simonds A, de Backer W, (Eds). UK: European Respiratory Society, Sheffield, UK; 2012. p. 136-46.
7. Bonsignore MR, McNicholas WT, Montserrat JM, Eckel J. The adipose tissue in obesity and obstructive sleep apnea. Eur Respir J. 2012;39:746-67.
8. Bordier P, Orazio S, Hofmann P, Robert F, Bourenane G. Short- and long-term effecys of nocturnal oxygen therapy on sleep apnea in chronic heart failure. Sleep Breath. 2015;19(1):159-68.
9. Borel JC, Borel AL, Monneret D, Tamisier R, Levy P, Pepin JL. Obesity hypoventilation syndrome: from sleep-disordered breathing to systmic comorbidities and the need to offer combined treatment strategies. Respirology. 2012;17: 601-10.
10. Burwell CS, Robin ED, Whaley RD, Bickelmann AG. Extreme obesity associated with alveolar hypoventilation: a Pickwickian Syndrome. Am J Med. 1956;21:811-8.
11. Campos-Rodriguez F, Martinez-Garcia MA, de la Cruz-Moron I, Almeida-Gonzales C, Catalan-Serra P, Montserrat JM. Cardiovascular mortality in women with obstructive sleep apnea with or without continuous positive airway pressure treatment. A cohort study. Ann Intern Med. 2012;156:115-22.
12. Campos-Rodriguez F, Matinez-Garcia MA, Reyes-Nunez N, Caballero-Martinez I, Catalan-Serra P, Almeida-Gonzales CV. Role of sleep apnea and continuous positive airway pressure therapy in the incidence of stroke or coronary

heart disease in women. Am J Respir Crit Care Med. 2014;189:1544-50.
13. Chesson AL, Berry RB, Pack A, American Academy of Sleep Medicine; American Thoracic Society; American College of Chest Physicians. Practice parameters for the use of portable monitoring devices in the investigation of suspected obstructive sleep apnea in adults. Sleep. 2003;26:907-13.
14. Contal O, Vignaux L, Combescure C, Pepin JL, Jolliet P, Janssens JP. Monitoring of noninvasive ventilation by built-in software of home bilevel ventilators: a bench study. Chest. 2012;141:469-76.
15. Deary V, Ellis JG, Wilson JA, Coulter C, Barclay NL. Simple snoring: not quite so simple after all? Sleep Med Rev. 2014;18(6):453-62.
16. Dempsey JA, Xie A, Patz DS, Wang D. Physiology in Medicine: Obstructive sleep apnea pathogenesis and treatment considerations beyond anatomy. J Appl Physiol. 2014;116:3-12.
17. Domingo C, Blanch L, Murias G, Luján M. State-of-the-art sensor technology in Spain: invasive and non-invasive techniques for monitoring respiratory variables. Sensors (Basel). 2010;10:4655-74.
18. Gold AR, Schwartz AR. The pharyngeal critical pressure: the whys and hows of using nasal continuous positive airway pressure diagnostically. Chest. 1996;110:1077-88.
19. Gonzales-Bermejo J, Perrin C, Janssens JP, Pepin JL, Mroue G, Léger P, et al. on behalf of the Somno NIV Group. Proposal for a systematic analysis of polygraphy or polysomnography for identifying and scoring abnormal events occurring during non-invasive ventilation. Thorax. 2012;67:546-52.
20. Guilleminault C, Stoohs R, Clerk A, Cetel M, Maistros P. A cause of excessive daytime sleepiness. The upper airway resistance syndrome. Chest. 1993;104:781-7.
21. Guilleminault C, Stoohs R, Shiomi T, Kushida C, Schnittger I. Upper airway resistance syndrome, nocturnal blood pressure monitoring, and borderline hypertension. Chest. 1996;109:901-8.
22. Iftikhar IH, Hays ER, Iverson MA, Magalang UJ, Maas AK. Effect of oral appliances on blood pressure in obstructive sleep apnea: a systematic review and meta-analysis. J Clin Sleep Med. 2013;9:165-74.
23. International Classification of Sleep Disorders, 3rd edition. [online] Available from www.aasmnet.org, Darien, Illinois: American Academy of Sleep Medicine. [Accessed December 2015]
24. Janssens JP, Borel JC, Pepin JL; SomnoNIV Group. Nocturnal monitoring of home non-invasive ventilation: the contribution of simple tools such as pulse oximetry, capnography, built-in ventilator software and autonomic markers of sleep fragmentation. Thorax. 2011;66:438-45.
25. Javaheri S, Simbartl LA. Respiratory determinants of diurnal hypercapnia in obesity hypoventilation syndrome: what does weight have to do with it? Ann Am Thorac Soc. 2014;11(6):945-50.
26. Johns MW. A new method for measuring daytime sleepiness: the Epworth sleepiness scale. Sleep. 1991;14:540-5.
27. Macavei VM, Spurling KJ, Loft J, Makker HK. Diagnostic predictors of obesity-hypoventilation syndrome in patients suspected of having sleep disordered breathing. J Clin Sleep Med. 2013;9:879-84.
28. Marik PE, Desai H. Characteristics of patients with the "malignant obesity hypoventilation syndrome" admitted to an ICU. J Intensive Care Med. 2012;28:124-30.
29. Marik PE. The malignant obesity hypoventilation syndrome (MOHS). Obes Rev. 2012;13:902-9.
30. Marin JM, Agusti A, Villar I, Forner M, Nieto D, Carrizo SJ, et al. Association between treated and untreated obstructive sleep apnea and risk of hypertension. J Am Med Assoc. 2012;307:2169-76.
31. Marin JM, Carrizo SJ, Vicente E, Agusti AGN. Long-term cardiovascular outcomes in men with obstructive sleep apnea-hypopnea with or without treatment with continuous positive airway pressure: an observational study. Lancet. 2005;365:1046-53.
32. Marklund M, Verbraecken J, Randerath W. Non-CPAP therapies in obstructive sleep apnoea: mandibular advancement device therapy. Eur Respir J. 2012;39:1241-7.
33. Martínez-García MA, Campos-Rodriguez F, Durán-Cantolla J, de la Peña M, Masdeu MJ, González M, et al. Obstructive sleep apnea is associated with cancer mortality in younger patients. Sleep Med. 2014;15:742-8.
34. Martínez-García MA, Campos-Rodríguez F, Catalán-Serra P, Soler-Cataluña JJ, Almeida-Gonzalez C, De la Cruz Morón I, et al. Cardiovascular mortality in obstructive sleep apnea in the elderly: role of long-term continuous positive airway pressure treatment: a prospective observational study. Am J Respir Crit Care Med. 2012;186: 909-16.
35. McNicholas WT. Impact of sleep in respiratory failure. Eur Respir J. 1997;10:920-33.
36. Montesi SB, Edwards BA, Malhotra A, Bakker JP. The effect of continuous positive airway pressure treatment on blood pressure: a systematic review and meta-analysis of randomized controlled trials. J Clin Sleep Med. 2012;8: 587-96.
37. Oldenburg O. Cheyne-Stokes respiration in chronic heart failure. Trreatment with adaptive servoventilation therapy, Circ J. 2012;76:2305-17.
38. Parati G, Lombardi C, Hedner J, Bonsignore MR, Grote L, Tkacova R, et al, Position paper on the management of patients with obstructive sleep apnea and hypertension: joint recommendations by the European Society of Hypertension, by the European Respiratory Society and by the members of European COST (Cooperation in Scientific and Technological research) ACTION B26 on obstructive sleep apnea. Eur Respir J. 2013;41(3):523-38.
39. Pinna GD, Robbi E, Pizza F, Taurino AE, Pronzato C, La Rovere MT, et al. Can cardiorespiratory polygraphy replace portable polysomnography in the assessment of sleep-disordered breathing in heart failure patients? Sleep Breath. 2014;18(3):475-82.

40. Piper AJ, Grunstein RR. Big breathing: the complex interaction of obesity, hypoventilation, weight loss, and respiratory function. J Appl Physiol. 2010;108:199-205.
41. Piper AJ. Obesity hypoventilation syndrome: the big and the breathless. Sleep Med Rev. 2011;15:79-89.
42. Polo O, Berthon-Jones M, Douglas NJ, Sullivan CE. Management of obstructive sleep apnoea/hypopnoea syndrome. Lancet. 1994;344:656-60.
43. Quadri S, Drake C, Hudgel DW. Improvement of idiopathic central sleep apnea with zolpidem. J Clin Sleep Med. 2009;5:122-9.
44. Redline S, Yenokyan G, Gottlieb DJ, Shahar E, O'Connor GT, Resnick HE, et al. Obstructive sleep apnea-hypopnea and incident stroke: the Sleep Heart Health Study. Am J Respir Crit Care Med. 2010;182:269-77.
45. Standards of Practice Committee of the American Sleep Disorders Association. Practice parameters for the use of portable recording in the assessment of obtructive sleep apnea. Sleep. 1994;17:372-7.
46. Sánchez-de-la-Torre M, Campos-Rodriguez F, Barbé F. Obstructive sleep apnoea and cardiovascular disease. Lancet Respir Med. 2013;1:61-72.
47. Teschler H, Döring J, Mang Y, Berthon-Jones M. Adaptive pressure support servo-ventilation. A novel treatment for Cheyne-Stokes respiration in heart failure. Am J Respir Crit Care Med. 2001;164:614-9.
48. Tregear S, Reston J, Schoelles K, Phillips B. Continuous positive airway pressure reduces risk of motor vehicle crash among drivers with obstructive sleep apnea: systematic review and meta-analysis. Sleep. 2010;33:1373-80.
49. Wang D, Teichtahl H. Opioids, sleep architecture and sleep-disordered breathing. Sleep Med Rev. 2007;11:35-46.
50. Young T, Palta M, Dempsey J, Skatrud J, Weber S, Badr S. The occurrence of sleep-disordered breathing among middle-aged adults. N Engl J Med. 1993;328:1230-5.
51. Yumino D, Bradley TD. Central sleep apnea and Cheyne-Stokes respiration. Proc Am Thorac Soc. 2008;5:226-36.

Section 3

Diagnostic Imaging

Chapter

16

Chest Radiograph: Technical Aspects, Normal Findings and Extrapulmonary Structures

Ali Nawaz Khan, Klaus L Irion, Prabhakar Rajiah, Carolyn Allen, Durr-e-Sabih, Koteyar Shyamsunder Radhakrishna, Hamdan Al-Jahdali, Syahminan Suut, Zeid Al-Ani, Claudio Sorino

OVERVIEW

The chest X-ray (CXR) is the most common radiological examination undertaken. To obtain a good quality radiograph is vital to the interpretation. The patient's history is important to narrow down the differential diagnosis. The radiologist should be familiar with the standard anatomy seen on a CXR. A CXR should be read in a systematic way. A suggested approach is to read the radiograph from the central to peripheral regions: the heart is looked at first, and then the mediastinum, major airways, lungs, pleura and the chest wall in that order. When interpreting the CXR, it is important precisely to view all structures on the image. Even interpreter develops a unique process for doing this. It is also important that the physician is familiar with various artifacts that can be encountered. A standard CXR is undertaken with X-ray tube at the back and X-ray film against the anterior chest wall [posteroanterior (PA)]. A good radiograph should have sufficient penetration (exposure) although the latter is not now as relevant in the digital age. The patient is instructed to take a deep inspiration, and the technologist is making sure that the patient is not rotated. It is important to examine particular areas where lesions are commonly missed such as the apical regions of the lung, the lung periphery, the pleura, the area under the diaphragm and the posterior mediastinum. Comparison with old films can be crucial as it can save the patient from further unnecessary radiation exposure and investigations that can be expensive in terms of finance and creates unwarranted patient worry and stress.

NOTES ON TECHNICAL ASPECTS

It is very important that each radiograph is properly associated to the right patient.

To check the patient's identity (name, date of birth, hospital number, and gender) makes sure that the correct CXR is being read. The date and time when it is taken should be also verified.

The side must be correctly marked to avoid an erroneous diagnosis of a dextrocardia.

CXR should be also labeled to indicate other important features such as anteroposterior (AP) projection or supine position.

Projection

In a standard PA CXR, the cathode ray is placed 1.5–1.8 m posterior to the patient and the X-ray plate positioned immediately anterior to the patient's chest. With immobile and very ill patients, X-rays may be exposed in AP projection.

The heart size and the mediastinal structures cannot be accurately assessed in an AP projection as these structures are magnified by the divergence of the X-ray beam. If on a PA CXR, the *cardiothoracic ratio* (= cardiac width/thoracic width, Fig. 16.1) is less than or equal to 50% (1:2), then the heart size can be considered to be normal. Any comment regarding heart size is not accurate if the projection is AP (the heart shadow is magnified because it is an anterior structure), or if the patient is rotate, or if the breath in is incomplete (Fig. 16.2). On a PA view, the scapulae always clear the lungs.

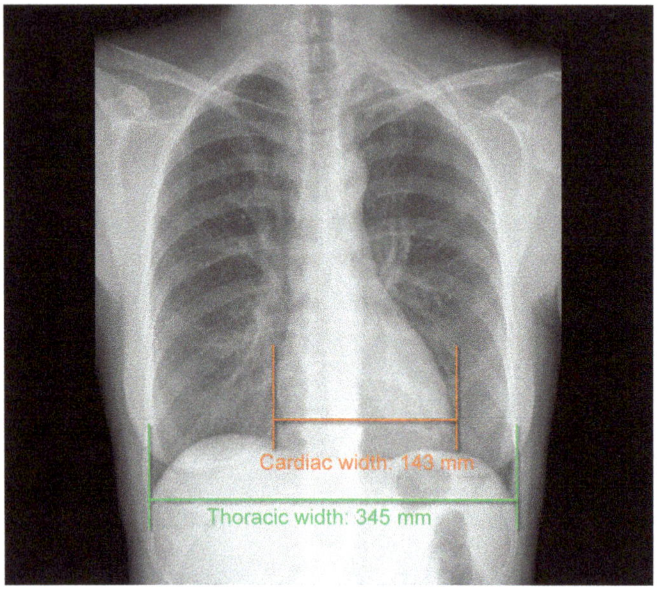

Fig. 16.1: Cardiothoracic ratio (CTR) and heart contours. Cardiac width is measured by drawing parallel lines down both sides of the heart shadow, at the most lateral points on each side, and measuring the distance between them. Thoracic width is measured by drawing parallel lines down the inner aspect of the widest points of the rib cage, and measuring the distance between these. The cardiothoracic ratio can then be stated. In this example, CTR is approximately 143/345 (= 41.5%).

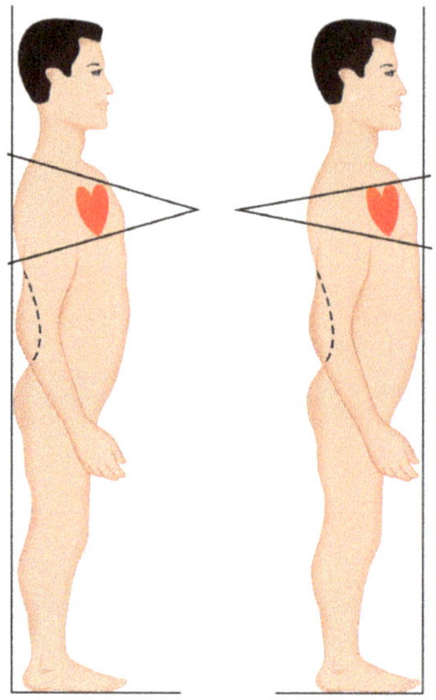

Fig. 16.2: Magnification of the heart shadow in anteroposterior (AP) chest X-ray (CXR).

Patient Positioning

All standard departmental PA CXRs are taken in the optimal erect position. Positioning is an important factor when assessing the appearance of air, fluid and vascular structures. As air rise to the highest point within the thorax, an ideal location for detection of pneumothorax is at the lung apices on the standard PA CXR. On an AP CXR, the highest point lies adjacently to the heart and mediastinum. Thus, pneumothorax may cause increased lucency adjacent to mediastinal structures, which appear well-defined, often with no lung edge visible. A suspected pneumothorax on an AP radiograph may be confirmed by a decubitus view.

Pleural fluid tends to collect at the lung base and appears as increased density obscuring adjacent structures. Pleural fluids reach the highest point along the lateral chest wall producing the *meniscus sign*. On a supine AP CXR, fluid will accumulate along the posterior chest wall, creating a veil-like opacification of the affected hemithorax. Vessels are visible anterior to the lung/effusion and should not be confused with consolidation.

The caliber of the blood vessels is different on an AP and PA radiographs. The upper lobe vessels appear smaller on a PA because of gravity (Figs. 16.3A and B). On the contrary, an AP CXR shows equal size vessels in the upper and lower lobes.

Rotation

Over-rotation can produce artifacts and hilar distortion. The degree of rotation can be assessed by examining the medial ends of the clavicles, which should be equidistant from the thoracic spinous processes (Figs. 16.4A and B).

Exposure

Penetration/exposure is less of a problem with digital radiography. With ideal penetration, the end plates of the lower thoracic vertebral bodies should be just visible through the heart shadow/lower mediastinum. An underpenetrated film appears diffusely dense obscuring retrocardiac structures. A left lower lobe collapse/consolidation may be easily missed. An overpenetrated CXR appears lucent, and the lung vessels and the lung detail are poorly seen (Figs. 16.5A to C).

Inspiratory Effort

To expose a good quality CXR, an adequate inspiratory effort is required. A good inspiration is said to have occurred when the diaphragm is seen at the level of the eighth to tenth posterior ribs or the right sixth anterior rib. Poor inspiration

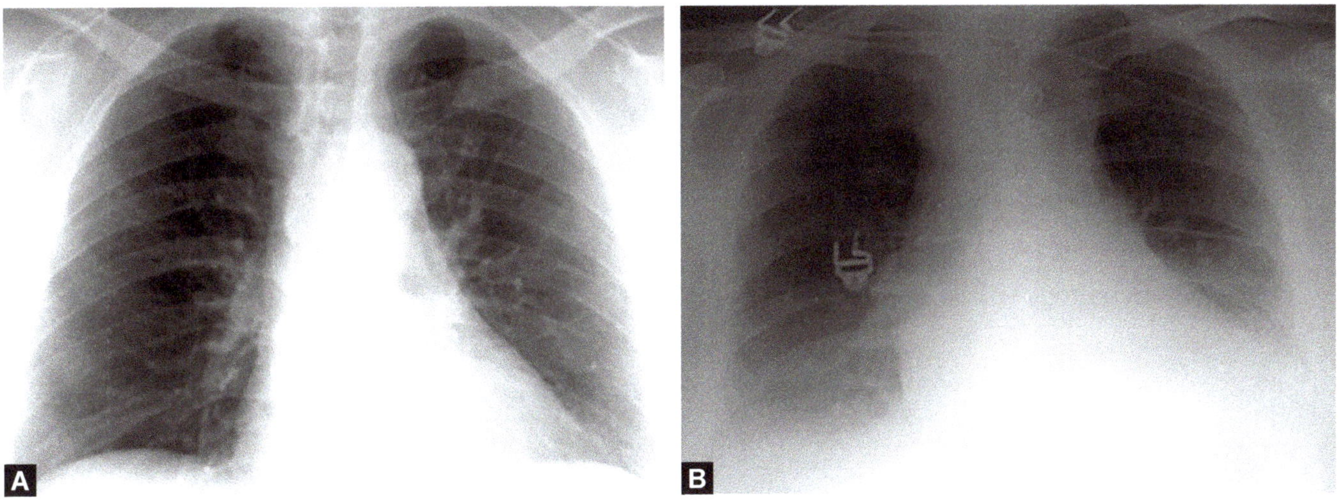

Figs. 16.3A and B: Comparison of (A) a posteroanterior chest X-ray (PA CXR) with (B) an anteroposterior (AP) supine CXR. The AP projection shows magnification of the heart and widening of the mediastinum.

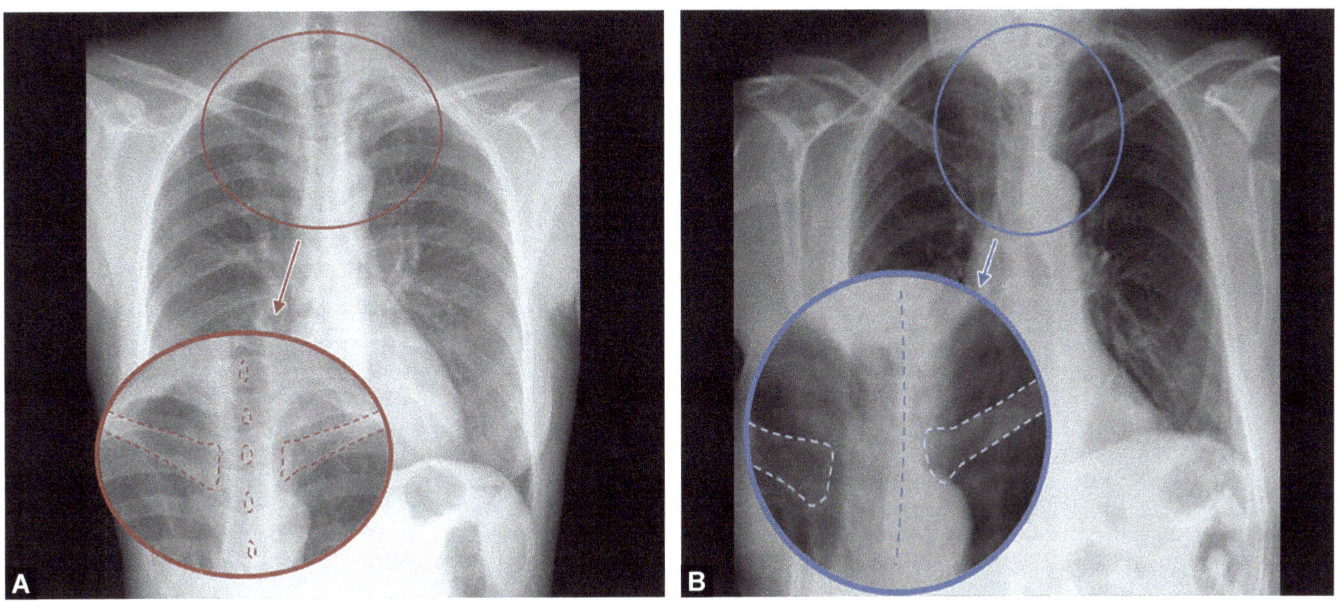

Figs. 16.4A and B: (A) Normal PA CXR without any rotation: medial ends of bilateral clavicles are equidistant from the midline of vertebral bodies. (B) Partially rotated film: the medial ends of the clavicles are not equidistant. Note the tracheal deviation and an impression of right superior mediastinal widening due either to the patient's chin or unfolded innominate vessel.

may cause increased opacification of the lungs particularly at the lung bases because of atelectasis (Figs. 16.6A and B).

Artifacts

Beware of electrocardiogram (ECG) leads stickers, hair plaits, bedding, skin folds, and clothing producing pseudopneumothorax. An unusual opacity with well-defined borders should prompt visual inspection of the chest wall.

NORMAL LUNG AND LUNG PARENCHYMA

For the purpose of interpretation, the lungs are divided into the upper, middle, and lower zones. The areas above the clavicles are often referred as apical zones (Fig. 16.7). With this approach lung densities can be assessed and compared as increased or reduced density. When a density variation is detected, the next step is to decide as to which side is abnormal. An area that appears different than the surrounding lung is the likely abnormal lung.

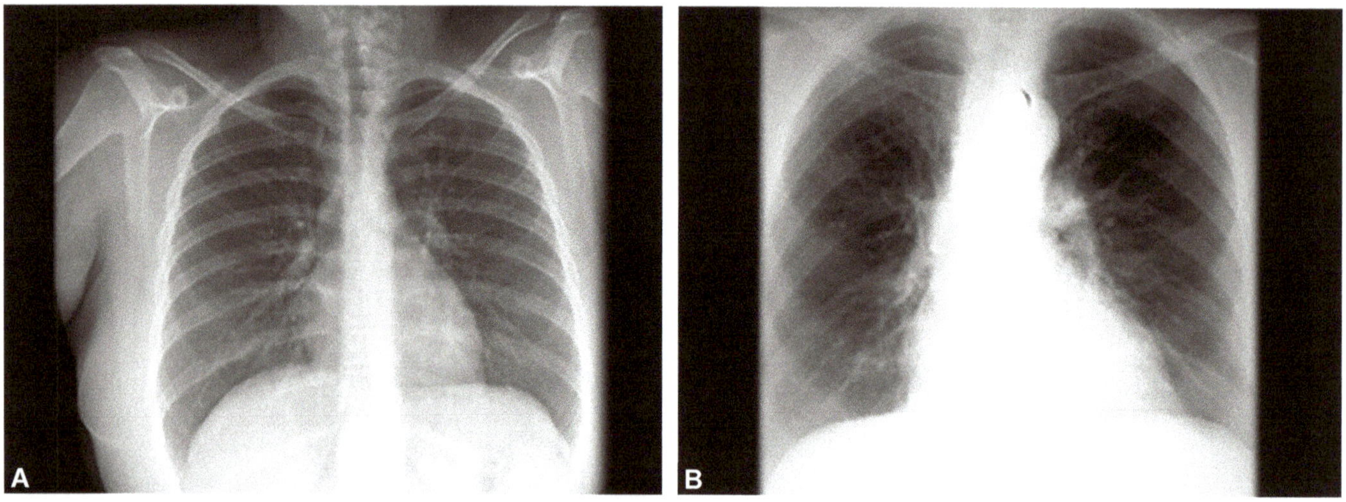

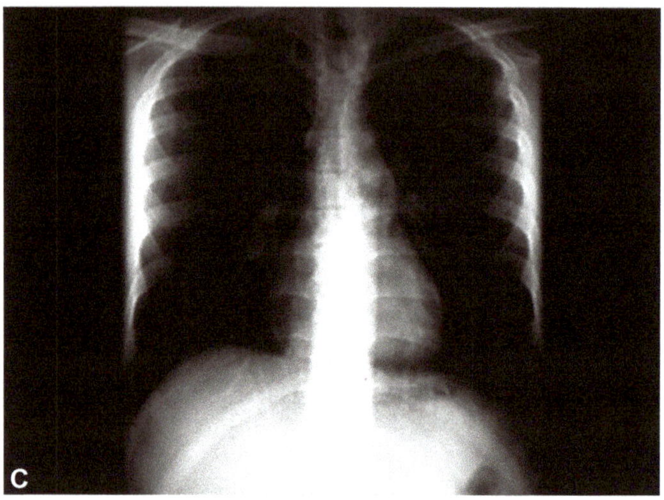

Figs. 16.5A to C: (A) Posteroanterior chest X-ray (PA CXR) with adequate penetration; (B) Underpenetrated film. (C) Overpenetrated film.

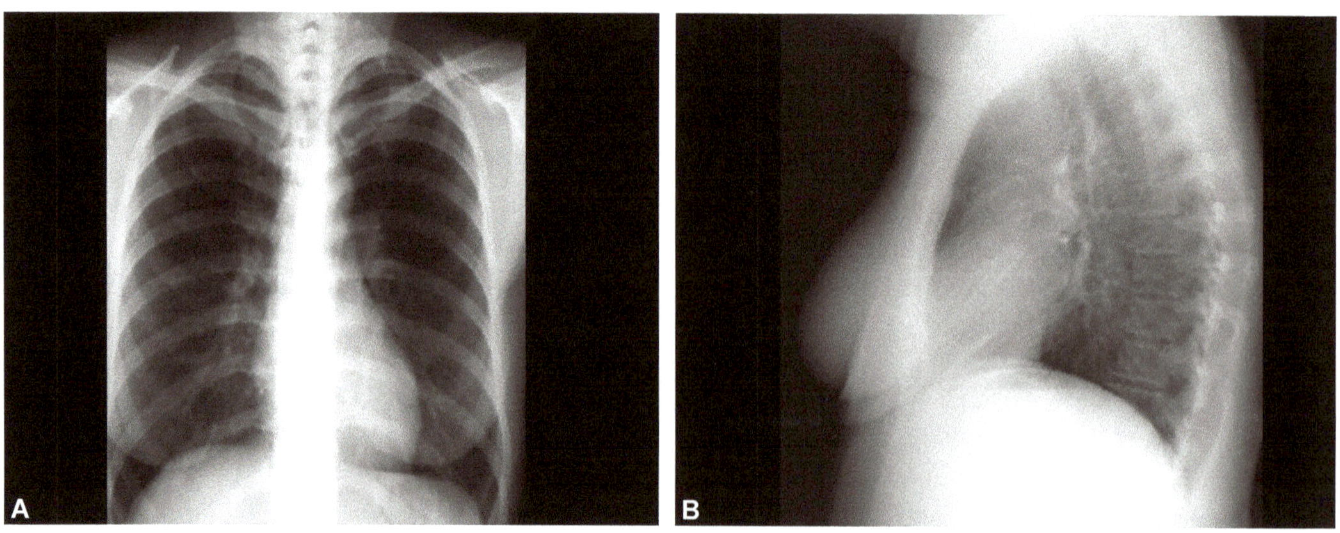

Figs. 16.6A and B: (A) Posteroanterior chest X-ray (PA CXR) with good inspiratory effort; the film is adequately penetrated, note the right hemidiaphragm is at the eleventh rib posteriorly and the seventh rib anteriorly. The lower dorsal spine and disk spaces are visible through the heart. (B) The lateral view is obtained with the left chest against the cassette, which diminishes the effect of magnification on the heart.

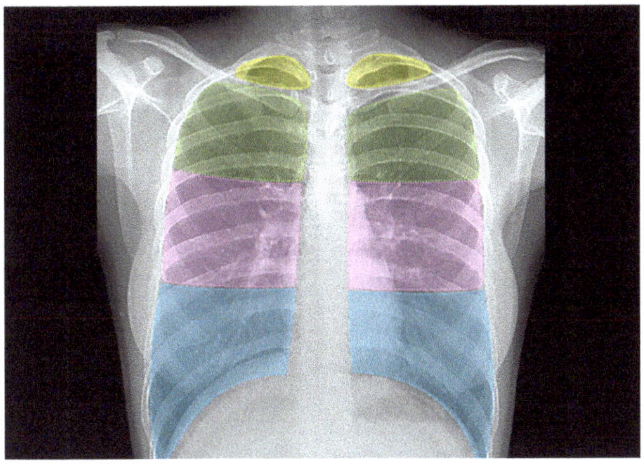

Fig. 16.7: The chest radiograph zones on a PA film. Yellow: apical zones (above the clavicles); green: upper zones (below the clavicles and above the cardiac silhouette); pink: mid zones (at the level of the hilar structures); light blue: lower zones (corresponding to the lung bases).

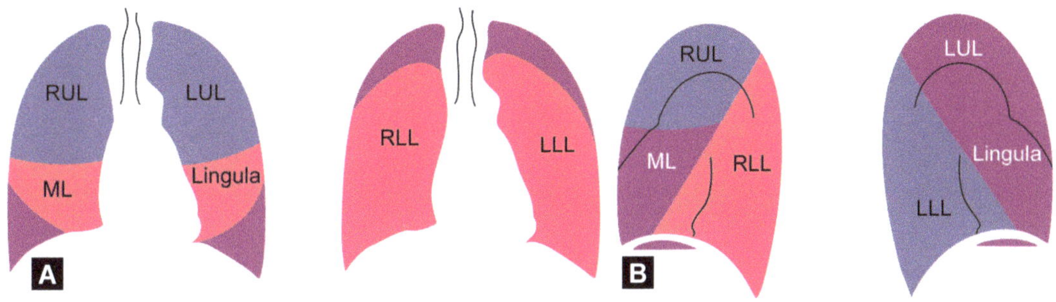

Figs. 16.8A and B: Extent and distribution of the lung lobes and fissures on (A) Posteroanterior (PA) and (B) lateral chest X-ray (CXR). (RUL: Right upper lobe; LUL: Left upper lobe; ML: Middle lobe; RLL: Right lower lobe; LLL: Left lower lobe).

The lungs are divided into lobes by fissures; the right lung has three lobes and left has two lobes. These divisions are important when describing collapse consolidations. The oblique fissures, separating the upper from the lower lobes, are not usually seen on a standard PA CXR, unless there is a distortion by lung scarring, thickening of the fissure due to pleural thickening or pleural effusions. A part of the lesser fissure is seen in approximately 50–60% of patients. Most commonly, the lateral portion of the lesser fissure is seen in contact with the chest wall at the level of the right sixth rib. The peripheral, pleural line is not usually visible, unless there is a pneumothorax or pleural thickening such as in asbestos-related pleural disease (Figs. 16.8A and B).

Subsequently, the rib cage is observed, looking for asymmetry, fractures, and areas of destruction, bone sclerosis, widening or narrowing of intercostal spaces. The intercostal spaces should be symmetrical.

Knowledge of the anatomy of the mediastinum and normal vascular structures is important to accurately interpret a CXR (Fig. 16.9).

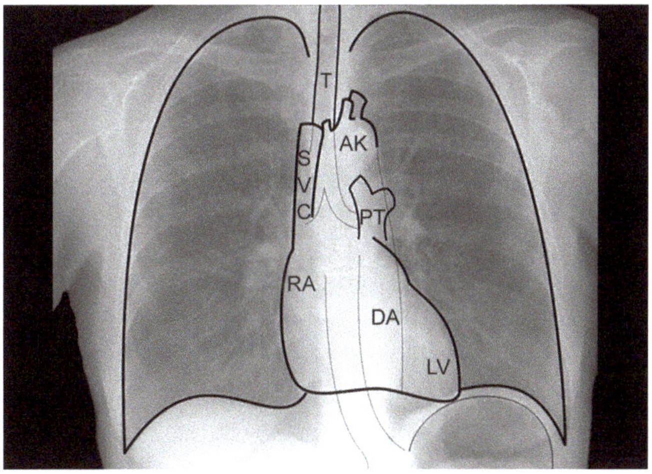

Fig. 16.9: Normal cardiomediastinal contours on posteroanterior (PA) chest X-ray. (SVC: Superior vena cava; PT: Pulmonary trunk; RA: Right atrium; AK: Aortic knuckle; LV: Left ventricle; DA: Descending aorta; T: Trachea).

The superior surfaces of the hemidiaphragms should be crisp, convex upward and the costophrenic and cardiophrenic angles well-defined. The right hemidiaphragm is usually 1–3 cm higher than the left. Look for fluid at the lung bases and air/air-fluid levels under the diaphragms.

It is important to recognize certain lines at the lung-soft tissue interface. These lines include the normal right paratracheal stripe, the silhouette of the aortic knuckle

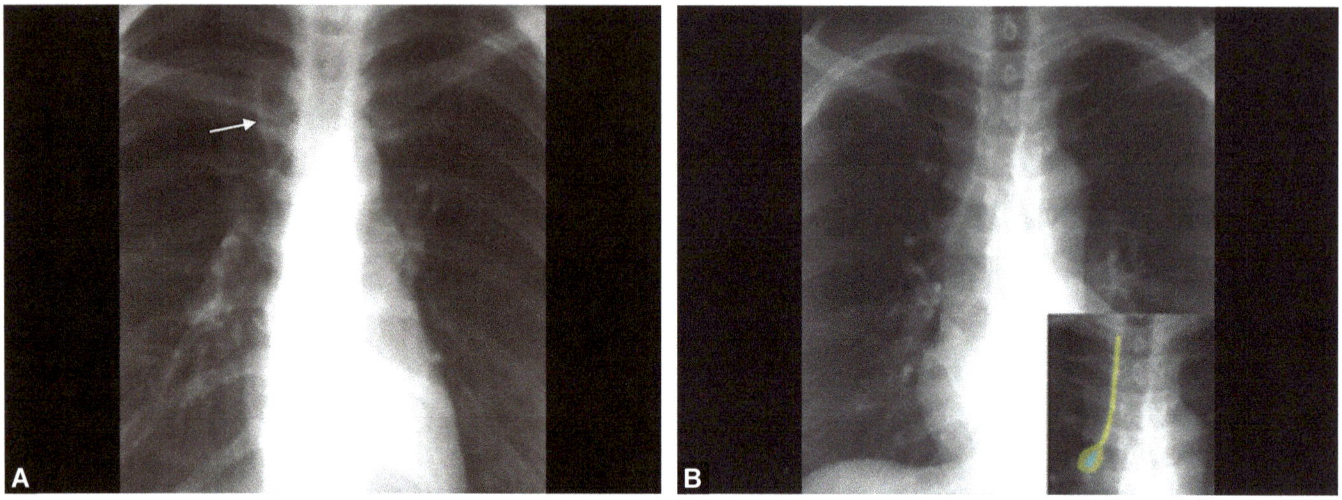

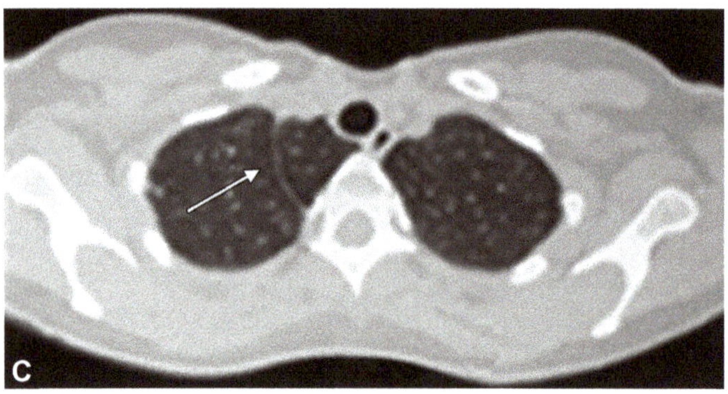

Figs. 16.10A to C: (A) Posteroanterior chest X-ray (PA CXR) shows a linear opacity in the left upper zone (arrow) suggestive of an azygos lobe. (B) This image is a line diagram depicting the position of an azygos vein. (C) An axial CT scan of the patient in image (A) confirms the presence of an azygos lobe (arrow).

and the left ventricle. Displacement push/pull of these lines indicates pathology. Recognizing the silhouette sign as described by Felson forms the basis for recognizing many lungs and mediastinal pathologies. Lymphadenopathy, pleural thickening and pleural effusions/pleural blood are some pathologies that may displace the paratracheal line (>2–3 mm). Similarly, the paraspinal line may be displaced by tumor, abscess or hemorrhage. An unfolded aorta, aortic aneurysm, aortic rupture and aortic dissection can displace the para-aortic line. Another important line to recognize is the azygoesophageal line or recess, as it is the site for the azygos accessory lobe not to be confused with pathology (Figs. 16.10A to C).

TRACHEA AND CENTRAL AIRWAYS

The trachea should lie in the midline in a well-centered radiograph. It ussually lies at fourth thoracic vertabra (T4) at expiration and T6 in inspiration. In children, the main bronchial division is symmetrical but, in adults the right main bronchus lies at a steeper angle. The trachea is shown as an air attenuation tubular structure that lies in the midline and slightly to the right. The carina and the main bronchi can be followed to the hila and the carina assessed for splaying. If the trachea is deviated, it is important to establish that the patient is not rotated. The trachea can deviate from push or pull from the adjacent pathology such as a mass or fibrosis or loss of lung volume. The trachea divides into the left and the right main bronchi, at the level of the sternal angle of and about the fifth thoracic vertebra. However, there is a minor variation of the exact level as the division may be two dorsal vertebrae higher or lower. The level of division is also affected by the phase of respiration and the inspiratory effort. The right main bronchus is wider, shorter, and more vertical than the left main bronchus. Thus, most aspirated foreign bodies lodge in the right main bronchus. The right main bronchus enters the right lung at about the fifth dorsal vertebral body. The right main bronchus subdivides into three lobar branches. The azygos vein arches over the origin of the right main bronchus from behind. The right main pulmonary artery lies first inferior and then anterior to the right bronchus. In 0.1–5% of the human population, there is an accessory right superior lobe bronchus (the tracheal or the pig bronchus) arising from the main stem bronchus prior to the carina. Known as a tracheal bronchus, and is regarded as an anatomical variation. It is usually asymptomatic but can become symptomatic from recurrent infections and resection may be required. The left main bronchus is shorter and enters the left lung at the level of the sixth dorsal vertebral body. It lies inferior to the arch of aorta and passes in front of the esophagus, the descending aorta and the thoracic duct. The left pulmonary artery lies above the left main bronchus and then in front of it. The left main bronchus divides into two secondary or lobar bronchi supplying the two lobes of the left lung (Figs. 16.11 to 16.24).

Accidental aspiration is a rare complication, but rarely, large amounts of barium sulfate are inadvertently aspirated into the lung. Neuromuscular conditions affecting the functional integrity of the oropharynx and esophagus are predisposing factors. Barium sulfate is nonirritant and severe lung injury is unusual. On the other hand, acute inflammation or even death attributed either to high or to low density preparations of barium sulfate have been reported.

PLEURA

Pleural Effusion

On average, more than 150 mL must be present for a pleural effusion to be detected on an erect CXR. However, a decubitus fluid quantity less than 75 mL may be detected on a lateral decubitus radiograph with the patient lying

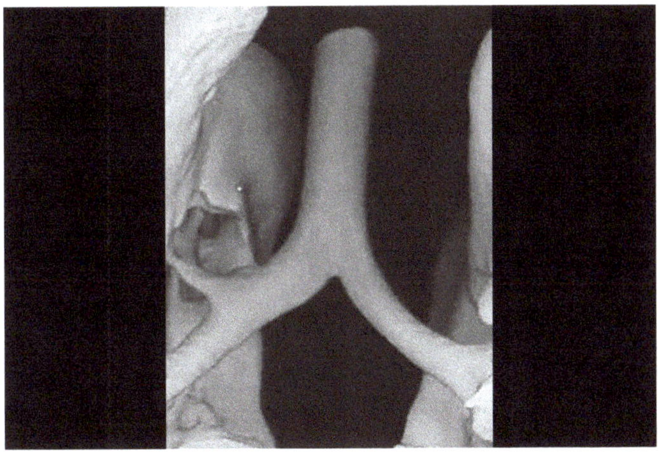

Fig. 16.11: Three-dimensional (3D) reconstruction of a coronal CT scan, showing the trachea and the right and left main bronchi. Note the wider right main bronchus and the steeper decent making the preferential site of lodgment of foreign bodies particularly children.

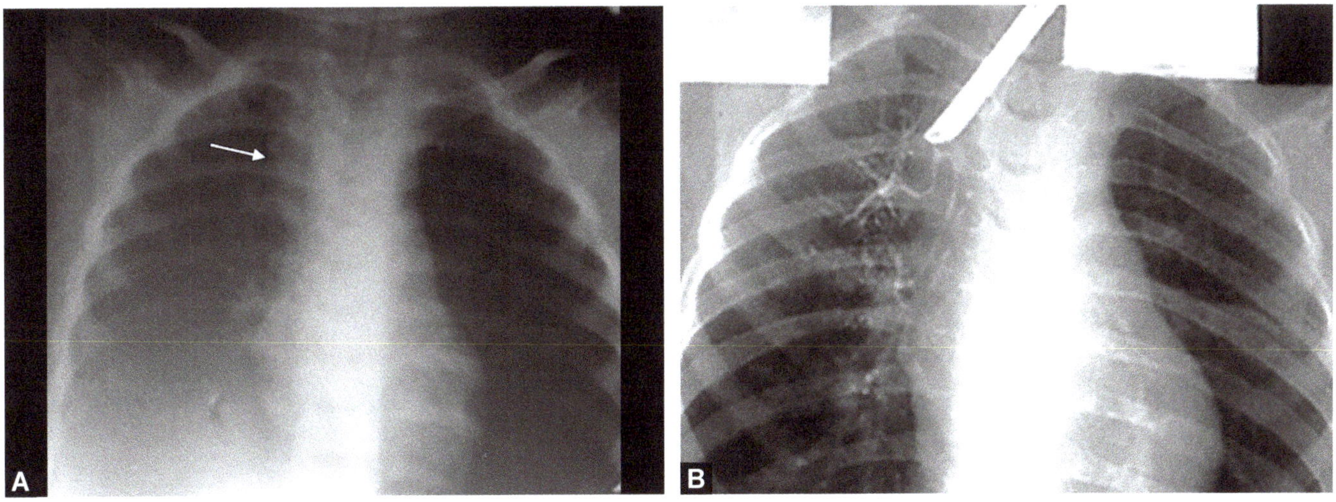

Figs. 16.12A and B: (A) Posteroanterior chest X-ray (PA CXR) showing a right upper lobe pneumonia (arrow). (B) Bronchography reveals a tracheal bronchus or "pig bronchus". This is an accessory bronchus that originates directly from the supracarinal trachea. The accessory bronchus is often incidentally discovered, and most patients are asymptomatic. Occasionally patients may have recurrent upper lobe pneumonia.

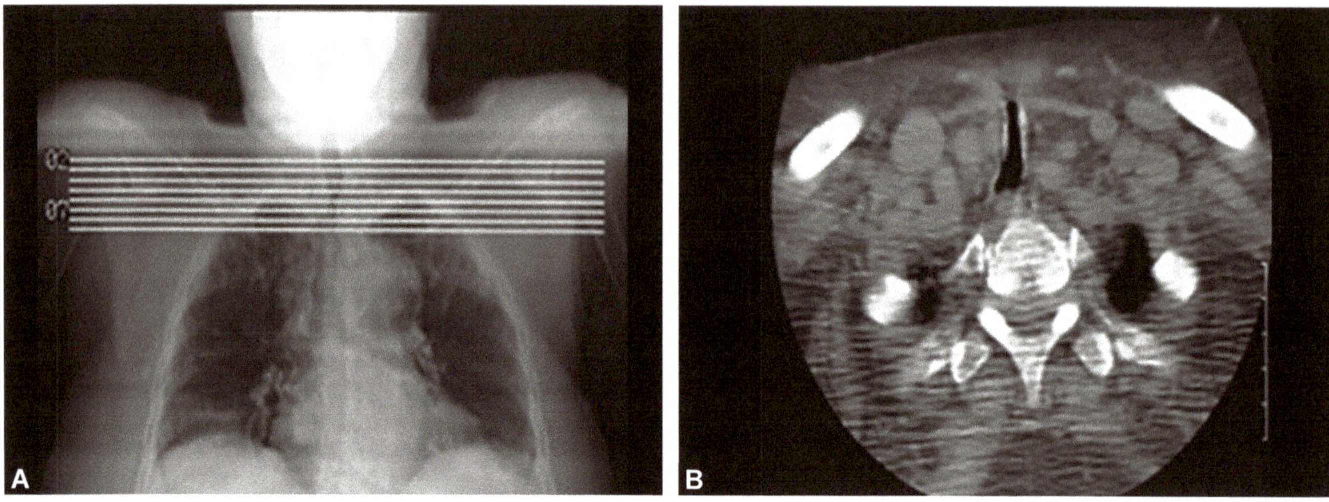

Figs. 16.13A and B: (A) A digital radiograph and (B) an axial computed tomography (CT) scan through the upper trachea show a significant tracheal stenosis in a patient with a history of prolonged intubation and subsequent stridor.

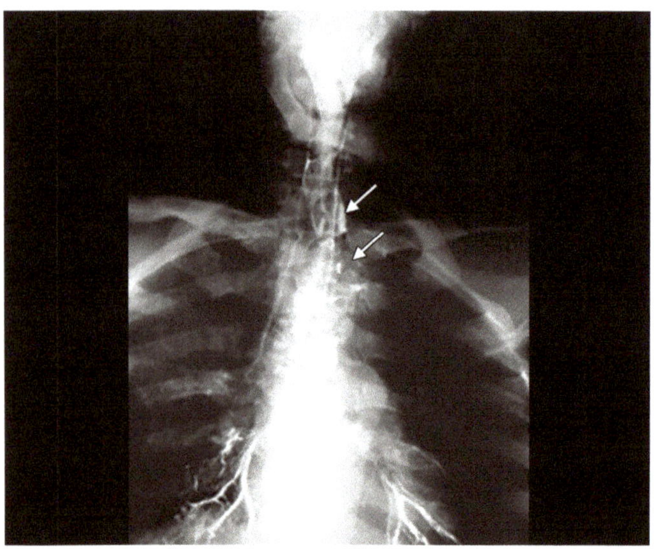

Fig. 16.14: A coned off view of the upper thorax of a patient with a history of swallowed dentures and subsequent dysphagia. The denture could not be retrieved by endoscopy. A barium swallow shows the metallic component of the denture (lower arrow) with a sharp cut-off at level of the esophagus above the impacted dentures (upper arrow). Aspiration of barium has occurred, the barium outlining the trachea and lower bronchi. The dentures were removed surgically.

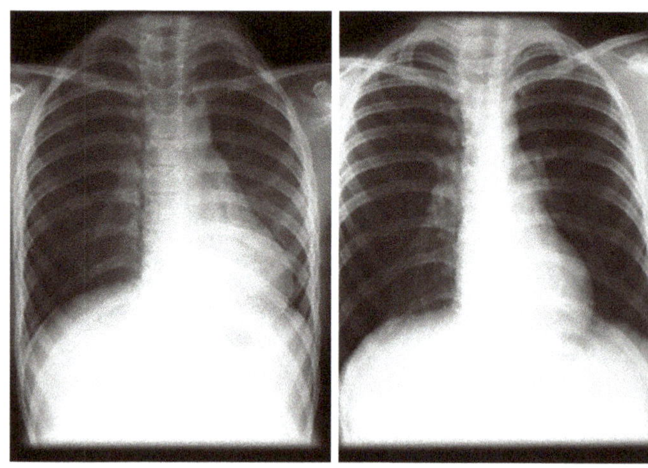

Fig. 16.15: Inspiratory and expiratory posteroanterior chest X-rays (PA CXRs) on a 16-year-old, who was juggling with peanuts, throwing them in the air and then catching them in the mouth, a peanut was accidently inhaled. The patient did not think much about it at the time but presented with a wheezy chest a few weeks later. The CXR shows right-sided air trapping (obstructive emphysema) due to partial obstruction (check valve mechanism). The left side deflates during expiration, whilst the right side cannot deflate. There is a mediastinal shift toward the obstructed side. Over 80%, foreign bodies are demonstrated on inspiratory and expiratory PA CXRs.

on the suspected side of the effusion on the radiograph as shown in Figure 16.22.

Feldman in 1951 has described localized interlobar pleural effusion as a reversible entity and typically occurred during congestive heart failure. The effusion can either clear spontaneously or with treatment response. The disease thought to provoke this response was termed obliterative pleuritis.

A loculated interlobular pleural effusion or pulmonary pseudotumor is a term frequently used to describe focal fluid collections trapped in the pleural fissures. Particularly on chest radiographs, these entities can cause confusion and appear as a solid pulmonary mass. The opacities are typically elongated along the direction of the fissures and may have tapered ends. A lateral chest radiograph is often

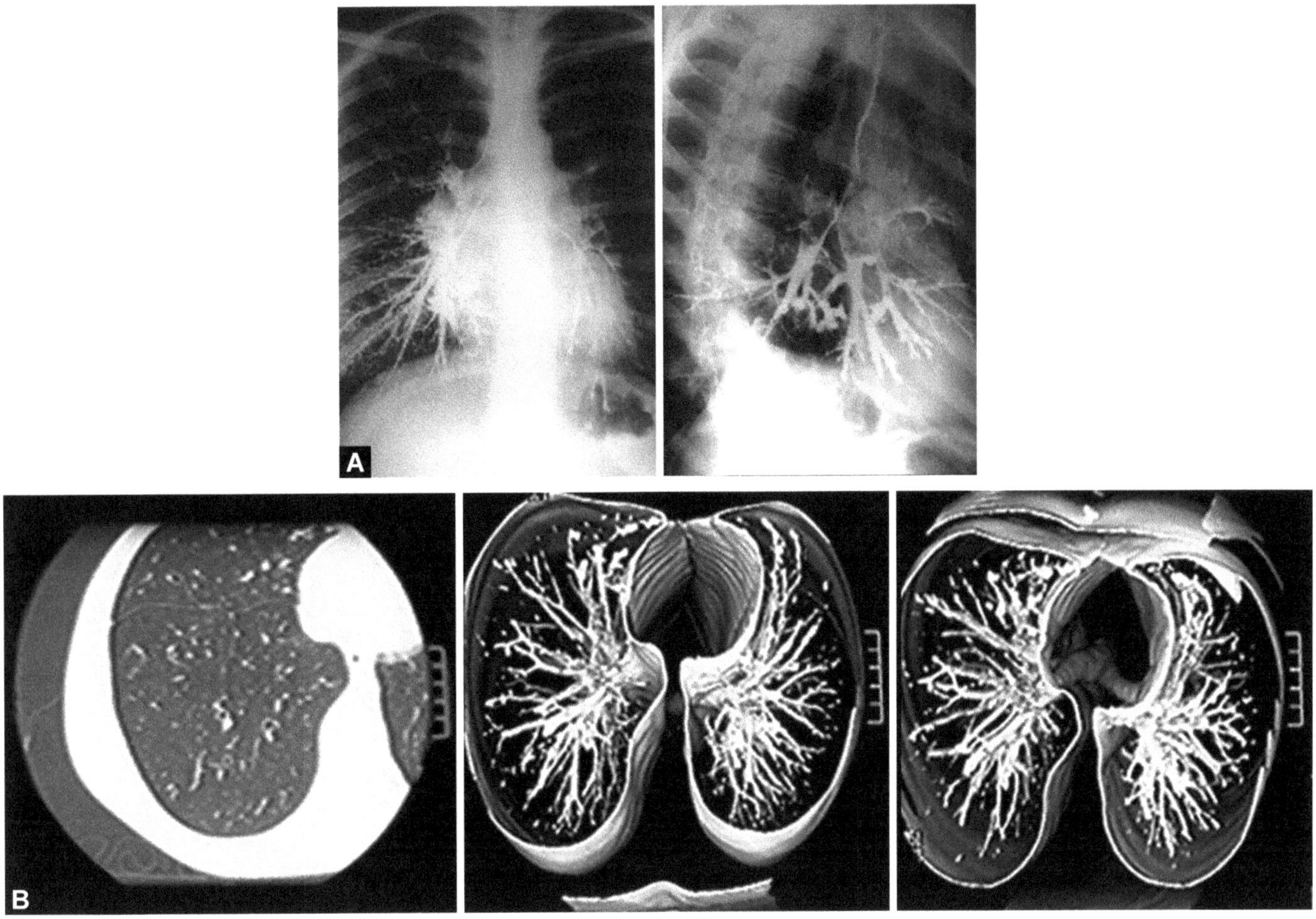

Figs. 16.16A and B: (A) Images from historical archives showing the now obsolete bronchography. It was undertaken for the diagnosis of bronchiectasis. The images delineate exquisitely the anatomy of trachea and the main bronchi, with bronchiectasis in both lower lobes. (B) High-resolution computed tomography (HRCT) of the chest showing a mild degree of bronchiectasis. HRCT is the imaging of choice in the modern era to depict bronchiectasis. Images can be enhanced by three 3D reconstructions, which show a mild bronchiectasis with retention of secretion in bronchomucoceles.

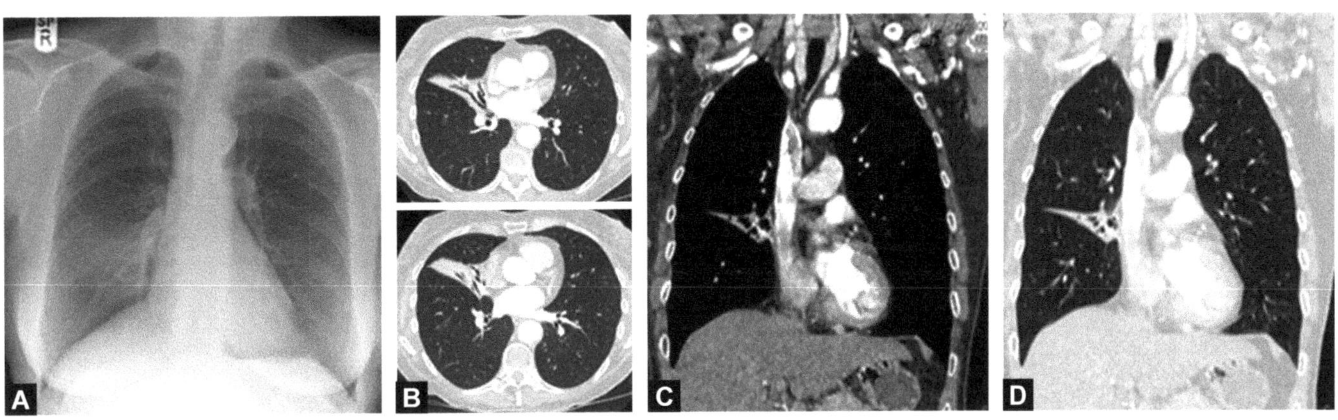

Figs. 16.17A to D: (A) Posteroanterior chest X-ray (PA CXR) and (B to D) Computed tomography (CT) findings showing a right middle lobe collapse and bronchiectasis in a patient with right middle lobe syndrome (RMLS). This refers to chronic right middle collapse, without an endobronchial obstructive lesion, often associated with bronchiectasis and occurs at all ages. In the older population-lesion, it has a predilection for females as in the case shown. RMS is often asymptomatic, but chronic cough, hemoptysis, chest pain and dyspnea may occur.

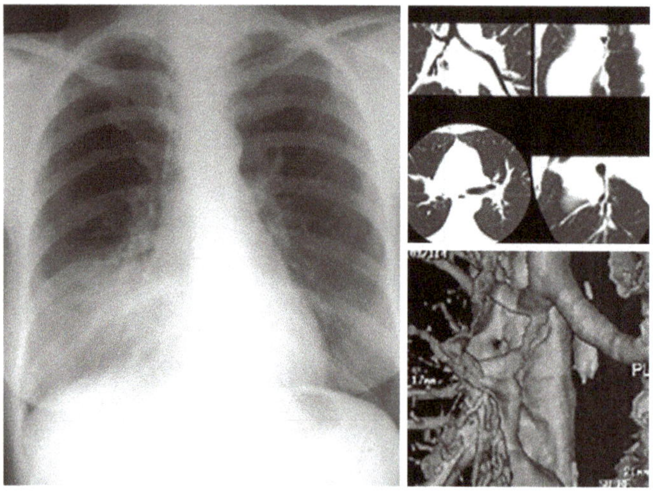

Fig. 16.18: Three-dimensional (3D) reconstructions showing an RMS may follow a post-tuberculous intermedius bronchus stenosis.

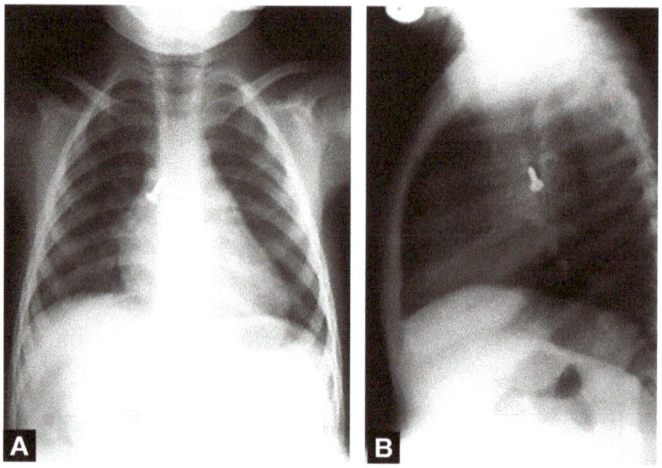

Figs. 16.19A and B: Posteroanterior (PA) and lateral chest X-rays (CXRs) showing an inhaled metal screw impacted into the right main bronchus removed via a bronchoscope.

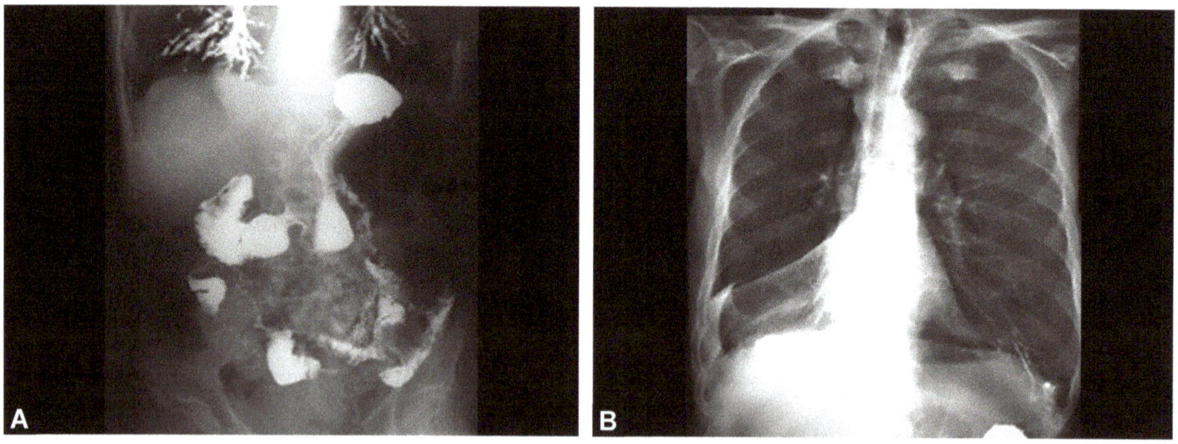

Figs. 16.20A and B: An abdominal radiograph on a patient that accidentally inhaled the barium during barium swallow. Note the unrelated bronchiectasis at the left lung base. No harm pursued and the patient eventually coughed up the barium. Barium sulfate is a relatively insoluble salt of barium used as a radiographic contrast medium. A barium swallow is used routinely to examine the oropharynx and esophagus, often combined with videofluoroscopy.

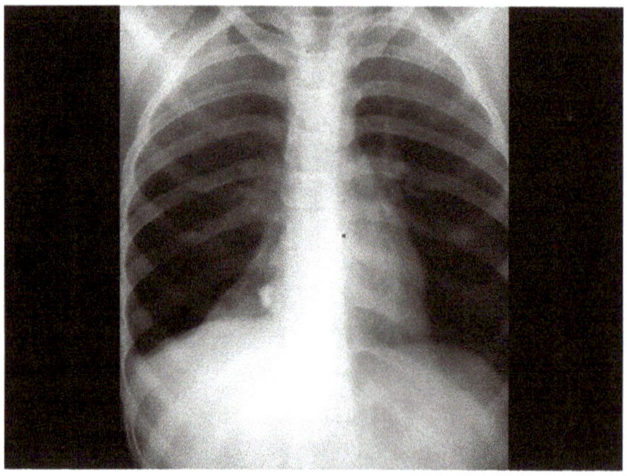

Fig. 16.21: A posteroanterior (PA) chest radiograph shows an inhaled tooth filling causing collapse of the right lower lobe.

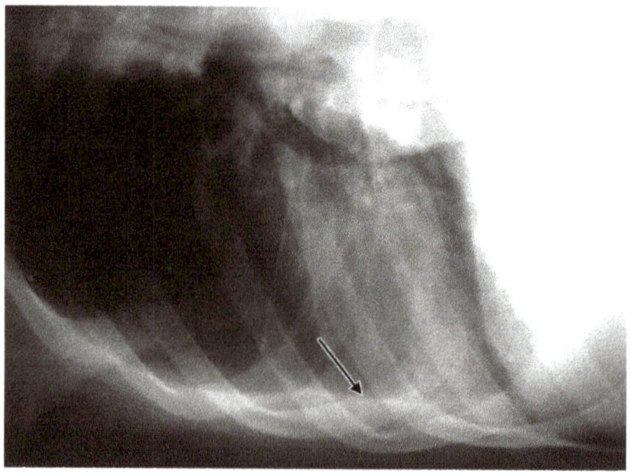

Fig. 16.22: A left lateral decubitus chest X-ray (CXR) shows a small pleural effusion not apparent on a PA CXR (arrow).

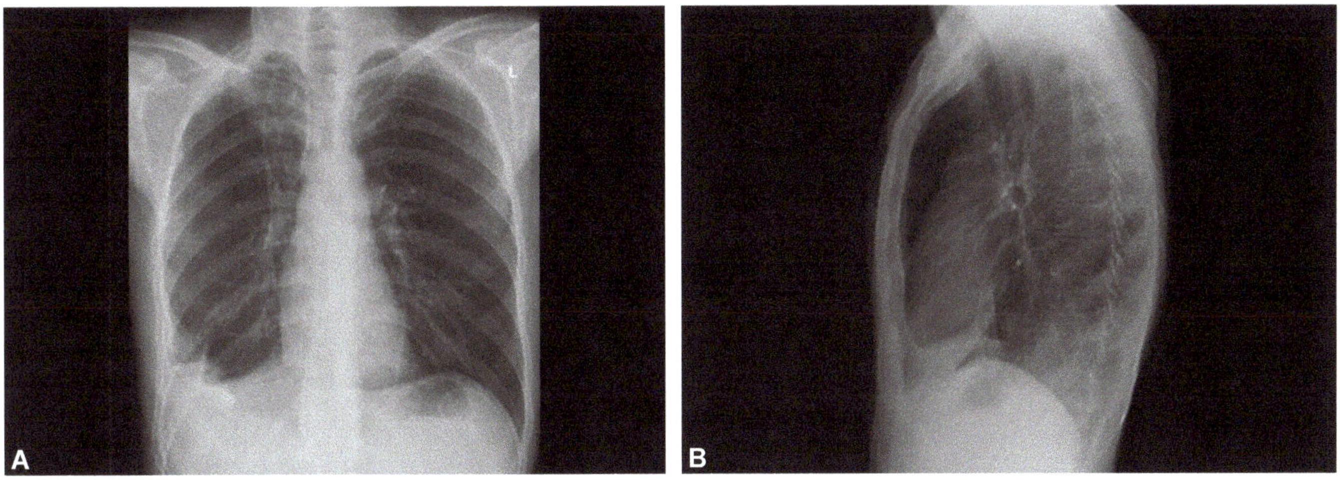

Figs. 16.23A and B: (A) Posteroanterior (PA) and (B) right lateral chest X-rays (CXRs) show either pleural thickening or pleural effusion tracking up the right greater fissure. An ultrasound examination (not shown) showed a pleural effusion. Also note the greater opacity of the right hemithorax related to pleural effusion. The patient has a jugular-peritoneal shunt for hydrocephalus. A diagnostic pleural tap revealed infective etiology.

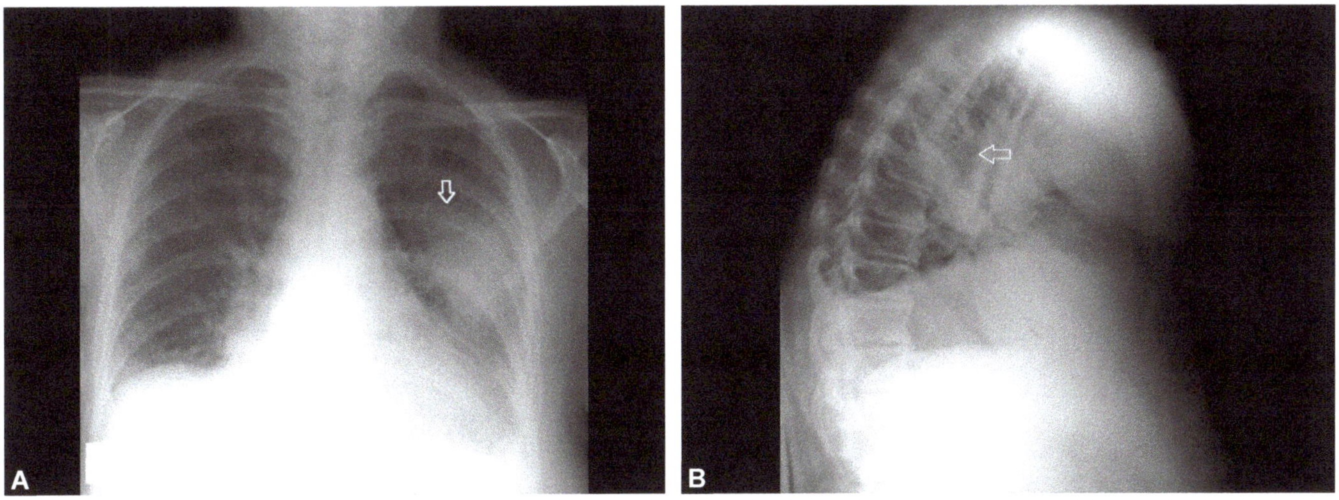

Figs. 16.24A and B: Vanishing tumor: (A) Posteroanterior chest X-ray (PA CXR) shows a ill-defined opacity (arrow). (B) Lateral CXR shows an elliptical opacity highly suggestive of loculated pleural effusions (arrow).

useful for further characterize these masses. In equivocal cases, CT would help establish the fluid density of the apparent mass and its location within a minor or major fissure.

These vanishing tumors are often seen in patients presenting with congestive cardiac failure. As the patient's disease begins to improve, radiological features would sometimes lag, and the resorption of the interlobar pleural fluid would be slower to show resolution than the other signs of cardiac failure. An eventual chest radiograph would however show resolution of the fluid (Figs. 16.23 to 16.29).

Pneumothorax

A pneumothorax is easily missed on a standard PA CXR, which is readily apparent on a film at the end of expiration in lateral decubitus (Fig. 16.30). A pneumothorax does not have the same characteristics on AP/supine CXR. However, there are certain features that suggest the presence of a pneumothorax on a supine CXR, which include: (1) relative hyperlucency on the involved side; (2) a deep costophrenic sulcus; (3) sharp mediastinal and heart borders; (4) visualization of the anterior costophrenic

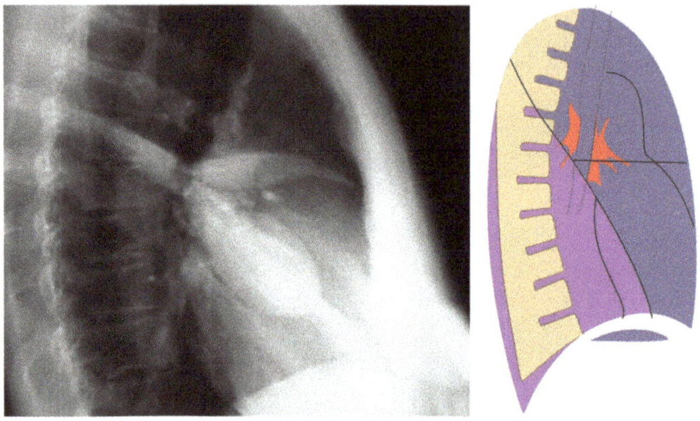

Fig. 16.25: Vanishing tumor: lateral chest X-ray (CXR) showing a pleural fluid within the fissures.

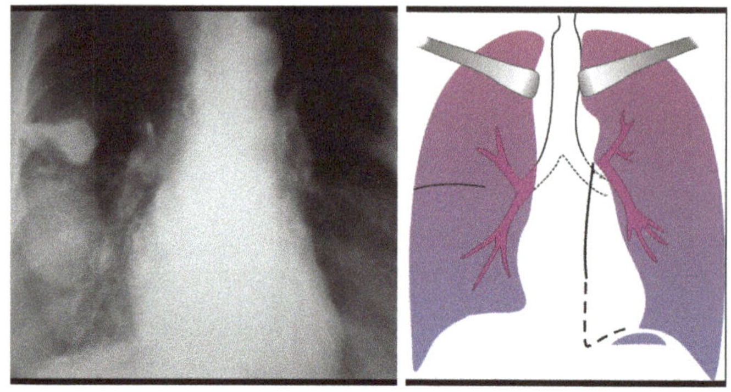

Fig. 16.26: Posteroanterior chest X-ray (PA CXR) showing a pleural fluid encysted within the fissures, giving rise to an impression of a mass, the so-called "vanishing tumors" as these disappear following treatment with diuretics.

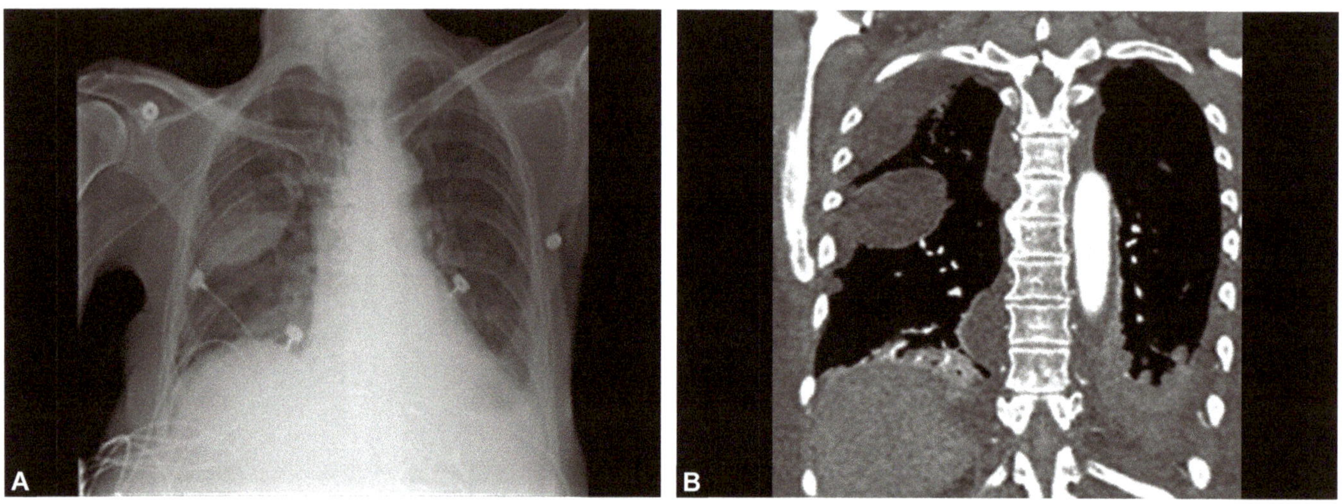

Figs. 16.27A and B: (A) Loculated pleural effusion: a smoothly defined right pleural-based mass is demonstrated on the chest radiograph. (B) On computed tomography (CT), this "mass" was noted to be of fluid density. The appearances are in keeping with a loculated pleural effusion.

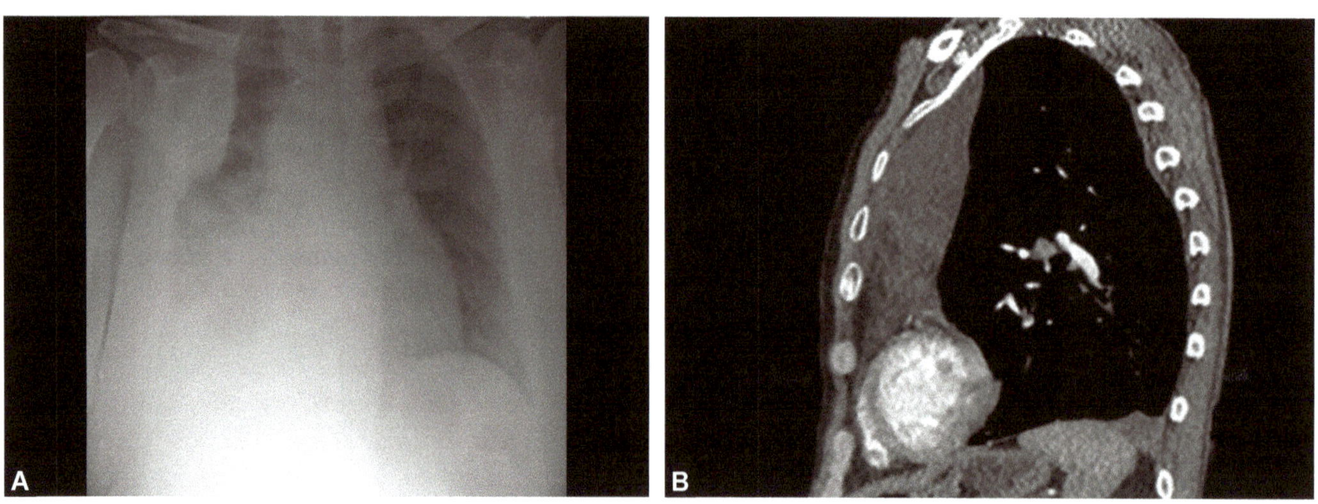

Figs. 16.28A and B: (A) An anteroposterior chest X-ray (AP CXR) shows an ill-defined opacity in the right upper zone, suggestive of a loculated pleural effusion. (B) The coronal CT scan shows bilateral pleural effusions with loculation in the right upper zone with some loculation around the mediastinum, left basal pleural effusion and a bilateral basal passive atelectasis.

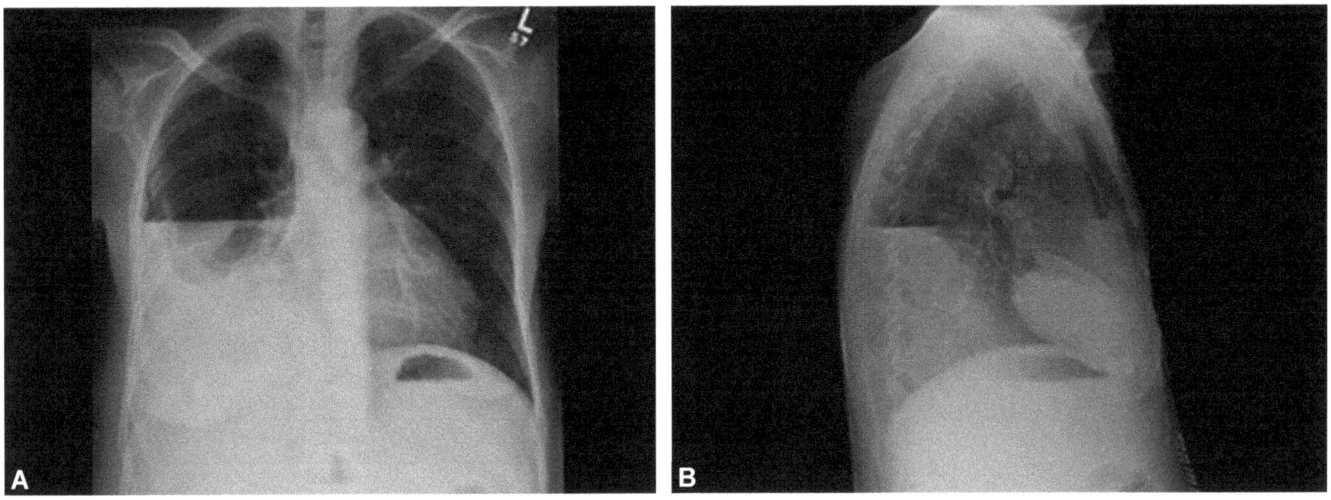

Figs. 16.29A and B: A chest X-ray (CXR) shows a left-sided hydrothorax, following aspiration of a right-sided pleural effusion as indicated by the straight upper border.

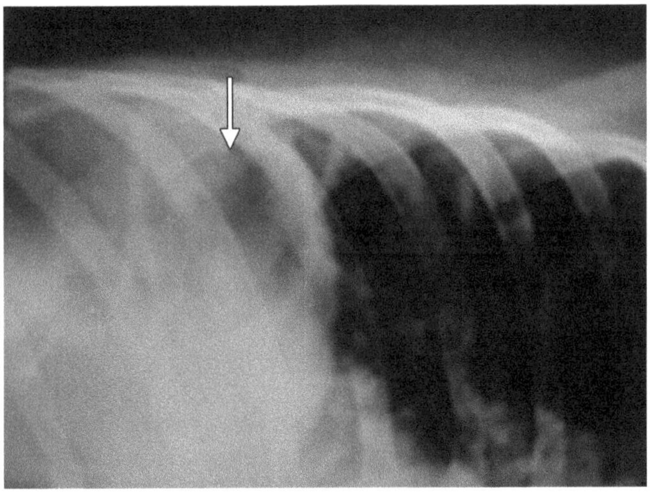

Fig. 16.30: Posteroanterior chest X-ray (PA CXR) right side raised decubitus radiograph on a patient with a sudden onset of right pleuritic chest pain. On a PA CXR, no pneumothorax was apparent. The decubitus radiograph, right side up shows a small pneumothorax (arrow).

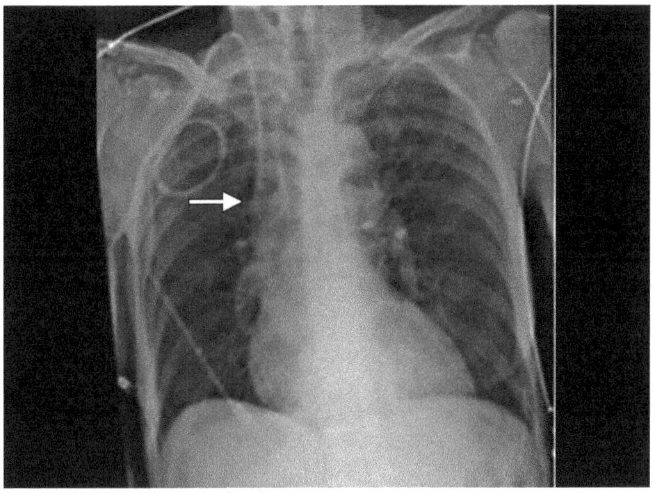

Fig. 16.31: An AP portable CXR shows a deep sulcus sign (arrow) also note the mediastinal lucency secondary to a pneumothorax.

sulcus (depression of the ipsilateral hemidiaphragm; (5) visualization of edge of the collapsed lung above the diaphragm. Pseudopneumothorax secondary to a skin fold or bedding should not be confused with a pneumothorax (Figs. 16.30 to 16.54).

Pleural Masses

Round atelectasis represents a folding atelectatic lung tissue with fibrous bands and adhesions to the visceral pleura. There is a high incidence in asbestos-related pleural disease (Figs. 16.32A and B).

The most common benign alteration of soft tissue at the level of the pleura is a *pleural lipoma* (Figs. 16.33A and B). These soft, fatty and encapsulated tumors are slow growing and originate from the submesothelial layers of the parietal pleura and may extend into the subpleural/pleural/extrapleural space. They can become extremely large. Patients often remain asymptomatic or present with nonproductive cough, exertional dyspnea, chest heaviness or back pain. Radiographic features include fat attenuation and homogeneity on CT [approximately –100 Hounsfield Unit (HU)]. It is important to differentiate a pleural lipoma from a liposarcoma. Liposarcomas may arise in all thoracic

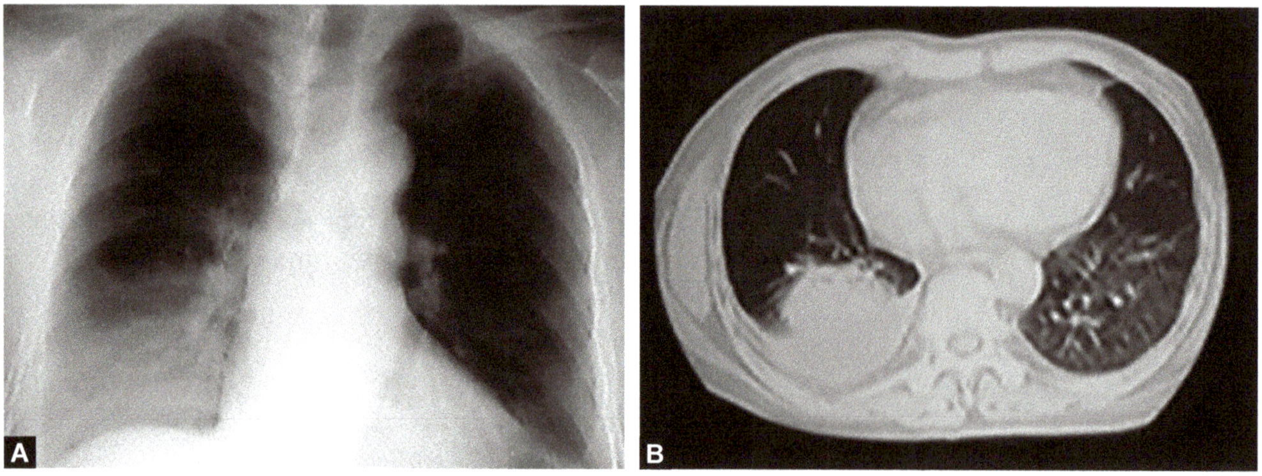

Figs. 16.32A and B: Round atelectasis represents a folding atelectatic lung tissue with fibrous bands and adhesions to the visceral pleura. There is a high incidence in asbestos-related pleural disease.

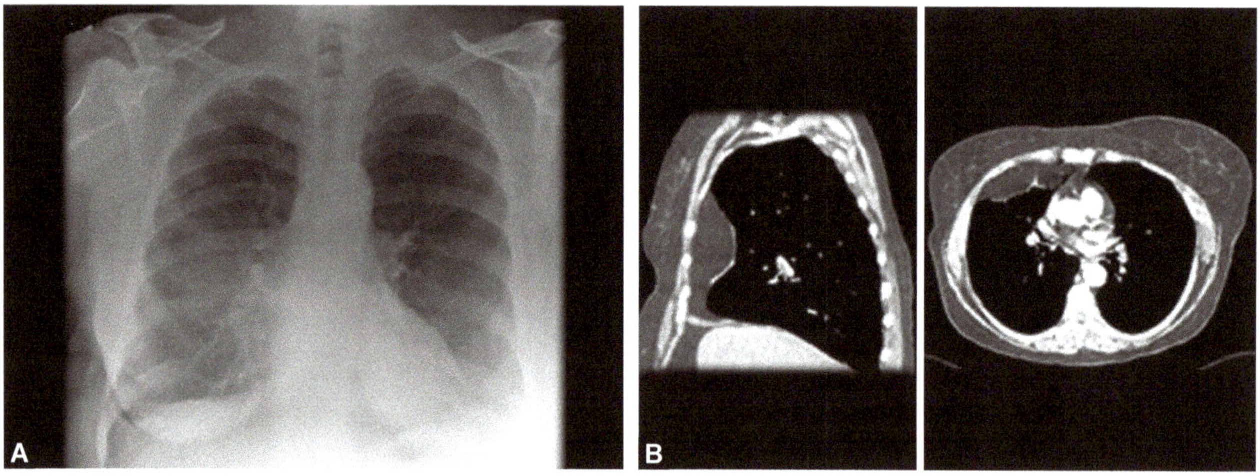

Figs. 16.33A and B: (A) Chest radiograph showed a hazy opacification in the right mid zone. (B) CT shows well-defined pleural-based mass with homogeneous fat content in keeping with a pleural-based lipoma.

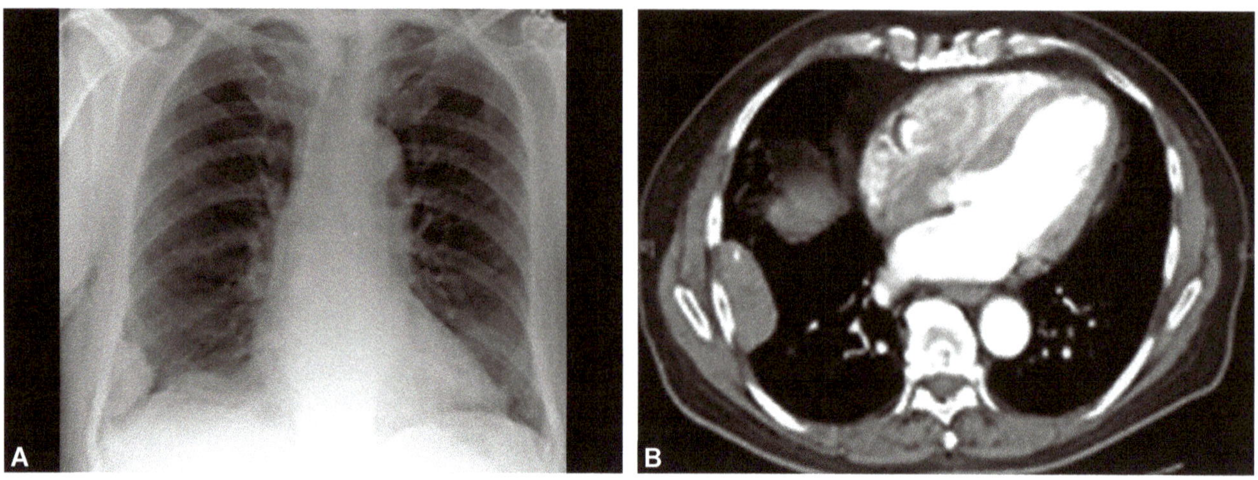

Figs. 16.34A and B: (A) Pleural fibroma: incidental pleural-based mass in the right costophrenic angle in a 65-year-old male presenting with shortness of breath. (B) CT confirms the presence of a well-defined homogeneous right lower parietal pleural mass measuring 6 cm × 3 cm with foci of calcification.

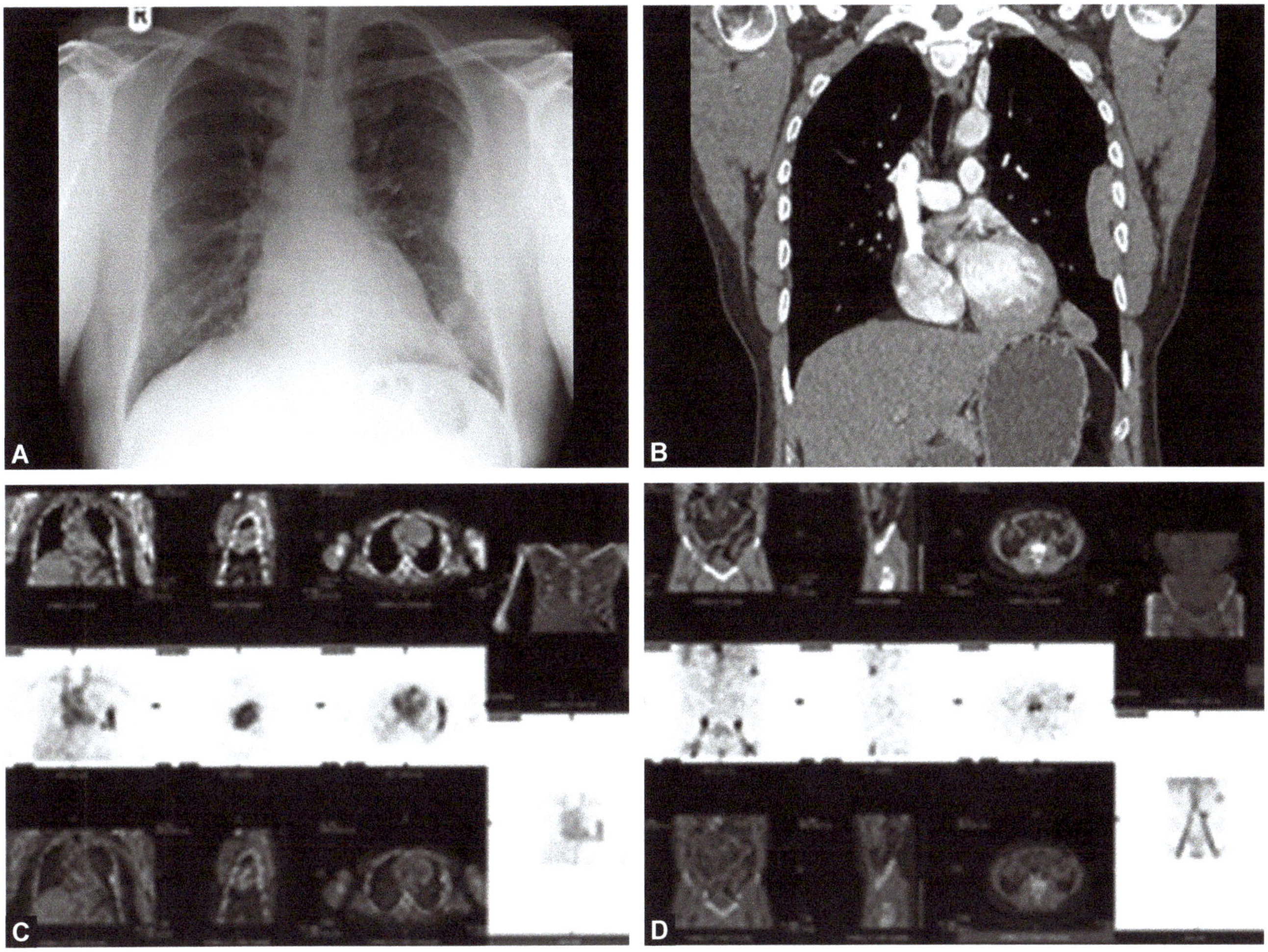

Figs. 16.35A to D: (A) Splenosis: incidental finding on a chest radiograph of a left-sided pleural-based mass. (B) CT scan confirms this and also other pleural nodularities, with the absence of a spleen. Further history was obtained and this patient was noted to have been involved in a blast injury. Splenic injuries were therefore suspected. (C and D) Splenic scintigraphic scans confirm intense uptake in the left hemithorax pleural nodularities. The appearances are those post-traumatic abdominal and intrathoracic splenosis.

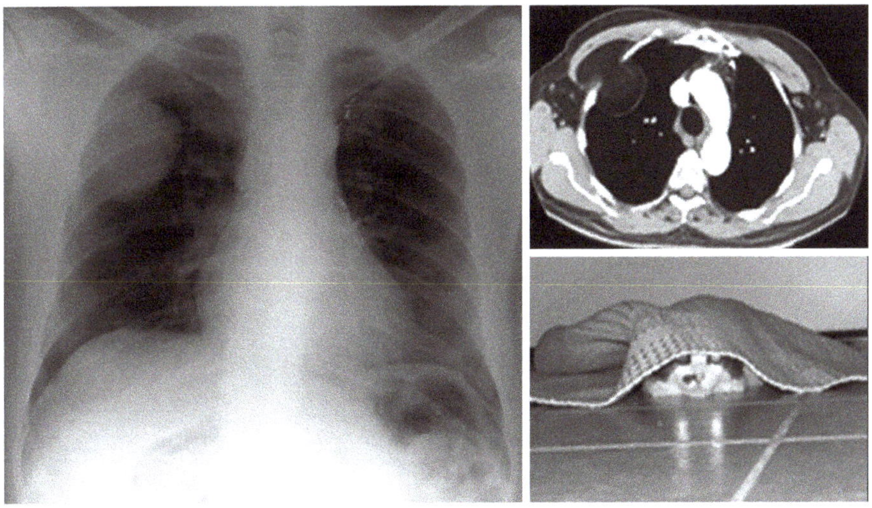

Fig. 16.36: An extrapleural sign is thoracic wall-based expanding density. The opacity is peripheral in location with a "cat under the rug appearance". The edges are concave, with sharp inner border but indistinct peripheral edge. The opacity is of equal length and width in the early stages.

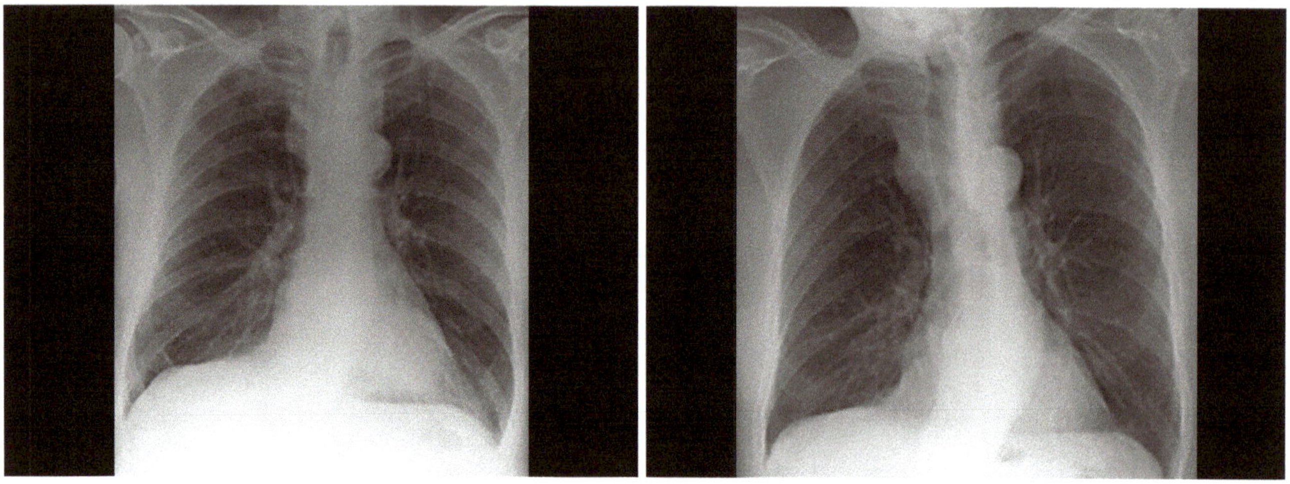

Fig. 16.37: Posteroanterior chest X-rays (PA CXRs) on a patient with known prostatic cancer presented with increasing dysphagia.

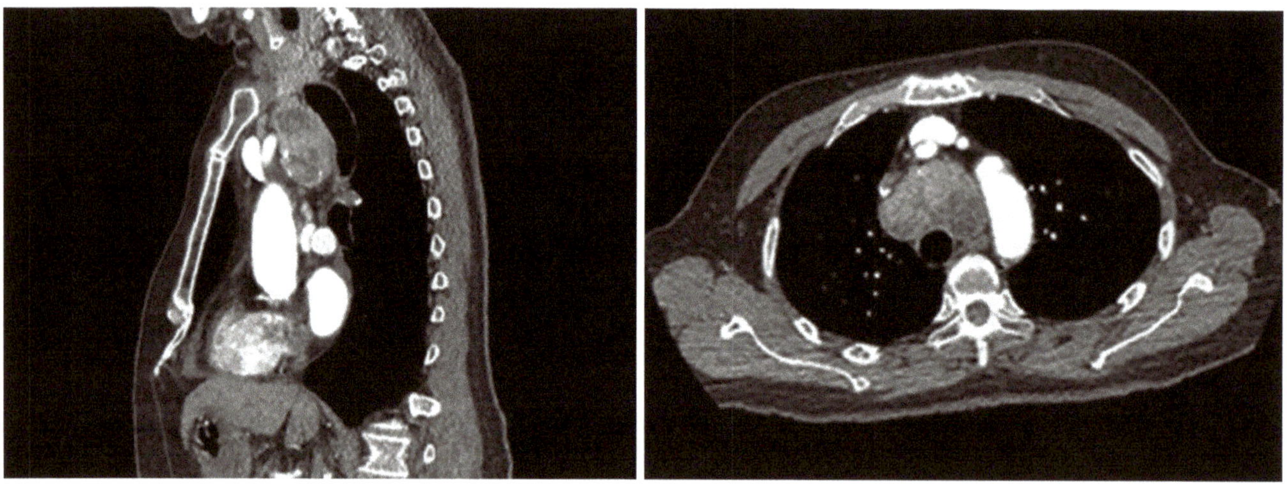

Fig. 16.38: The sagittal and axial CT scans on the same patient of Figure 16.37 shows a large retrosternal goiter compressing the esophagus.

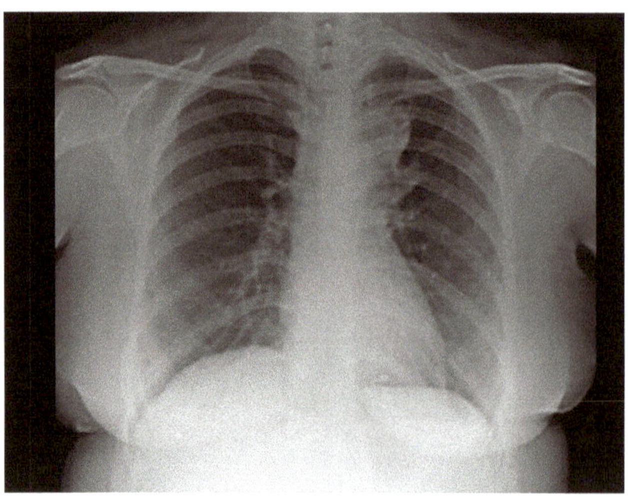

Fig. 16.39: A posteroanterior chest X-ray (PA CXR) on a 19-year-old woman shows lobulated left superior mediastinal mass subsequently proved tuberculous adenopathy.

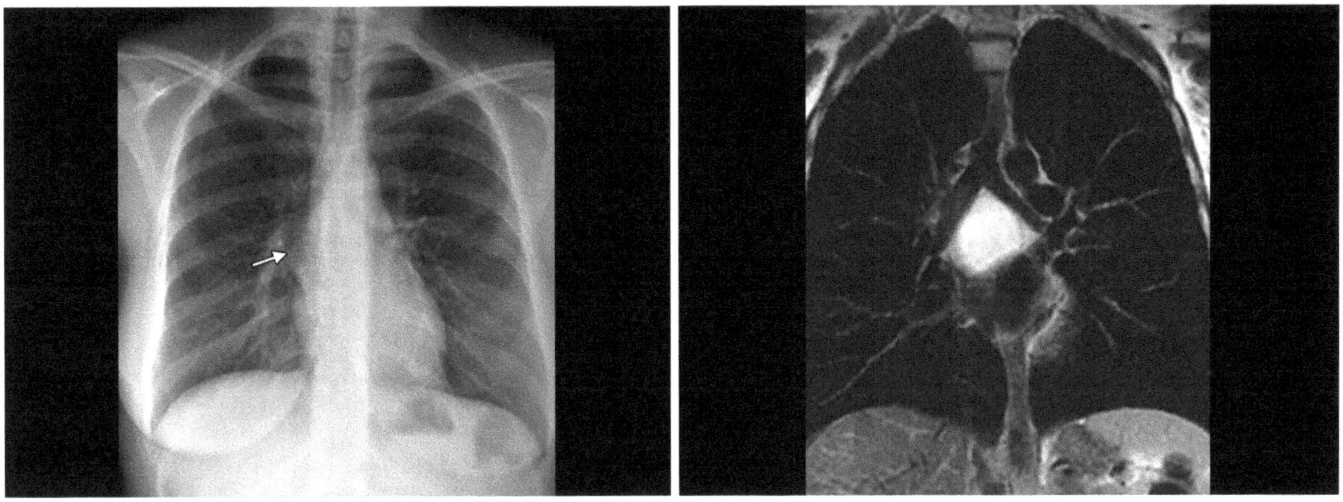

Fig. 16.40: Bronchogenic cyst: A posteroanterior chest X-ray (PA CXR) shows a triangular opacity in the carina; the right lateral border is visible (arrow). The short-tau inversion recovery (STIR) sequence MR scan shows a fluid-filled structure.

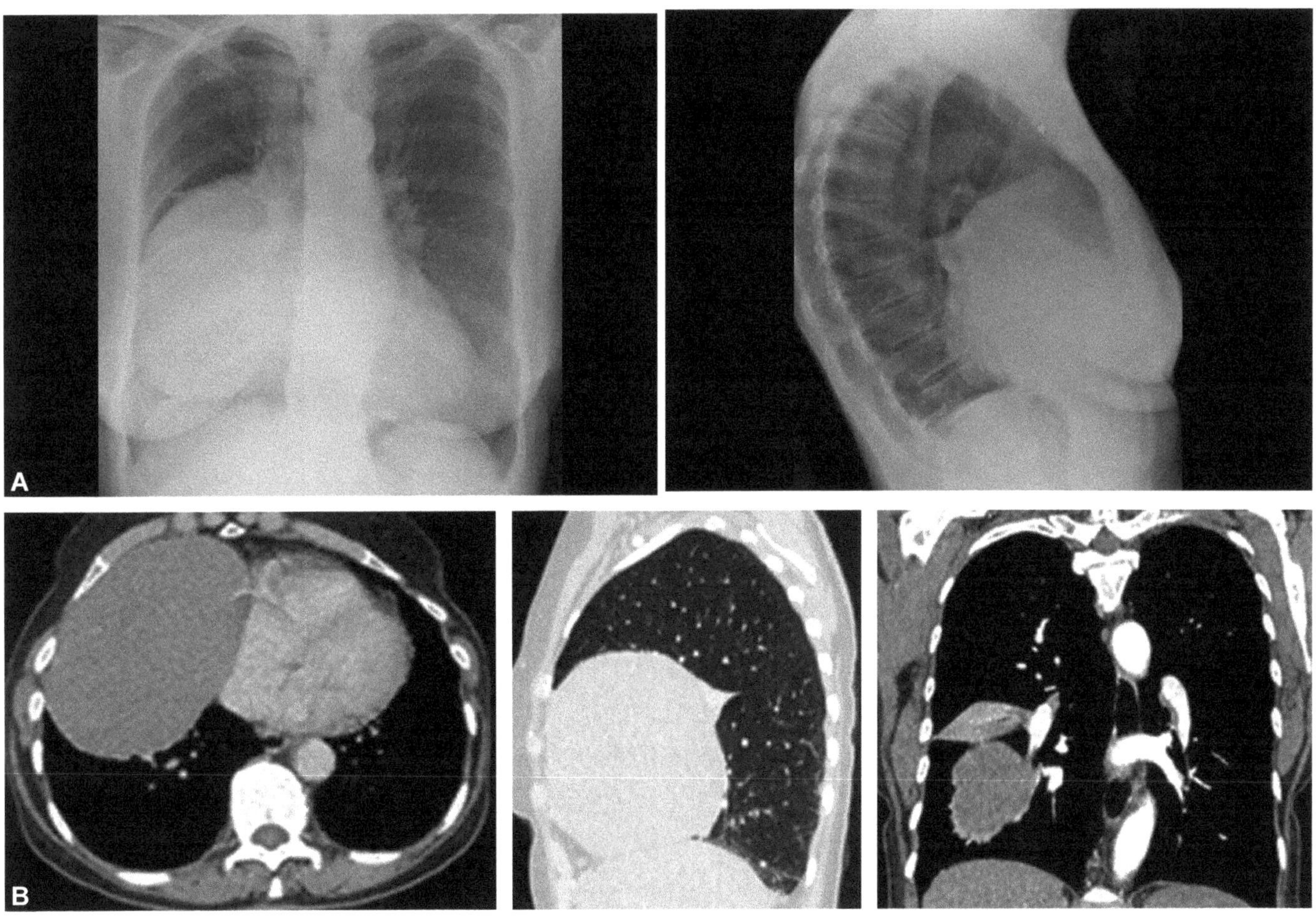

Figs. 16.41A and B: (A) Posteroanterior (PA) and right lateral CXRs showing an anterior mediastinal mass of nonspecific nature. (B) CT images in axial, coronal, and sagittal planes allowed to further characterize the lesion. A biopsy revealed non-Hodgkin's lymphoma.

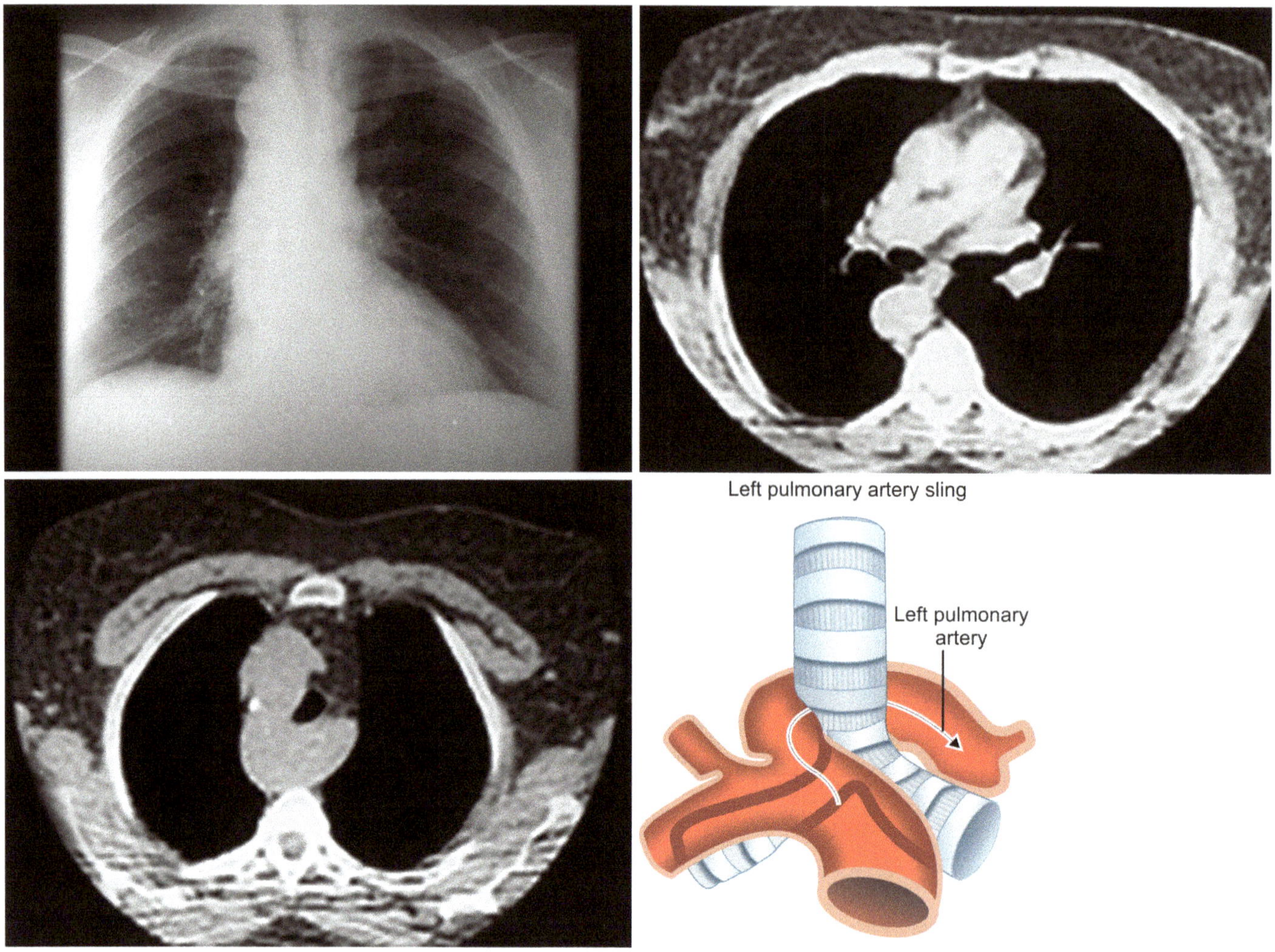

Fig. 16.42: A posteroanterior chest X-ray (PA CXR) shows lobulation of the superior mediastinal. On further questioning, the patient admitted to mild dysphagia. Axial CT scans show aortic arch duplication with descending right-sided aorta.

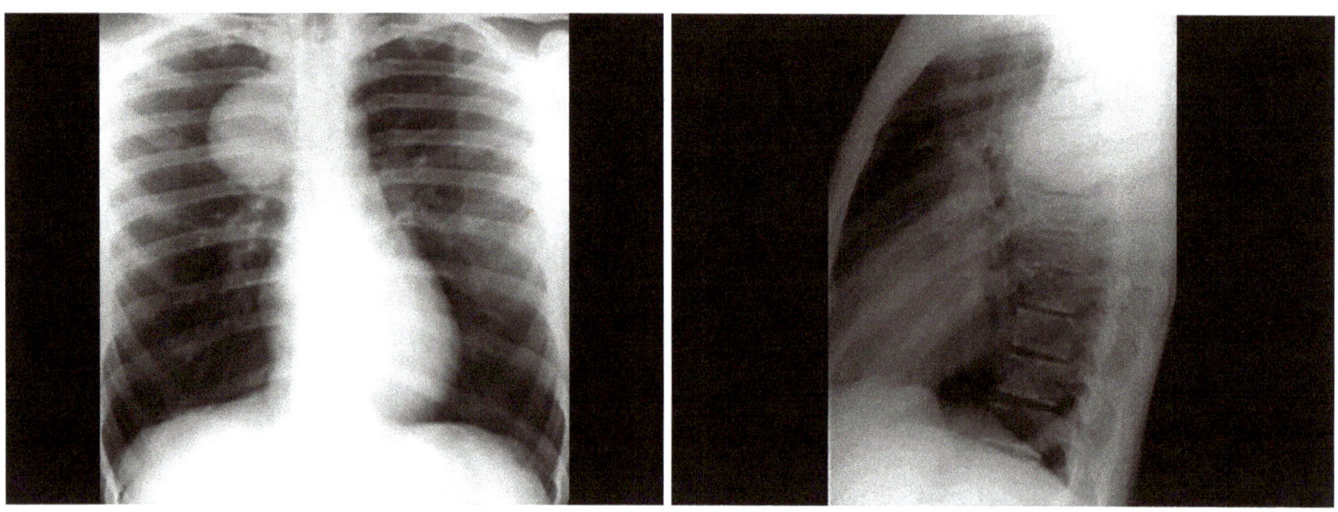

Fig. 16.43: Posteroanterior (PA) and lateral CXRs on a 32-year-old man showing a well-defined mass in the superior mediastinum located in the posterior paravertebral gutter in a patient with known neurofibroma NF1. The appearance suggests a neurofibroma.

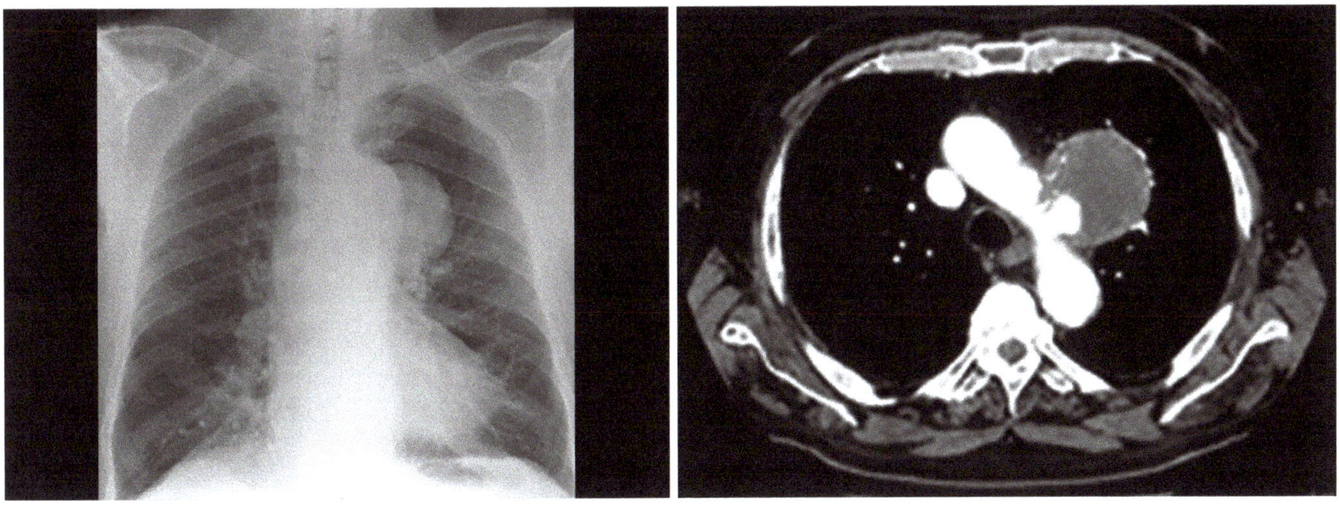

Fig. 16.44: A chest X-ray (CXR) on a patient with nonspecific symptoms shows a well-defined superior mediastinal mass. A postcontrast axial CT at the level of the aortic arch shows a pseudoaneurysm of the aorta.

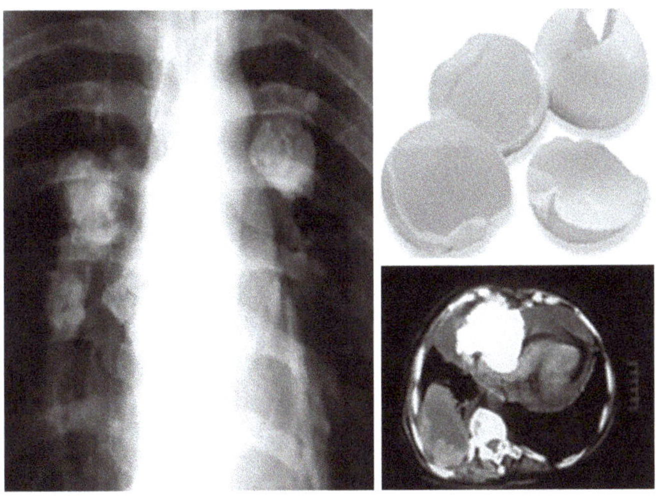

Fig. 16.45: Posteroanterior chest X-ray (PA CXR) conned to the mediastinum shows "eggshell calcification" in hilar lymph nodes secondary to old sarcoidosis. The axial CT scan from a different patient shows a calcified/ossified metastatic deposit from an osteosarcoma.

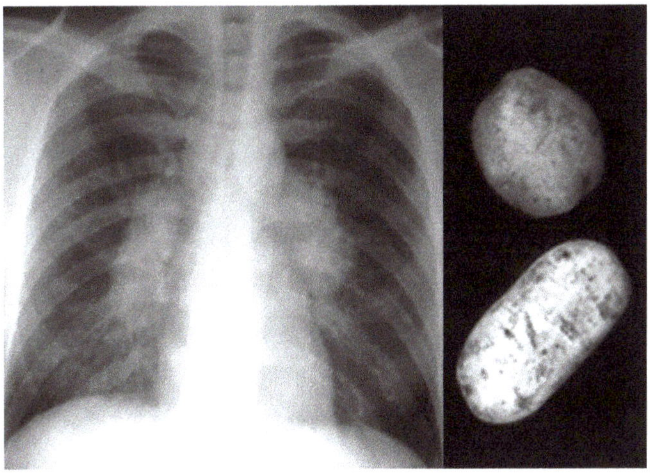

Fig. 16.46: Potato nodes in sarcoidosis: Massive, symmetrical hilar lymphadenopathy in sarcoidosis is referred to as "potato nodes", which do not merge with the cardiac border an appearance that distinguish the nodes that accompany lymphomatous nodes. The right paratracheal lymphadenopathy is more frequently seen because of the ease of identification on a posteroanterior chest X-ray (PA CXR). The left paratracheal nodes are equally involved but more difficult to see on a PA CXR.

regions which contain adipose tissue. The inhomogeneity of these tumors on either CT or Magnetic resonance imaging (MRI) helps differentiate liposarcomas from lipomas. Irregular areas of enhancing soft tissue would also suggest a malignant nature. If in doubt, fluorine-18-labeled fluorodeoxyglucose positron emission tomography (^{18}F-FDG PET) may be valuable in the differentiation of lipomas from liposarcomas.

Pleural fibromas [localized fibrous tumors of the pleura (LFTPs)] are usually discovered incidentally on a CXR of asymptomatic individuals. There is no gender predilection or association with prior asbestos exposure. Symptoms are usually nonspecific and include cough, dyspnea, chest pain and hypertrophic pulmonary osteoarthropathy.

LFTPs can be rounded, oblong, or lobulated. They are often found in the dependent portions of the thorax, and if large, they will displace rather than invade adjacent structures. On unenhanced CT scans, LFTP may appear as soft tissue attenuation; on MRI they appear as intermediate to low signal on T1 and also T2 hypointensity. Marked

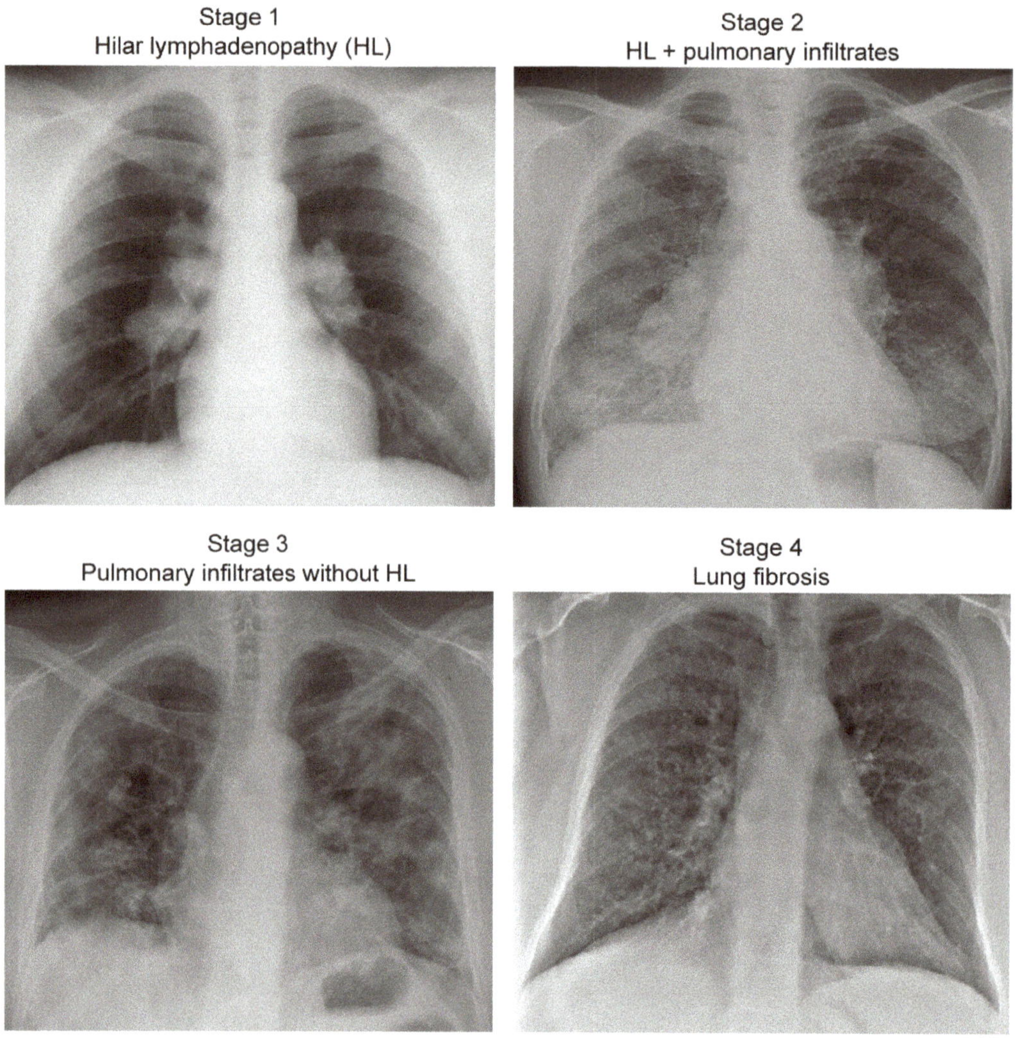

Fig. 16.47: Staging of sarcoidosis on the basis of chest X-ray.

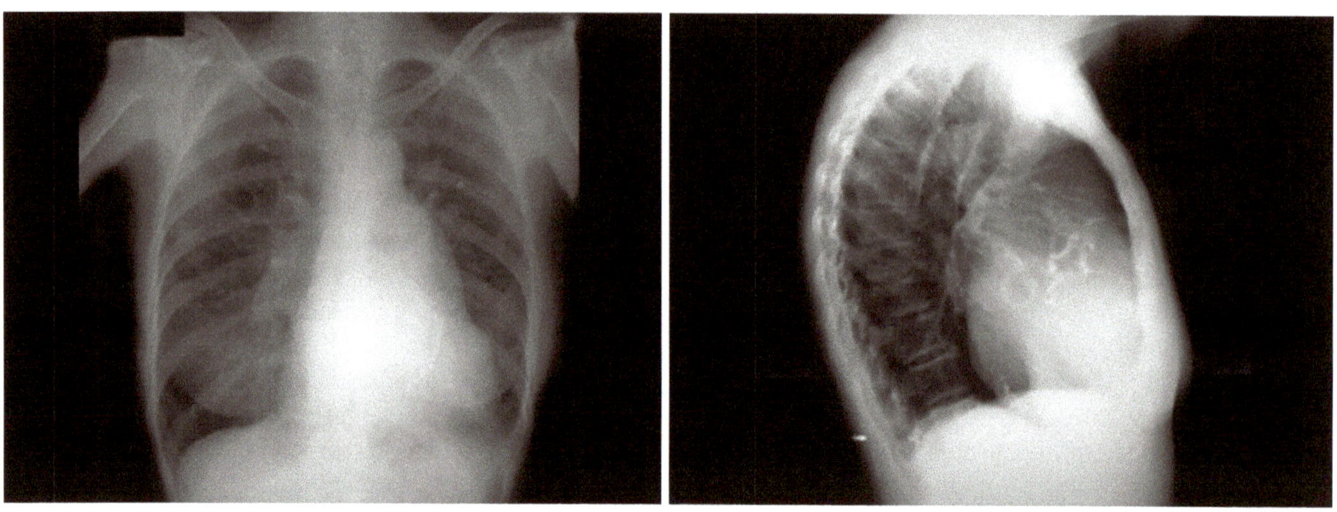

Fig. 16.48: Posteroanterior (PA) and lateral chest X-ray (CXR) showing a mitralization of the heart.

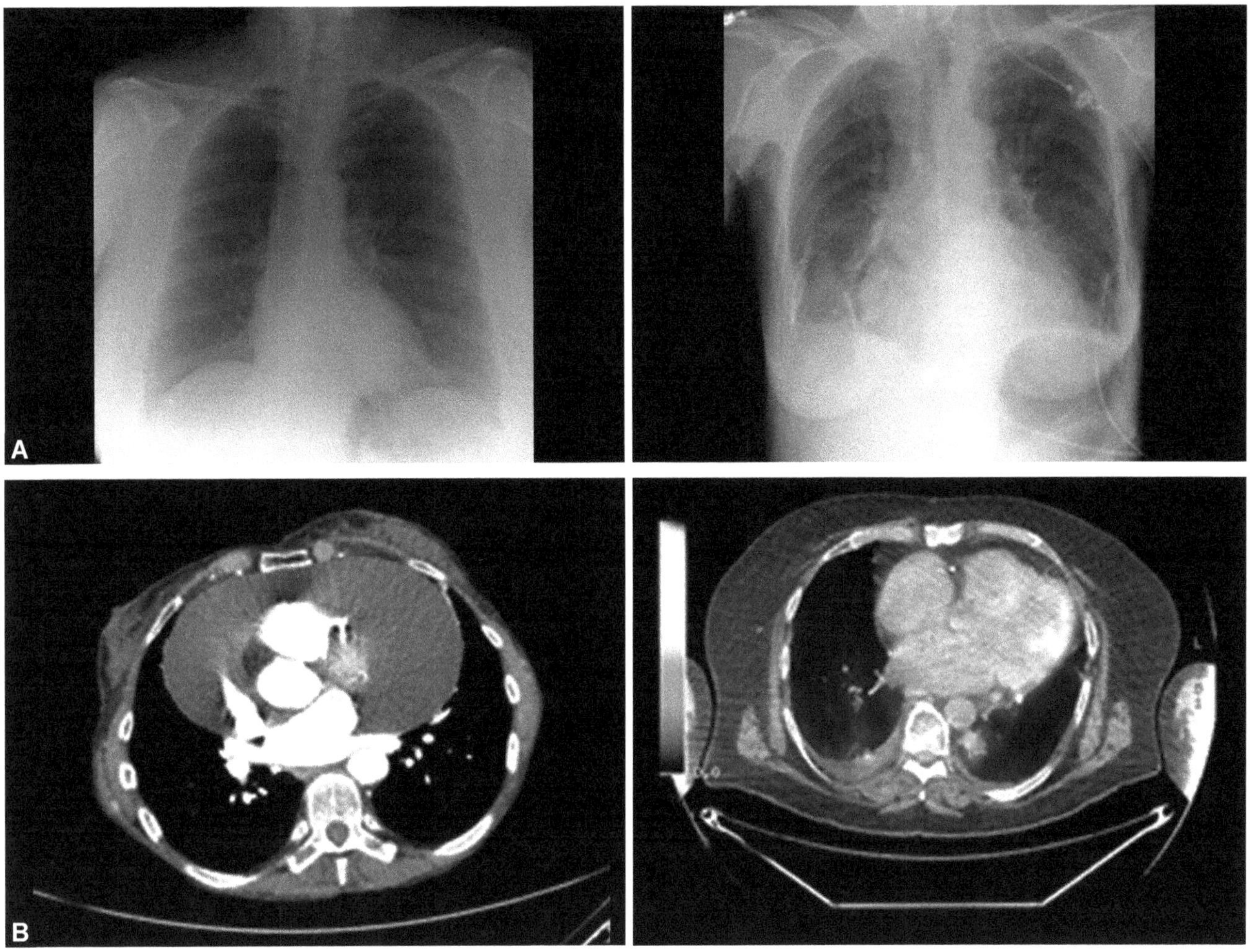

Figs. 16.49A and B: (A) Two PA CXRs 3 weeks apart show a rapidly enlarging cardiac size and pleural effusions. (B) The PET/CT on the same patient shows a tumor in the posterior sulcus and pericardial metastatic disease.

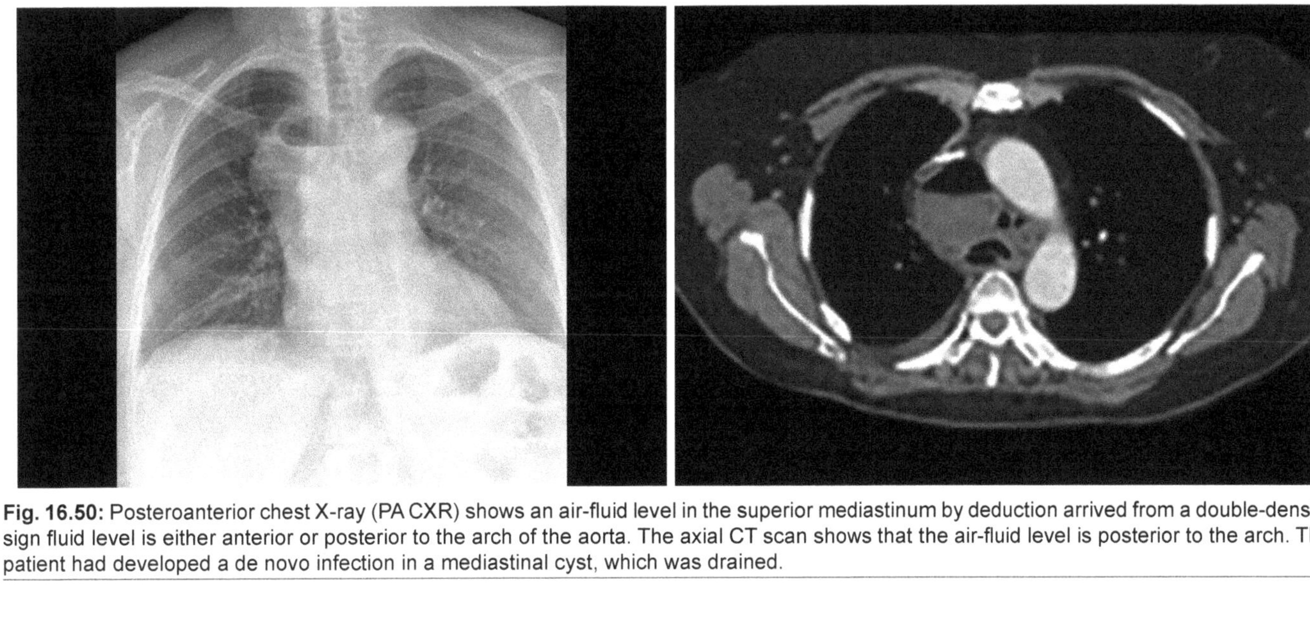

Fig. 16.50: Posteroanterior chest X-ray (PA CXR) shows an air-fluid level in the superior mediastinum by deduction arrived from a double-density sign fluid level is either anterior or posterior to the arch of the aorta. The axial CT scan shows that the air-fluid level is posterior to the arch. The patient had developed a de novo infection in a mediastinal cyst, which was drained.

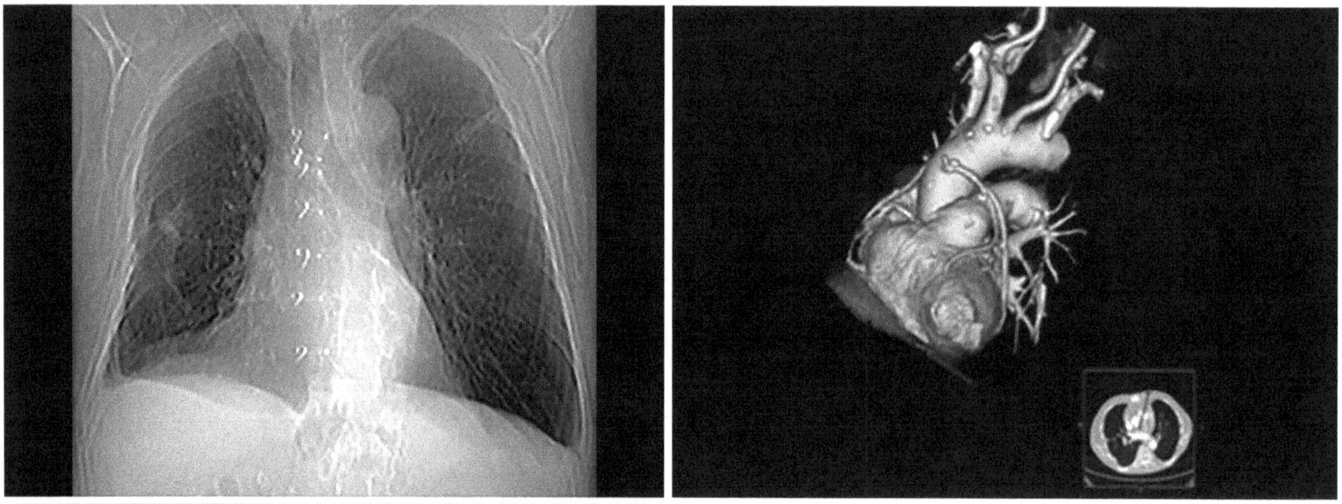

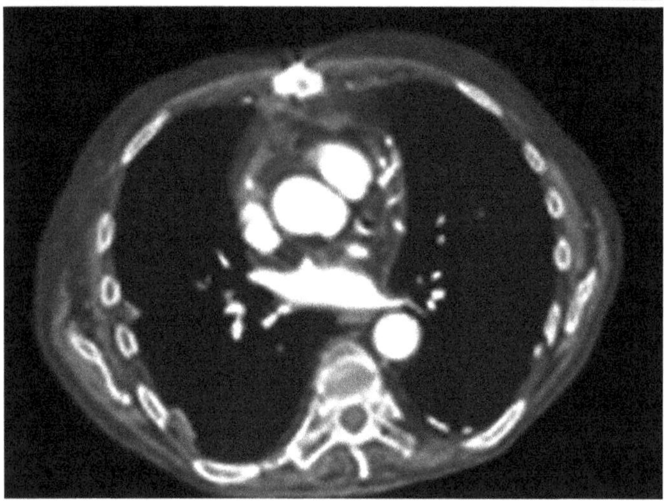

Fig. 16.51: Mediastinal hematoma following coronary bypass surgery: Posteroanterior chest X-ray (PA CXR) of a patient that presented with retrosternal discomfort following coronary bypass surgery. The CXR shows sternotomy clips but nothing else significant. However, an axial CT showed a soft tissue anterior mediastinal mass with blood attenuation. The 3D reconstructions elegantly show extension of the hematoma.

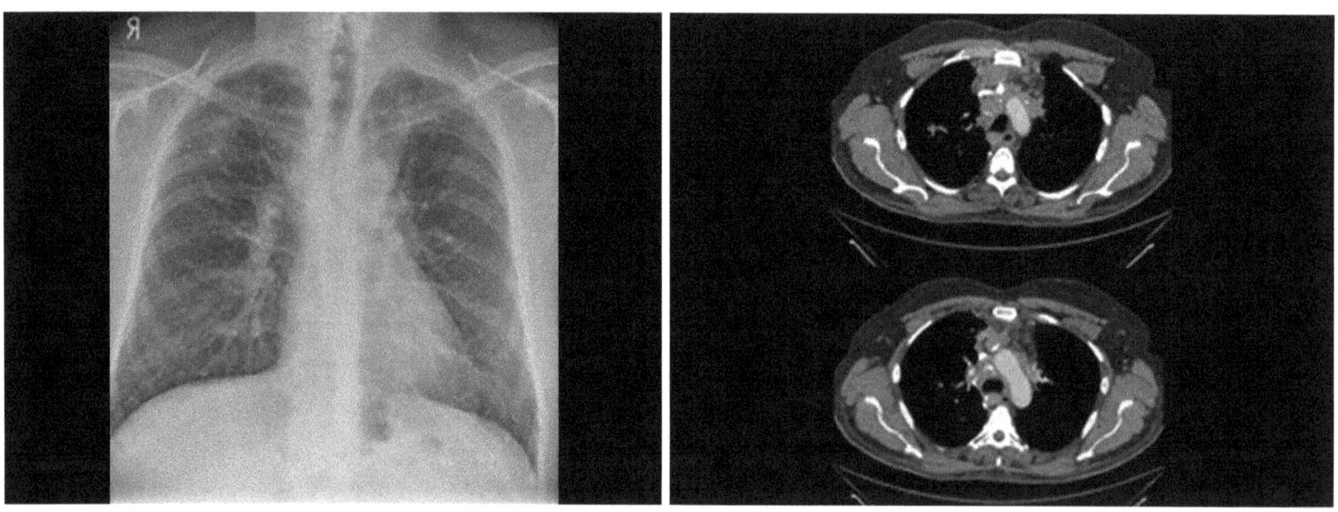

Fig. 16.52: Fibrosing mediastinitis. This patient with known dental technician pneumoconiosis developed a pyrexial illness with raised inflammatory markers. The CXR shows widening of the superior mediastinum with "whiskery borders". A biopsy revealed MAI mycobacterium avium fibrosing mediastinitis.

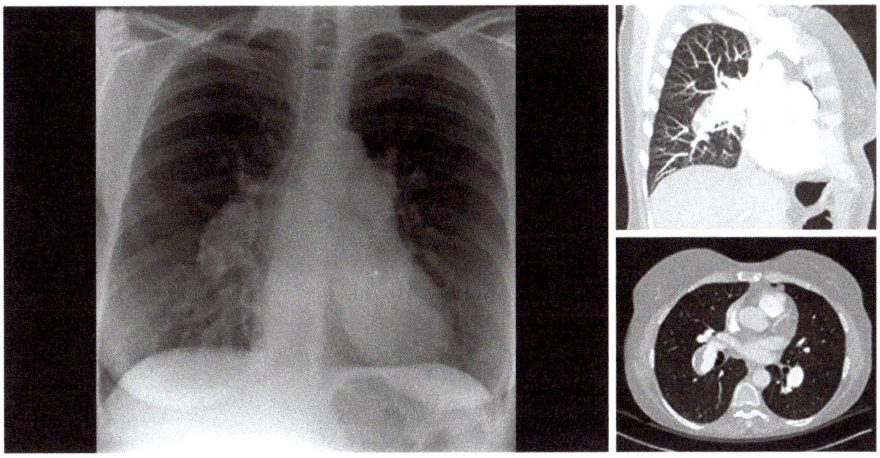

Fig. 16.53: Posteroanterior chest X-ray (PA CXR) showing a pulmonary artery aneurysm; there were no echocardiographic or clinical features of pulmonary, note the partially thrombosed left pulmonary artery on the axial and coronal CT scans. The appearances are in keeping with Behçet's disease.

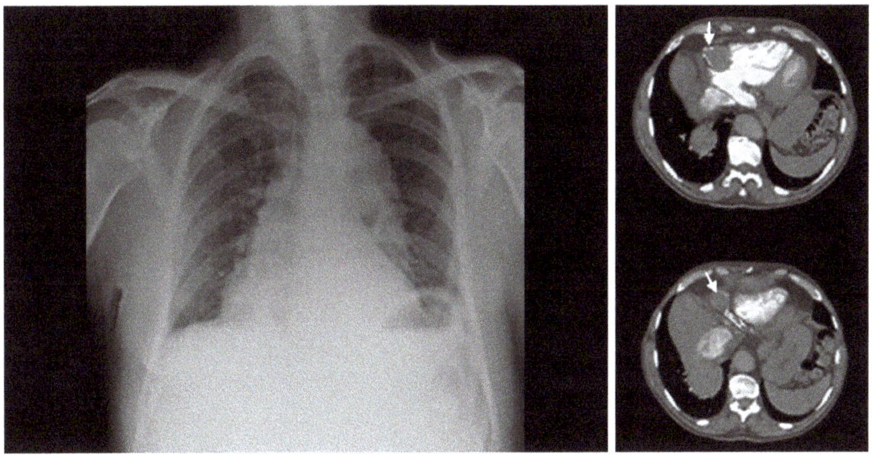

Fig. 16.54: Posteroanterior chest X-ray (PA CXR) showing a mass at the right cardiophrenic angle, shown to be a right coronary artery aneurysm on the axial CT images (arrows).

enhancement is demonstrated with contrast because of rich vascular supply. Cysts and hemorrhagic necrosis may be associated. Surgical excision is usually curative with a 16% risk of local recurrence (Figs. 16.34A and B).

Intrathoracic splenosis is rare and involves the autotransplantation of splenic tissue into the pleural cavity (Figs. 16.35A to D). Commonly, secondary to diaphragmatic and splenic rupture following blunt or penetrating abdominal trauma. Thourani et al. described the chest radiographic findings of a pleural-based mass (confirmed on CT). Surgically they observed numerous purplish implants throughout the thoracic cavity which covered the pleural, pericardial and hemidiaphragmatic surfaces. The presence of Howell-Jolly bodies on postoperative blood smear confirmed the diagnosis of intrathoracic splenosis.

Intrathoracic splenosis is usually a benign condition, in comparison to abdominal splenosis whereby patients may present with pain and bowel obstruction. Radiographic diagnosis can be made by technetium 99m Tc-labeled heat-damaged erythrocyte scan, 99mTc sulfur colloid scintigraphy, or indium 111-labeled platelet scan.

Extrapleural Sign

Expanding lesions of chest wall structures include:

- Peripheral location
- Cat under the rug
- Concave edges
- Sharp inner edge and indistinct outer edge
- Equal length and width.

An extrapleural sign is thoracic wall-based expanding density. The opacity is peripheral in location with a "cat under the rug appearance". The edges are concave, with sharp inner border but indistinct peripheral edge. The opacity is of equal length and width in the early stages. A lipoma of the thoracic wall presenting an "extrapleural sign" is shown in Figure 16.36.

MEDIASTINUM

Enlargement of the thyroid gland *(goiter)* is one of the causes of superior mediastinal mass. Although there is no clear definition but thyroid gland enlargement is considered as a goiter that requires surgical removal when there is retrosternal extension with intrathoracic component appears to extend more than 3 cm from the thoracic inlet.

Ultrasound with Doppler studies is the imaging modality of choice when there is clinical suspicion of enlarged thyroid gland. The latter modality usually demonstrates diffuse enlargement/nodularity of the gland with possible colloid content. It is also useful to evaluate retrosternal extension. CT can evaluate the degree of intrathoracic extension in larger goiters. They usually demonstrate contrast enhancement and may contain calcification (Figs. 16.37 and 16.38).

Unilateral superior mediastinal lymphadenopathy has a wide differential, including infectious etiologies (e.g. tuberculous adenopathy, Fig. 16.39) and malignancy.

Bronchogenic cyst is a rare congenital malformation of the bronchial tree; however, it is considered the commonest of foregut duplication cysts. It accounts for 5–10% of pediatric mediastinal masses. Most bronchogenic cysts are asymptomatic and found incidentally on imaging. However, mediastinal cysts can present as a mediastinal mass that may enlarge and cause local compression and respiratory distress. Infection of bronchogenic cysts is also reported.

Bronchogenic cyst forms as an abnormal budding of the bronchial tree during embryogenesis that is lined by secretory respiratory epithelium (cuboid or columnar ciliated epithelium). The wall is made up of tissues similar to that of the normal bronchial tree, including cartilage, elastic tissues, mucous glands and smooth muscle. They contain water; variable amounts of proteinaceous material, blood products, and calcium oxalate and hence can be confused with solid lesions due to their high attenuation content. They do not usually communicate with the bronchial tree and therefore typically are nonaerated. Occasionally a communication may develop following infection or intervention, resulting in and air-filled cystic structure with an air-fluid level.

Bronchogenic cysts can be classified as mediastinal and intrapulmonary types. The most common location is the middle mediastinum (65–90%). Parenchymal (intrapulmonary) bronchogenic cysts are typically perihilar with lower lobes predilection.

On plain radiographs, the cysts usually appear as soft tissue density rounded structures, sometimes with a compression effect of surrounding structures. On CT, they appear as well-circumscribed spherical or ovoid masses of variable attenuation.

Approximately 50% are fluid density (0–20 HU), with the remaining cysts being of soft tissue density (> 30 HU) or even hyperdense compared to the mediastinal soft tissue. CT can also detect calcium oxalate (milk of calcium) layering dependently. No solid contrast enhancement is the general rule.

Treatment options include surgical excision of the cyst considering the chance of developing complications like infection, hemorrhage, bronchial obstruction and rarely, to undergo malignant transformation. Increasingly, these lesions are treated with transbronchial or percutaneous CT-guided aspiration that will confirm the diagnosis and treat/reduce their size. Small lesions can be followed however they do have a tendency to increase in size over time, sometimes rapidly (Fig. 16.40). Malignant transformation is very rare, but reported, with primaries including: rhabdomyosarcoma, pleuropulmonary blastoma, anaplastic carcinoma, leiomyosarcoma, and adenocarcinoma.

A lower mediastinal mass (Figs. 16.41 to 16.43) is best characterized by a combination of a CXR and CT, supported by clinical input. A right descending aorta is a rare, but a known cause of dysphagia. Well-defined posterior mediastinal masses, associated with rib notching can be a feature of neurofibromas.

A *pseudoaneurysm* of the aorta (Fig. 16.44) is a possible cause of mediastinal mass observed at CXR. This is a hematoma that forms as the result of trauma with a leaking hole in the aorta, also known as a false aneurysm, and can be acute or chronic.

Fine calcifications at the periphery of a mass are usually referred as "eggshell calcification". This is commonly seen in hilar lymph nodes secondary to old sarcoidosis (Fig. 16.45) or silicosis, but they can also be calcified/ossified metastatic deposit from an osteosarcoma.

A massive, symmetrical hilar lymphadenopathy can be observed in sarcoidosis. This finding is referred to as "potato nodes", which do not merge with the cardiac border an appearance that distinguish the nodes that accompany lymphomatous nodes (Figs. 16.46 and 16.47). The right paratracheal lymphadenopathy is more frequently seen because of the ease of identification on a PA CXR. The left paratracheal nodes are equally involved but more difficult to see on a PA CXR. Sarcoidosis is a noncaseating granulomatous multisystem chronic inflammatory condition of unknown etiology. Most of patients (90%) present with lung and mediastinal/hilar lymphadenopathy. Often patients below the age of 40 years old are affected, and the incident peaks in the third decade of life. Half of the patients remain asymptomatic, but symptoms such as cough and dyspnea may occur. CT findings in the chest include paratracheal, mediastinal and bilateral hilar lymphadenopathy. Pulmonary nodules if present would typically be in a peribronchovascular distribution or along fissures. Sarcoidosis can be staged even on the basis of chest radiographs.

Mitral stenosis can result in a straightening of the left border of the cardiac shadow. This is often referred as *mitralization of the heart,* with prominent pulmonary conus, dilated left atrium and extensive mitral valve calcification. Mitral valve calcification is common in the elderly and not all calcification is symptomatic (Fig. 16.48).

A rapidly enlarging heart on a PA CXR may indicate a pericardial effusion, which may be further characterized by CT. Figures 16.49A and B show an example of a rapidly enlarging pericardial effusion shown on a PET/CT to be secondary to a metastatic pericardial disease.

An air/fluid level in the mediastinum in appropriate clinical setting is suggestive of an infected cyst (Fig. 16.50). A widened mediastinum can also be due to mediastinal hematoma, i.e. the presence of blood within the mediastinum (Fig. 16.51). This can be caused by aortic injury, tearing of mediastinal vessels, sternal injury or thoracic spine injury. In patients with blunt chest trauma, early diagnosis of mediastinal hematoma is important, because it could be associated with thoracic vessel injury. Signs of mediastinal haematoma due to aortic injury include widened mediastinum, indistinct or abnormal aortic contour, deviation of trachea to the right, depression of left main bronchus, widened paraspinal stripe, left apical pleural cap.

Pleuropericardial cysts are uncommon congenital cysts of the anterior and middle mediastinum that result from abnormalities in the development of the coelomic cavities. Rarely can they occur as a result of previous pericarditis. Most cases are diagnosed incidentally on imaging and remain asymptomatic.

Pericardial cysts are typically seen as right cardiophrenic angle mass but can be found anywhere adjacent to the heart. On CT, they appear as well-defined, nonenhancing, low (water) attenuating, rounded mass next to the pericardium. MR examination usually shows typical fluid signal content with occasional high signal on T1-weighted images due to proteinaceous material and there is no enhancement with intravenous contrast on CT or MR (Fig. 16.55).

Figure 16.56 shows the value of a CT scan in confirming a fat density pericardial lipoma as a cause of apparent right diaphragmatic hump seen on a PA and lateral chest radiographs.

Benign nerve sheath tumors are usually seen as posterior mediastinal or paraspinal masses. On CT, schwannomas are frequently heterogeneous with areas of low attenuation secondary to cystic degeneration, hypercellularity,

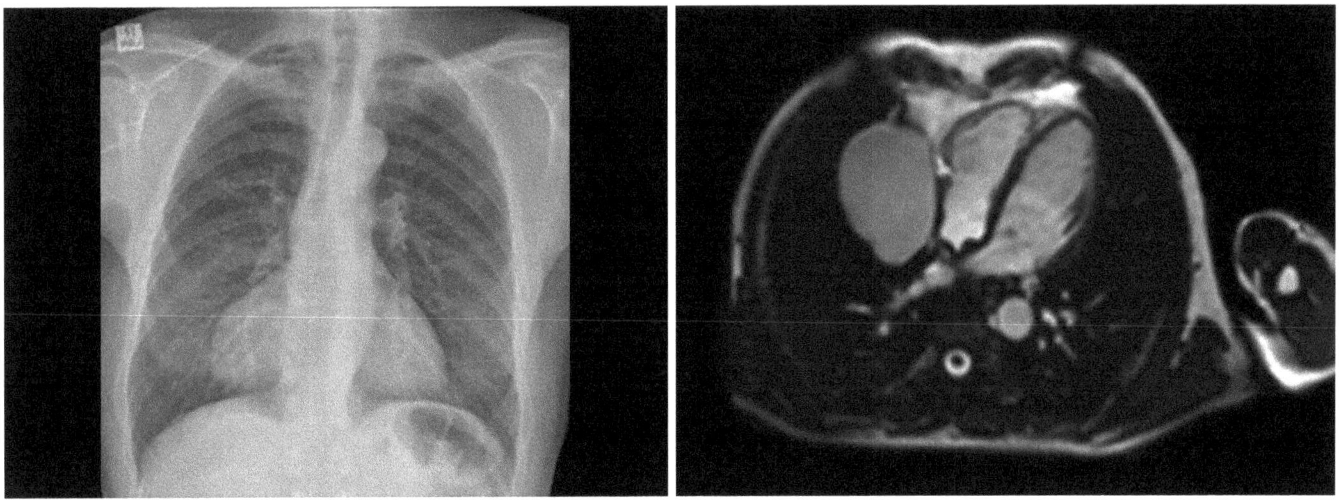

Fig. 16.55: A posteroanterior chest X-ray (PA CXR) shows a well-defined mass at the right cardiophrenic angle. An axial MR image shows a fluid signal mass suggestive of a pleuropericardial cyst (spring water cyst), and no further imaging was undertaken.

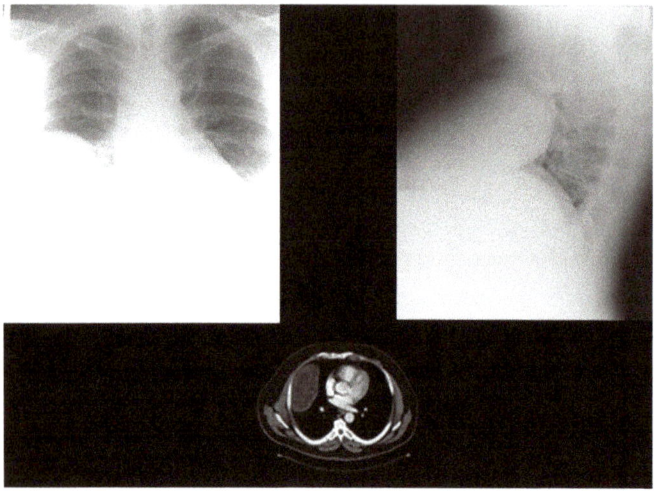

Fig. 16.56: Posteroanterior (PA) and lateral CXRs showing a mass in close relationship with right hemidiaphragm shown to be a mass of fat density suggestive of a pericardial lipoma.

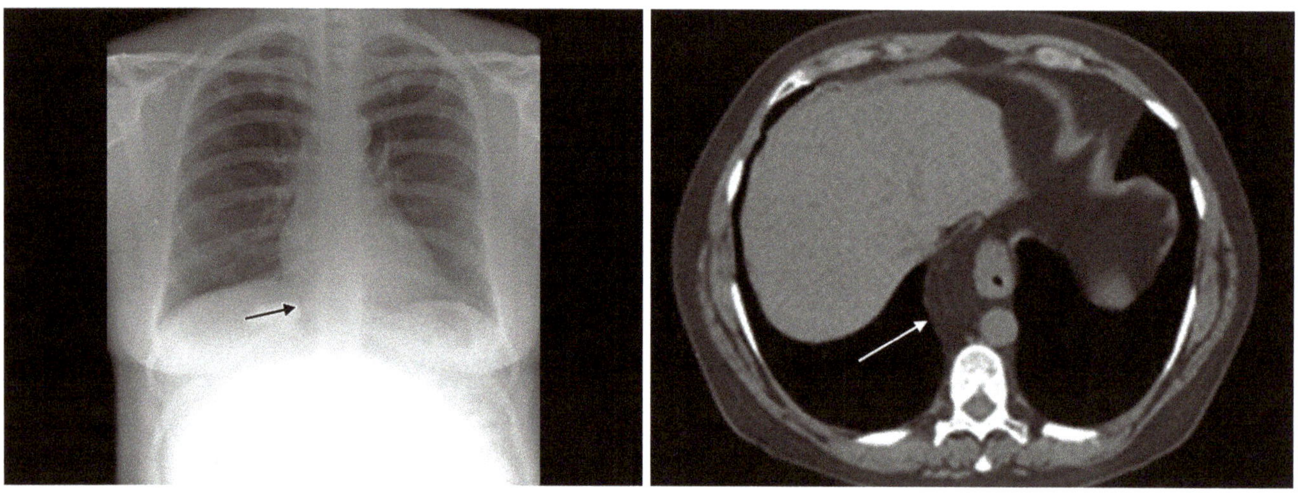

Fig. 16.57: A posteroanterior chest X-ray (PA CXR) shows a biopsy proved schwannoma in the posterior vertebral gutter note the well-defined benign nerve sheath tumor.

hemorrhage, lipid, or myelin (Fig. 16.57). Punctate calcifications may also be detected on CT.

Enhancement pattern can be variable (homogeneous, heterogeneous, or peripheral). They may extend through the adjacent intervertebral foramen to the spinal canal with a "dumb-bell" configuration. MRI typically exhibits low-to-intermediate signal intensity on T1-weighted imaging and may show areas of intermediate-to-high signal intensity on T2-weighted imaging.

Other examples of mediastinal abnormal findings on CXR are shown in Figures 16.57 to 16.59.

CHEST WALL

Chest X-ray can show chest wall anomalies such pectus excavatum and pectus carinatum, as well as asymmetry, rib fractures, or more rarely costal chondroma and chondrosarcoma (Figs. 16.60 to 16.67). Pectus excavatum is a depression of the sternum due to an abnormal development of the rib cage, resulting in a sunken chest wall deformity. On the contrary, pectus carinatum, also called pigeon chest, is a deformity of the chest characterized by a protrusion of the sternum and ribs. CXR remains the primary imaging technique in the study of chest wall diseases; however, CT and MRI allow today to better define their localization and nature.

Many extrathoracic masses can mimic intrathoracic lesions (Figs. 16.63 and 16.64).

Thoracoplasty was used in early 1900s to 1950s as a collapse therapy to obliterate the pleural cavity. This form of collapse therapy was employed in cases of empyema and lung cavities. Many upper ribs were resected, and

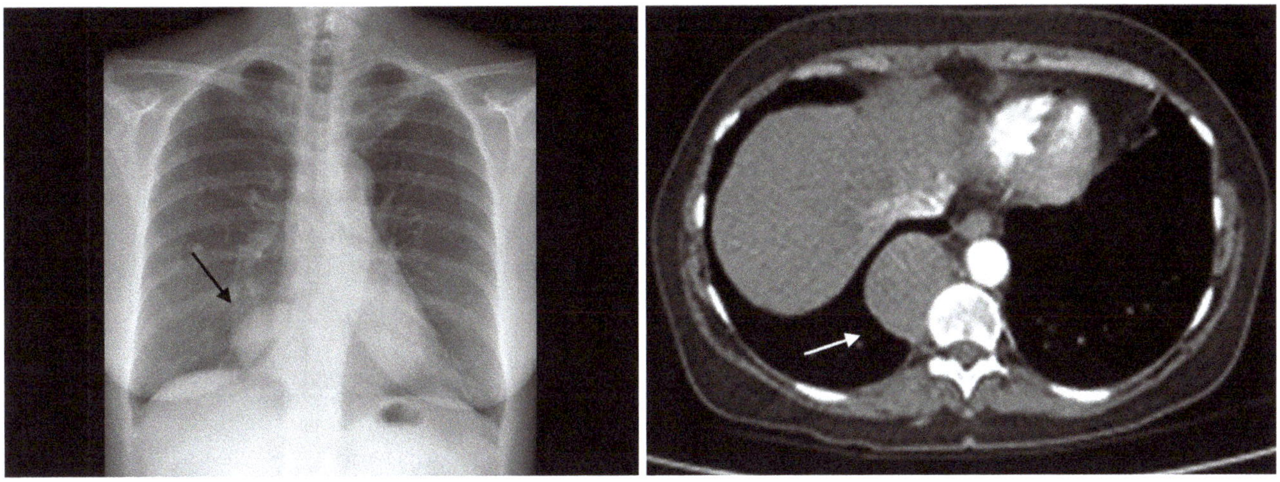

Fig. 16.58: A posteroanterior chest X-ray (PA CXR) showing a lower dorsal smooth paravertebral mass (black arrow); axial CT confirms the presence of fat in the said location (white arrow).

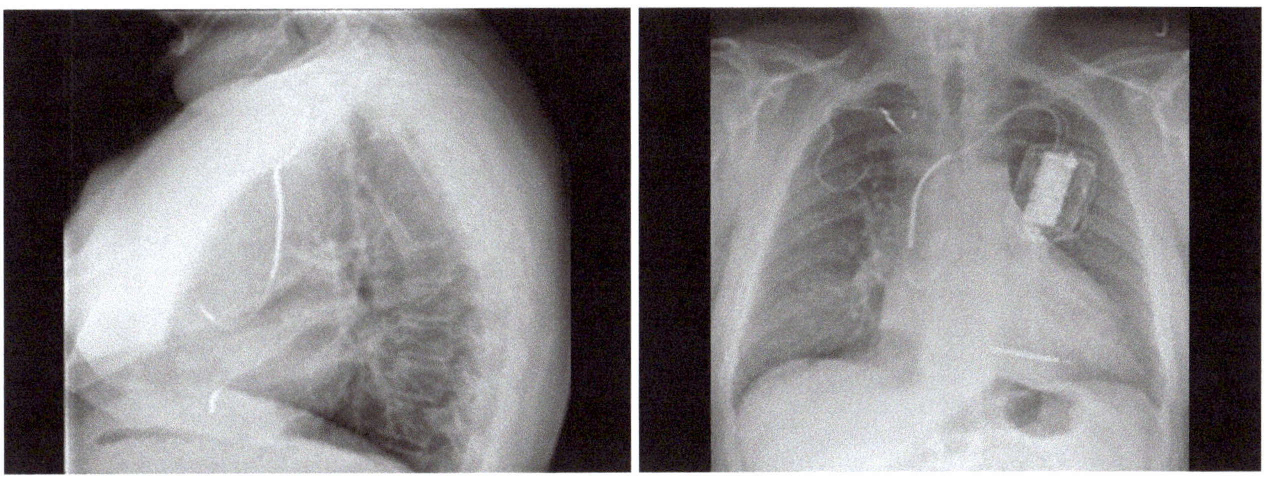

Fig. 16.59: The PA and lateral CXR show one of the complications of cardiac pacing. The cardiac catheter has sheared and has embolized into the upper-lobe pulmonary artery, attempts to retrieve the sheared catheter were unsuccessful.

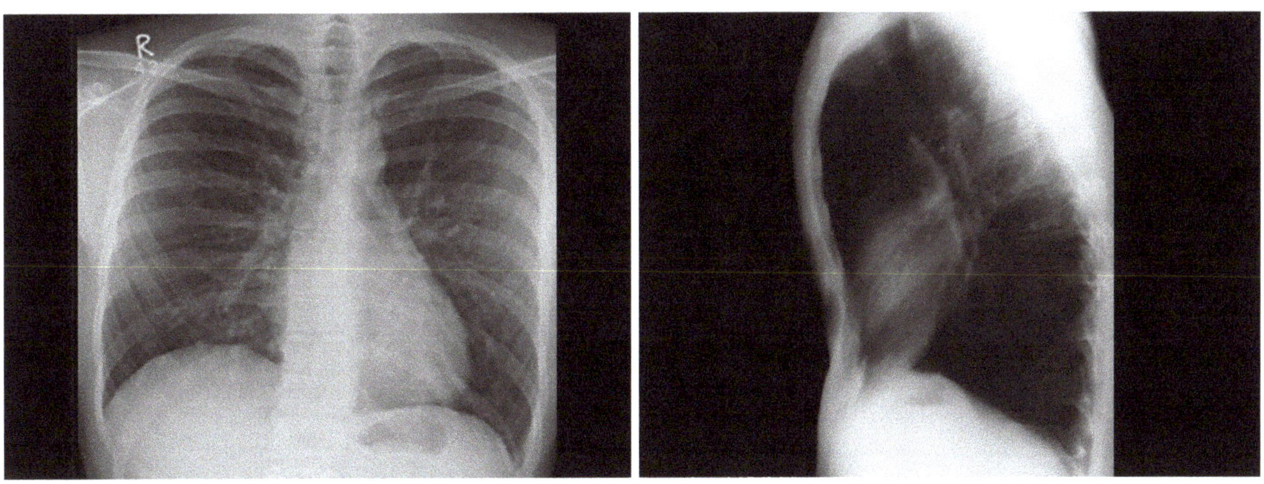

Fig. 16.60: A posteroanterior chest X-ray (PA CXR) shows characteristic features of a pectus excavatum. Note upward slopping of the posterior ribs and sharp anterior decent of the anterior ribs. No lateral radiograph is required; the lateral image nevertheless confirms the pectus.

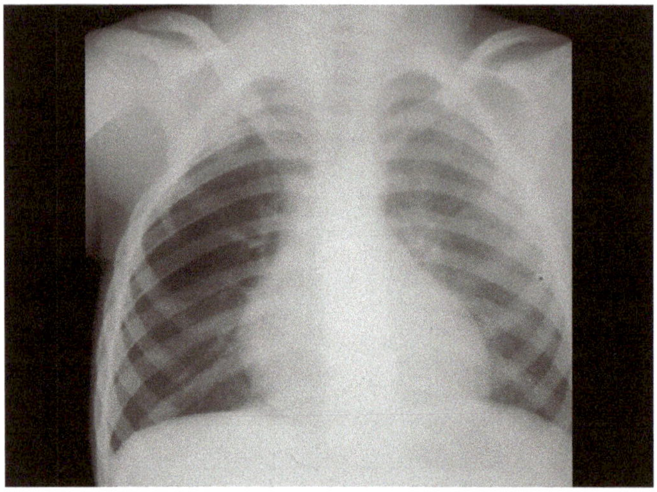

Fig. 16.61: One of the features of Poland syndrome as shown by a unilateral transradiancy due to absent right pectoralis major muscle.

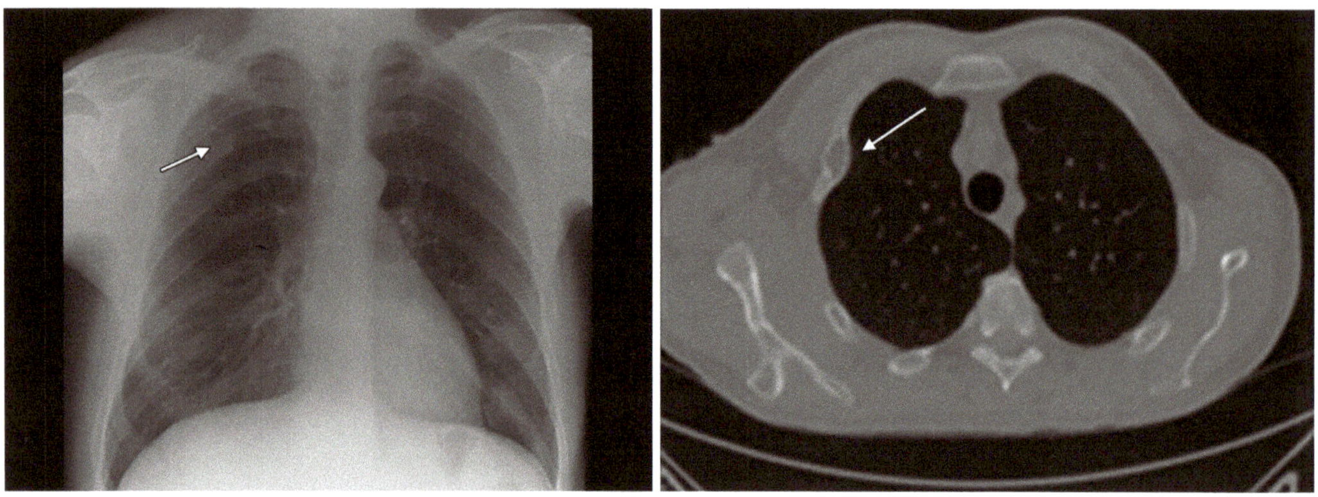

Fig. 16.62: Posteroanterior chest X-ray (PA CXR) and axial CT of a fibrous rib lesion that remained stable for 6 years and no further observation was undertake.

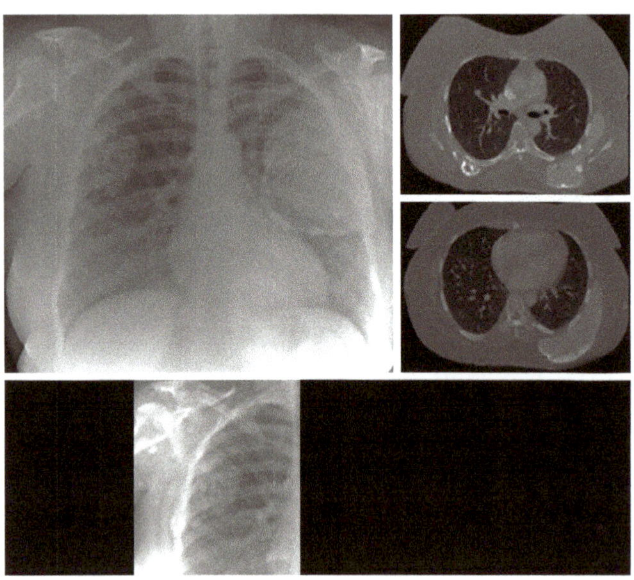

Fig. 16.63: Posteroanterior chest X-ray (PA CXR), radiograph of the left shoulder and axial CT scans show extensive myositis ossificans mimicking pleural lesions that mimic pleural calcification on the PA CXR.

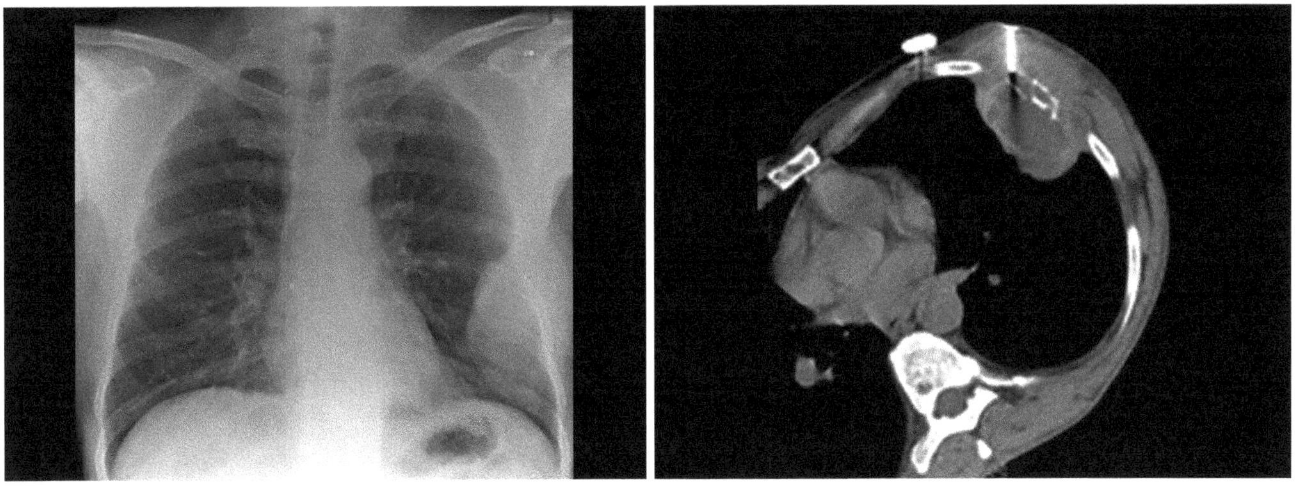

Fig. 16.64: Posteroanterior chest X-ray (PA CXR) showing an extrapleural sign secondary to a plasmacytoma of the rib that presented with pleural rub on auscultation. The CT scan shows placement of a biopsy needle in the affected rib.

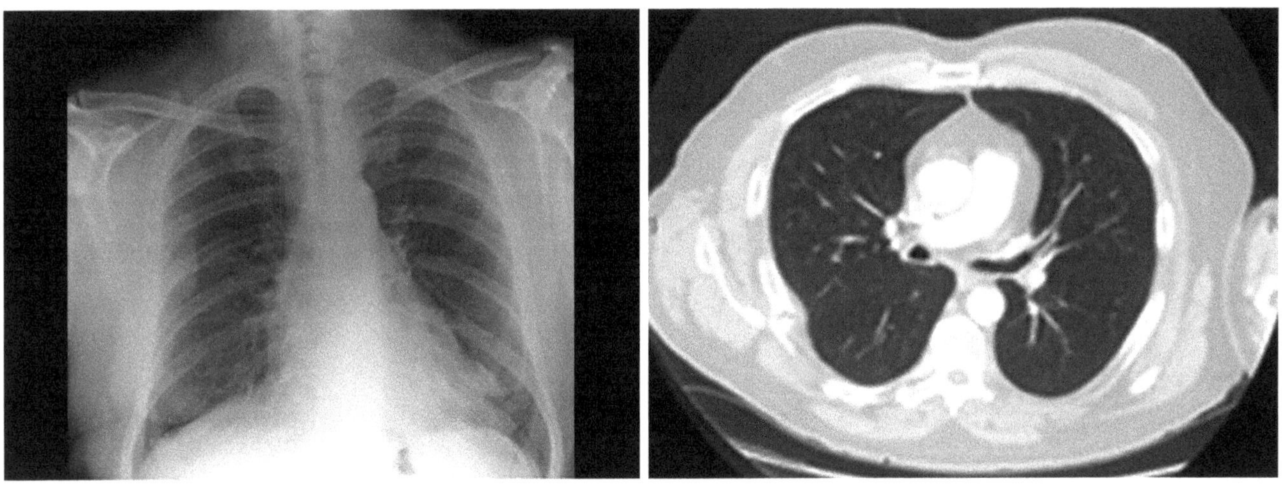

Fig. 16.65: Posteroanterior chest X-ray (PA CXR) shows an extrapleural/pleural shadow in a patient that presented with right-sided pleuritic chest pain. Axial CT scan shows a fibrous union/nonunion of a fractured rib.

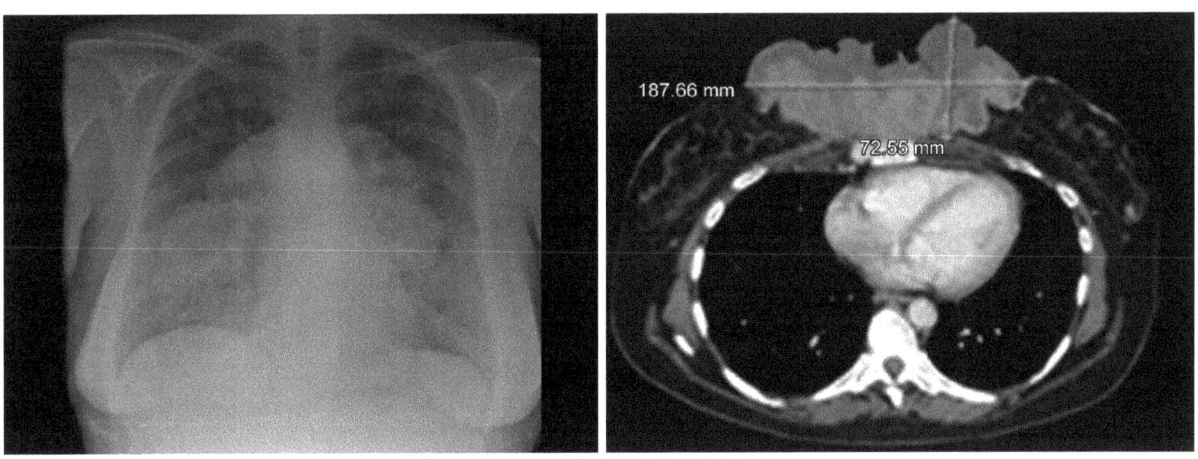

Fig. 16.66: Posteroanterior chest X-ray (PA CXR) showing a large mass from a biopsy proved Ewing's sarcoma. Note the hilum overlay sign implying that the mass is either anterior or posterior to the heart. The axial CT shows the mass arising from the sternum.

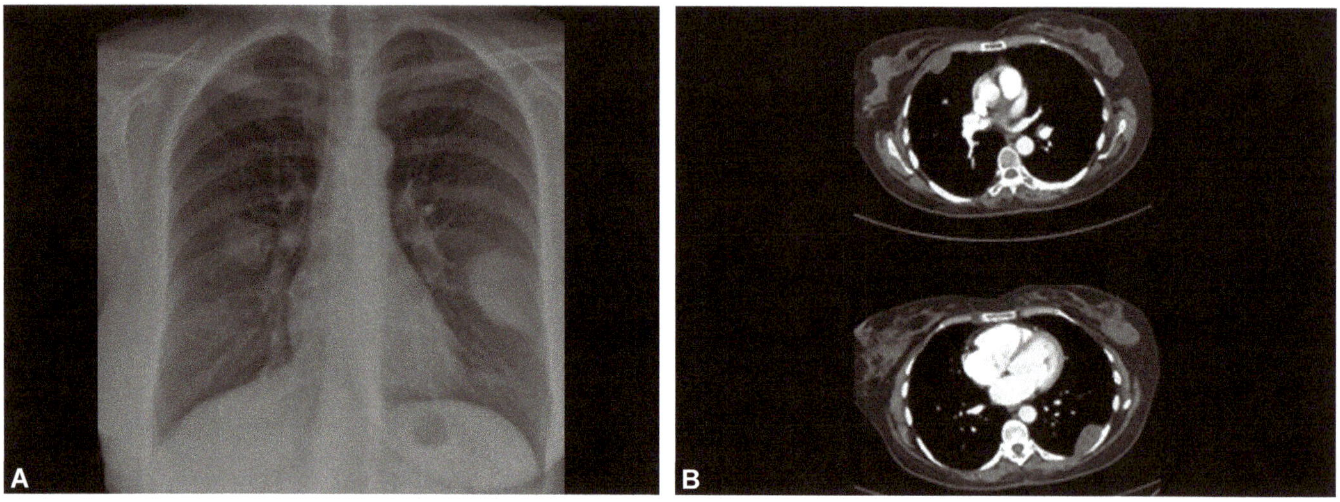

Figs. 16.67A and B: Posteroanterior chest X-ray (PA CXR) showing rib notching in a patient with neurofibromatosis type 1. The axial CT scans confirm rib notching.

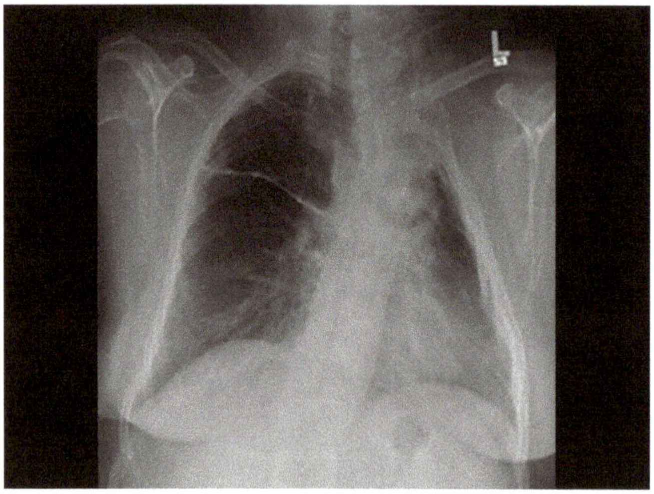

Fig. 16.68: Posteroanterior chest X-ray (PA CXR) showing the effects of a left-sided thoracoplasty.

the lung was allowed to collapse resulting in a characteristic deformity of the upper thoracic cage in which the first several ribs are displaced toward the mediastinum (Fig. 16.68).

Plombage involved the extrapleural insertion of a "plombe" to collapse the lung. The "plombe" is solid paraffin or plastic ping pong balls used in the1940s (Figs. 16.69A and B).

Review Areas

A systemic approach should be used to look at a CXR. Some areas are worth a second look as these are areas where lesions are often missed. These review areas include the lung apices, the posterior mediastinum, below the diaphragm, the thorax and having a second look for an apical pneumothorax, which can be subtle. The position of catheters/intrathoracic tubes should be carefully monitored. Also look at soft tissues especially at the breast shadows or mastectomy and surgical emphysema.

A mycetoma is solid, round or oval mass with soft tissue opacity. Its name derives from the tumor-like mass it forms. Mycetomas are often due to local infections caused by *fungi and* occur in pre-existing cavities (Figs. 16.70 and 16.71). A Mycetoma can be easily missed at the lung apices, particularly on an overexposed radiograph.

Steering column impact injuries may be forgotten and diaphragmatic hernias may present years after the injury and discovered incidentally (Fig. 16.72).

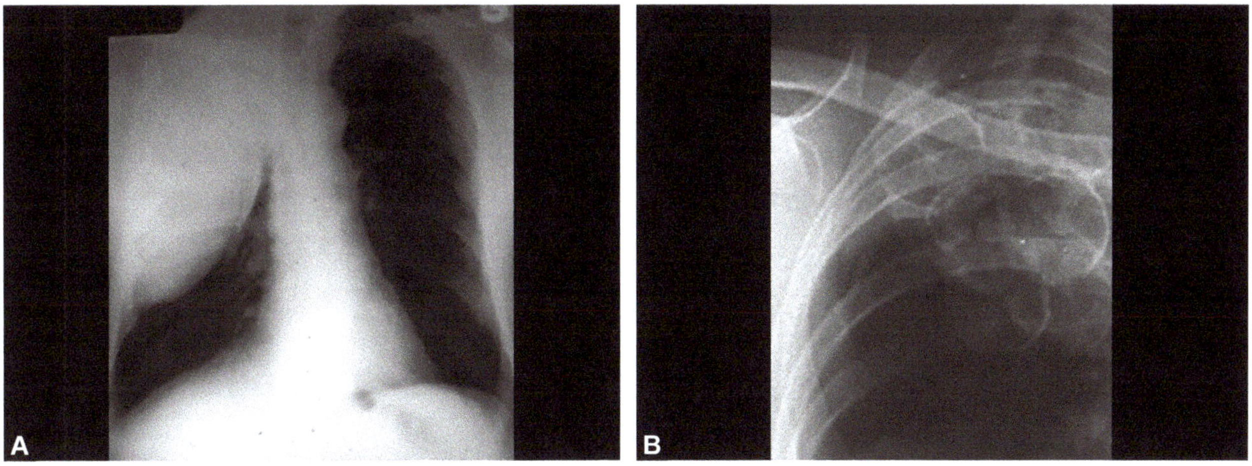

Figs. 16.69A and B: Plombage involved the extrapleural insertion of a "plombe" to collapse the lung. The "plombe" in (A) is solid paraffin and (B) plastic ping pong balls (1940s).

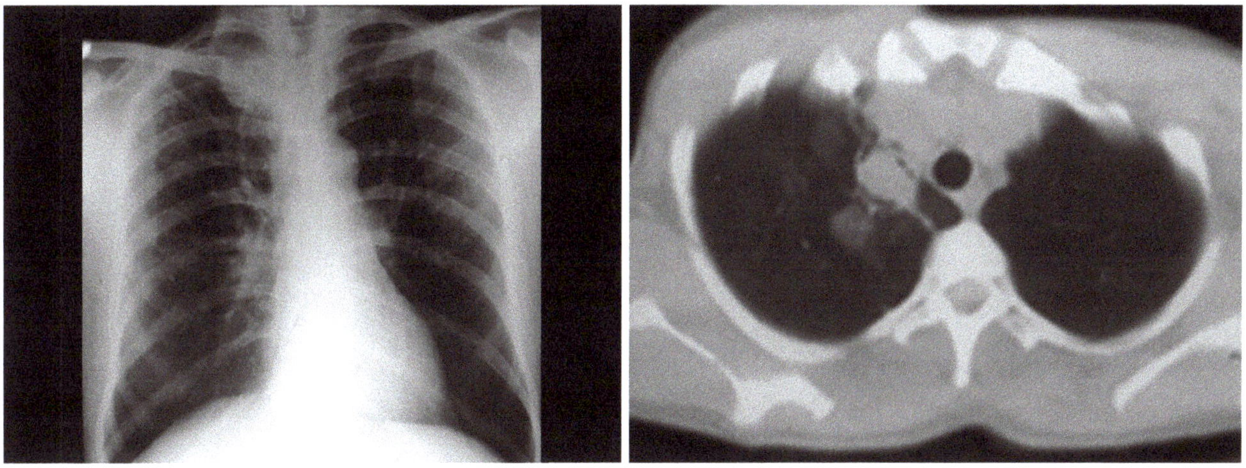

Fig. 16.70: Posteroanterior (PA) chest X-ray and CT showing a mycetoma at right lung apex.

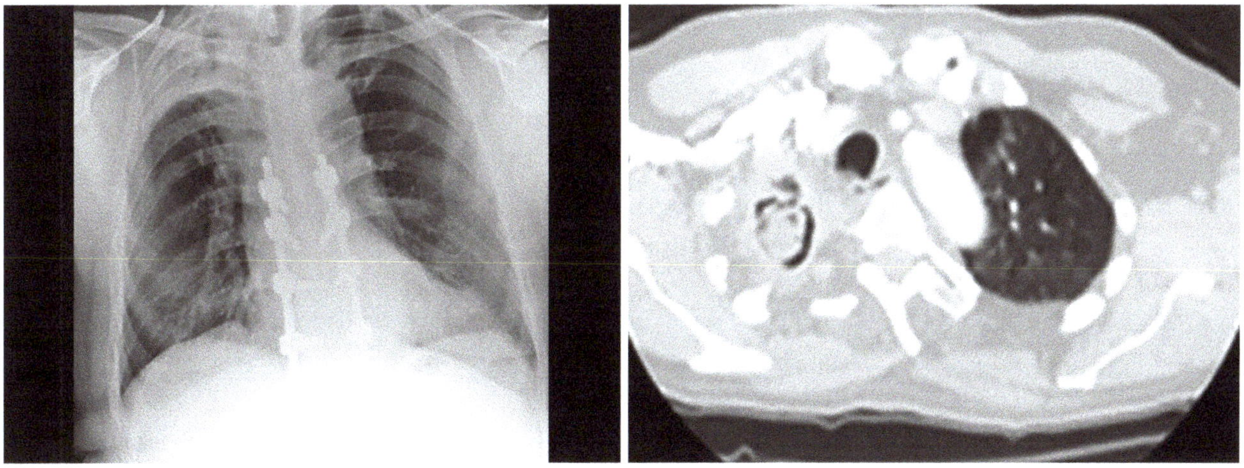

Fig. 16.71: A mycetoma can be easily missed at the lung apices, particularly on an over exposed radiograph.

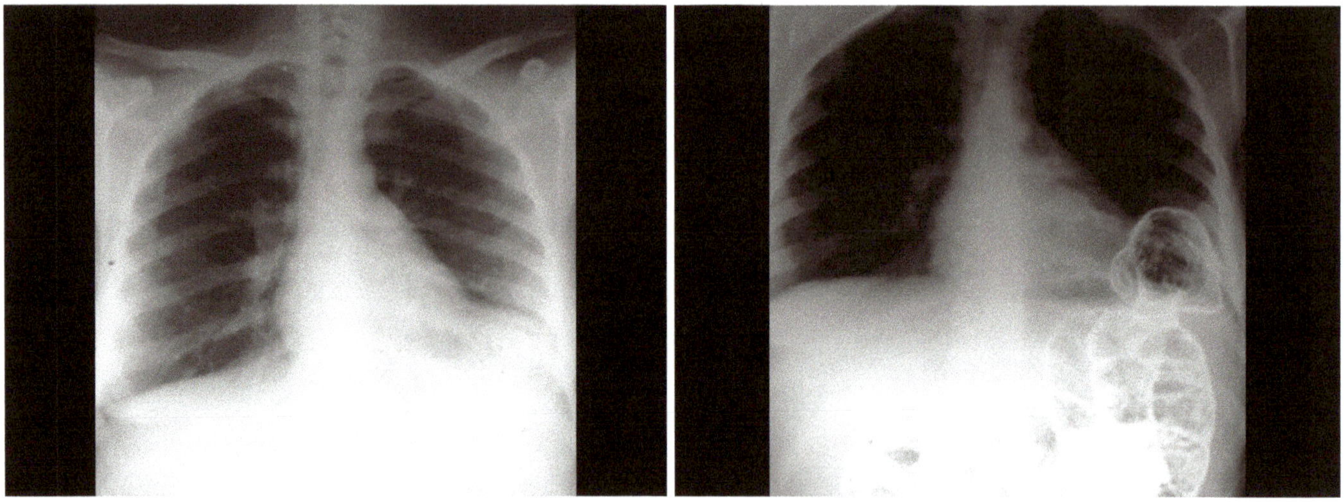

Fig. 16.72: A posteroanterior (PA) chest radiograph showing a hump on the right hemidiaphragm, which it proved to be a diaphragmatic hernia. The patient had nonspecific symptoms, a further probe into the patient's history revealed that the patient had sustained a steering column injury a few years ago.

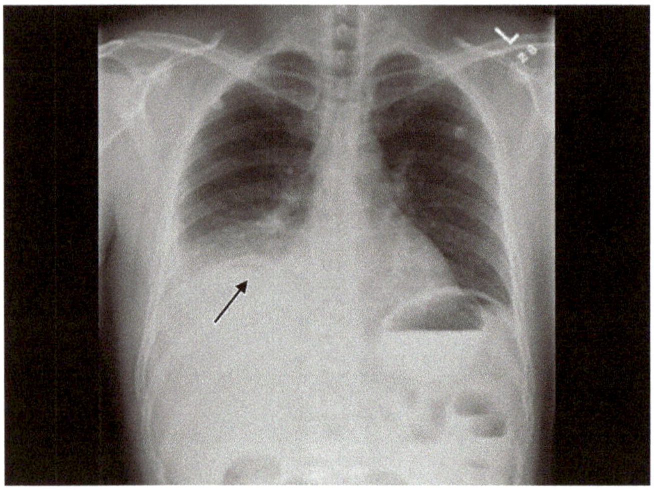

Fig.16.73: A posteroanterior chest X-ray (PA CXR) on a 45-year-old man with a long history of dyspepsia that presented with a right pleuritic chest pain. The CXR shows a right basal pleural effusion and air under the diaphragm (arrow), suggestive of a pneumoperitoneum. At surgery, a perforated duodenal ulcer was repaired.

In Figure 16.73, a PA CXR on a 45-year-old man with a long history of dyspepsia that presented with a right pleuritic chest pain.

CONCLUSION

The CXR remains the radiological examination of choice for any suspected intrathoracic and extrathoracic pathology. A CXR is cost effective, quick and available universally. The procedure is portable and can be undertaken at the patient's bedside, on the field and even in an ambulance or operating theater. Most pathology that needs urgent attention is accurately identified such as a large pneumothorax and cardiac tamponade to name just a few. Despite innovations in chest imaging, the CXR is here to stay.

BIBLIOGRAPHY AND FURTHER READING

1. Armstrong P. Basic patterns in lung disease. In: Armstrong P, Wilson AG, Dee P, Hansell DM (Eds). Imaging of Diseases of the Chest, 3rd edition. St. Louis: Mosby; 2000.
2. Brown JC, Chapman T, Klein EJ, Chisholm SL, Phillips GS, Osincup D, et al. The utility of adding expiratory or decubitus chest radiographs to the radiographic evaluation of suspected pediatric airway foreign bodies. Ann Emerg Med. 2013;61(1):19-26.
3. Cardillo G, Facciolo F, Cavazzana AO, Capece G, Gasparri R, Martelli M. Localized (solitary) fibrous tumors of the pleura: an analysis of 55 patients. Ann Thorac Surg. 2000;70(6):1808-12.
4. Collins J. Stern EJ. Chest Radiology: The Essentials. Philadelphia: Lippincott Williams & Wilkins; 2012.
5. Deepak D, Shah A. Thoracic sarcoidosis: the spectrum of roentgenologic appearances. Indian J Radiol Imag. 2001;11:191-8.

6. Ho ML, Gutierrez FR. Chest radiography in thoracic polytrauma. AJR Am J Roentgenol. 2009;192(3):599-612.
7. Jeung MY, Gasser B, Gangi A, Bogorin A, Charneau D, Wihlm JM, et al. Imaging of cystic masses of the mediastinum. Radiographics. 2002;22:S79-93.
8. Lucaya J, Baert AL, Strife JL. Pediatric Chest Imaging: Chest Imaging in Infants and Children. New York: Springer-Verlag; 2007.
9. Miller WT. Diagnostic Thoracic Imaging. New York: McGraw-Hill Professional; 2006.
10. Molinari F, Bankier AA, Eisenberg RL. Fat-containing lesions in adult thoracic imaging. AJR Am J Roentgenol. 2011;197(5):W795-813.
11. Müller NL, Silva CI. Imaging of the Chest, 1st edition. Philadelphia: Saunders; 2008.
12. Terris DJ, Gourin CG. Thyroid and Parathyroid Diseases: Medical and Surgical Management, 1st edition. New York: Thieme Medical Publishers; 2008.
13. Thourani VH, Sharma J, Duarte IG, Miller JI Jr. Intrathoracic splenosis. Ann Thorac Surg. 2005;80(5):1934-6.
14. Truong M, Munden RF, Kemp BL. Localized fibrous tumor of the pleura. AJR Am J Roentgenol. 2000;174(1):42.
15. Webb WR, Higgins CB. Thoracic Imaging: Pulmonary and Cardiovascular Radiology. Philadelphia: Lippincott Williams & Wilkins; 2010.

Chapter

17

Chest Radiograph: Lung Pathological Findings and Main Signs

Ali Nawaz Khan, Klaus L Irion, Prabhakar Rajiah, Carolyn Allen, Durr-e-Sabih, Koteyar Shyamsunder Radhakrishna, Hamdan Al-Jahdali, Syahminan Suut, Zeid Al-Ani, Claudio Sorino

OVERVIEW

Despite advances in radiology, the chest X-ray (CXR) remains an extremely useful tool in the evaluation of lung diseases, and is the most frequently performed radiological examination. With current technology, a frontal CXR involve a radiation dose equivalent to only 3 days' exposure to natural background radiation.

A posteroanterior (PA) CXR is the initial procedure of choice in any patient presenting with pulmonary symptoms, but a correlation with history, biochemical and serological examinations, and lung function tests is usually required.

Whenever possible, PA CXR should be associated to a lateral CXR, although the latter is less frequently performed. Lateral CXR provides a lot of information and may help to localize lesions and to explore the retrosternal and retrocardiac regions.

Pathological findings often require the correlation with computed tomography (CT) or high-resolution CT (HRCT). Nevertheless, a CXR remains a useful and cost-effective tool for flow-up imaging having carried out a CT or HRCT.

Lung abnormalities may present on a CXR as areas of increased density or as areas of decreased density.

Lung abnormalities with an *increased density* (also called opacities) can be divided into four types:

1. Interstitial lung pattern
2. Nodules
3. Lung consolidations
4. Atelectasis.

A *decreased density* (or hyperlucency), of the lung may be caused by:

1. Hyperinflation due to an obstructive lung disease without parenchymal damage (e.g. asthma)
2. Air trapping with reduction of lung parenchyma (e.g. emphysema)
3. Diseases affecting pulmonary vasculature (e.g. pulmonary embolism)
4. Cavitations.

Lung anomalies with decreased density should be differentiated from diseases involving extrapulmonary structures which may occur with unilateral hyperlucencies (e.g. pneumothorax, mastectomy).

Interstitial Lung Pattern

Many radiologists are less confident in interpretation of interstitial lung disease on standard radiographs and are relying more on the exquisite detail provided by HRCT. However, when approached systematically, the plain radiograph remains a valuable modality, shortening the differential diagnosis and in many instances it is the only imaging required, particularly when good supporting history is available. Many centers use the lung pattern approach. This pattern approach relies on peripheral linear, reticular, nodular, cystic, and ground glass shadowing (Figs. 17.1 to 17.6). *Linear shadows* that criss-cross produce a polygonal network which is classed as *reticular pattem*, whilst focal interstitial thickening results in *nodular opacities.* The picture is not always well defined and in many instances nodules and reticular shadowing may coexist, resulting in *reticulonodular pattern* confusing the issue. The *cystic pattern* is difficult to appreciate on a CXR. When the cysts have thick walls like in Langerhans cell histiocytosis or honeycombing, they frequently

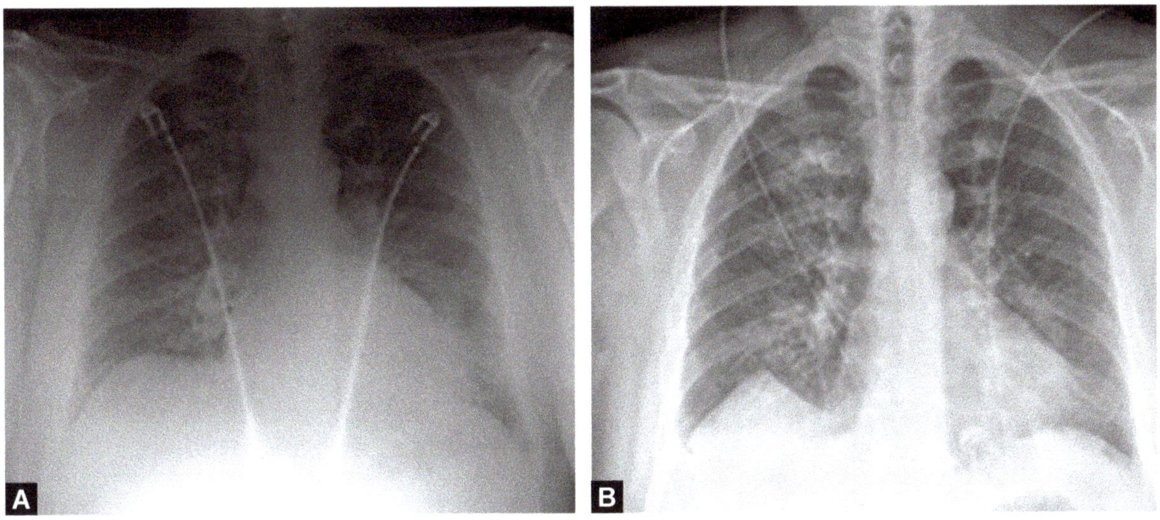

Figs. 17.1A and B: Linear interstitial pattern: images from a patient that developed pulmonary edema due to acute myocardial infarction and heart block. (A) Posteroanterior chest X-ray at hospital admission; (B) Posteroanterior chest X-ray 18 hours later showing higher extension of interstitial pulmonary edema.

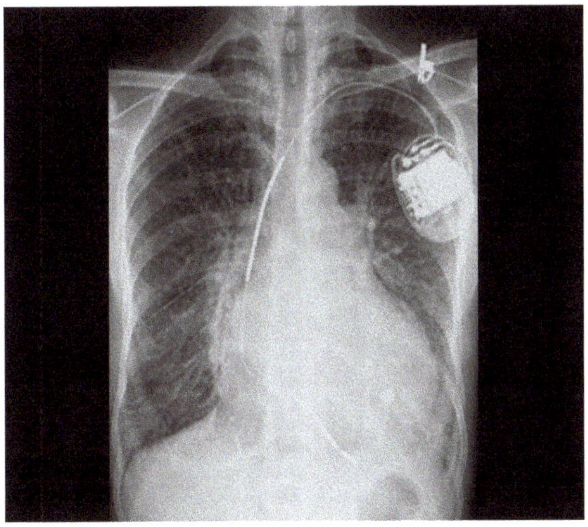

Fig. 17.2: Linear interstitial pattern: Posterior chest X-ray showing cardiomegaly with extensive interstitial pulmonary edema. Note the Kerley lines a (from the periphery to the hila) and b (horizontal, perpendicularly to the pleural surface at the lung base) secondary to heart failure.

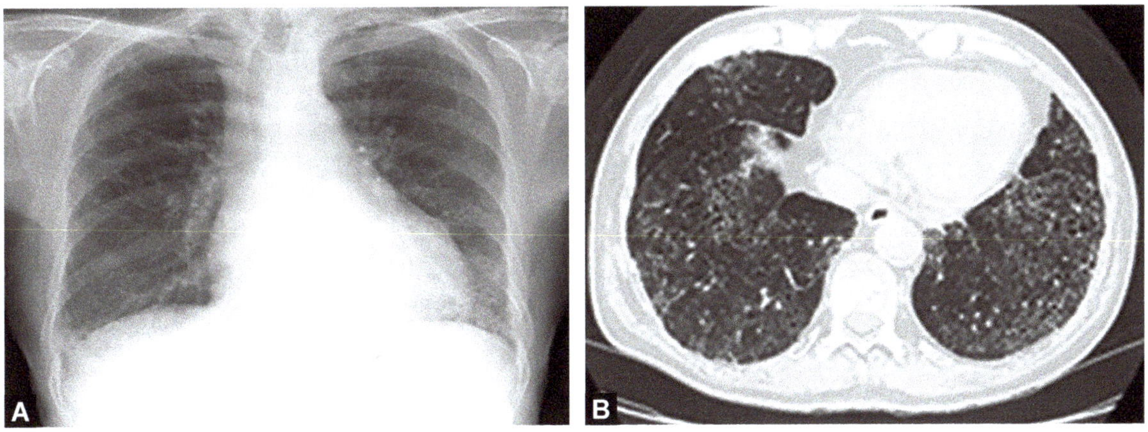

Figs. 17.3A and B: Linear interstitial pattern: Posteroanterior chest X-ray in a patient with congestive cardiac failure. Axial CT shows a honeycomb appearance.

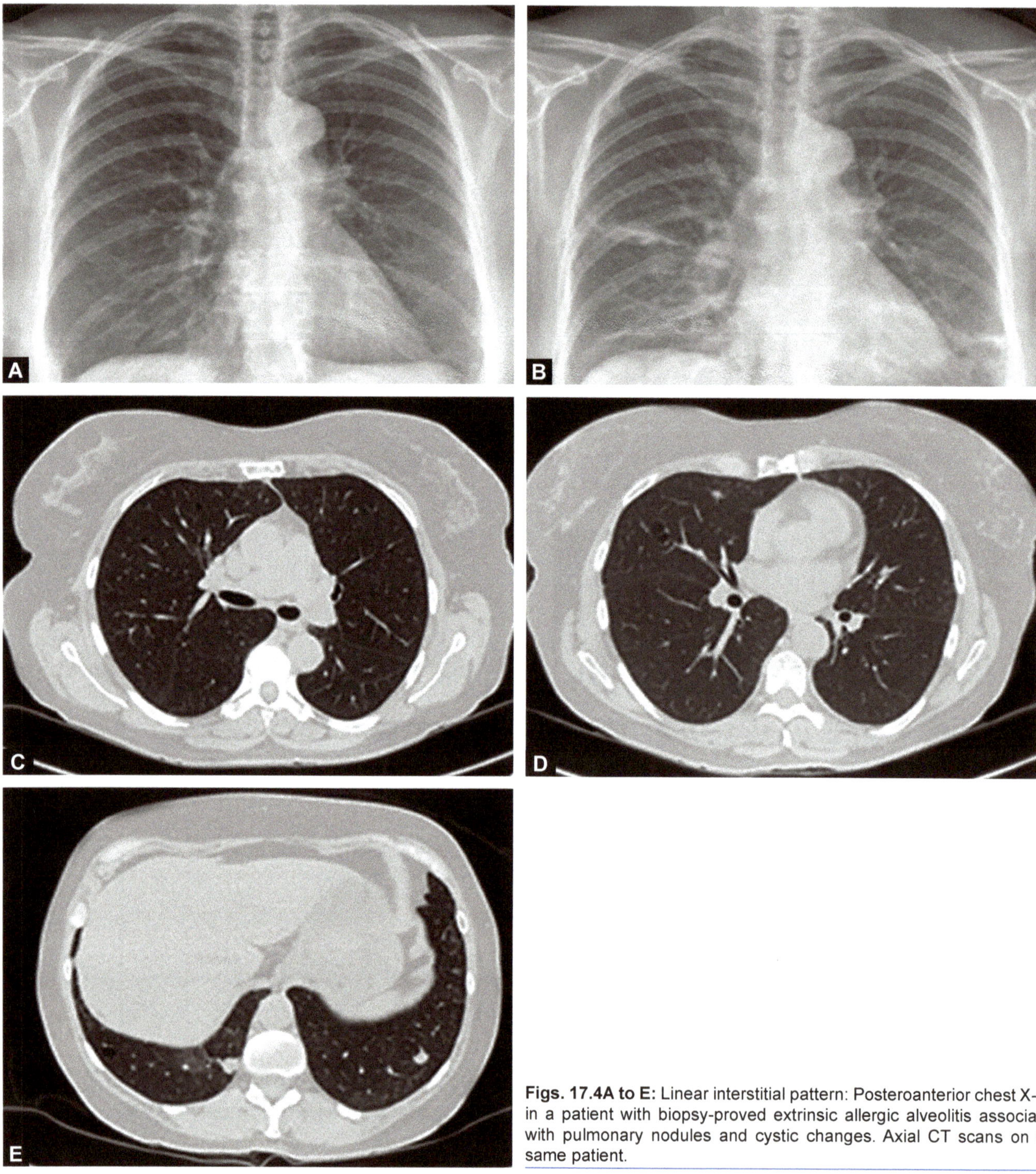

Figs. 17.4A to E: Linear interstitial pattern: Posteroanterior chest X-ray in a patient with biopsy-proved extrinsic allergic alveolitis associated with pulmonary nodules and cystic changes. Axial CT scans on the same patient.

presents as a reticular pattern. *Ground glass* opacification is a nonspecific appearance found in a multitude of pulmonary pathologies. This appearance can be focal or diffuse and present as ill-defined increased lung attenuation. The pulmonary vasculature is usually indistinct, although sometimes the blood vessels can still be identified. Subtle air bronchograms may be seen giving rise to the dark bronchus sign on HRCT. Ground glass attenuation is readily

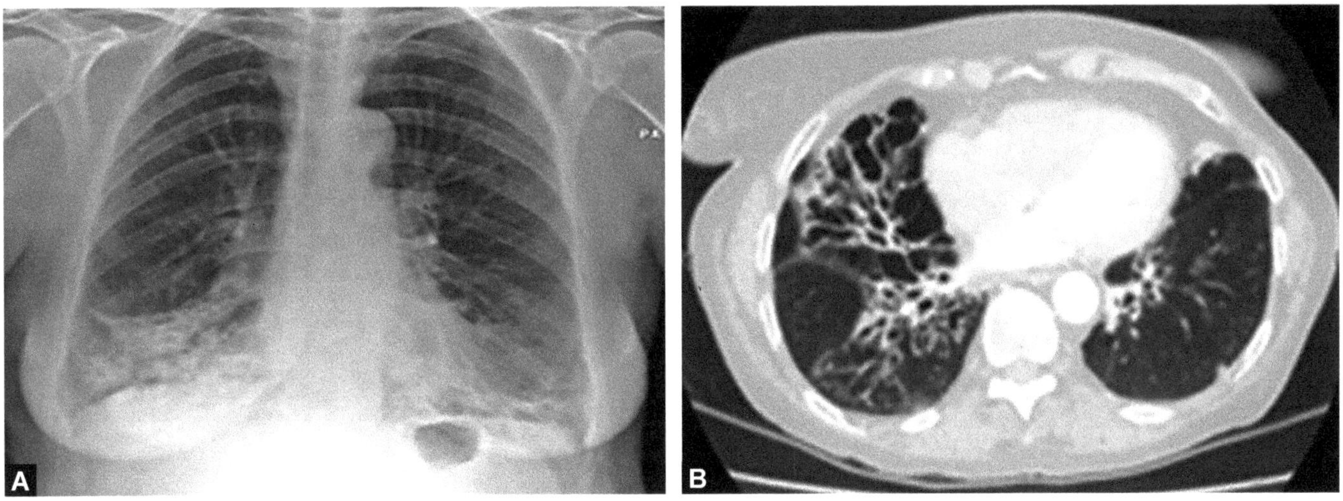

Figs. 17.5A and B: Linear interstitial/cystic pattern: Posteroanterior chest X-ray and axial CT scan showing thickened bronchi and large cystic spaces due to cystic bronchiectasis.

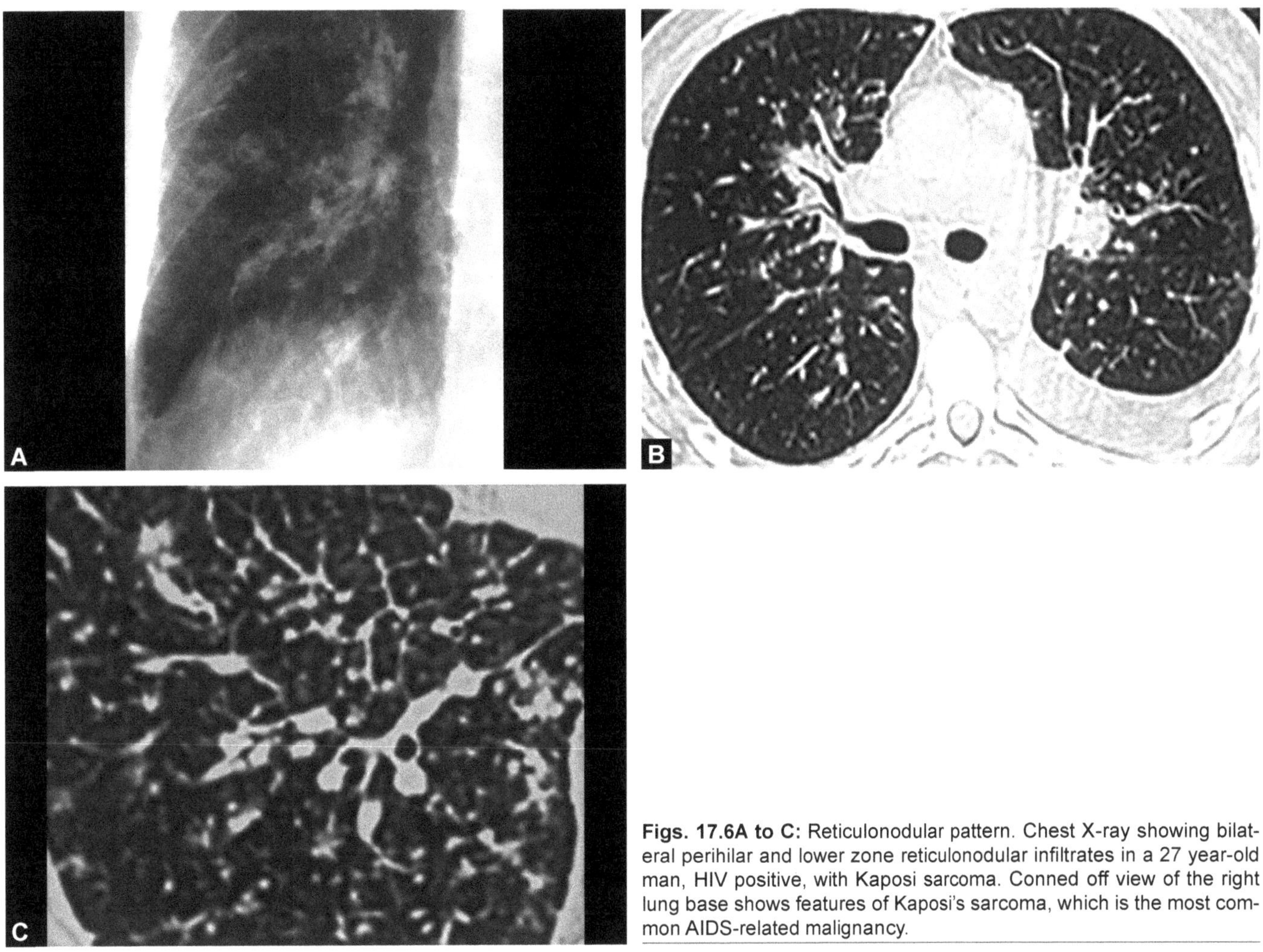

Figs. 17.6A to C: Reticulonodular pattern. Chest X-ray showing bilateral perihilar and lower zone reticulonodular infiltrates in a 27 year-old man, HIV positive, with Kaposi sarcoma. Conned off view of the right lung base shows features of Kaposi's sarcoma, which is the most common AIDS-related malignancy.

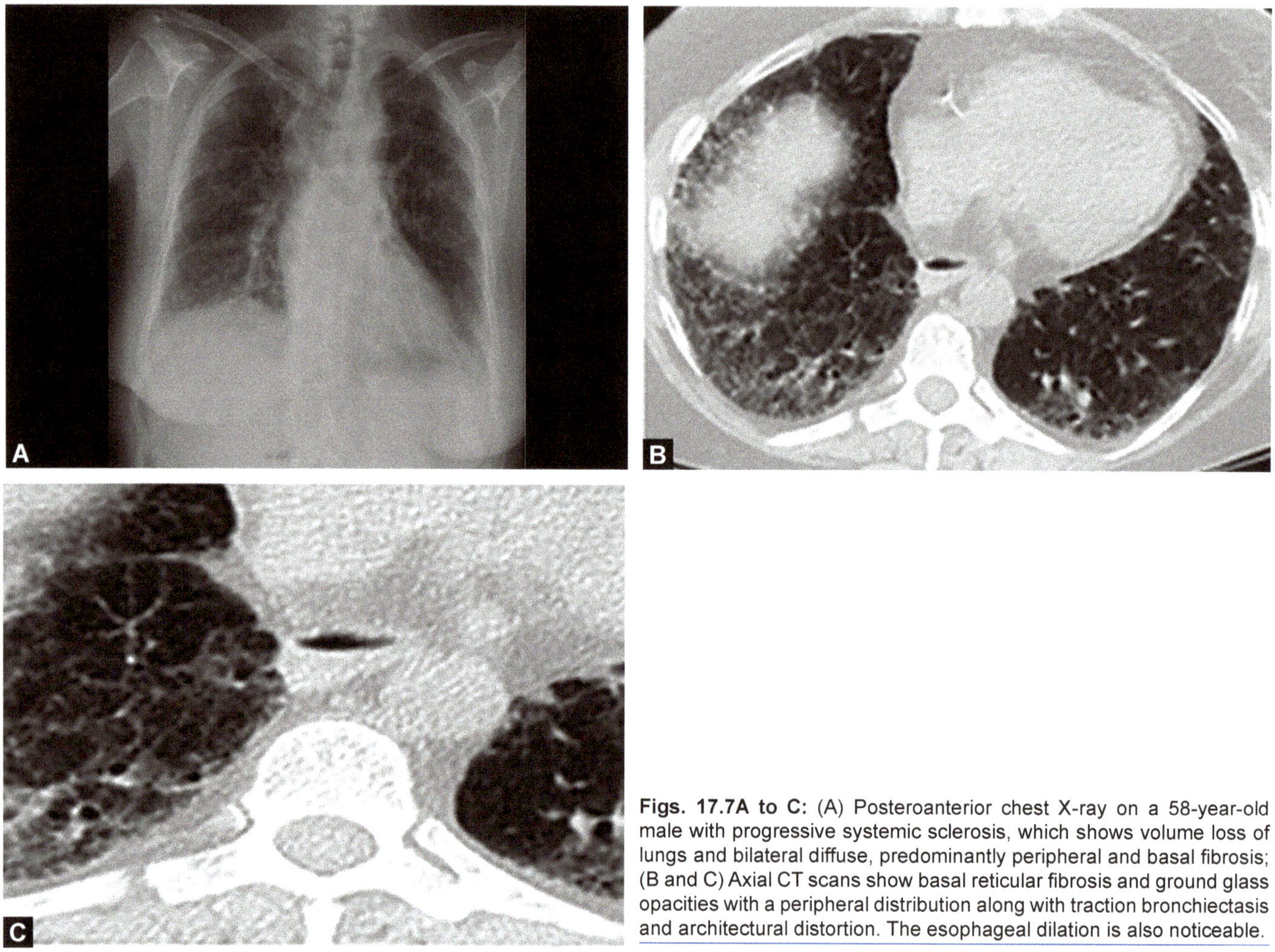

Figs. 17.7A to C: (A) Posteroanterior chest X-ray on a 58-year-old male with progressive systemic sclerosis, which shows volume loss of lungs and bilateral diffuse, predominantly peripheral and basal fibrosis; (B and C) Axial CT scans show basal reticular fibrosis and ground glass opacities with a peripheral distribution along with traction bronchiectasis and architectural distortion. The esophageal dilation is also noticeable.

seen on HRCT, but mild forms may be difficult to see on conventional radiographs. Zonal distribution also plays an important role in distinguishing interstitial disease as specific pathologies have a typical zonal distribution. It is not always possible to diagnose lung interstitial disease using the pattern approach, patient history and zonal distribution. In this instance HRCT usually adds accurate information, although there is significant overlap of various lung pathologies.

Reticular shadowing or small nodules have a wide differential diagnosis. Clinical input, signs and symptoms, the length of the history and other concomitant diseases such as rheumatoid arthritis, other autoimmune diseases, drug history and occupational history are important. *Peripheral reticular pattern* refers to a network of polygonal spaces that resembles a honeycomb. These polygonal spaces are less than 5 mm in diameter and have peripheral and basal distribution. The small cystic spaces are seen best at the costophrenic angles. The most common causes of a honeycomb appearance are (1) idiopathic interstitial pneumonia, (2) asbestosis, and (3) collagen vascular disease (Figs. 17.7A to C). Rarely the pattern is seen in bronchiolitis obliterans organizing pneumonia (BOOP), sarcoidosis and bleomycin lung toxicity. The CXR findings of bleomycin toxicity include bilateral, bibasilar alveolar infiltrates. Interstitial fibrosis and honeycombing may follow (Figs. 17.8 and 17.9). Heart failure/pulmonary edema are also a rare cause of linear and reticular pattern. Clinical history and presentation play an important role in the differentiation between these lung pathologies.

In asbestos-related lung disease, fibrotic change has a predilection of the lung periphery, subpleural lung with basilar distribution.

High-resolution CT show thickening of bronchovascular bundles reflecting the bronchocentric disease. Interlobular septal thickening due lymphatic obstruction

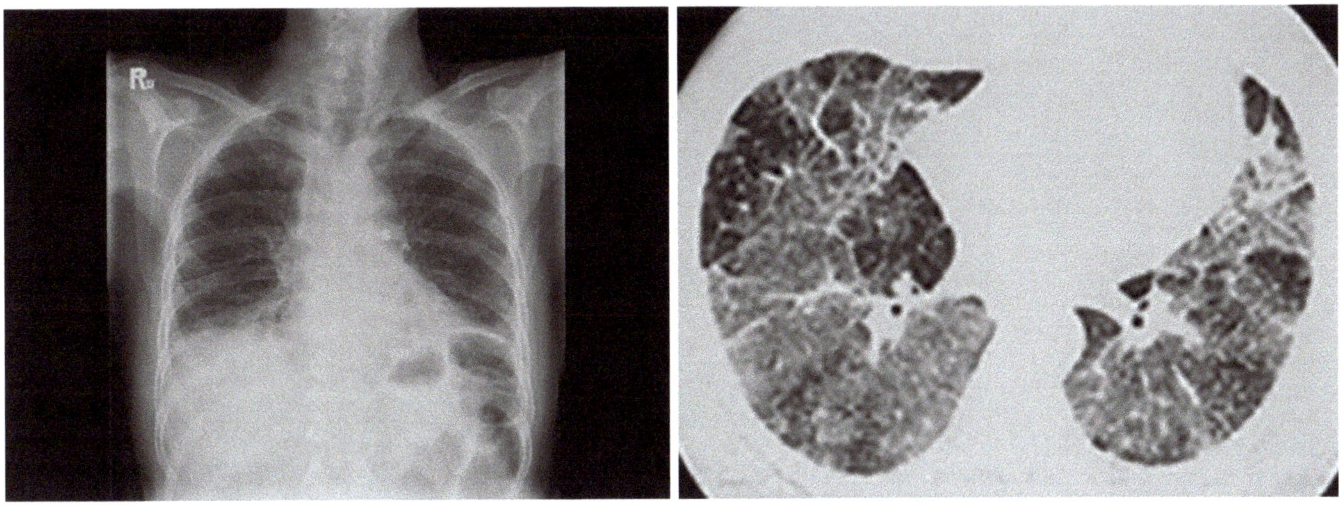

Fig. 17.8: A posteroanterior chest X-ray on a patient with bleomycin lung toxicity shows linear/reticular shadowing mostly bibasal and subpleural; note the blunting of the costophrenic angles. High-resolution CT better depicts diffuse alveolar damage, airspace and ground-glass opacification. End-stage fibrosis includes extensive reticular markings, traction bronchiectasis, and honeycombing. Organizing pneumonia with ground-glass opacification may represent a part of the spectrum.

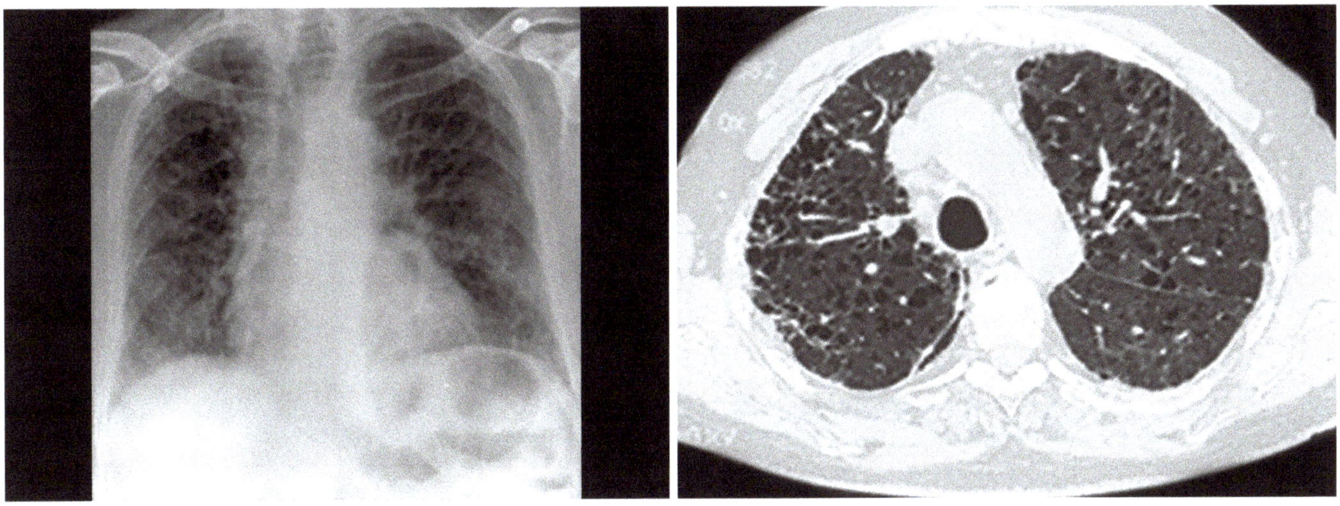

Fig. 17.9: A posteroanterior chest X-ray and high-resolution CT (HRCT) of a 38-year-old man who was treated with bleomycin for testicular cancer, developed dyspnea, nonproductive cough and weight loss. The chest X-ray shows extensive areas of fibrosis. HRCT shows scattered areas of ground glass opacity, subpleural reticular opacities and bands and areas of honeycombing indicating severe pulmonary fibrosis.

due to tumor invasion is also seen. Note the tree in bud appearance.

Nodules

Nodules are space-occupying lesions within the lung of varying sizes and varying distribution. They may be solitary or multiple. A solitary pulmonary nodule (SPN) is defined as a well-marginated, round or oval opacity smaller than or equal to 3 cm in diameter that is completely surrounded by lung parenchyma, does not touch the hilum or mediastinum and is not associated with lymphadenopathy, atelectasis, pneumonia or pleural effusion.

Most lesions smaller than 3 cm are benign, while lesions larger than 3 cm are called masses and treated as malignancies until proven otherwise.

Malignant lung nodules include lung cancers, lymphomas and hematogenous metastases. The latter are the most common cause of multiple pulmonary nodules. They

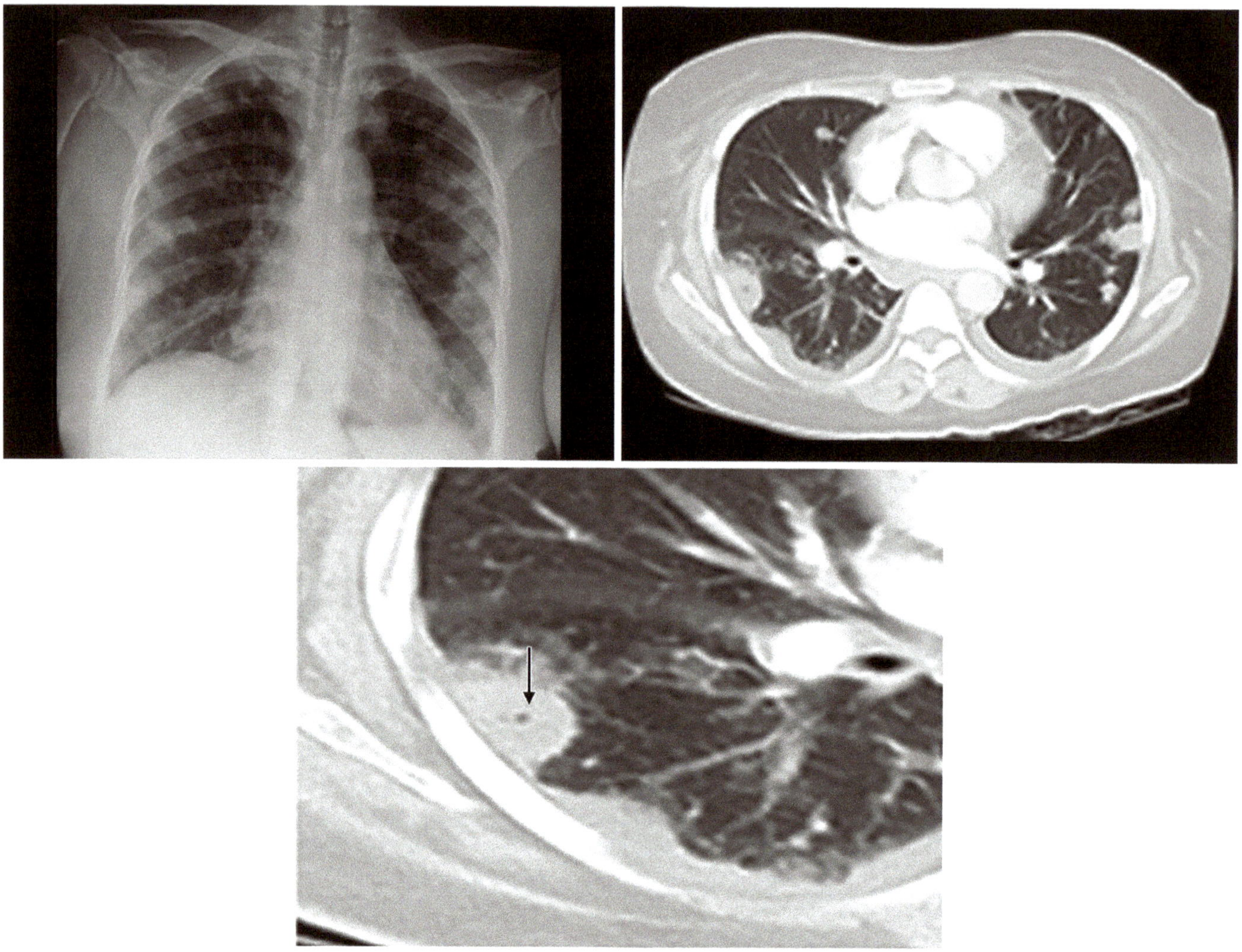

Fig. 17.10: Chest X-ray and high-resolution CT showing lower lobe opacities/nodules varying in size and with cavitations (arrow) in a patient with septic pulmonary emboli.

may vary in size, are usually smooth or lobulated, and prevail in the peripheral regions of lower lobes. The most common types of benign lung nodules include: granulomas, hamartomas, nodules from bacterial infections (e.g. tuberculosis), fungal infections (e.g. histoplasmosis, coccidioidomycosis, cryptococcosis, and aspergillosis), parasitic infections (e.g. pneumocystis jiroveci pneumonia in immune deficient patients). Septic emboli occur from infective foci and many primary sites have been described. They usually present as multiple ill-defined nodules, and about half of them have cavitation (Figs. 17.10 and 17.11).

Benign pulmonary nodules may also occur in conditions that cause lung inflammation and fibrosis, such as rheumatoid arthritis, sarcoidosis, Wegener's granulomatosis, healed pulmonary infarcts, focal hemorrhage, hemangiomas and multiple recurrent bronchopneumonias. Sometimes, mucus plugs can mimic the appearance of lung nodules.

The term miliary opacities refers to innumerable, small (1–4 mm) pulmonary nodules, scattered throughout the lungs. They can occur in hematogenous spread of tuberculosis (*miliary TB,* Figs. 17.12 to 17.14), but are also seen in metastatic cancer, sarcoidosis, pneumoconiosis and hypersensitivity pneumonitis (Figs 17.15 to 17.21).

Examples of these nodules are provided with hints how to differentiate as to the cause, on the bases of clinical presentation and history, including occupational history and other concomitant diseases.

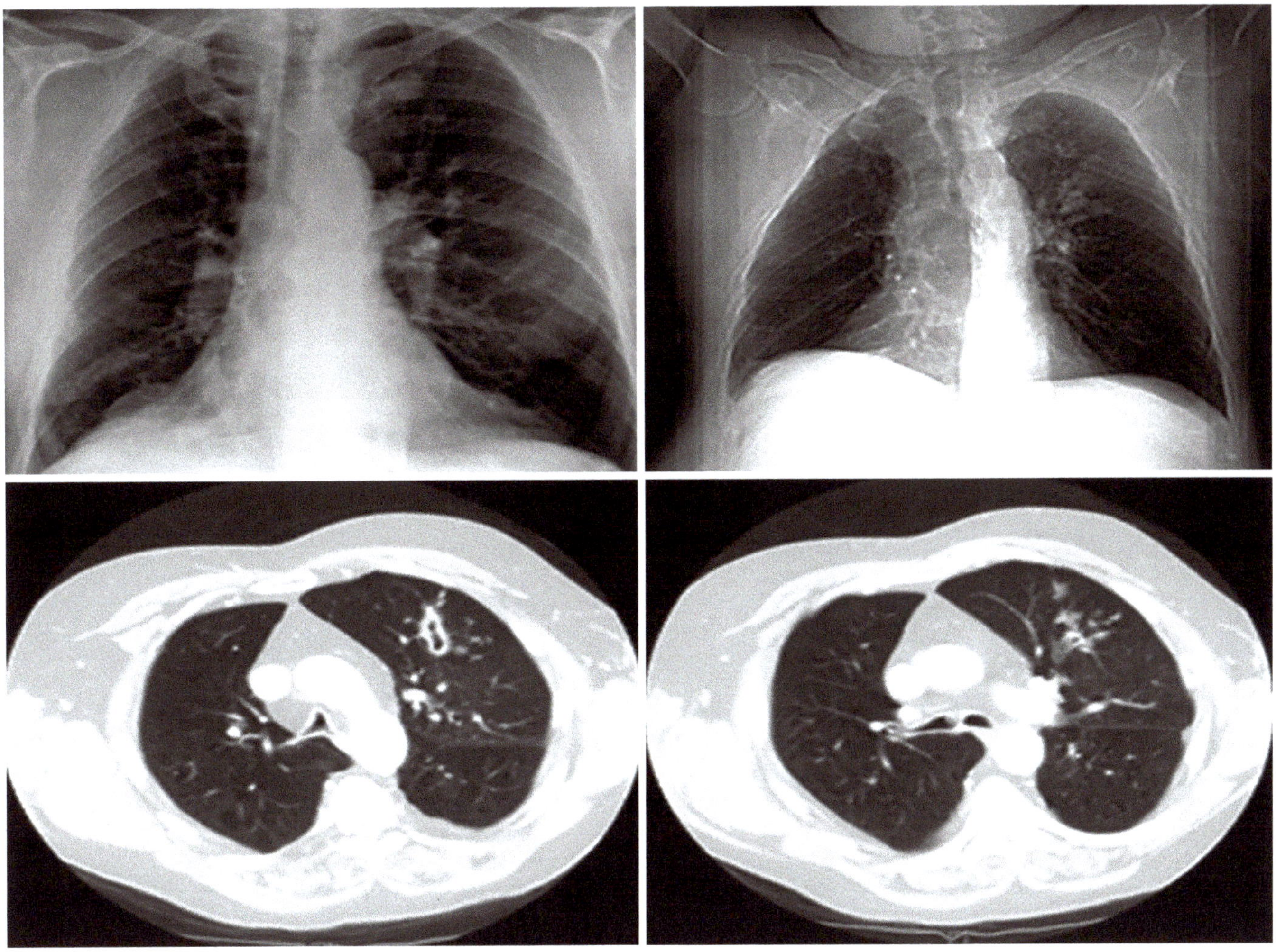

Fig. 17.11: Septic pulmonary emboli. Posteroanterior Chest X-ray showing vague nodular shadowing in the left upper zone in a patient that presented acutely with cough, fever, and shortness of breath. A scanogram prior to a CT scan shows patchy shadowing in the left upper zone suggestive of pneumonia. Axial CT scans on the same patient show not only nodular shadowing but also cavitation in some of the nodules.

Lung Consolidations

Lung consolidations correspond to areas of increased lung density (thus increased attenuation) seen on a CXR and/ or CT (Figs. 17.22 to 17.27). Consolidations obscure the underlying pulmonary vessels. The differential diagnosis of lung consolidations is wide and includes any pathologic process that fills the alveoli with fluid (in pulmonary edema), pus (in infection), blood (in hemorrhage), tumor cells or other substances, resulting in lobar, diffuse or multifocal ill-defined opacties. As with any radiological finding of the chest, clinical data and a comparison with previos radiographs is essential.

The rapidity of onset can help to make a diagnosis. Acute consolidations may occur in pulmonary edema, pneumonia or hemorrhage

Less common causes of acute consolidations include radiation pneumonitis and acute eosinophilic syndrome. Chronic causes of consolidation include alveolar proteinosis, lymphoma, granulomatous pathology and bronchoalveolar carcinoma. Bronchiolitis obliterans organizing pneumonia should also be considered as a cause of a multifocal consolidation with subacute presentation. Some pathological processes can present with more than a single pattern. For instance, a lobar pneumonia caused by *Streptococcus pneumoniae* may become diffuse if the patient does not respond to the treatment.

When opacification of the lung appears spherical, the term mass, rather than consolidation, is often used, and malignancy is the main cause. A similar lesion smaller than 3 cm in diameter on a CXR or computed tomography

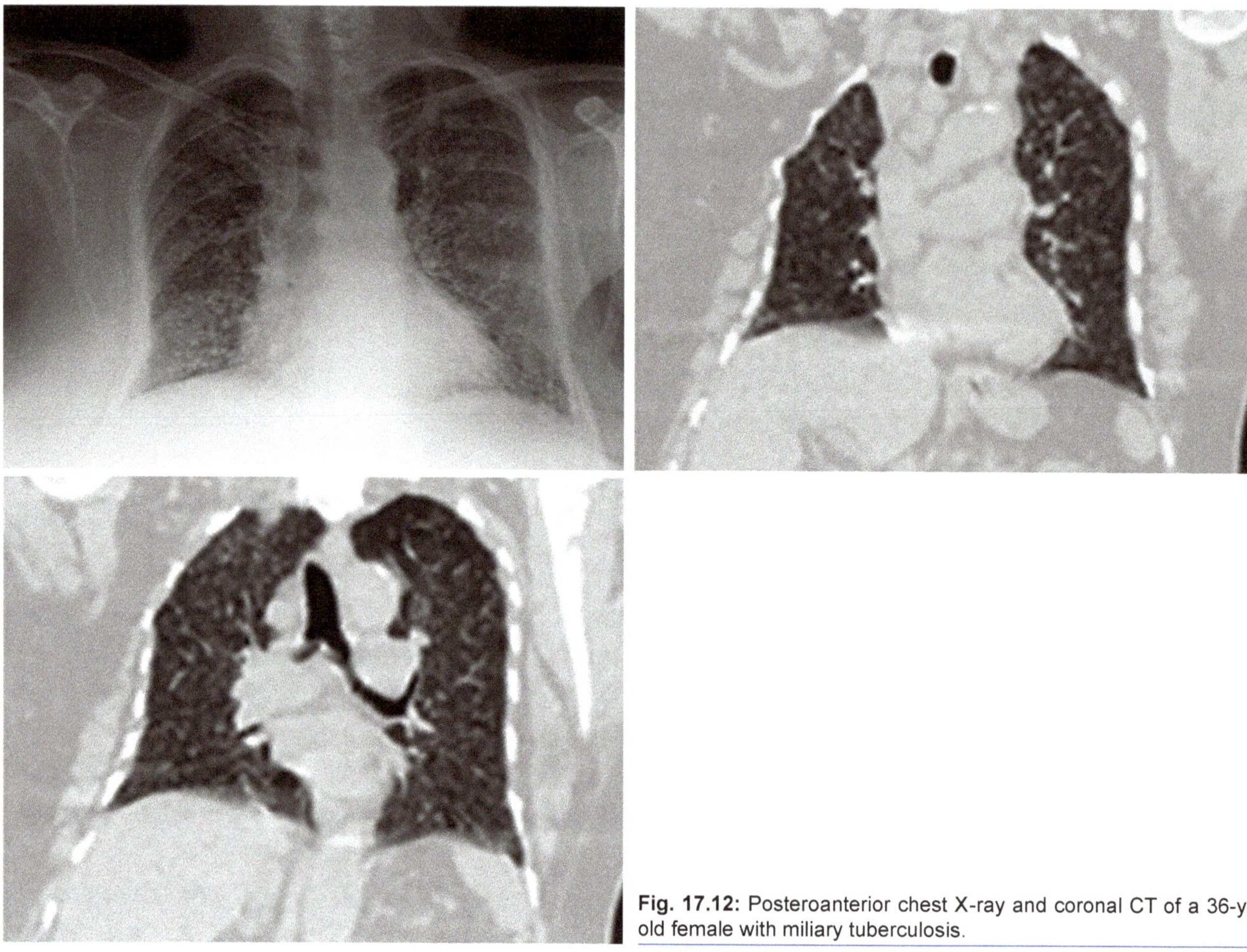

Fig. 17.12: Posteroanterior chest X-ray and coronal CT of a 36-year-old female with miliary tuberculosis.

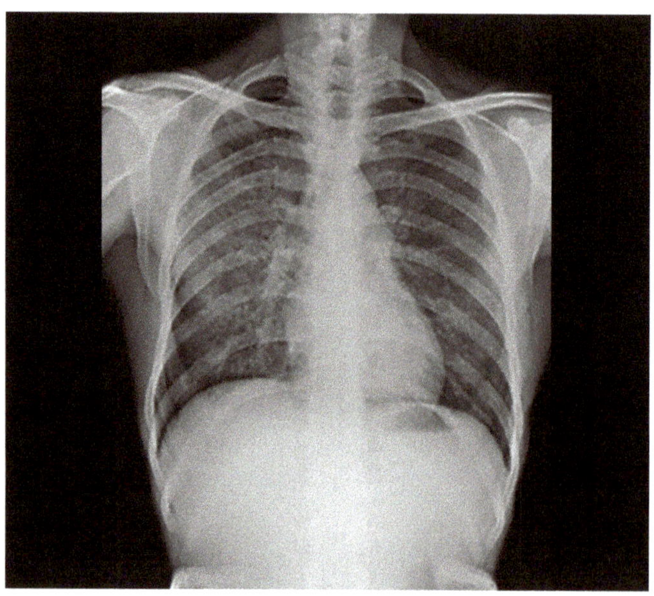

Fig. 17.13: Posteroanterior chest X-ray showing extensive miliary shadowing due to miliary tuberculosis in an HIV-positive patient.
Source: Dr Gunjan Puri, Surat-395017, Gujarat, India.

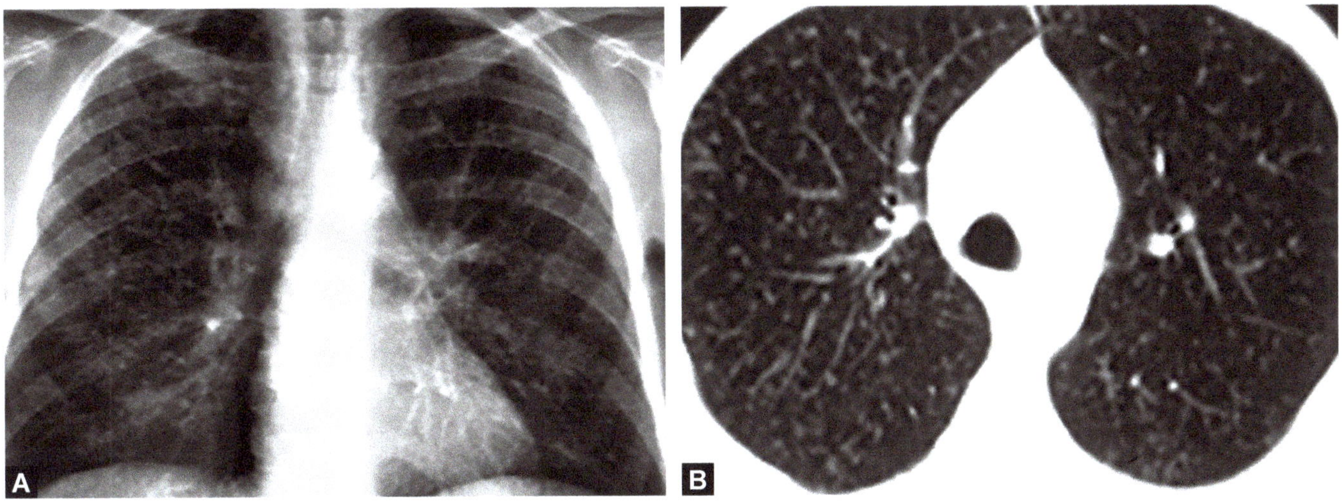

Figs. 17.14A and B: Chest X-ray and CT in a patient with reactivation MTB in HIV. "Primary" tuberculosis manifests as focal unilateral, often lower lobe consolidation and adenopathy. Cavitation is less common at lower CD4 counts. Patients in this range also have an increased incidence of miliary tuberculosis, with diffuse, randomly distributed nodules on CT.

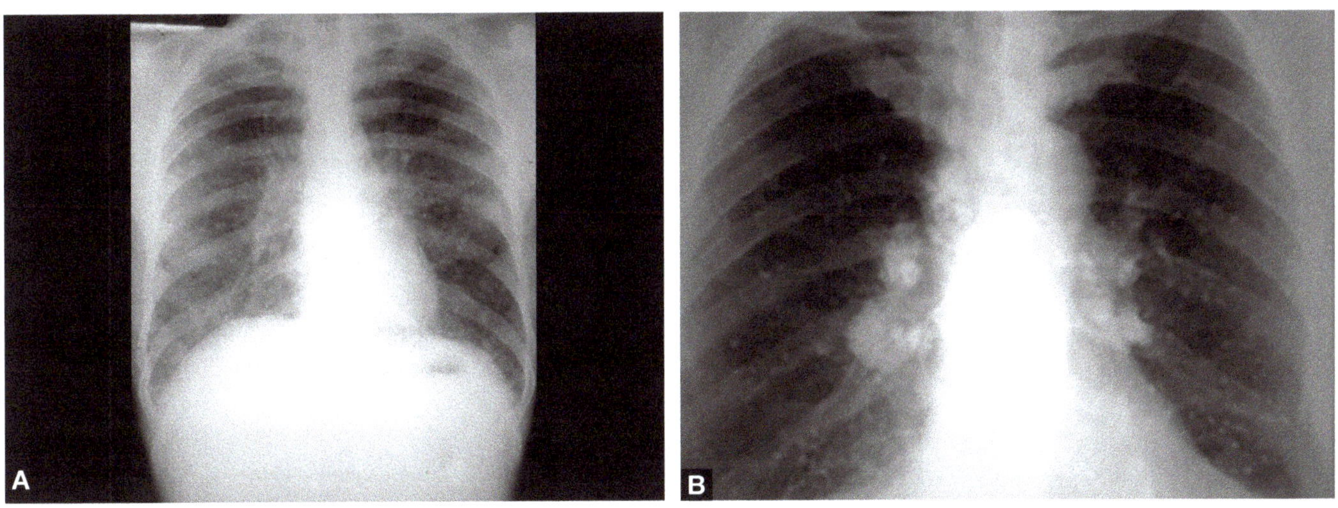

Figs. 17.15A and B: Posteroanterior chest X-rays from two patients with histoplasmosis showing (A) miliary shadowing and (B) calcified lymph nodes, clumpy calcification and calcified lung nodule.

is termed coin lesion or solitary pulmonary nodule (Figs. 17.28 to 17.30). A coin lesion has many causes and can be inflammatory or neoplastic. It can be an incidental finding found in up to 0.2% of CXR and around 1% of CT scans. Inflammatory tumors are rare benign tumors that may affect any organ, but are relatively common in lungs accounting for less than 1% of all lung tumors. These tumors usually occur in children and young adults. They typically present with symptoms of an inflammatory airway disease, including cough, pyrexia, shortness of breath. On a CXR they present with a coin lesion or solitary mass, indistinguishable from other lung masses. Calcification within the mass is rare. The mass may invade the mediastinum and rarely it is intrabronchial and multiple. The preferred treatment is surgical resection.

Pulmonary hamartomas are the most common but rare benign tumor-like lesions (Figs. 17.31A and B).

The majority of patients are asymptomatic and hamartomas are seen as coin lesions with popcom calcification in a chest radiograph.

Attention should be paid to "pseudo-coin lesion", which is caused by artifacts (e.g. button on patient's clothing, nipple shadow).

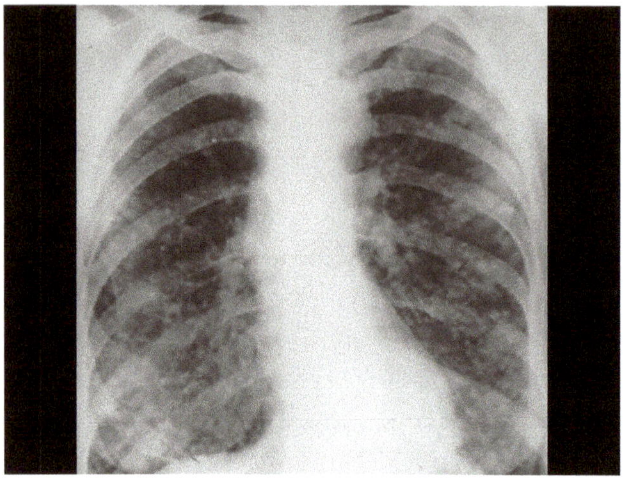

Figs. 17.16: Posteroanterior chest X-ray showing extensive miliary shadowing in a patient who underwent thyroidectomy for medullary thyroid carcinoma 2 years previously.

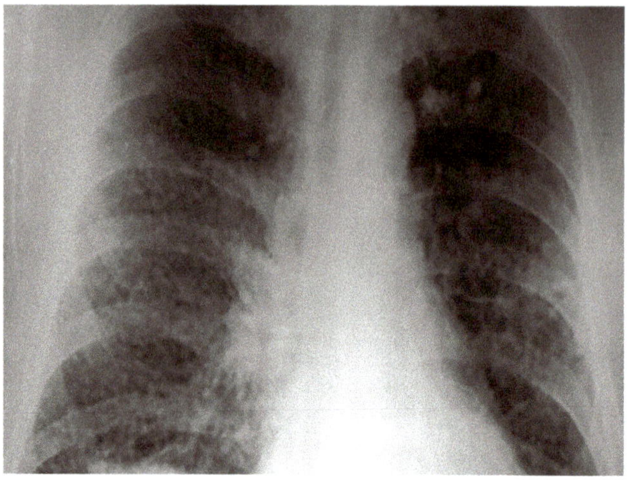

Fig. 17.17: Posteroanterior chest X-ray showing multiple high density micronodules secondary to silicosis.

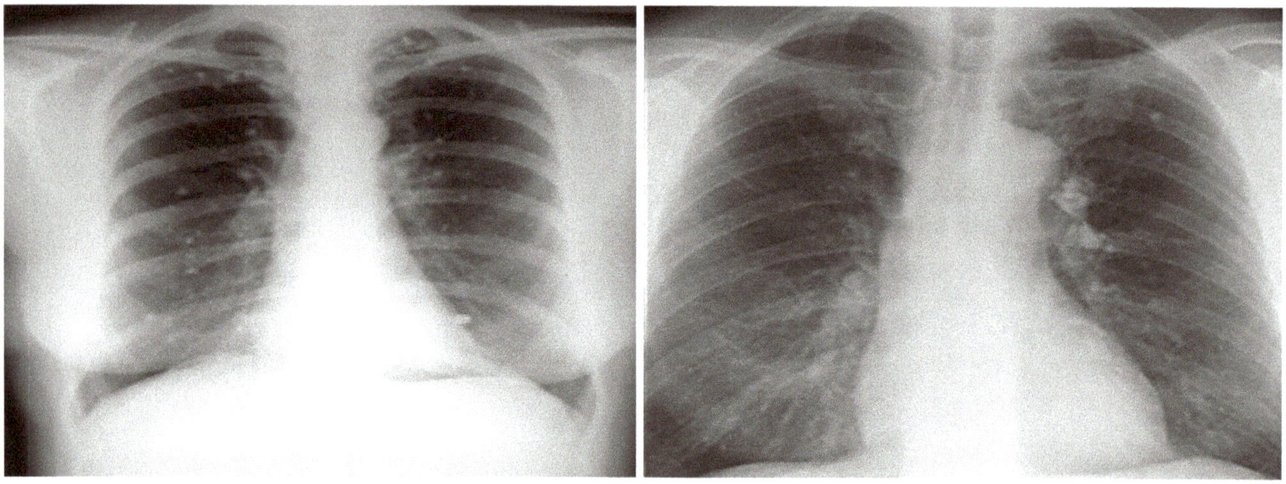

Fig. 17.18: Posteroanterior chest X-rays from two patients showing multiple calcified nodules secondary to old healed chickenpox pneumonia. When the density of a lung nodule is similar to that of the ribs, they can be presumed to be calcified.

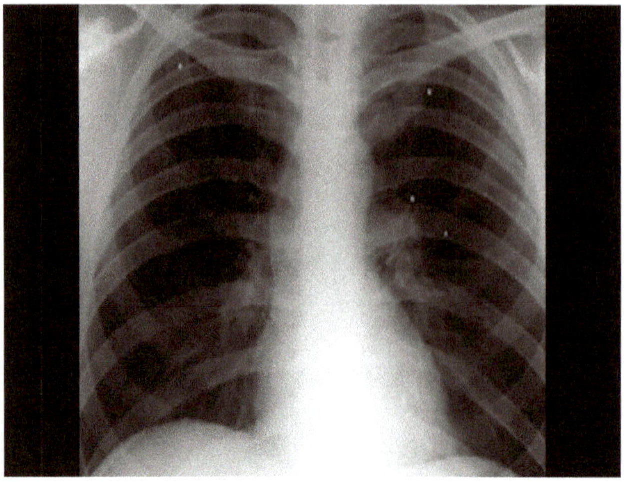

Fig. 17.19: Posteroanterior chest X-ray in a patient with accidental inhalation of dental fillings. Note the multiple metallic particles in the upper zones.

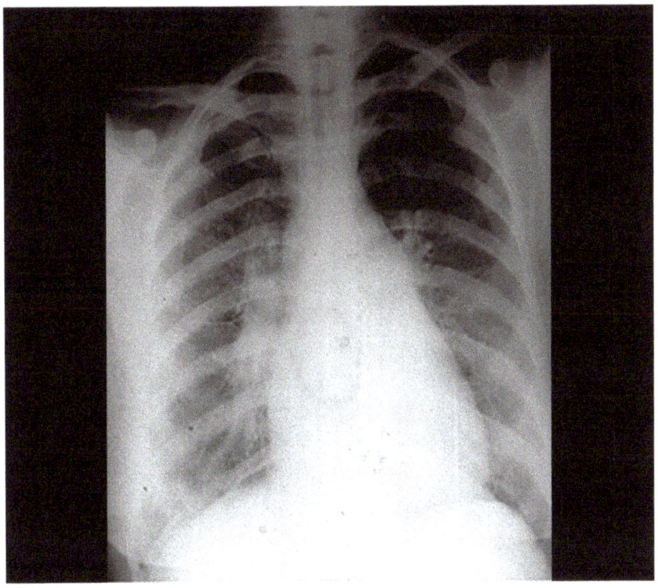

Fig. 17.20: Posteroanterior chest X-ray showing extensive miliary shadows and enlarged hila secondary to enlarged pulmonary arteries due pulmonary hypertension in a patient with primary hemosiderosis.

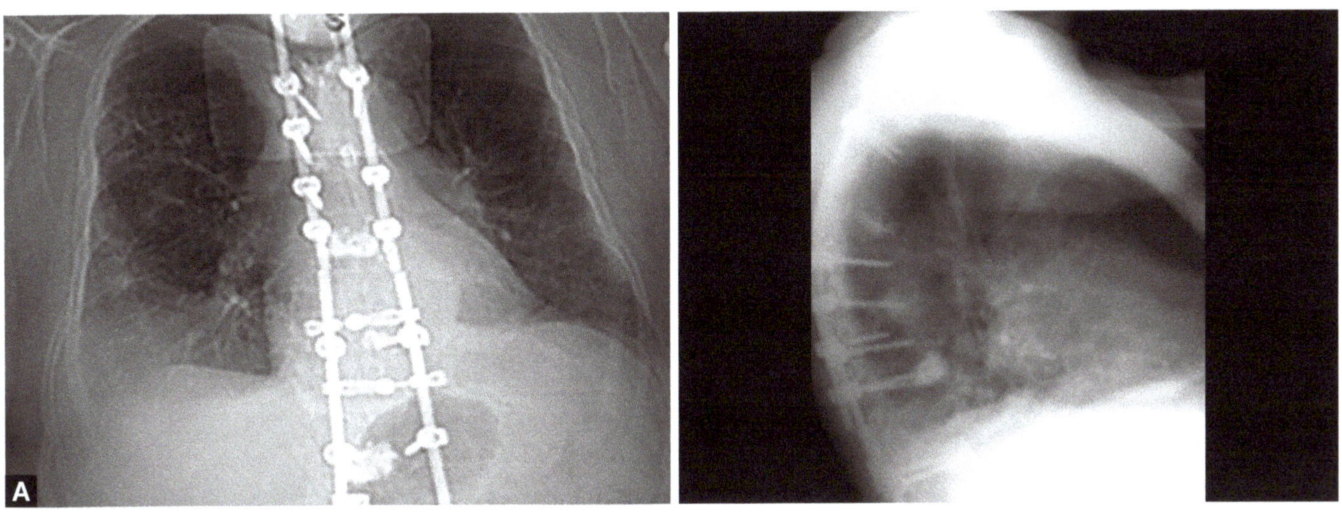

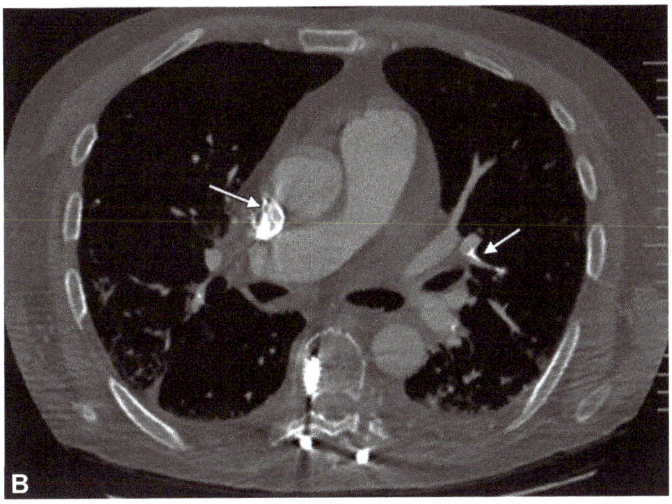

Figs. 17.21A and B: (A) Posteroanterior and (B) lateral chest X-ray on a 70-year-old man known to have pulmonary hypertension that presented with worsening dyspnea after a kyphoplasty for the treatment of osteoporotic compression fracture. The axial CT shows methyl methacrylate emboli (arrows). Methyl methacrylate is cement used for kyphoplasty.

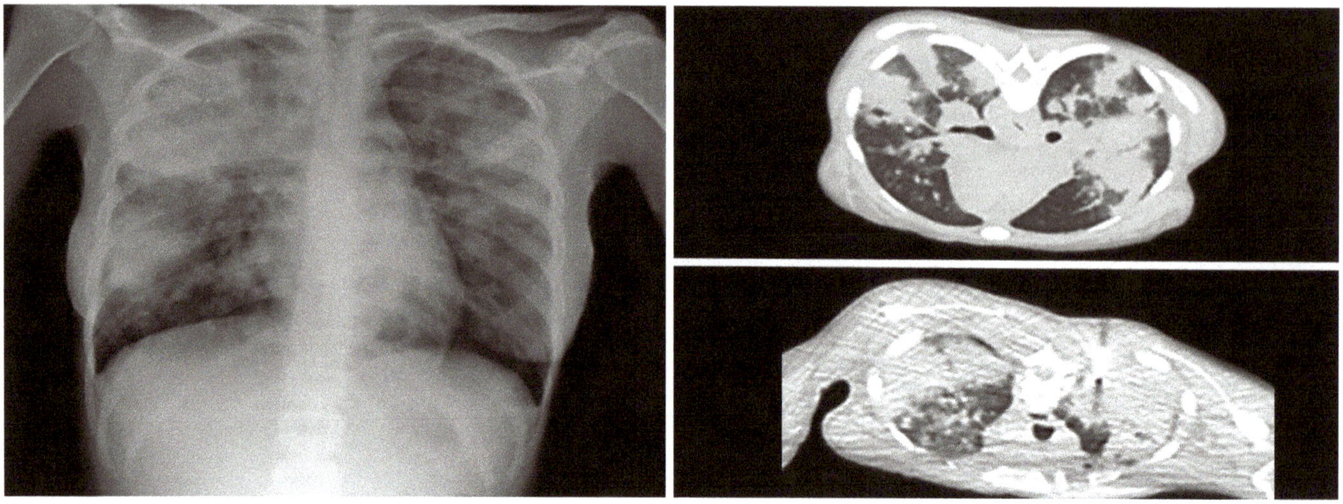

Fig. 17.22: Posteroanterior chest X-ray on a 35-year-old woman showing multifocal lung consolidations. (Metastasis from renal cell carcinoma).

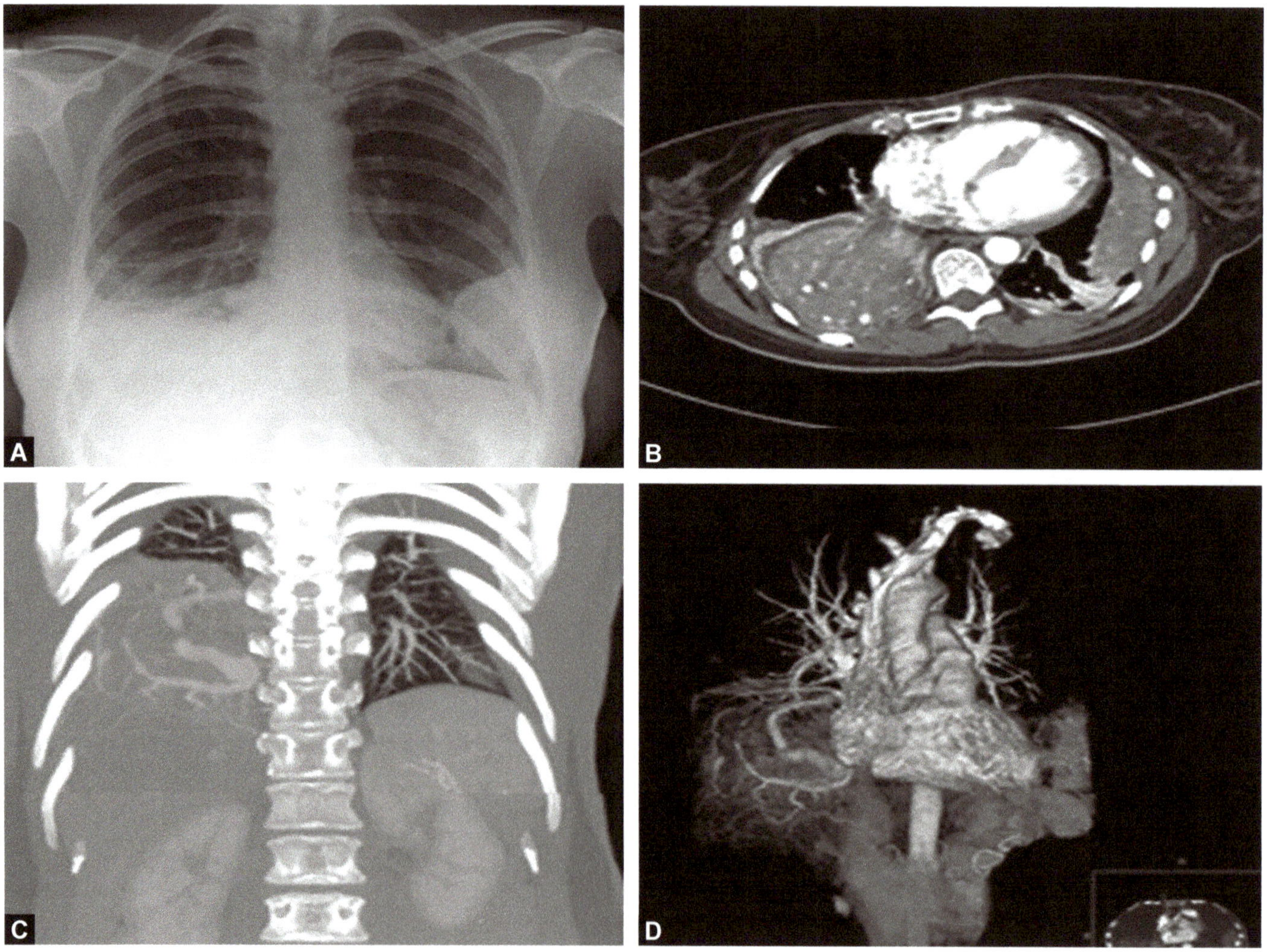

Figs. 17.23A to D: Pleural based tumors, histologically proved benign pulmonary metastasizing leiomyoma in a patient who underwent hysterectomy for leiomyoma 13 years previously. (A) Posteroanterior chest X-ray. (B) Axial CT scan. (C) Coronal CT scan. (D) Three-dimensional reconstructions.

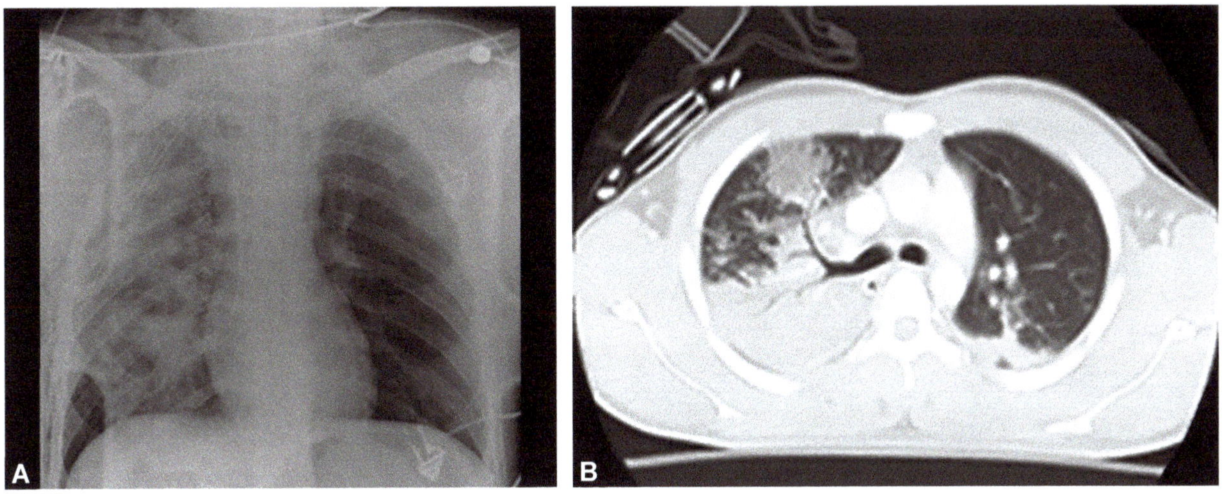

Figs. 17.24A and B: (A) Anteroposterior chest X-ray and (B) axial CT scan showing an extensive multifocal consolidation due to lung contusion following a road traffic accident.

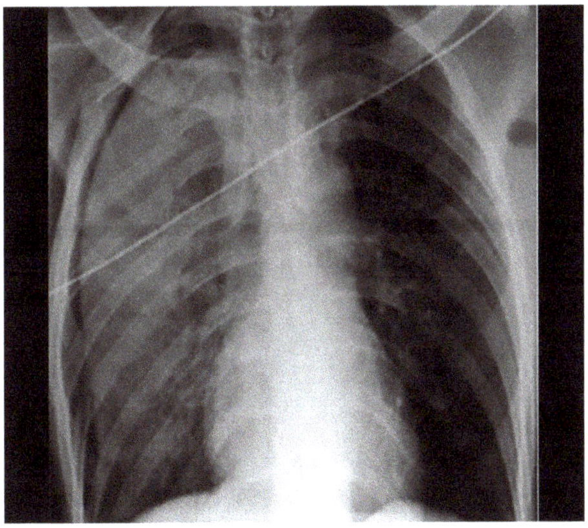

Fig. 17.25: Anteroposterior chest X-ray showing pulmonary hemorrhage and pneumothorax following blunt thoracic trauma.

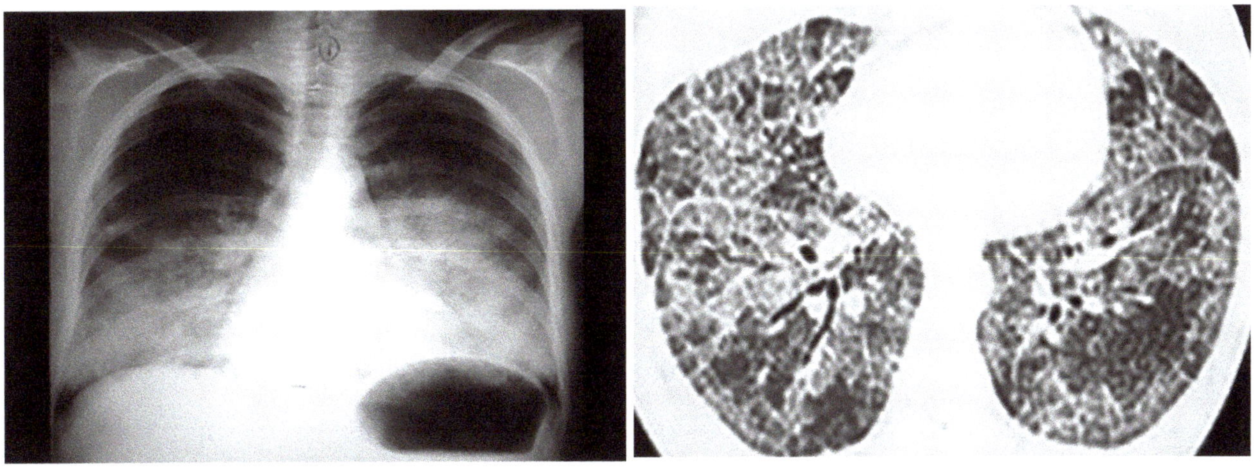

Fig. 17.26: Posteroanterior chest X-ray and axial CT scan showing extensive air space shadowing/consolidation in a patient with alveolar proteinosis.

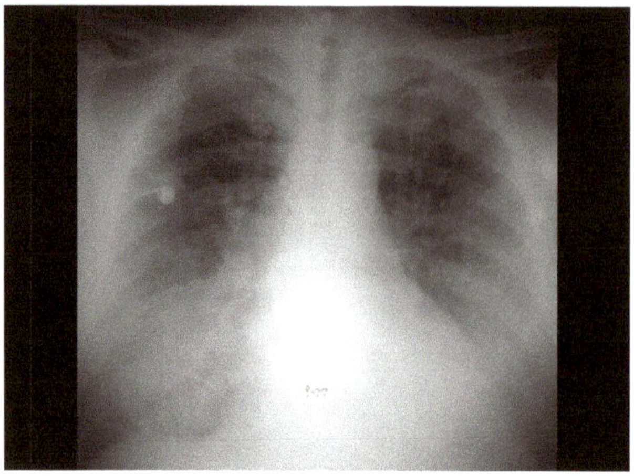

Fig. 17.27: Posteroanterior chest X-ray of a patient known to have Wegner's granulomatosis presented with acute shortness of breath and blood stained sputum due to pulmonary hemorrhage.

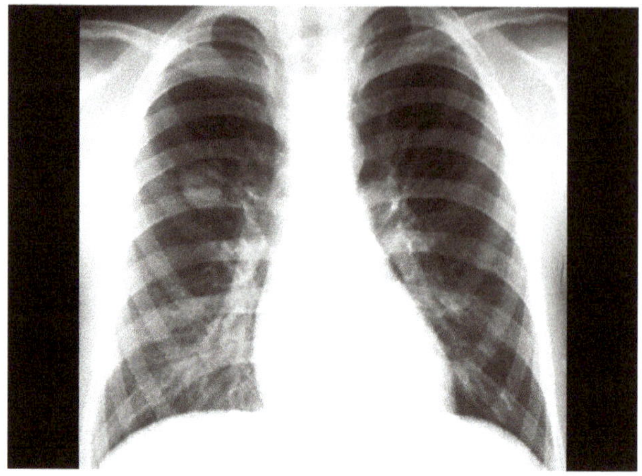

Fig. 17.28: A posteroanterior chest X-ray on a 26-year-old male shows a coin lesion in the right upper zone. The mass was resected and the histology showed an inflammatory myofibroblastic tumor.

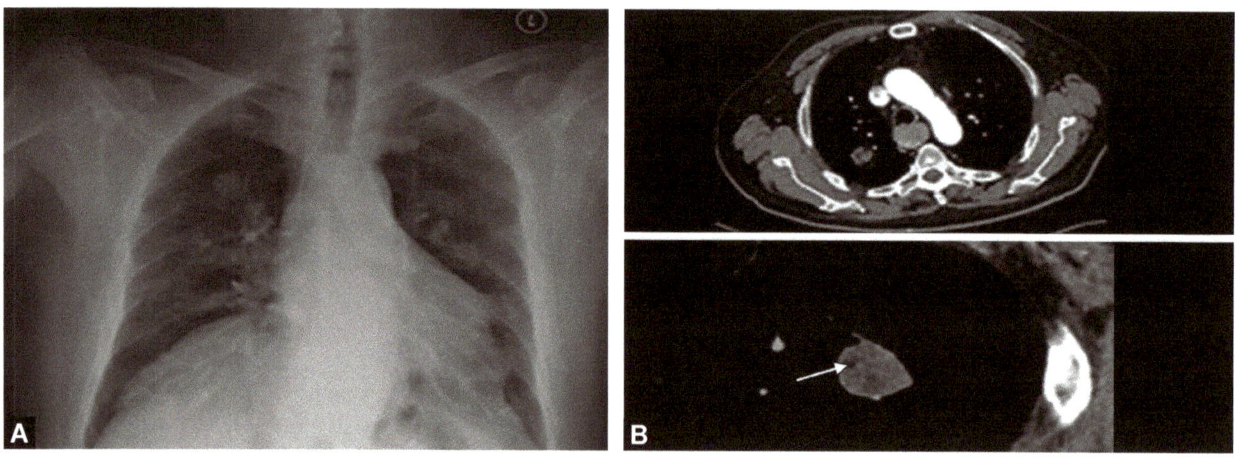

Figs. 17.29A and B: (A) Posteroanterior chest X-ray showing a coin lesion in the upper zone of the right lung. (B) Axial CT scan showed fat content with a well-defined tumor. The mass was observed and remained stable for five years.

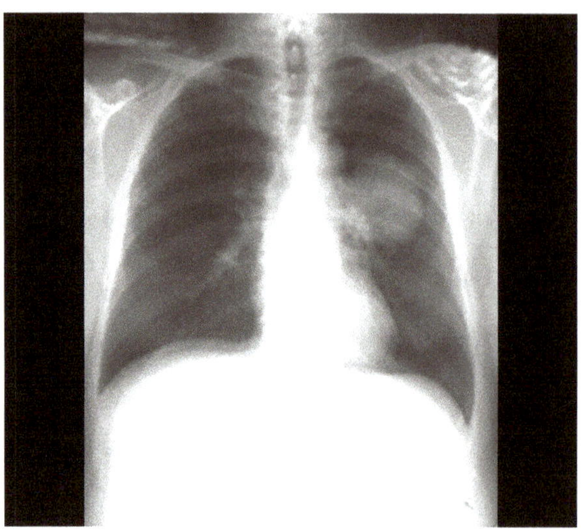

Fig. 17.30: A round mass of about 5 cm in diameter sited in the middle zone of the left lung. A bronchial biopsy revealed a small cell lung cancer.

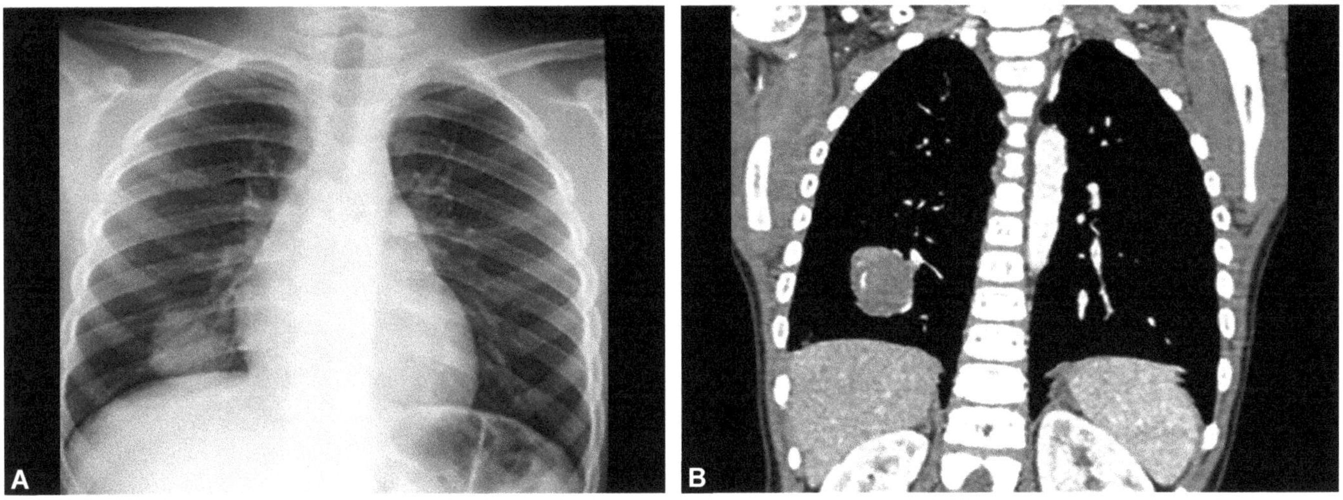

Figs. 17.31A and B: (A) Chest X-ray and (B) coronal CT scan showing a little mass with calcification fine-needle aspiration cytology (FNAC) showed features of hamartoma (benign bronchial cells, fibromyxoid stroma, cartilage, adipose tissue and bone), thus avoiding a surgical approach.

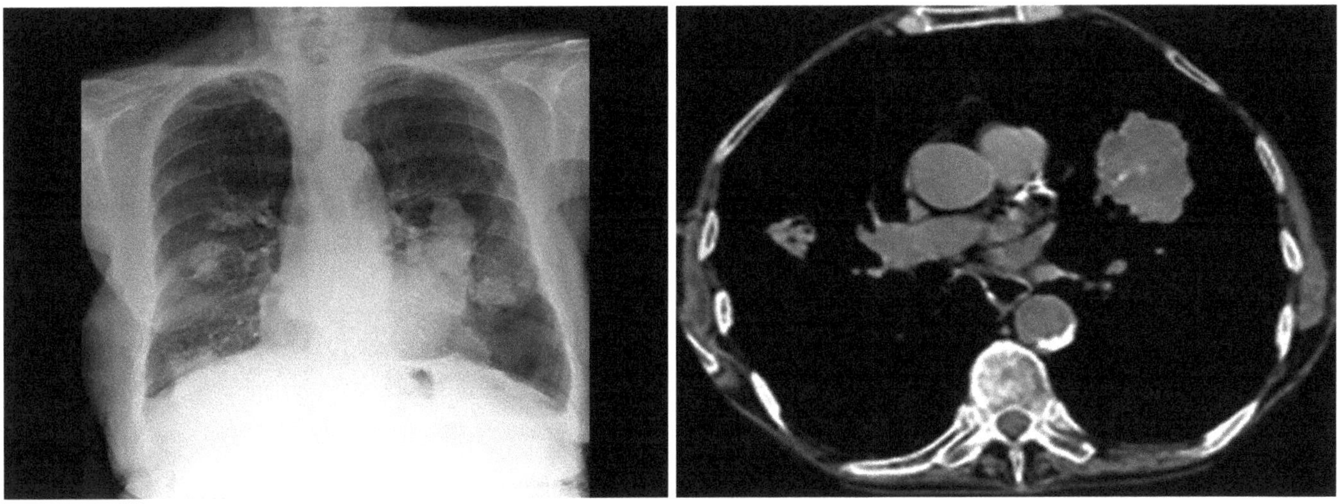

Fig. 17.32: Posteroanterior chest X-ray showing multiple calcified nodules of varying sizes (the same density as the ribs) proved nonmucinous adenocarcinoma from the sigmoid colon. An axial CT scan confirms calcification within one of the lobulated tumors.

Calcified lung metastases (Fig. 17.32) are from primary sarcomas such as osteogenic, chondrosarcoma, synovial sarcomas, giant cell tumor, malignant mesenchymoma and fibrosarcoma of the breast. Metastases from other primary carcinomas that may calcify are papillary and mucinous adenocarcinomas. Occasionally, pulmonary metastases from a medullary carcinoma of the thyroid may calcify.

Calcified pulmonary metastases have been reported on CT images from a breast malignant cystosarcoma phylloides. The metastases of a number of other tumors have calcified after anticancer therapy. A variety of mechanisms are involved in the genesis of calcified lung metastases: bone formation in tumor osteoid, calcification and ossification of tumor cartilage, dystrophic calcification and ossification of tumor cartilage, dystrophic calcification and mucoid calcification.

Atelectasis

Atelectasis or lung-collapse is the result of loss of air in a lung or part of the lung with subsequent loss of volume

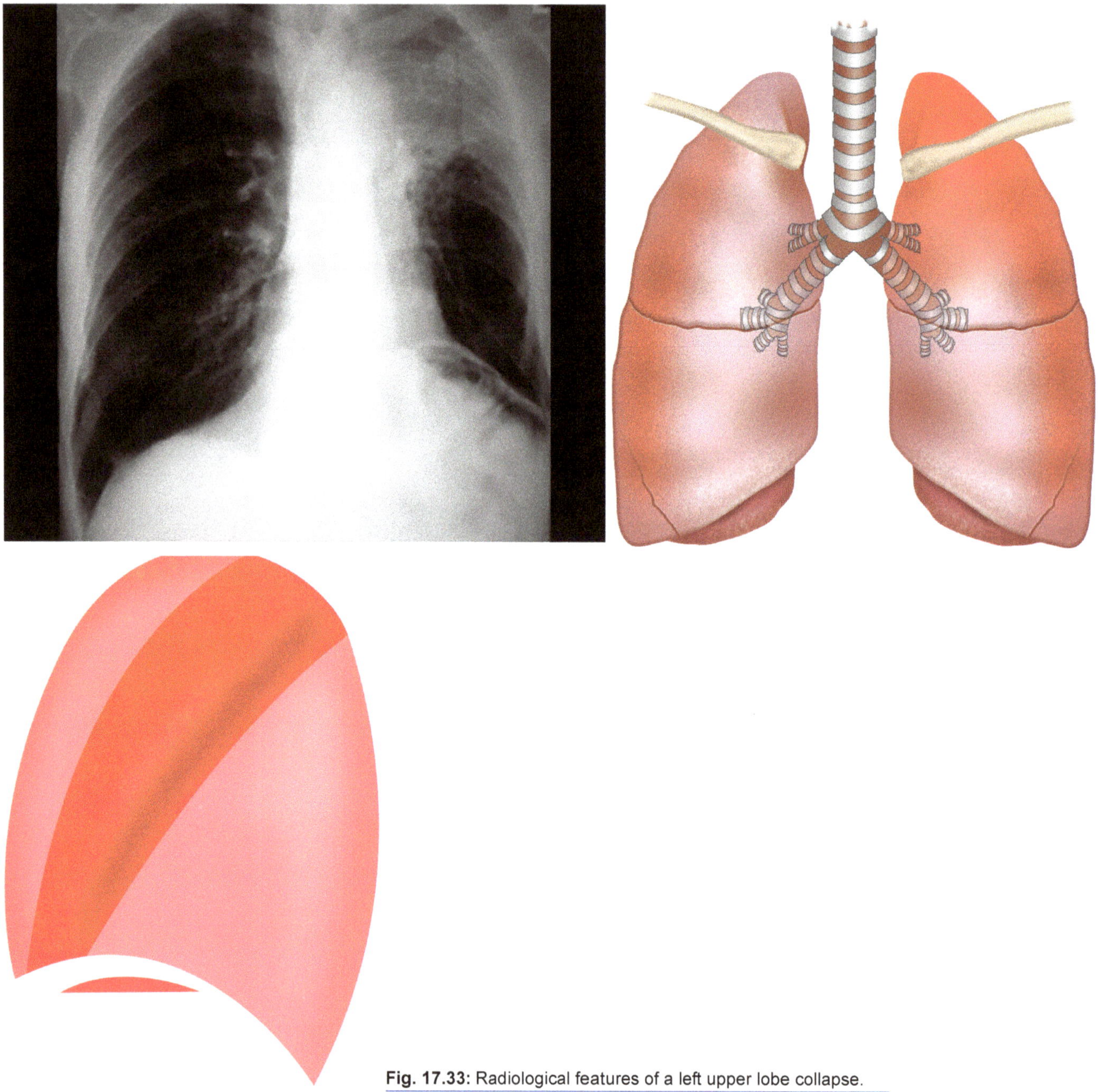

Fig. 17.33: Radiological features of a left upper lobe collapse.

and increased density. It may include a lung subsegment or the entire lung and is almost always a secondary phenomenon, due to airway obstruction or compression of the lung by pleural fluid or a pneumothorax. The collapse consolidation is often defined by the lung fissure with a characteristic appearance (Figs. 17.33 to 17.34).

The key-findings on the X-ray are:

- Sharply-defined opacity obscuring vessels without air bronchogram
- Volume loss resulting in displacement of diaphragm, fissures, hili or mediastinum.

Lobar atelectasis or lobar collapse is an important finding on a CXR; it is often secondary to bronchial obstruction and has a limited differential diagnosis.

The most common causes of atelectasis are:

- Bronchial carcinoma in smokers
- Mucus plug in patients on mechanical ventilation or astmathics (ABPA)

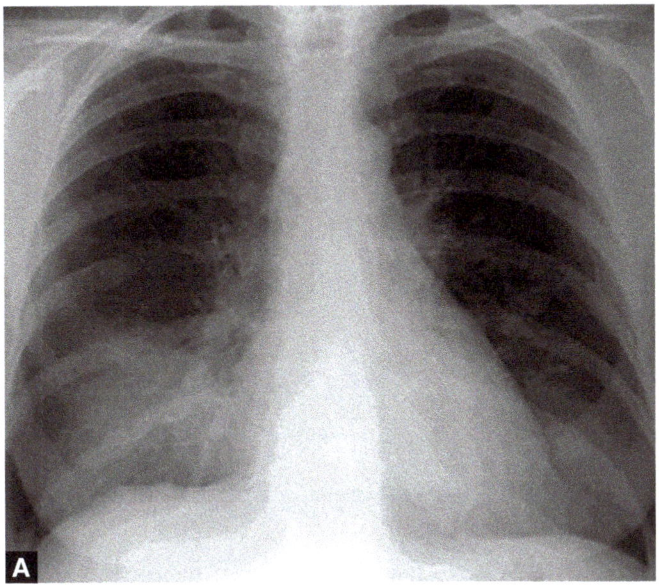
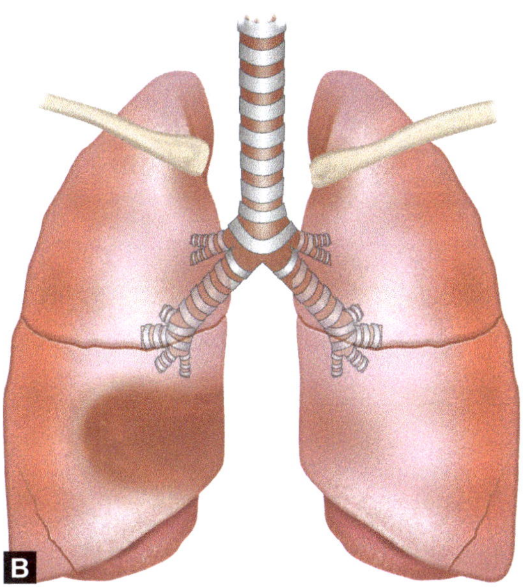

Figs. 17.34A and B: (A) Posteroanterior chest X-ray and (B) line diagram of a right middle lobe collapse/consolidation abutting the right border.

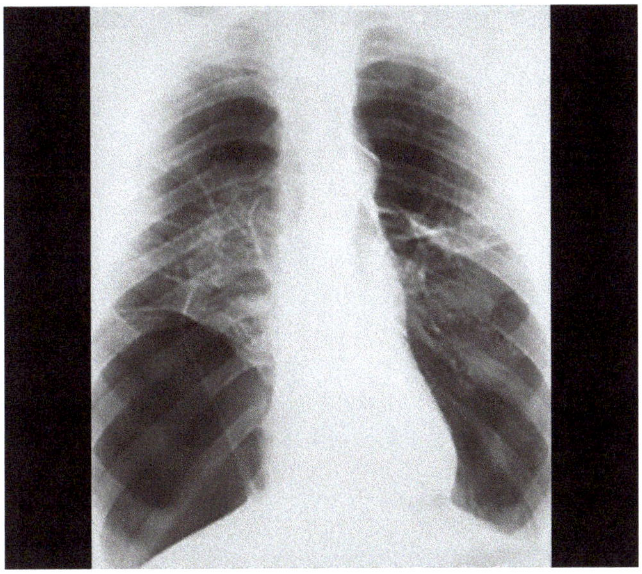

Fig. 17.35: Posteroanterior chest radiograph on a 49-year-old man with emphysema showing compression atelectasis secondary to lung bullae.

- Malpositioned endotracheal tube
- Foreign body in children.

Sometimes lobar atelectasis produces only mild volume loss due to overinflation of the other lung parts.

Compression atelectasis may occur in association with any pace-occupying lesion within the thorax (Fig. 17.35). The intrathoracic mass compresses the adjacent lung, which forces air out of the alveoli.

Replacement atelectasis occurs with the loss of volume in a lung lobe when the alveoli are filled by tumor such as in, bronchioalveolar cell carcinoma (Figs. 17.36 and 17.37).

A passive atelectasis occurs when a pneumothorax eliminates contact between the parietal and visceral pleurae. The uniform elasticity of normal lung leads to the preservation of shape even when volume is decreased in a passive atelectasis (Fig. 17.38).

Postoperative atelectasis is a frequent occurrence in patients following thoracic and upper abdominal procedures. General anesthetic and surgical manipulation lead to diaphragmatic splinting and reduced surfactant activity. Postoperative atelectasis is typically basilar and segmental in distribution (Fig. 17.39). Adhesive atelectasis results from surfactant deficiency, which reduces surface tension of the alveoli, thereby decreasing the tendency alveoli to collapse. This is observed particularly in acute respiratory distress syndrome and similar disorders (Fig. 17.40).

The right middle lobe syndrome (Figs. 17.41A to C) is a disorder of recurrent or fixed atelectasis involving the right middle lobe. It can result from either extra luminal (bronchial compression by surrounding lymph nodes) or by intraluminal bronchial obstruction. It may develop in the presence of a patent lobar bronchus without identifiable obstruction. Inflammatory processes and defects in the bronchial anatomy and collateral ventilation have been designated as the nonobstructive causes of middle lobe syndrome. Timely medical intervention in patients

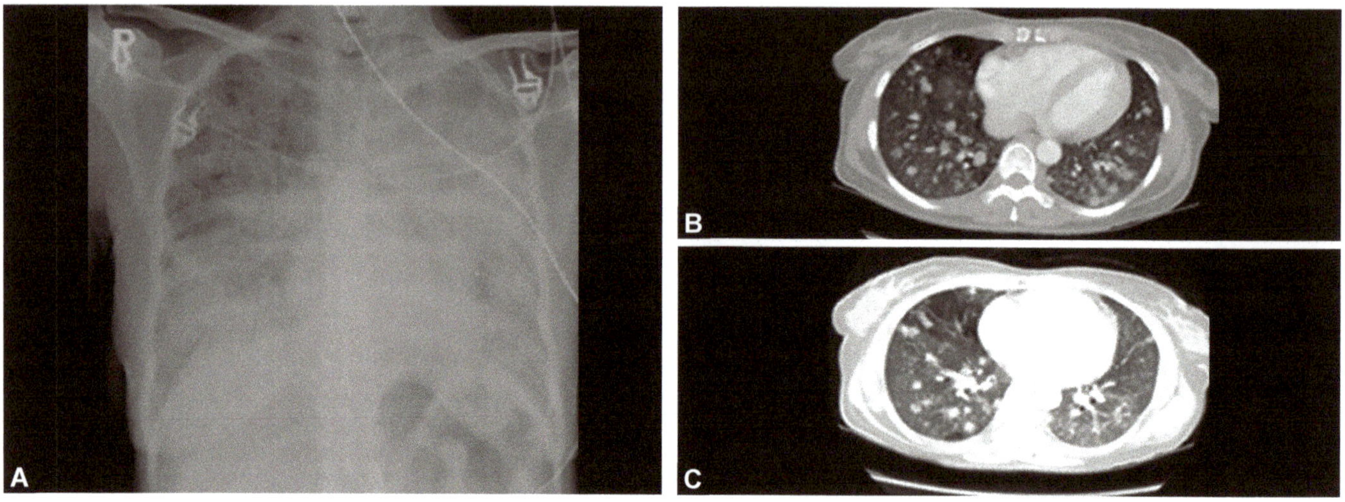

Figs. 17.36A to C: Replacement atelectasis. (A) Portable radiograph and (B and C) computed tomograms show the loss of volume due to alveoli filled by bronchioalveolar cell carcinoma.

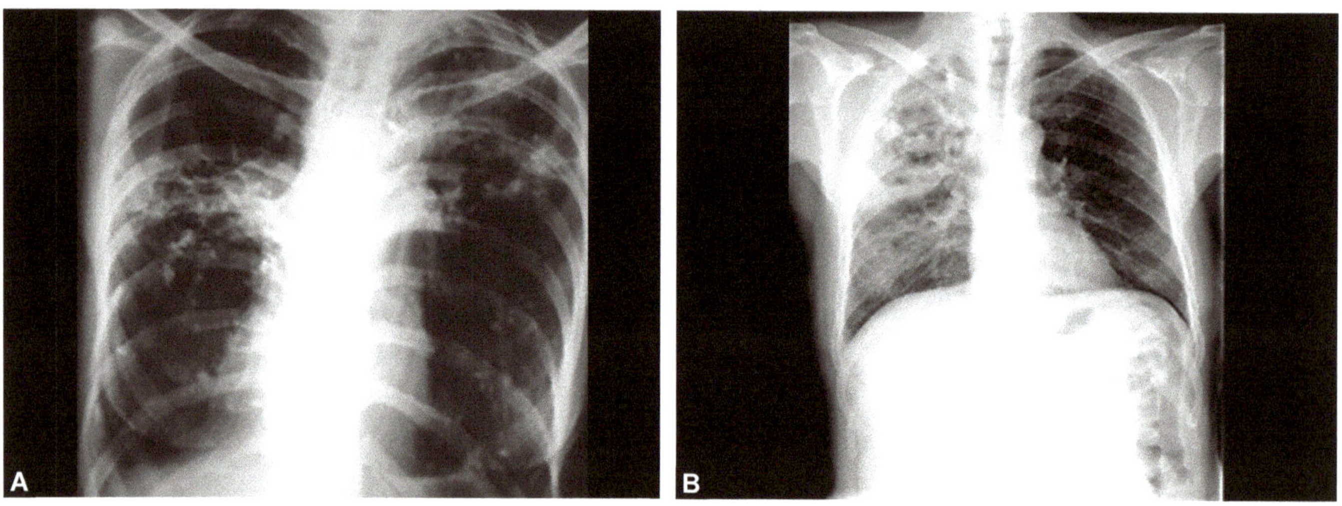

Figs. 17.37A and B: Cicatrization/replacement atelectasis, which occurs secondary to severe lung parenchymal scarring, such as from (A) granulomatous disease or (B) necrotizing pneumonia.

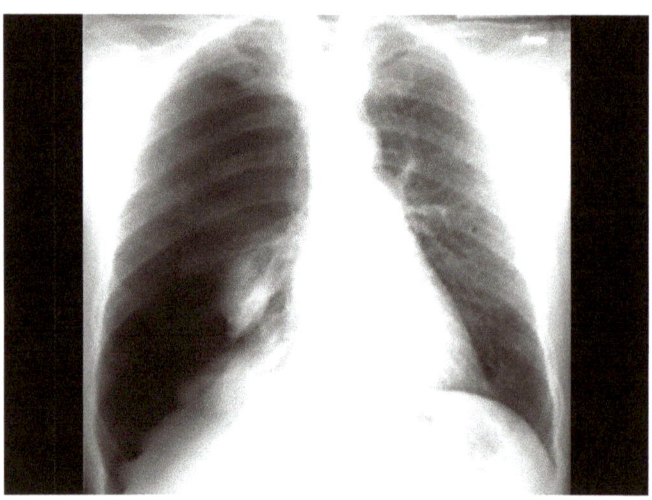

Fig. 17.38: Posteroanterior chest X-ray showing a passive atelectasis of the right lower lobe secondary to a pneumothorax.

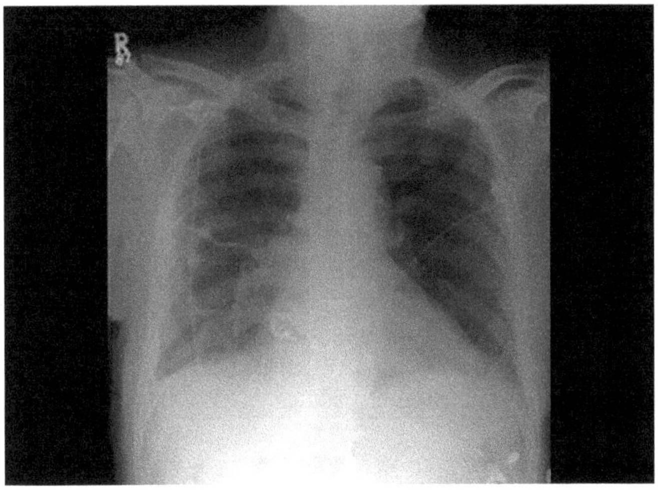

Fig. 17.39: Postoperative atelectasis.

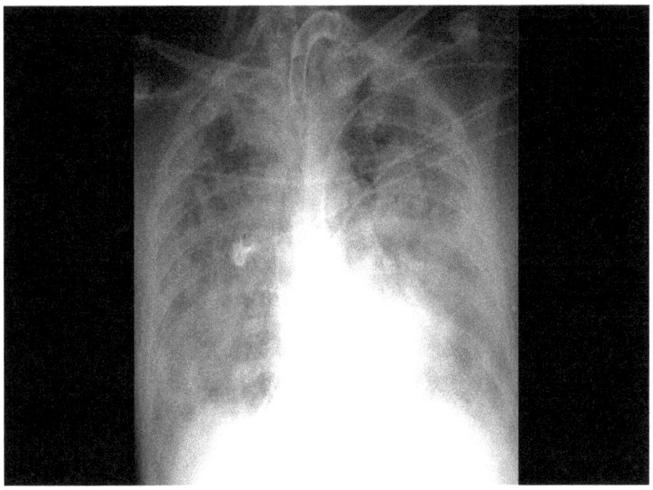

Fig. 17.40: Adhesive atelectasis resulting from surfactant deficiency.

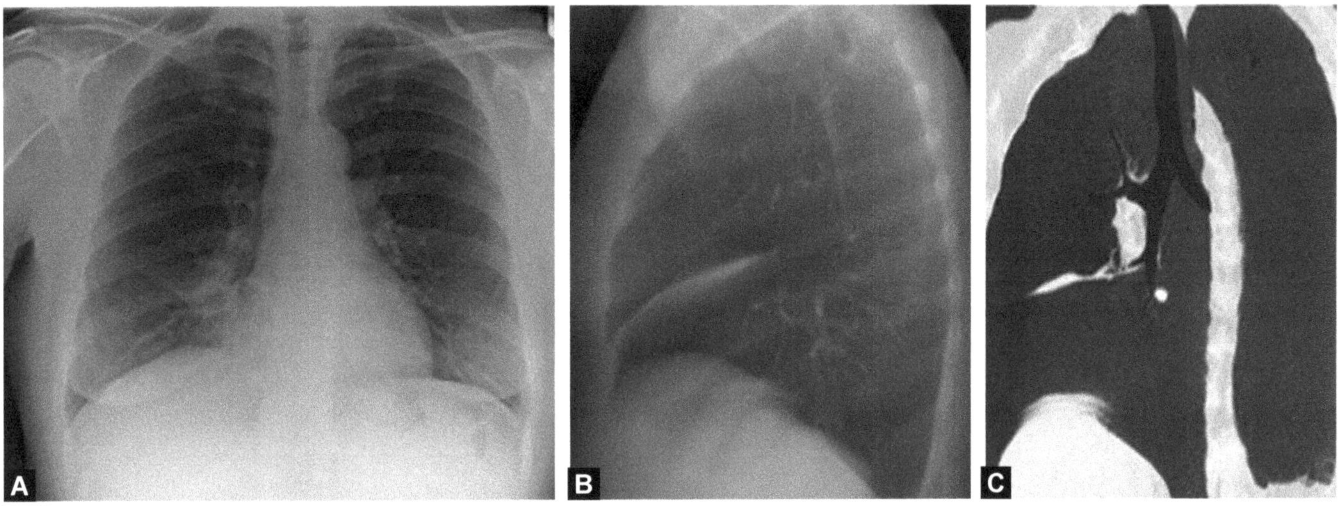

Figs. 17.41A to C: Features of a right middle lobe syndrome: (A) Posteroanterior chest X-ray. (B) Lateral chest X-ray. (C) Coronal CT scan.

(especially children) with middle lung syndrome, including fiberoptic bronchoscopy with bronchoalveolar lavage, prevents bronchiectasis that may be responsible for recurrent infections and an ultimately unfavorable outcome of chronic atelectasis.

Middle lobe syndrome has been reported as a pulmonary manifestation of primary Sjögren syndrome. Transbronchial biopsies performed in such patients revealed lymphocytic bronchiolitis in the atelectatic lobes. Atelectasis responds well to glucocorticoid treatment, suggesting that the peribronchiolar lymphocytic infiltrates may play an important role in the development of middle lobe syndrome in these patients.

A right lower lobe collapse is easily identified on a frontal radiograph (Fig. 17.42). A triangular opacity at the medial base of the right lung is apparent associated with the loss of the medial dome of the right hemidiaphragm. The right hilum is displaced downwards, and the descending lower lobe pulmonary artery cannot be identified. The right heart border is clearly seen. Nonspecific signs include elevation of the hemidiaphragm, crowding of the left-sided ribs and mediastinal shift to the right. On lateral radiographs, the right hemidiaphragmatic outline is lost posteriorly, and the lower thoracic vertebrae appear denser than normal.

Subsegmental atelectasis (Fig. 17.43) is the most common atelectasis seen on chest radiographs. It may be plate, discoid or subsegmental, and occurs probably because of obstruction of a small bronchus and is seen in conditions that result in hypoventilation, pulmonary embolism or

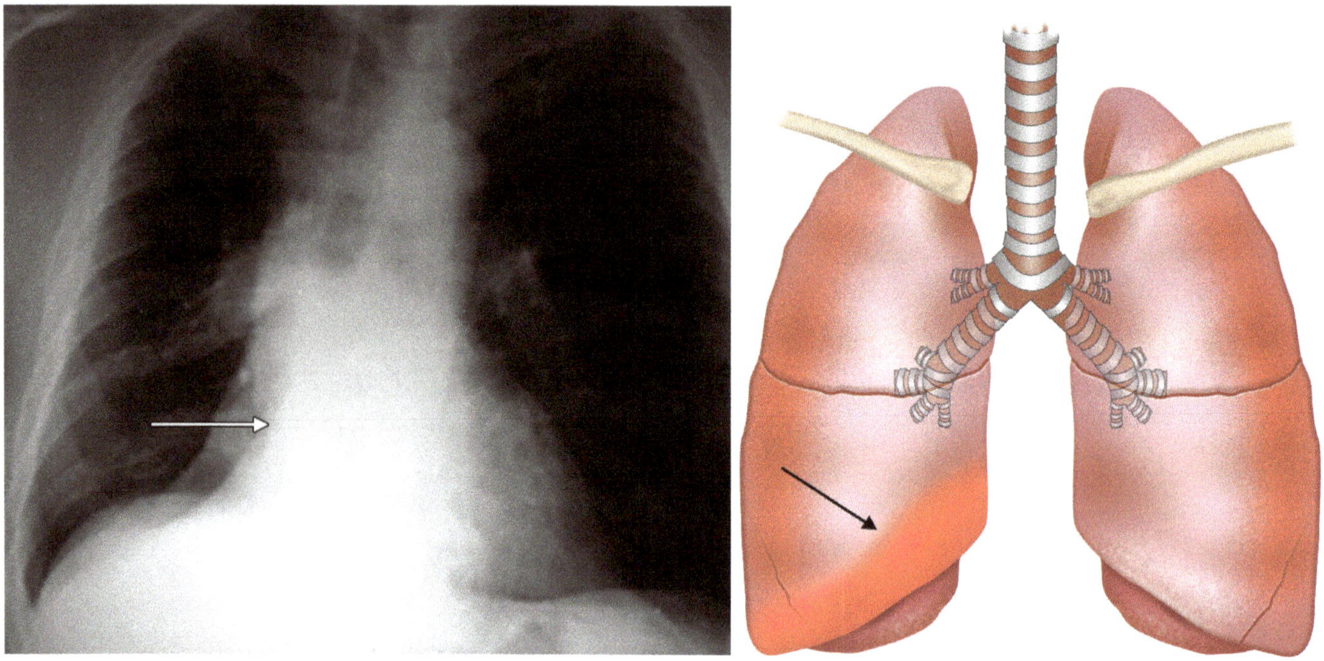

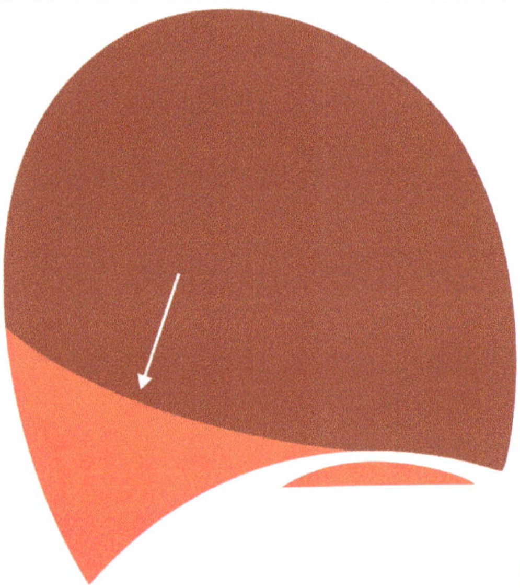

Fig. 17.42: Right lower lobe collapse (arrow).

lower respiratory tract infection. Small areas of atelectasis occur because of inadequate regional ventilation and abnormalities in the surfactant formation from hypoxia, ischemia, hyperoxia and exposure to various toxins. There is an associated gas exchange abnormality because of ventilation-perfusion mismatch and intrapulmonary shunt.

DECREASED PULMONARY DENSITY

Airway obstruction due to asthma is a cause of hyperinflation without parenchymal damage, with subsequent decreased density of the lung at CXR. Characteristics of hyperinflation of the lungs in CXR include hyperleucent lungs and flattened diaphragm.

Patients with emphysema often have hyperinflation associated with destruction of parenchymal structures. CXR in such individuals may also show abnormally increased chest diameter, enlargement of the pulmonary arteries, bullae, and areas of damaged pulmonary tissue that makes up the large air sacs.

An increase of lucency in CXR may occur in diseases with reduction of the vascular component, such as pulmonary embolism. However, in most cases of acute pulmonary

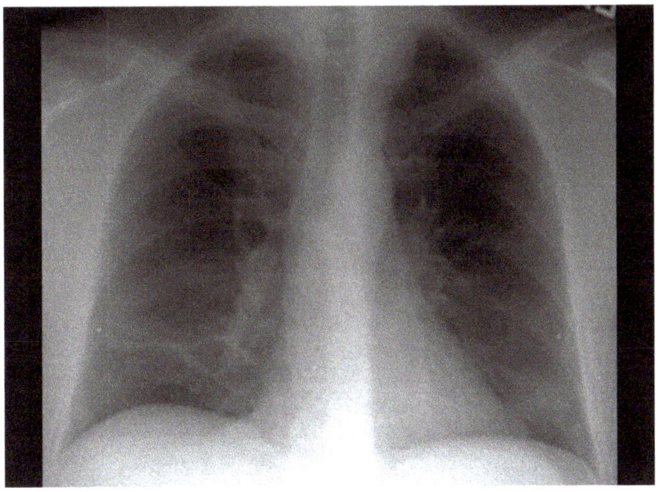

Fig. 17.43: Subsegmental atelectasis.

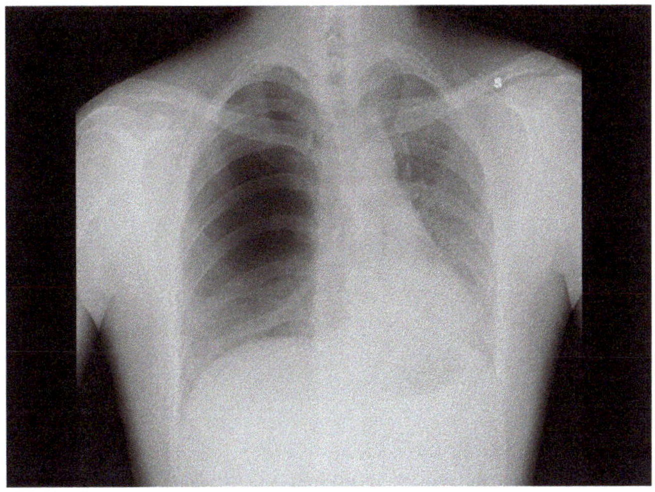

Fig. 17.44: Posteroanterior chest X-ray showing an enormous bulla in the in the right upper and middle zone, which compresses the adjacent lung parenchyma and displaces contralaterally the mediastinum.

thromboembolism CXR is normal or with nonspecific features such as atelectasis and patchy pulmonary opacity.

Pulmonary bullae are focal regions of emphysema with no discernible wall which measure more than 1 cm in diameter. The term bleb is sometimes used for 1–2 cm lesion. Subpleural bullae may result in spontaneous pneumathorax. In some cases bullae can be very large and result in compression of adjacent lung (Fig. 17.44).

A lung cavitation is a gas-filled space within a zone of pulmonary consolidation or within a mass or nodule, and appears radiographically as a lucent area within the lung. It is surrounded by a wall of varied thickness and may contain a fluid level.

Cavities are present in a wide variety of infectious and noninfectious processes.

The radiographic appearance of cavitary lesions can help to identify the cause. Wall thickness is one of the most used methods to classify cavitary lesions, but this is easily done by CT scan.

Cavities with a wall thickness lower than 4 mm have a higher than 90% likelihood to be caused by nonmalignant processes. More than 90% of cavities with a wall thickness of 15 mm or higher are malignant.

Lucencies without a visible wall or with visible walls that measure less than 1 mm are called bullae and occur mainly in emphysematous lungs. Lucencies with a thin wall (<3 mm) are usually named cysts. The term is mostly used to describe enlarged thin-walled airspaces in patients with lymphangioleiomyomatosis or Langerhans cell histiocytosis. Langerhans cell histiocytosis results from clonal proliferation of Langerhans cells, derived from bone marrow capable of migrating from skin to lymph nodes. Clinically, its manifestations range from unifocal bone lesions to multisystem involvement isolated bone lesions to multisystem disease. Thicker-walled honeycomb cysts are seen in patients with end-stage fibrosis.

However, the global aspect on CXR of diseases with multiple cysts or honeycombing is an increased density with interstitial reticular pattern with distortion of the underlying parenchymal architecture (Figs. 17.45 and 17.46).

MAIN SIGNS IN RADIOLOGY

Silhouette Sign

The "Silhouette Sign" (Fig. 17.47), first described in 1950 by Dr Benjamin Felson, is an important and extremely useful sign in chest radiography. The sign describes the loss of normal lung/soft tissue interface or "silhouette", caused by disease processes that either replaces or displaces normal air-filled lung. This sign can be applied mediastinal structures, the thoracic wall and the diaphragm. Examples of these are shown in various collapse/consolidations of lung lobes. The outlines and edges seen on a CXR depend on the presence of two areas of different density. Only, four densities are seen on plain radiographs; air, fat, soft tissue and calcium. If two soft tissue densities lie adjacent, then

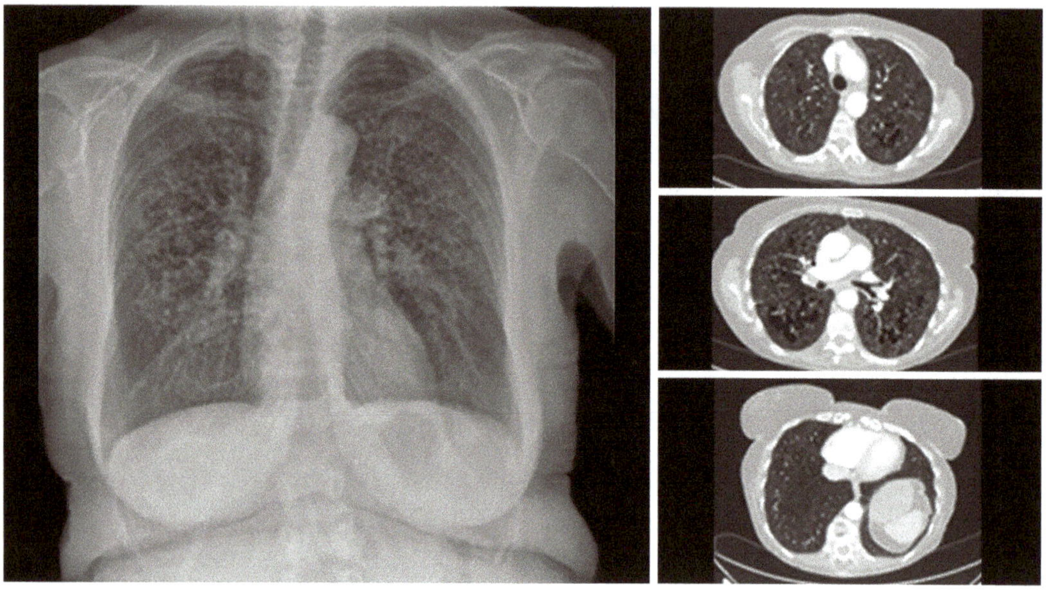

Fig. 17.45: Langerhans cell histiocytosis.

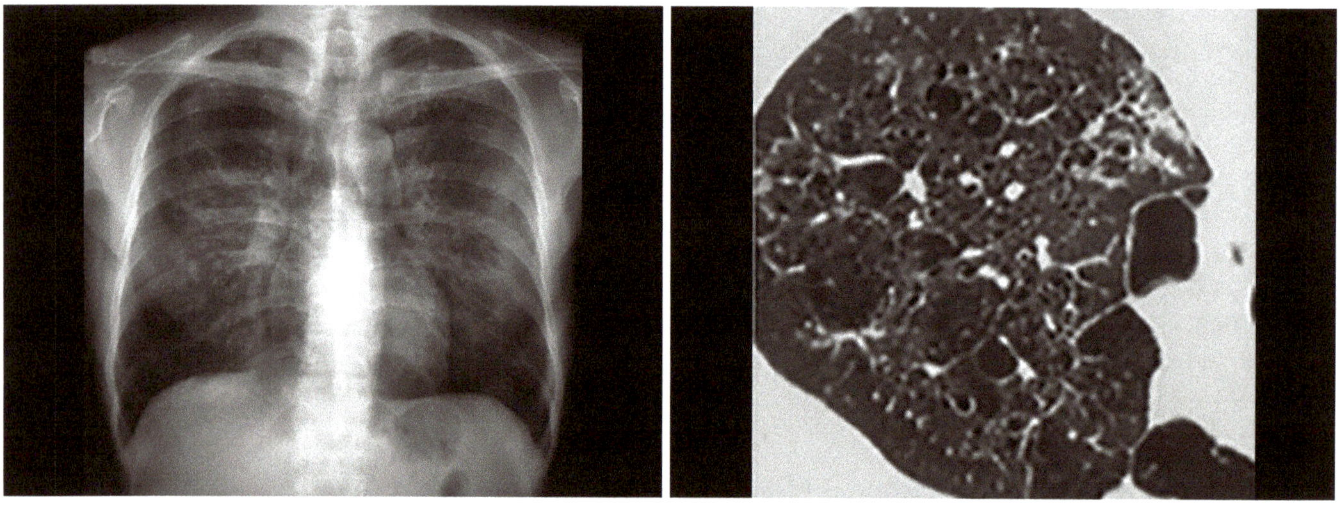

Fig. 17.46: Pneumocystis pneumonia (PCP) is a common manifestation in HIV patients. A chest X-ray usually shows multiple lung cysts, which range in size, shape and distribution. They may develop in the acute or postinfective chest X-ray but have been reported to remain for up to 3 years. The cysts are better depicted on high-resolution CT and seen in up to a third of patients.

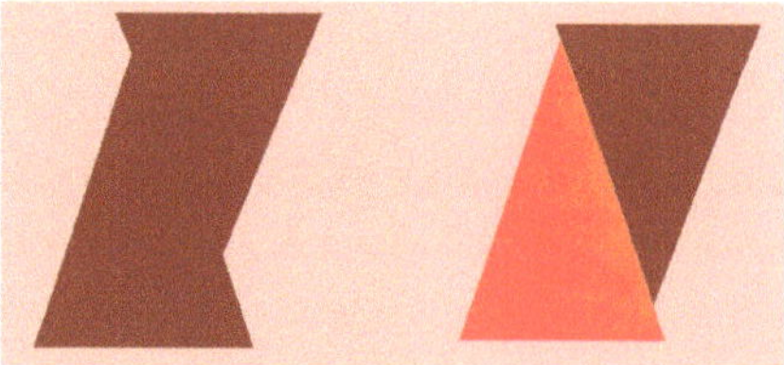

Fig. 17.47: The silhouette sign: if two soft tissue densities lie adjacent, then they will not be visible separately. If, however, they are separated by air, the boundaries are clearly seen.

they will not be visible separately. If, however, they are separated by air, the boundaries are clearly seen.

A left paravertebral line represents a normal reflection of the mediastinal pleura over descending aorta and esophagus (Fig. 17.48). However, the presence of a right paravertebral line is always abnormal and related to a dilated esophagus, posterior mediastinal lymphadenopathy and osteophytes amongst other pathologies (Fig. 17.49).

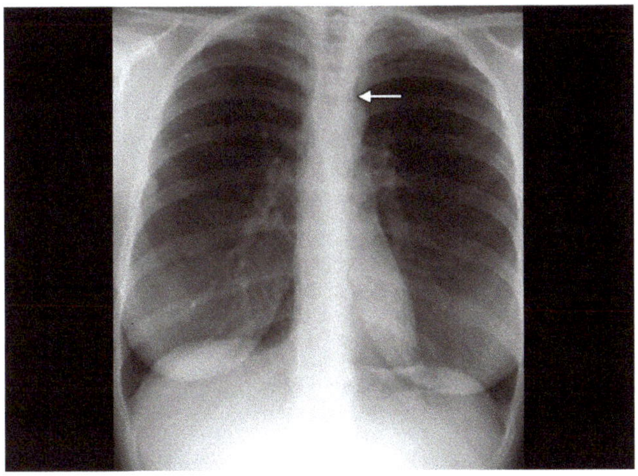

Fig. 17.48: Left paravertebral line: due to the normal reflection of the mediastinal pleura over descending aorta and esophagus (arrow).

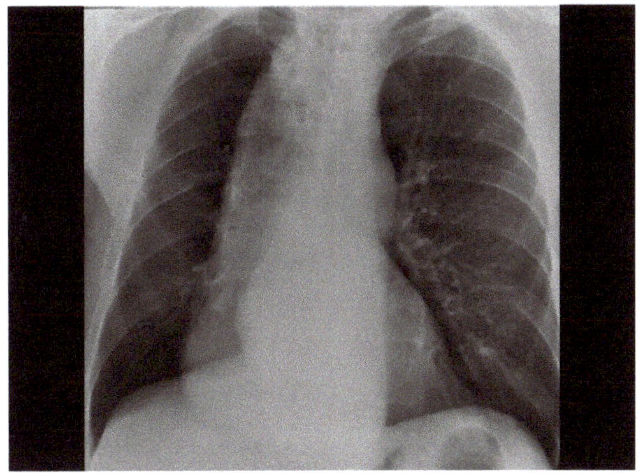

Fig. 17.49: A posteroanterior chest X-ray (PA CXR) of a patient with dysphagia shows an inlet to outlet shadow due to esophageal achalasia.

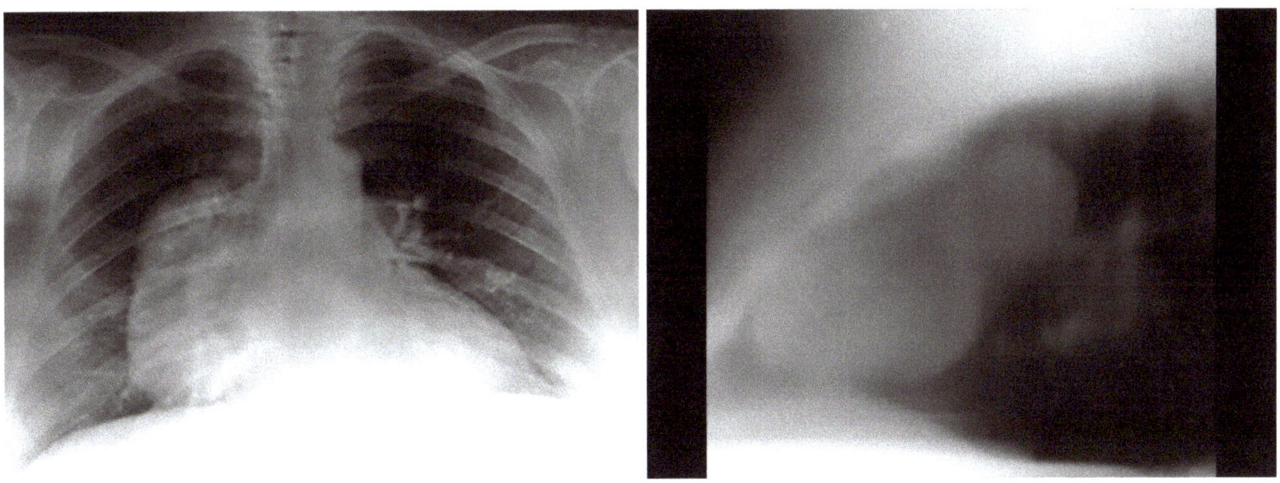

Fig. 17.50: Double density sign: Chest X-ray shows a double density sign due to a dermoid cyst. The cyst is shown in the anterior mediastinum by conventional tomography.

Pulmonary Artery Overlay Sign/Double Density Sign

The pulmonary artery overlay sign occurs when the pulmonary artery is seen through a mass. This implies that the mass is either in front or behind the pulmonary artery (Figs. 17.50 to 17.52).

Left lower lobe, disease, hiatus hernia and posterior mediastinal masses give a double density over the left side of the heart (Figs. 17.53 and 17.54).

The heart is of uniform density, except over vertebrae and the descending aorta. Increased density in one portion of the heart means an abnormal density lies either in front or behind the heart. The circular double density can recognize a left atrial enlargement. Any other increased density in one portion compared to the rest of the heart is abnormal and suggests a mass either in front or behind the heart.

The Golden S sign derive its name from the resemblance to a reverse "S" shape", thus it is also referred to as the reverse S sign of Golden (Figs. 17.55A to C).

It is visible both on PA CXR and CT scans, and typically seen with right upper lobe collapse, due to a central mass, most often primary lung cancer, which obstructs the upper lobe bronchus. However, the S sign can also be seen with the collapse of other lobes and can also be caused by other kind of central masses such as metastases, primary mediastinal tumors, or enlarged lymphnodes.

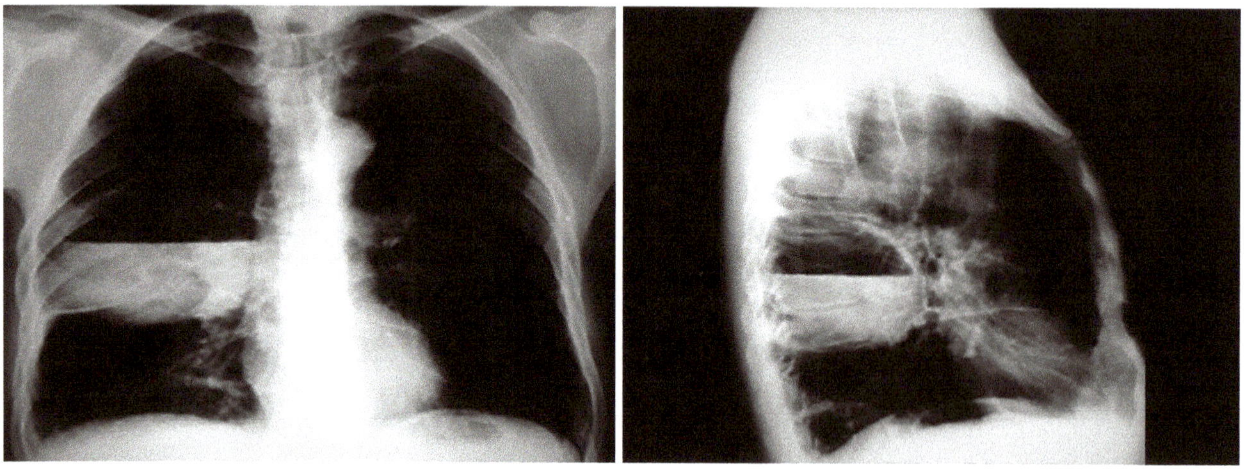

Fig. 17.51: Pulmonary artery overlay sign in a patient with a right lung abscess. The pulmonary artery can be seen through the abscess cavity implying that the abscess is either in front or behind the pulmonary artery.

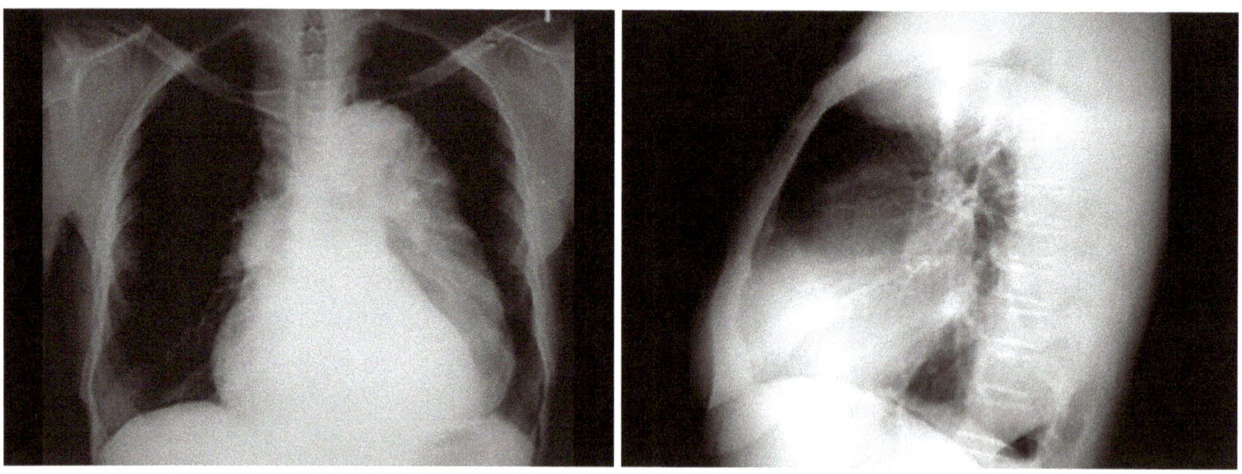

Fig. 17.52: Pulmonary artery overlay sign in a patient with descending aortic aneurysm. The pulmonary artery can be seen through the descending aortic aneurysm shadow implying that it is either in front or behind the pulmonary artery.

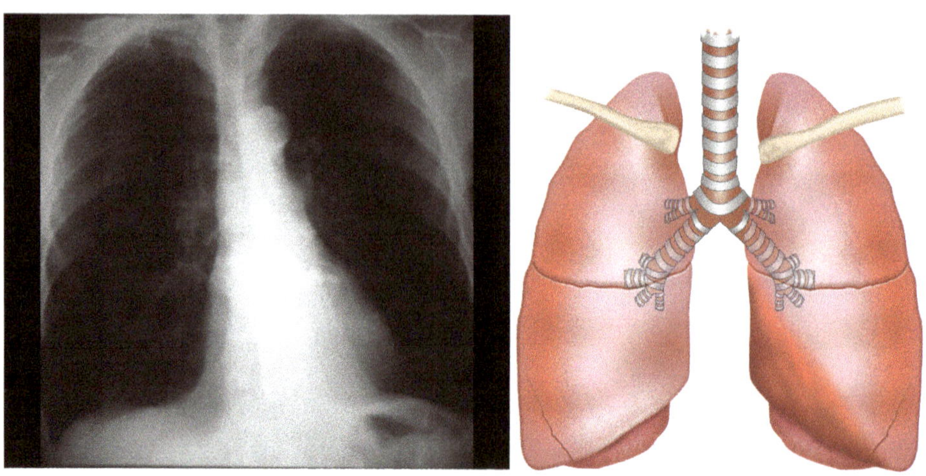

Fig. 17.53: A left lower collapse with a double density sign and a silhoette signe.

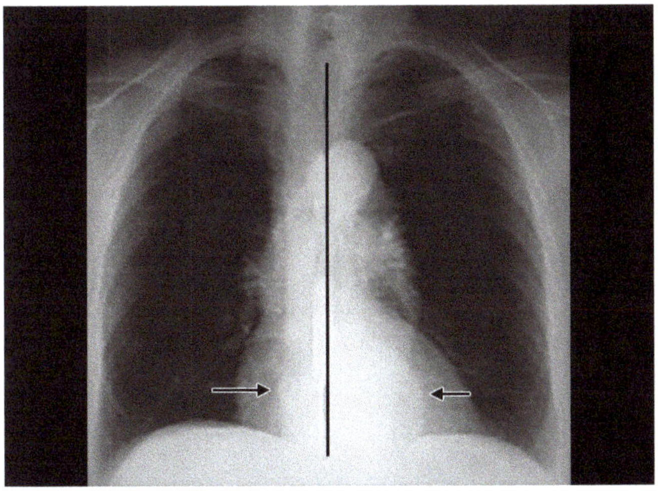

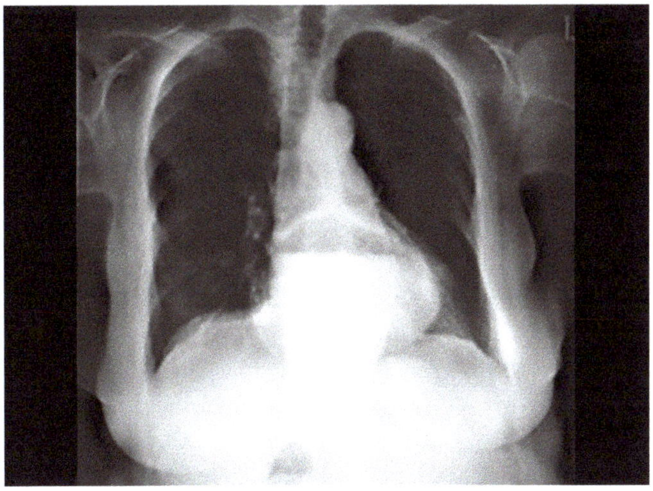

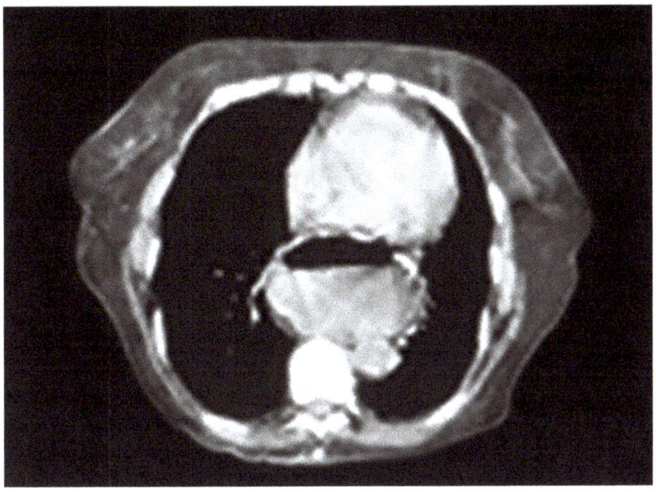

Fig. 17.54: A double density sign due to a hiatus hernia (arrows): If the mediastinal density crosses midline most likely it is a hiatus hernia.

Double Lesion Sign

Double lesion sign refers to the collapse of two or more segments which are not contiguous (Fig. 17.56). For example, when an atelectasis of the right upper lobe and left lower lobe occur sparing the middle lobe, it is unlikely that a single endobronchial lesion is the cause of both lesions. There has to be two independent endobronchial lesions; hence, it was proposed that this finding is unlikely to be due to a central primary bronchogenic cancer. However, the sign does not rule out lung cancer. It just suggests to look for an alternate explanation for the second lesion. For example, it could be due to aspiration of blood from the first lesion.

The Halo Sign

In a cavity with fungus ball there is a crescentic lucent space along the upper portion of a density giving the appearance of a halo. This phenomenon is seen with two clinical presentations of pulmonary aspergillosis, fungus ball and necrotizing subacute pneumonia during the recovery phase from leucopenia episodes (Fig. 17.57).

Inlet-to-Outlet Shadow

The esophagus, aorta and thoracic duct traverse from inlet to outlet of mediastinum. Dilatation of any one of the above-described structures gives rise to inlet-to-outlet shadows. A mediastinal shadow to the right of the midline is due to esophageal dilatation, and on the left is due to dissecting aneurysm (Fig. 17.58).

Air Bronchogram

Air bronchogram appears as air filled bronchi (black on X-rays) in the context of lung consolidation (white on X-rays), and indicate patent airways. It may occur when the

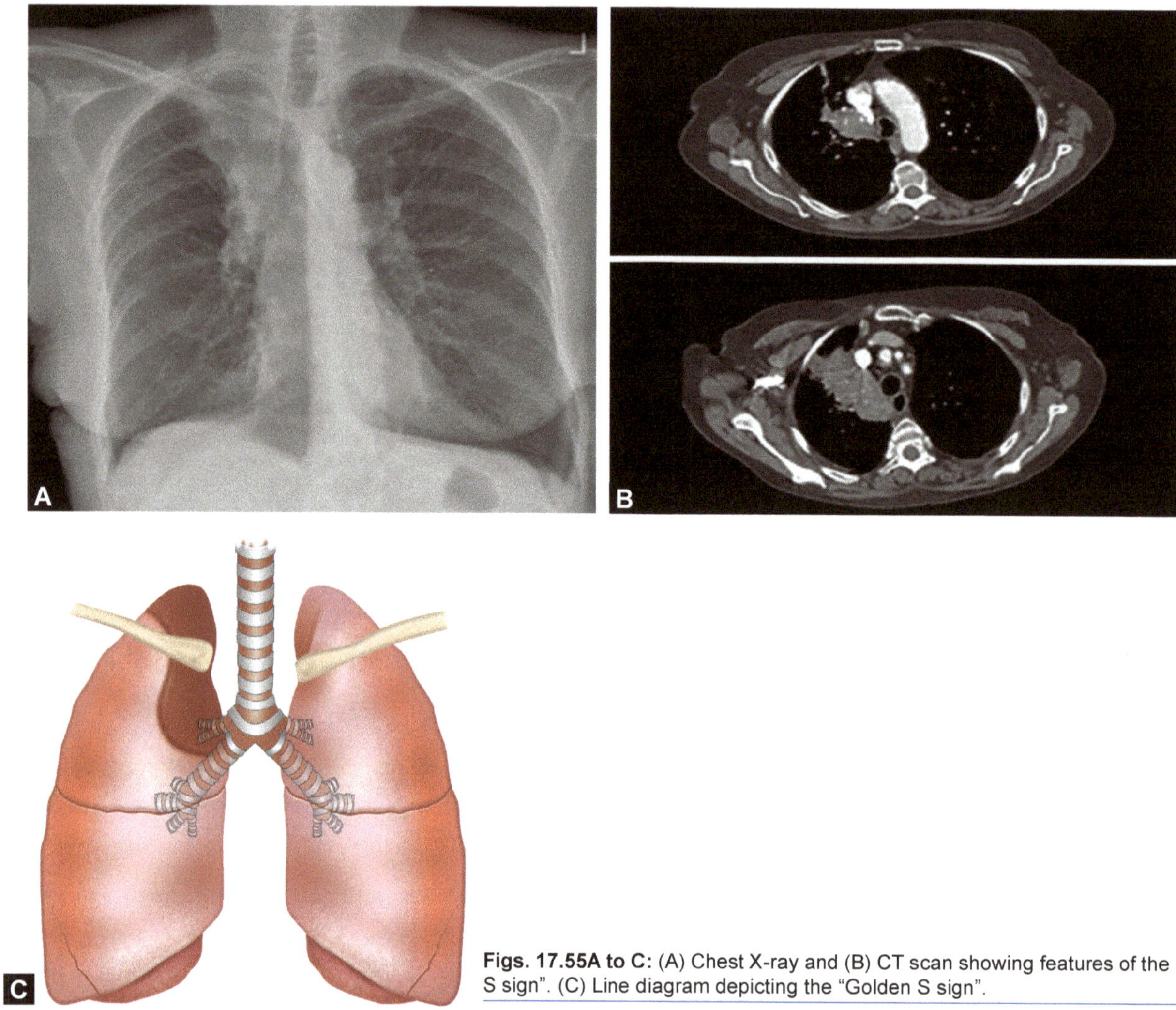

Figs. 17.55A to C: (A) Chest X-ray and (B) CT scan showing features of the "Golden S sign". (C) Line diagram depicting the "Golden S sign".

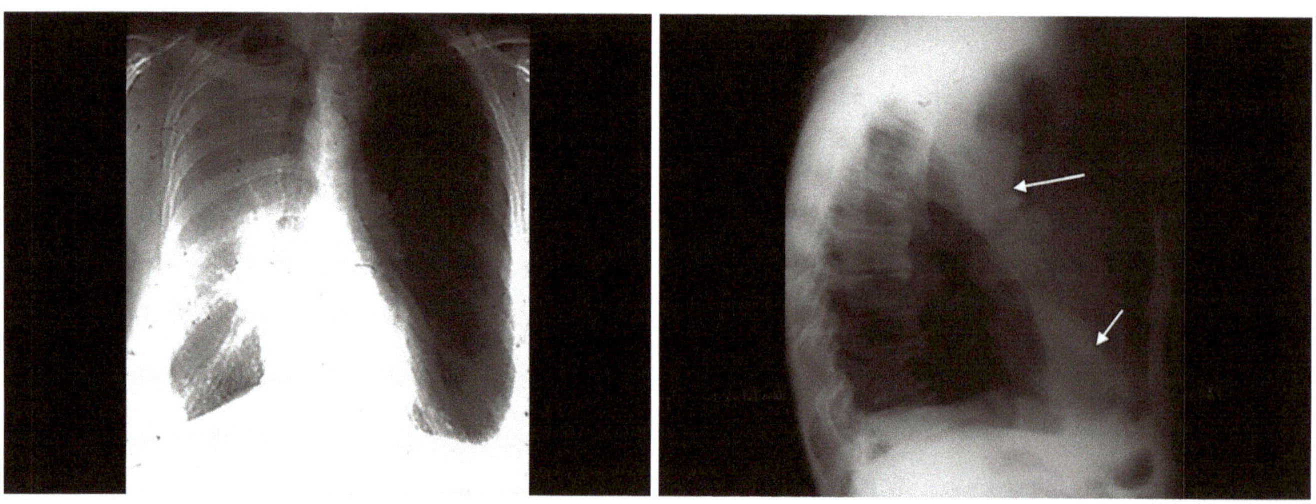

Fig. 17.56: Posteroanterior and right lateral chest X-rays showing features of a right upper (arrow) and right lower (arrow) lobe collapse (double lesion sign).

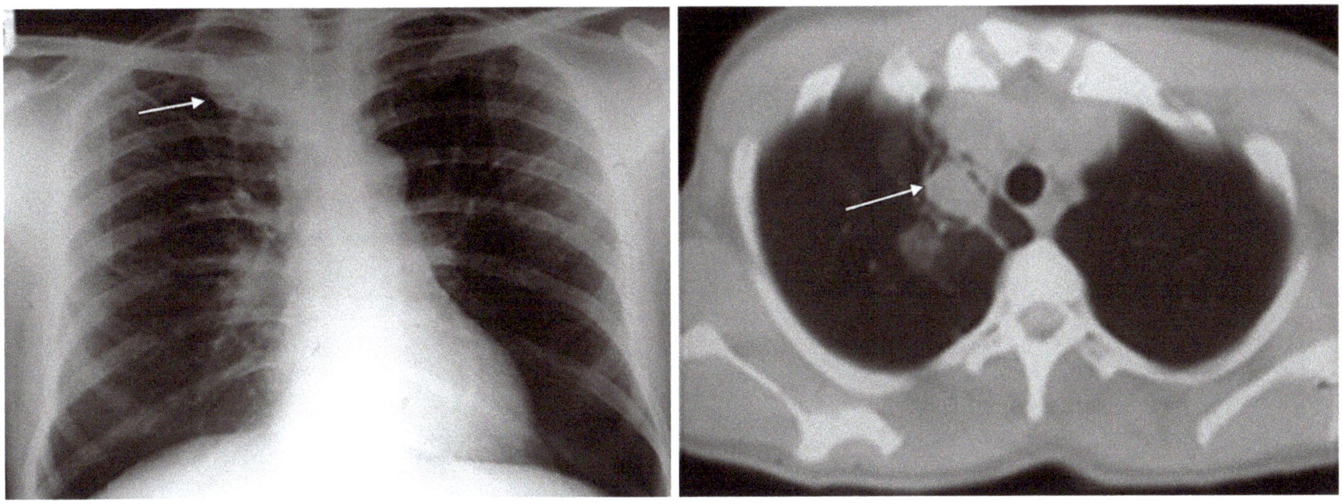

Fig. 17.57: Right lateral chest X-ray showing a fungus ball surrounded by a halo (arrow). An axial CT scan from a different patent shows a fungus ball surrounded by a halo (Mycetoma).

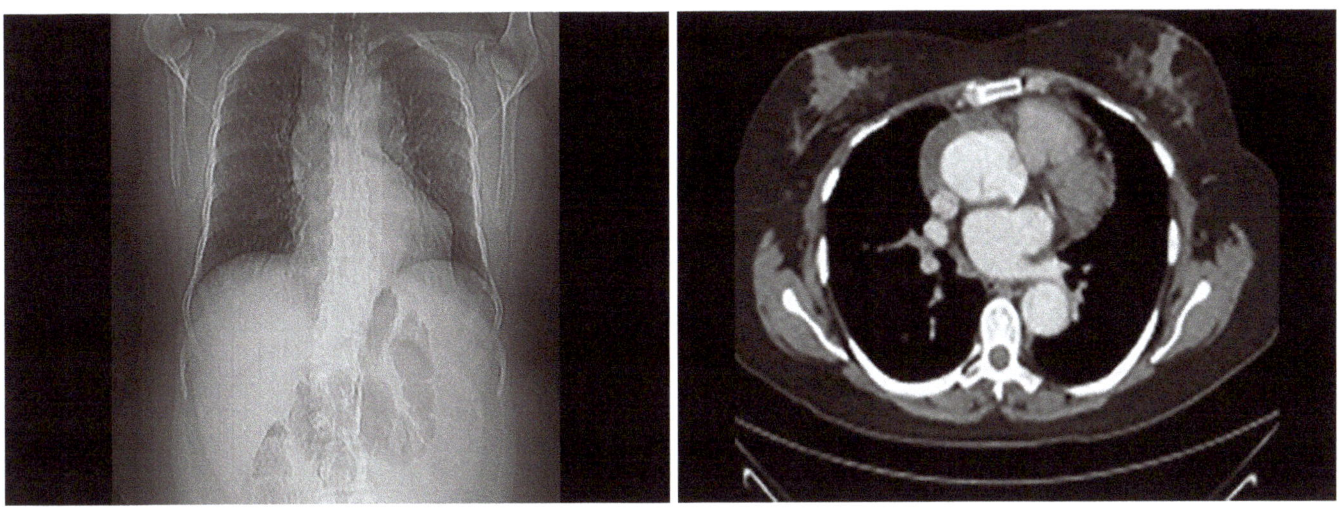

Fig. 17.58: Inlet-to-outlet shadow: aortic aneurysm with dissection extending to subclavian arteries, carotid arteries, coronary arteries, celiac trunk, superior mesenteric artery, iliac arteries, renal ischemia due to renal artery flap.

alveolar lung spaces are filled with fluid due to edema, inflammatory fluid, hemorrhage, pulmonary infarction, bronchoalveolar carcinoma lymphoma and atelectasis (Fig. 17.59).

Open Bronchus Sign

It corresponds to an air bronchogram, occurring when the air filled bronchus is seen within a lung consolidation, which is usually due to adhesive alveolar atelectasis. This finding indicates that the airways are patent (Fig. 17.60).

Luftsichel Sign

The Luftsichel sign is seen on a PA CXR in some cases of left upper lobe collapse. It derives its name from the German words *luft*—air, *sichel*—sickle, and literally describes an "air crescent" which may be observed between the aortic arch and the medial border of the collapse (Fig. 17.61). The signs are due to hyperinflation of the superior segment of the left lower lobe interposing itself between the mediastinum and the collapsed left upper lobe.

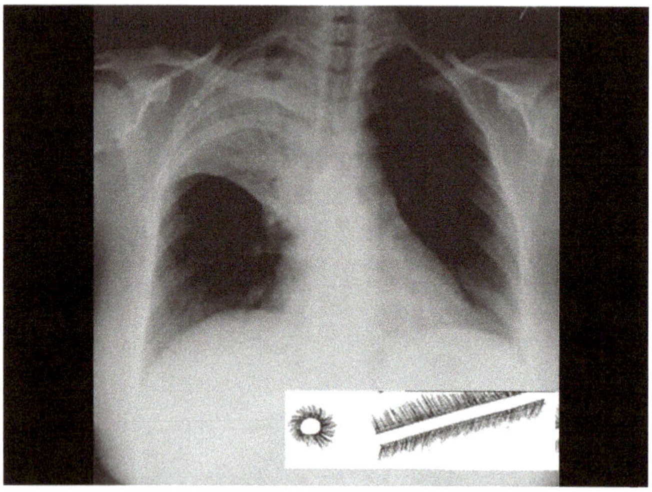

Fig. 17.59: Posteroanterior chest X-ray showing a consolidation in the upper right zone with air bronchogram.

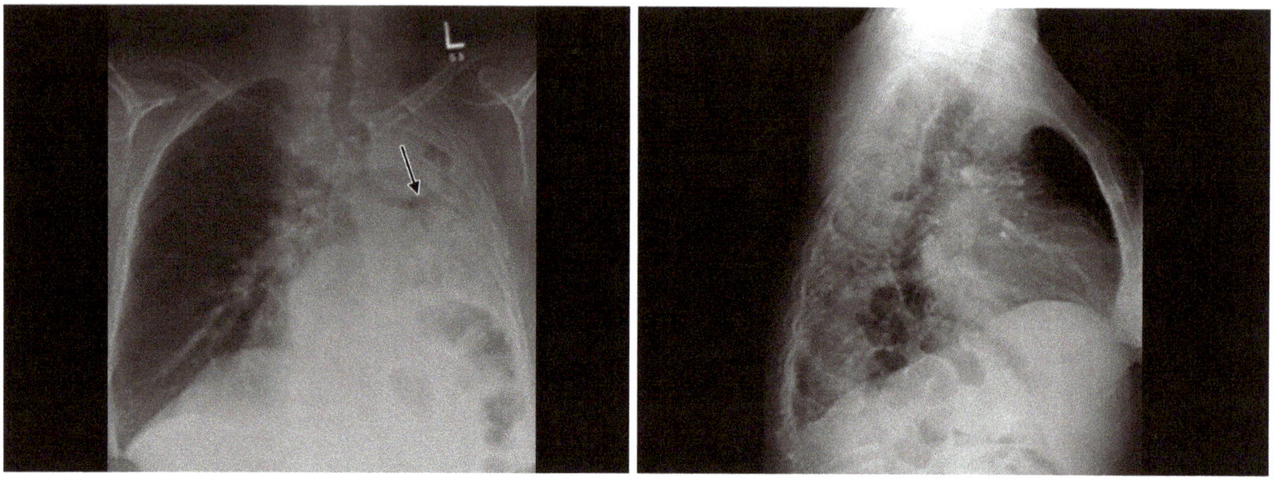

Fig. 17.60: Open bronchus sign (arrow). If the bronchi within the opacified lung are open, an obstructing lesion completely occluding a more central bronchus is unlikely.

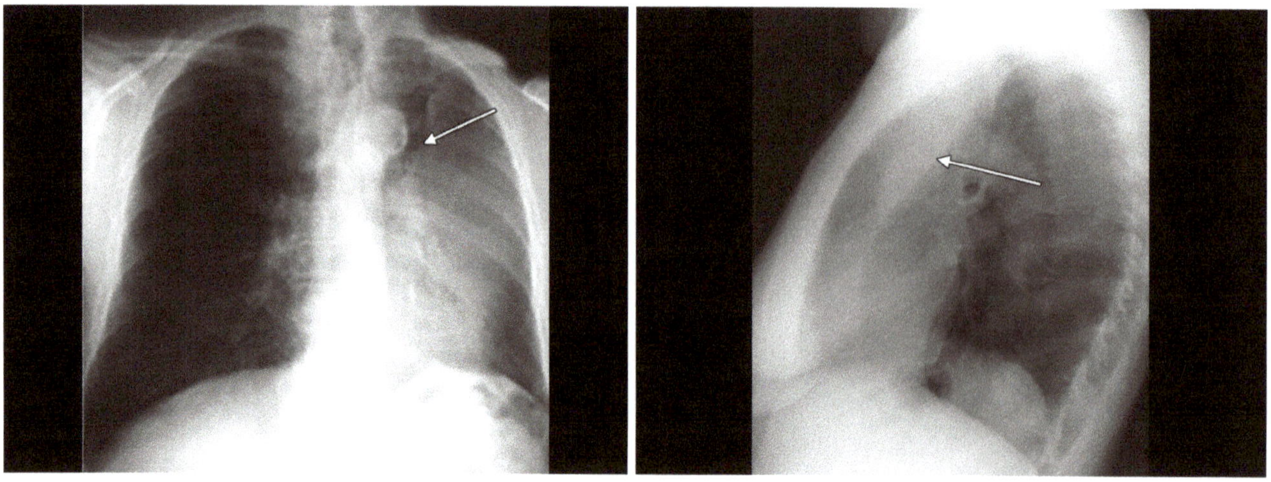

Fig. 17.61: Luftsichel sign, which occurs with the collapse of the left upper lobe when the left lower lobe migrates superiorly causing a lucency abutting the aorticknuckle due to volume loss. The lucency is related to migration of the right upper lobe herniating across the superior mediastinum.

BIBLIOGRAPHY AND FURTHER READING

1. Abu-Rustum NR, Curtin JP, Burt M, Jones WB. Regression of uterine low-grade smooth-muscle tumors metastatic to the lung after oophorectomy. Obstet Gynecol. 1997;89:850-2.
2. Agrons GA, Rosado-de-Christenson ML, Kirejczyk WM, Conran RM, Stocker JT. Pulmonary inflammatory pseudotumor: radiologic features. Radiology. 1998; 206:511-8.
3. Almadi A, Rami M, Khattala K, Chater L, Harmouch T, Atmani S, et al. Pseudotumeur inflammatoire pulmonaire chez un enfant. J Pediatr Puericulture. 2011;24:69-71.
4. Carney JA, Stratakis CA. Familial paraganglioma and gastric stromal sarcoma: a new syndrome distinct from the Carney triad. Am J Med Genet. 2002;108(2):132-9.
5. Chien-Kuang C, Chia-Ing J, Jian-Shun T, Hsu-Chih H, Pin-Ru C, Yu-Sen L, et al. Inflammatory myofibroblastic tumor of the lung- a case report. J Cardiothorac Surg. 2010;5:55.
6. Craighead JE, Abraham JL, Churg A, Green FH, Kleinerman J, Pratt PC, et al.. The pathology of asbestos-associated diseases of the lungs and pleural cavities: diagnostic criteria and proposed grading schema. Report of the Pneumoconiosis Committee of the College of American Pathologists and the National Institute for Occupational Safety and Health. Arch Pathol Lab Med. 1982;106(11):544-96.
7. De boeck K, Willems T, Van gysel D Corbeel L, Eeckels R. Outcome after right middle lobe syndrome. Chest. 1995;108(1):150-2.
8. Engelke C, Schaefer-Prokop C, Schirg E, Freihorst J, Grubnic S, Prokop M. High-resolution CT and CT angiography of peripheral pulmonary vascular disorders. Radiographics. 2002;22(4):739-64.
9. Felson B, Felson H. Localization of intrathoracic lesions by means of the postero-anterior roentgenogram; the silhouette sign. Radiology. 1950;55:363-74.
10. Fraser RG, Peter Paré JA, Paré PD, Fraser RS, Genereux GP, (Eds). Diagnosis of Disease of the Chest, 3rd edition. Philadelphia: WB Saunders; 1999.
11. Hampton AO, Castleman B. "Correlation of postmortem chest teleroentgenograms with autopsy findings". Am J Roentgenol Radium Ther. 1940;34:305-26.
12. Hedlund GL, Navoy JF, Galliani CA, Johnson WH. Aggressive manifestations of inflammatory pulmonary pseudotumor in children. Pediatric Radiol. 1999;29:112-6.
13. Horstmann JP, Pietra GG, Harman JA. Spontaneous regression of pulmonary leiomyomas during pregnancy. Cancer. 1977;39:314-21.
14. Jautzke G, Muller-Ruchholtz E, Thalmann U. Immunohistological detection of estrogen and progesterone receptors in multiple and well differentiated leiomyomatous lung tumors in women with uterine leiomyomas. Pathol Res Pract. 1996;192:215-23.
15. Khan AN, Al-Jahdali HH, Irion KL, Arabi M, Koteyar SS. Solitary pulmonary nodule: A diagnostic algorithm in the light of current imaging technique. Avicenna J Med. 2011;1(2):39-51.
16. Knollmann FD, Hummel M, Hetzer R, Felix R. CT of heart transplant recipients: spectrum of disease. Radiographics. 2000:20:1637-48.
17. Knollmann FD, Mäurer J, Bechstein WO, Vogl TJ, Neuhaus P, Felix R. Pulmonary disease in liver transplant recipients. Spectrum of CT features, Acta Radiol. 2000;41:230-6.
18. Lipton JH, Fong TC, Burgess KR. Miliary pattern as presentation of leiomyomatosis of the lung. Chest. 1987;91:781-2.
19. Maile CW, Rodan BA, Godwin JD, Chen JT, Ravin CE. Calcification in pulmonary metastases. Br J Radiol. 1982;55:108-13.
20. Maschmeyer G. Pneumonia in febrile neutropenic patients: radiographic diagnosis. Curr Opin Oncol. 2001;13:229-35.
21. Miller WT, Gefter WB, Miller WT. Asbestos-related chest diseases: plain radiographic findings. Semin Roentgenol. 1992;27(2):102-20.
22. Miller WT. Diagnostic thoracic imaging. McGraw-Hill Professional. 2006.
23. Narla LD, Newman B, Spottswood SS, Narla S, Kolli R. Inflammatory pseudotumor. RadioGraphics. 2003;23:719-29. Erratum in: RadioGraphics. 2003;23:1702.
24. Ochs K, Hoksch B, Frey U, Schmid RA. Inflammatory myofibroblastic tumour of the lung in a five-year-old girl. Interact Cardiovasc Thorac Surg. 2010;10(5):805-6.
25. Pinillaa I, Herreroa Y, Torresa MI, Nistalb M, Pardoa M. Tumor inflamatorio miofibroblástico pulmonary. Radiologa. 2007;49:53-5.
26. Platt OS, Brambilla DJ, Rosse WF, Milner PF, Castro O, Steinberg MH, et al. Mortality in sickle cell disease. Life expectancy and risk factors for early death. N Engl J Med. 1994;330:1639-44.
27. Reed JC. Chest radiology, plain film patterns and differential diagnoses. Mosby. 1997.
28. Samuels T, Kerenyi N, Hamilton P. Cystosarcoma phylloides: calcified pulmonary metastases detected by computed tomography. Can Assoc Radiol J. 1990;41:217-8.
29. Shin MS, Fulmer JD, Ho KJ. Unusual computed tomographic manifestations of benign metastasizing leiomyomas as cavitary nodular lesions or interstitial lung disease. Clin Imaging. 1996;20:45-9.
30. Thomas AN, Pattison C, Serjeant GR. Causes of death in sickle-cell disease in Jamaica. Br Med J (Clin Res Ed). 1982;285:633-5.
31. Ward S, Heyneman L, Lee MJ, Leung AN, Hansell DM, Müller NL. Accuracy of CT in the diagnosis of allergic bronchopulmonary aspergillosis in asthmatic patients. Am J Roentgenology. AJR Am J Roentgenol. 1999;173(4): 937-42.
32. Webb WR, Higgins CB. Thoracic Imaging: Pulmonary and Cardiovascular Radiology. Philadelphia: Lippincott Williams and Wilkins; 2010.
33. Wolff M, Silva F, Kaye G. Pulmonary metastases (with admixed epithelial elements) from smooth muscle neoplasms. Report of nine cases, including three males. Am J Surg Pathol. 1979;3:325-42.
34. Zhang Y, Dong ZJ, Zhi XY, Liu L, Hu M. Inflammatory myofibroblastic tumor in lung with osteopulmonary arthropathy. Chin Med J (Engl). 2009;122(24):3094-6.

Chapter

18 Chest Computed Tomography for the Evaluation of Respiratory Diseases

Maria Bellia, Claudio Sorino, Mario Spatafora, Fabio Cannizzaro, Ali Nawaz Khan, Vincenzo Bellia

INTRODUCTION

In modern medicine, the comprehension of the relationship between the structure and the function of each body component may be considered as the foundation of any progress.

In particular, the assessment of structural changes of the respiratory system and the related alterations in function represents a fundamental approach to the clinical work-up and the ensuing clinical decisions. However, until recently the practical and extensive application of this approach has been hampered by the poor availability and limited acceptability of gold-standard methods, i.e. the invasive techniques aimed at providing tissue diagnosis.

Radiology has long been a partial response to this open question since it was able to provide gross morphological data, susceptible only of subjective and, at best, semiquantitative interpretation. In recent decades, the technical improvements in both hardware and software for acquisition and processing of images lead to a dramatic progress of imaging techniques. This has allowed a noticeable increase in diagnostic yield of the full spectrum of imaging techniques, which include digital radiography and *high-resolution computer tomography (HRCT)*. These procedures are instrumental in not only obtaining richer images in morphological details but also quantifying lung morphology and the various types of damage in a highly reproducible fashion.

The introduction of improved techniques of image analysis, pattern recognition, tomographic densitometry and morphometric assessment of airway alterations has radically modified the approach to a wide spectrum of respiratory disorders, including lung cancer, *chronic obstructive pulmonary disease (COPD)* and *diffuse lung parenchymal diseases (DLPD)*. Advances in CT have changed the "rules of the game", anticipating and refining the judgment at various steps, with obvious positive outcomes in terms of effectiveness, safety and acceptability of therapeutic strategies.

The present chapter will provide an account on some of the most important and updated applications of chest CT. The content of this chapter must be considered as complementary with other chapters of this book as concerns the role of CT in its relationship with the still valuable 2-projections chest radiography, in the study of the pulmonary arteries (*CT pulmonary angiography*), and in the anatomical and functional assessment of airways.

EVOLUTION OF CT AND APPLICATIONS TO THE RESPIRATORY TRACT

The history of CT follows the contemporary evolution of the complex techniques for image capturing, mainly aimed at obtaining a substantial reduction in acquisition time and an increase in spatial resolution. This evolution, started in the last decades of the 20th century, has been favored by the unexpectedly fast progress in electronic computational machines. It resulted in the computer breakthrough that has characterized the most recent years in terms of increase of velocity and complexity of elaboration. The wealth of data made available in this way resulted in the development of very effective post-processing and reconstruction of images.

In its early days, CT was a technique of sequential acquisition of transverse slices: images could be generated only on the axial plane and suffered two major quality limitations: firstly poor definition of details and secondly breathing-related artifacts. The introduction of spiral CT scanning was a major step forward, since it allowed faster acquisition and better quality image reconstructions along different planes, selected on the basis of diagnostic needs. Successively, dual slice spiral opened the way to the development of *multidetector CT (MDCT)* through the introduction of four-slice scanners, soon followed by systems of increasing complexity up to 128 detector arrays and over.

In comparison with conventional CT, MDCT has proved advantageous in terms of shorter scan duration, longer scan range and thinner collimation. With faster scans, procedures have become simpler, as in the case of CT angiography, for which the quantity of contrast medium needed for the opacification of the vascular bed has been reduced. In addition, artifacts due to breathing movements have been reduced to a minimum. As a consequence from the rich data volume, it is now possible to obtain different reconstructions on various section planes [*multiplanar reformations (MPR)*] to fulfill specific diagnostic needs, and excellent three-dimensional (3D) displays have become possible (Fig. 18.1).

The success of CT in the study of respiratory system lies in the anatomy itself of the respiratory structures. The respiratory system lends itself to easy characterization because of large lung air content, rich and complex vascular network, and well-differentiated tissues in terms of density values, with ease of measurement of air, bone, fluid and fat.

These well-defined contrasts make CT very effective in identifying various normal and abnormal components of lungs, pleura and mediastinum, showing the details of the shape, contours, and content of structures as well as their relationship with the other anatomical components placed nearby, without any superimposition (Figs. 18.2A to F).

Such a result is achieved by means of various techniques of multiplanar reconstruction, which give the

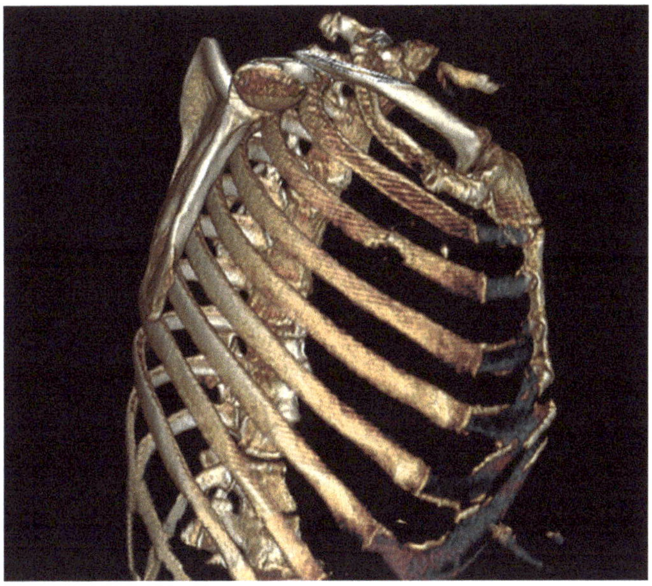

Fig. 18.1: Three-dimensional display of the rib cage, based on multiplanar reconstruction of CT data. The neoplastic erosion on the inferior aspect of the third right rib is clearly recognizable.

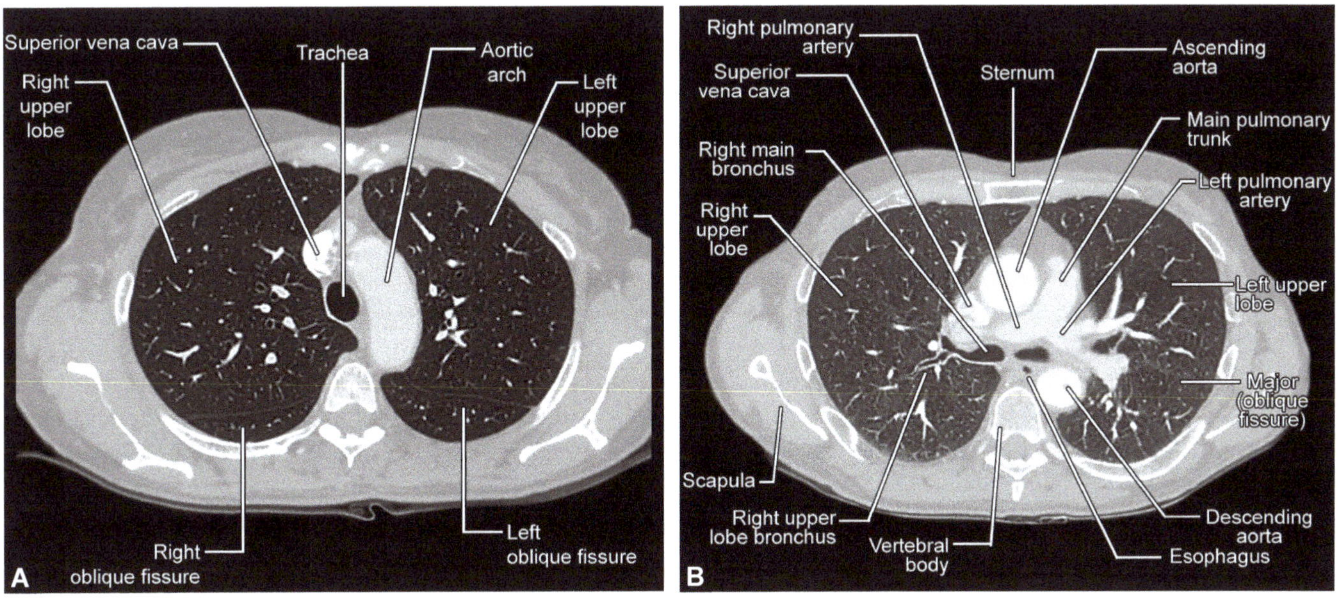

Figs. 18.2A and B

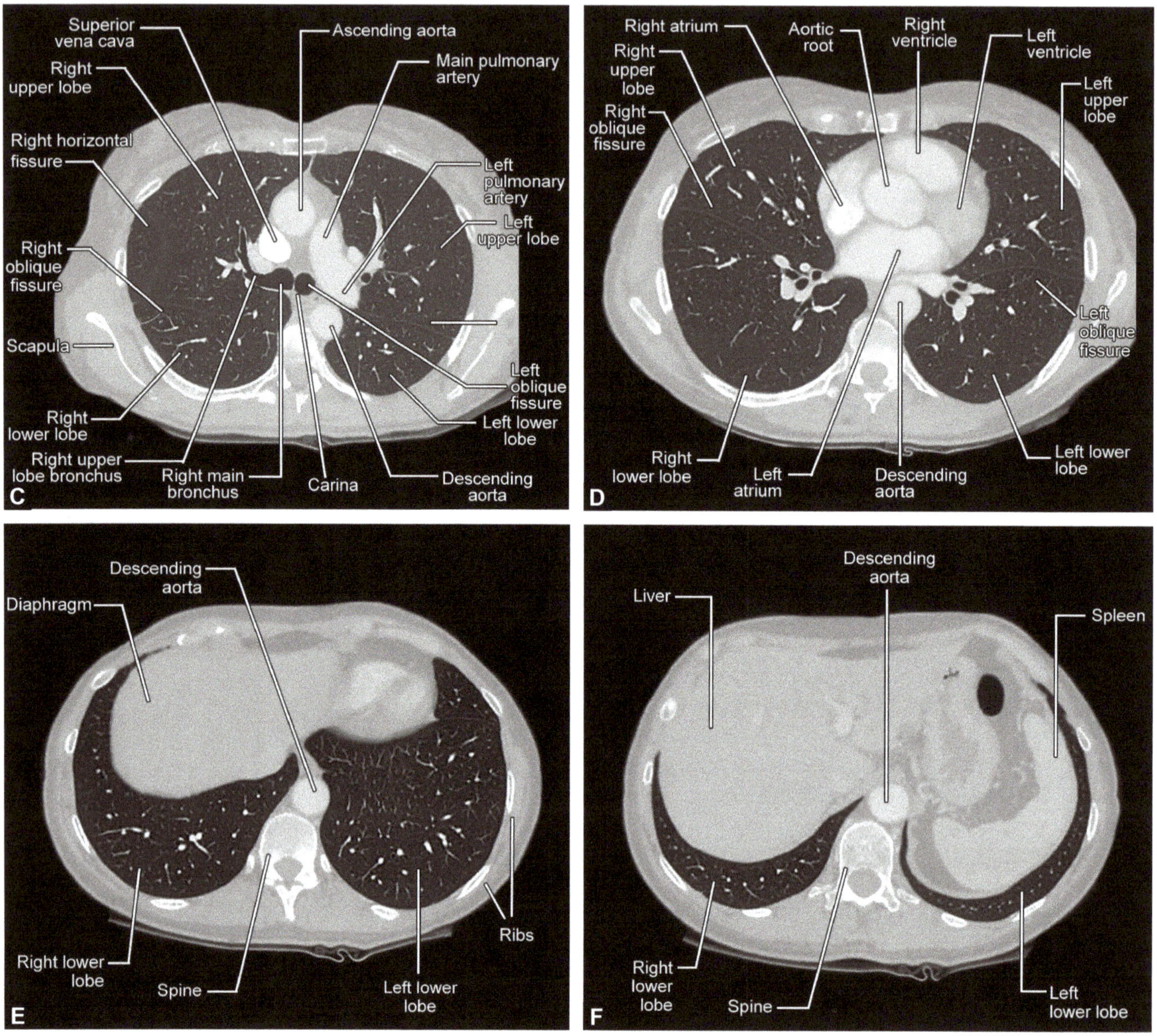

Figs. 18.2A to F: Axial CT scans showing normal anatomy in great detail at different levels.

possibility of changing the axial perspective into a sagittal and coronal one (Figs. 18.3A to C).

In addition, the spiral technique, by providing the acquisition of an entire region into a single set of data, allows 3D representation, particularly advantageous for the study of the mediastinum and for virtual bronchoscopy (*see* below).

The foundation of diagnostic application of CT in the respiratory system is the capacity of discriminating different tissues on the account of relevant densities. Density of soft tissues is extended over a narrow range of the full spectrum, i.e. between 10 and 90 *Hounsfield Units (HU)*; this range is very far from the density of air, placed at -1,000 HU. In this condition it is also possible to select a "window", i.e. a restricted range of density as close as possible to the mean density featured by the tissues under examination. By setting an adequate window, i.e. by selecting and applying appropriate parameters of representation, it is possible to obtain images differentiated on the basis of the anatomical structures to be evaluated, namely pulmonary parenchyma on one hand and mediastinum with its content on the other (Figs. 18.4A to C).

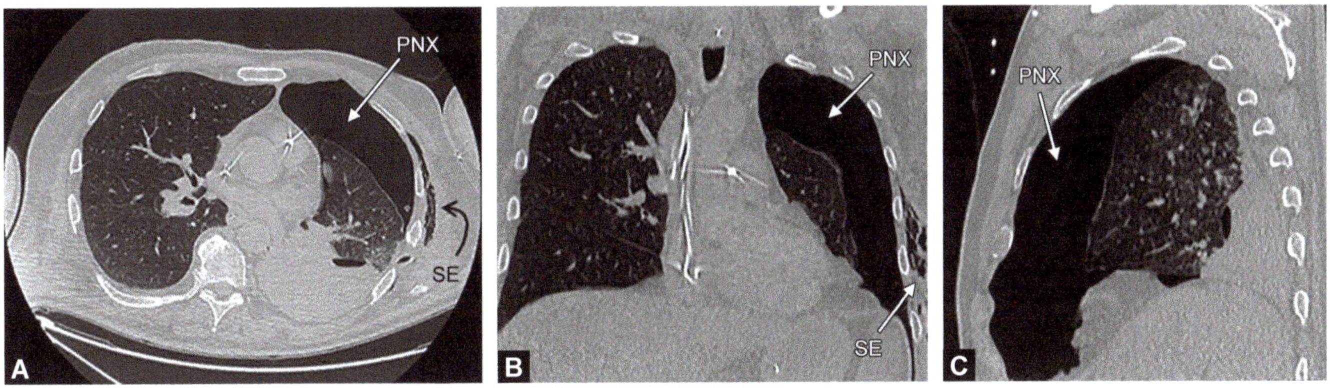

Figs. 18.3A to C: Multiplanar reconstruction of chest CT in a patient with traumatic pneumothorax (PNX) associated with subcutaneous emphysema (SE). (A) Transverse (or axial) plane. (B) Coronal (or frontal) plane. (C) Sagittal plane.

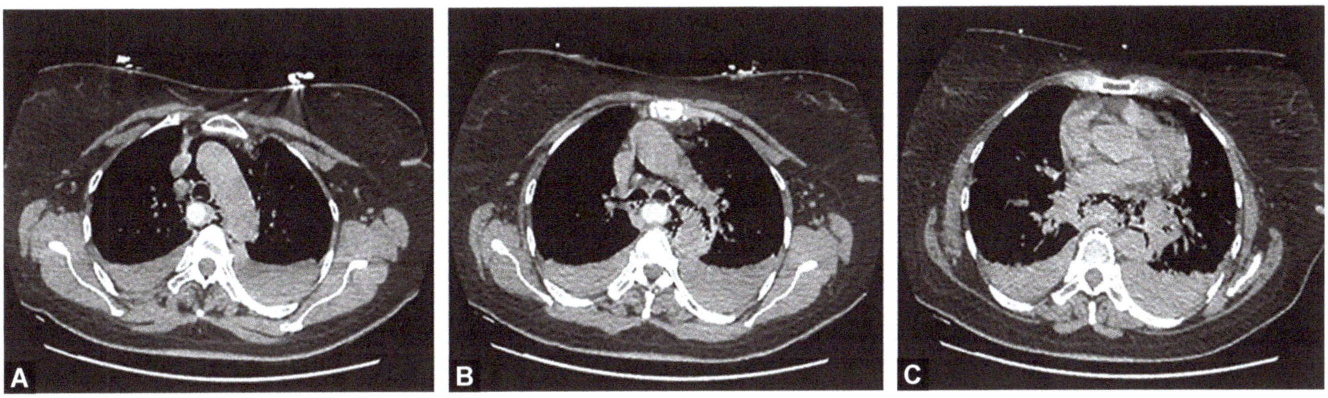

Figs. 18.4A to C: Soft tissue window of chest CT showing extraluminal gas within the mediastinum (pneumomediastinum or mediastinal-emphysema) at different levels.

Parenchymal window application allows the representation of lung fields as a background of uniform density corresponding to the air content, with the superimposed network of vascular markings.

A careful examination of the peripheral lung fields observed at high resolution (HR), i.e. on thin thickness sections, allows the identification of a fundamental anatomical structure, the *secondary pulmonary lobule*: it represents the basic element of the organization of the lung parenchyma, as well as the cornerstone for the interpretation of HRCT. The secondary lobule is the smallest lung unit that is surrounded by connective tissue septa. The lobule measures about 1–2 cm and includes 5–15 pulmonary acini, which, in turn, are composed of the gas exchanging structures of parenchyma, i.e. the alveoli. Air supply to the lobule is provided by a small bronchiole (*terminal bronchiole*) in the center of the structure that is paralleled by the centrilobular artery. Pulmonary veins and lymphatics run in the periphery of the lobule, close to the interlobular septa. The latter can be recognized as thin lines of uniform thickness, 2–3 cm long, better identified in the peripheral areas of the lungs. There are two lymphatic systems draining from the lobule: a central network, that is placed toward the center of the lobule, along the bronchovascular bundle, and a peripheral one, that is located within the interlobular septa and along the pleural linings. The full knowledge of this architecture is a key element for understanding the various routes and the modalities through which various lung diseases develop (*see* below).

Furthermore, the awareness of the complex organization of lung periphery, as ensured by CT, is the basis for the comprehension of the circulatory component of respiratory disorders. With the enhancement due to intravenous injection of contrast media, vessels may be optimally identified and followed along the route to their own territory of blood supply. In addition, contrast-enhanced imaging provides evidence of abnormal angiogenetic growth on the sites of neoplastic invasion. CT also plays a fundamental role in lung cancer staging, by allowing the assessment of the hila and mediastinum including the status of vascular and extravascular components. In this setting CT is very useful to detect enlarged lymph nodes, which in diagnostic protocols are assumed as reliable evidence of lymphatic spreading (*see* below).

Another very fruitful application of CT is for the study of pleural space, in particular for detection of irregularities, thickening areas, plaques, and fluid collection, to be differentiated from masses in adjacent parenchyma and from organized pleural tissue (Figs. 18.5 to 18.7).

Computed tomography is also very valuable in detecting and studying sites of reduced density compatible with the occurrence of air collections, allowing a differential diagnosis from parenchymal areas of reduced attenuation due to hyperinflation.

MAIN INDICATIONS

Because of the high contrast offered by the very large air content, lungs and respiratory diseases may be regarded as the ideal area of application of radiologic methods for diagnostic purposes. This statement, valid since the early introduction of plain radiograph, is even more appropriate in the era of CT.

The latter has become the reference diagnostic method in manifold fields, although in consideration of cost, time expenditure and risk due to exposure to X-rays, CT cannot

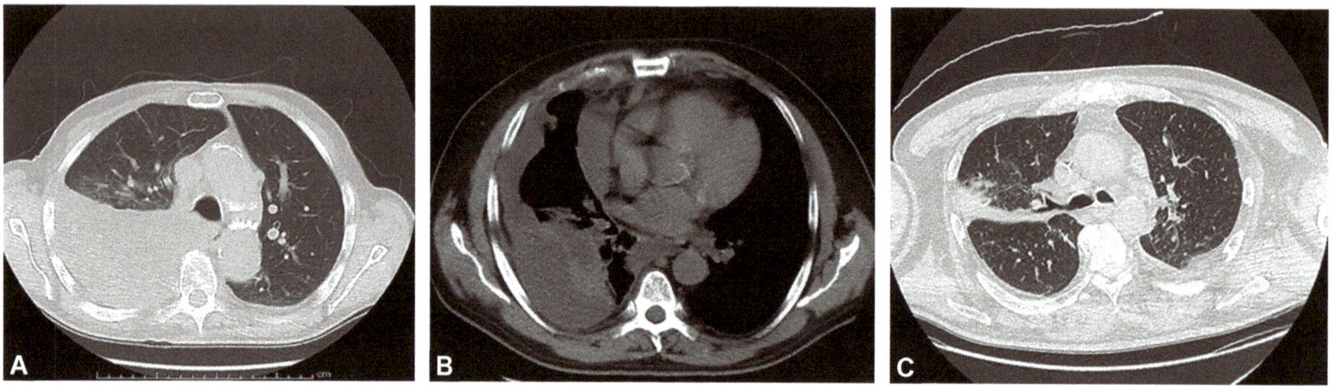

Figs. 18.5A to C: Application of CT in pleural diseases. (A) Right free-flowing pleural effusion. (B) Right loculated pleural effusion. (C) Right intrascissural pleural effusion.

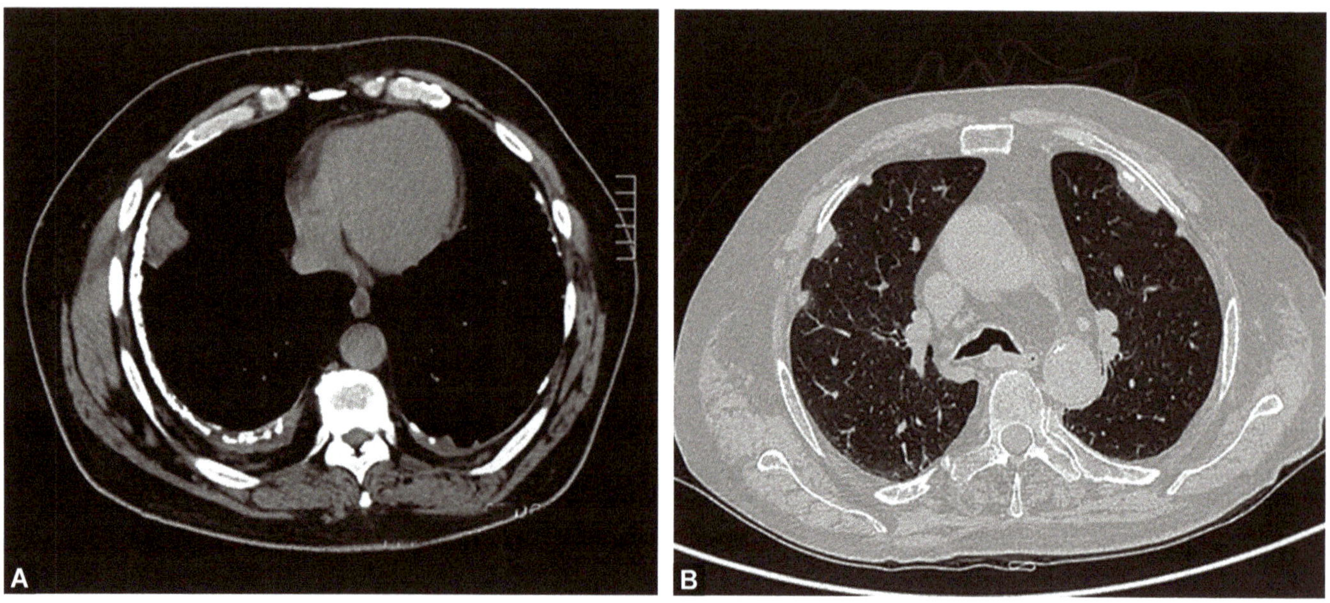

Figs. 18.6A and B: Application of CT in pleural diseases. Irregularities, thickening areas and diffuse calcifications on the pleural contour. Pleural plaques are deposits of hyalinized collagen fibers in the parietal pleura and may be calcified or not. They can be benign sequelae of pleural inflammation and are by far the most common indication of significant exposure to asbestos.

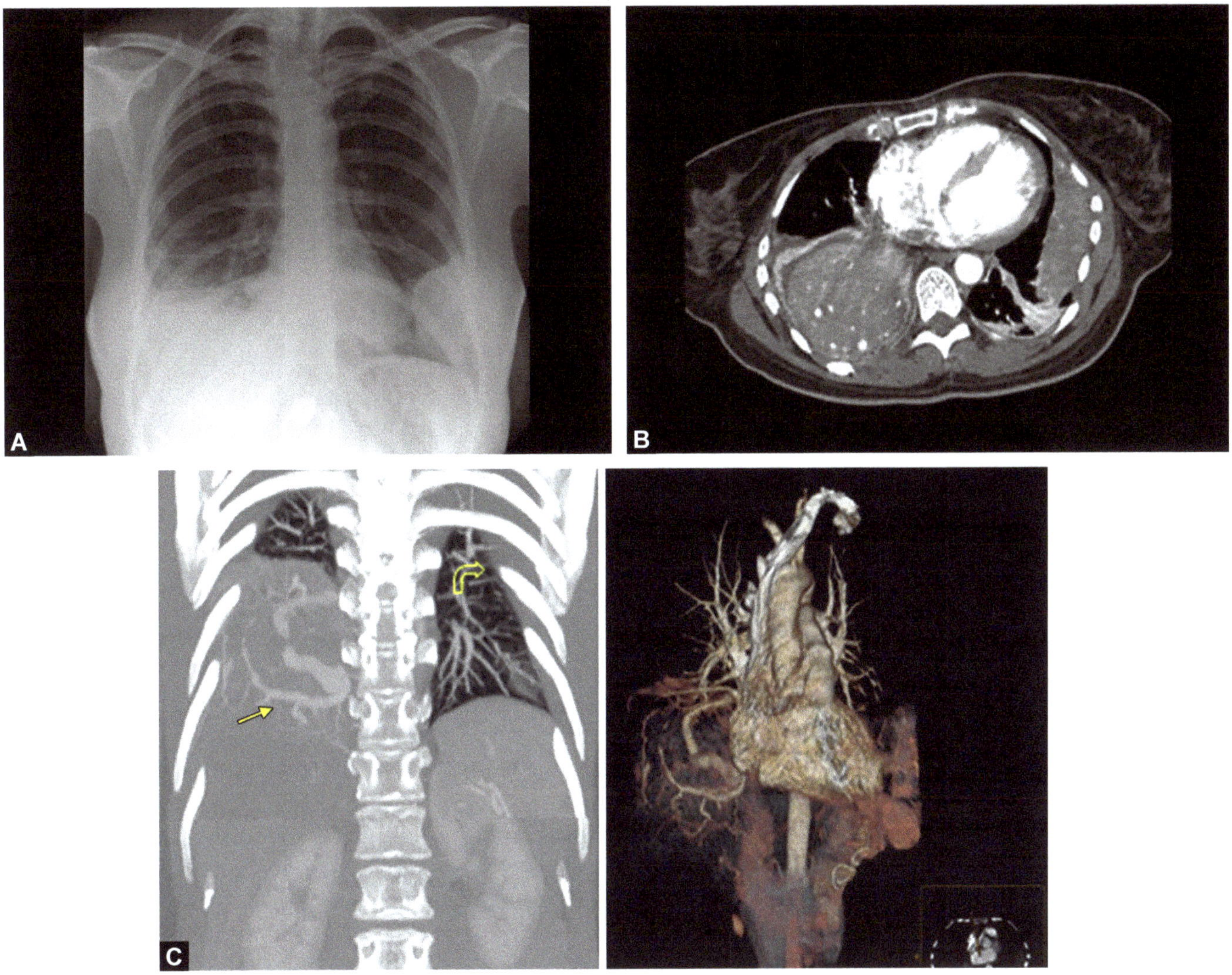

Figs. 18.7A to C: Series of images of 26-year-old woman that presented with cough. (A) Chest X-ray shows a pleural based mass at the left costophrenic angle and a right basal opacity not reliably characterized (suspected pleural effusion). (B) Axial chest CT scan shows a pleural effusion along the left lower chest wall and a solid enhancing mass at the right lung base associated with a small pleural effusion at the costophrenic angle. (C) Coronal reconstruction and a 3D depiction show anomalous pulmonary venous drainage right lower lobe and a solid mass at the right lung base in keeping with a sequestrated lung segment. The diagnosis was confirmed at surgery.

be considered as an all-purpose procedure: conversely, whenever based on precise indications, the yield of the technique is such as to warrant the relatively high cost-benefit ratio. Such a proper indication is most often based on a clinical history addressing respiratory apparatus, along with abnormal findings at two-projection radiography. Modern equipment with short scanning times (2–5 seconds) and the use of thin sections compare favorably with standard radiography as far as the examination of mediastinum and parenchyma are concerned.

In a limited group of diseases, CT may be virtually diagnostic, particularly if correlated to a compatible clinical picture, as in the case of idiopathic pulmonary fibrosis (Fig. 18.8).

Similarly, diagnosis may be based solely on CT in the case of bronchiectasis. In fact, CT has replaced bronchography as the gold standard for the diagnosis of this disease (Figs. 18.9A and B).

Conversely in others, like in parenchymal masses, although nonspecific, CT result proves to be a reliable foundation for the choice of the most effective further diagnostic steps.

In a restricted number of cases, CT is indicated in spite of a negative result of standard radiography in two projections. This may occur in case of blood or atypical/neoplastic cells in sputum or when the location of a primary tumor is searched for in patients with evidence of extrathoracic metastasis.

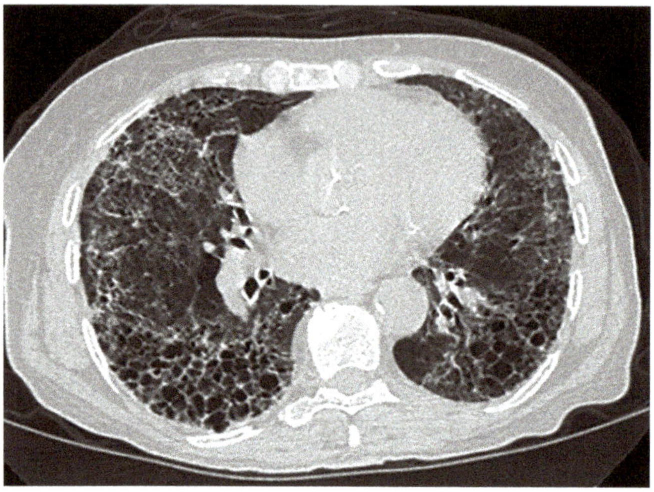

Fig. 18.8: Computed tomography appearance in a full blown picture of idiopathic pulmonary fibrosis. The heterogeneous combination of reticular opacities, often associated with traction bronchiectasis, honeycombing and ground-glass opacities, identifies the "usual interstitial pattern" (UIP) that is virtually diagnostic for the disease.

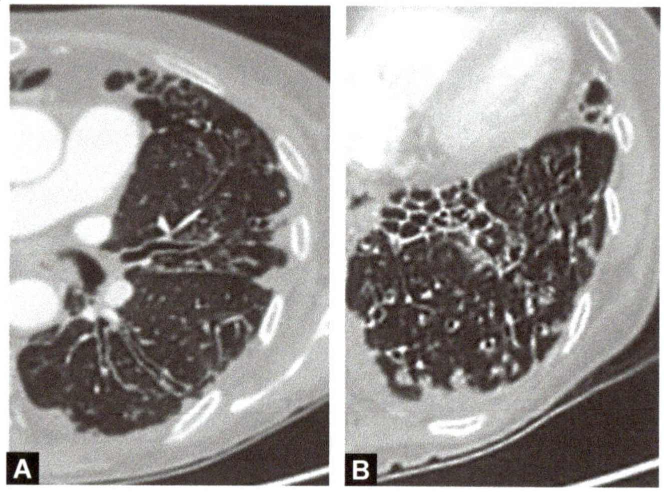

Figs. 18.9A and B: Bronchiectasis in the left lung. (A) In the proximal regions they are cylindrical and occur with a lack of bronchial tapering. (B) At the base of the lung they are cystic and have a honeycomb appearance.

APPLICATIONS TO LUNG CANCER

General Aspects

Lung neoplasms are the leading cause of death from cancer. Malignant neoplastic diseases of the lungs represent an increasingly common medical and social problem: its incidence is closely related to chronic exposure to tobacco smoke and to various environmental and occupational pollutants. Lung cancer is classified into two categories: *small cell lung cancer (SCLC)* and *non-small cell lung cancer (NSCLC)*.

The expression NSCLC is used to indicate a group of primary lung neoplasms (adenocarcinoma, squamous cell carcinoma, and large cell carcinoma) that share the same evolution pattern and the same responsiveness to treatment, including the possibility to be submitted to curative resection if diagnosed at an early stage. For these reasons cancers belonging to the NSCLC group can be staged according to the same staging system, namely the American Joint Committee on Cancer (AJCC) staging system. It is identified by the acronym TNM that refers to three variables: T for size and location of primary tumor, N for level of neoplastic spread to lymph nodes, M for the occurrence of metastases.

Small cell lung cancer accounts for 20–25% of pulmonary neoplasms: most often (70–80%) it has a central location. In comparison with NSCLC it is characterized by more severe aggression capacity with frequent and early metastases; in addition it carries a higher risk of paraneoplastic syndrome. For these reasons a diagnosis or suspicion of SCLC implies most invariably the prescription of CT investigations. In general they will be guided by signs and symptoms, as usual. However, the awareness of the high incidence of early aggression of distant organs (in particular brain, bones, and abdomen) often prompts the request of CT studies also in asymptomatic or minimally symptomatic patients. On this basis the staging system of SCLC is kept apart and pragmatically simplified with respect to NSLC. It divides SCLC into limited and extensive stage. The former refers to the possibility of applying radiotherapy by a single radiation field. Conversely the expression "extensive stage" refers to the widespread of tumor mono or bilaterally or at distance, preventing the applicability of limited field radiotherapy.

The poor outcome of lung cancer has been related to the fact that it is most often diagnosed at an advanced stage when no curative treatment is available anymore. The natural history of the disease may be heterogeneous, but in general the early presentation is marked by minor and non specific symptoms, with the consequence of high risk of late diagnosis or misdiagnosis.

In the field of lung malignancies CT plays a pivotal role practically in all the steps of diagnostic itinerary: actually with different modalities it is indicated in the screening for early detection of suspect opacities, as well as for diagnosis of alternative presentations of lung cancer, for staging of the disease and in the assessment of the response to treatments and for the monitoring for possible tumor recurrences or metastases.

For this reason extending, refining and optimizing the use of CT in the approach to thoracic neoplasms represent the most promising challenge for CT-based imaging techniques.

Central and Peripheral Lesions

From a topographic point of view, lung neoplasms may be divided into two large subsets, i.e. central and peripheral, on the basis of the location of neoplastic growth, as it appears according to the evidence produced by imaging investigations.

Peripheral neoplasms are often characterized by round shape, uneven contours with irregular extensions to surrounding parenchyma, dishomogeneities in attenuation: CT, also by means of multiplanar reconstruction, allows an accurate assessment of dimensions as well as of the anatomical relationship with proximal structures, including pleura, fissures, mediastinum and chest wall. In addition, it is possible to detect the occurrence of alterations in the blood supply of the mass, in particular if characterized by larger dimensions. This is due to irregularities in angiogenesis which are a frequent feature of neoplastic growth; these irregularities may result in necrosis with evidence of excavation. Conversely, in peripheral neoplasms of little dimensions, the density is usually homogeneous, and necrotic phenomena within the mass are absent or hardly distinguishable.

At CT central masses may develop either intraluminally, as endobronchial lesions (Figs. 18.10 and 18.11) or infiltrating and thickening the bronchial wall; alternatively the prevailing growth from the primary bronchial lesion is in extraluminal direction, possibly involving outer structures and, in particular lymph nodes. In these circumstances patency may be limited by compression exerted by the extrinsic growth of cancer or by enlarged nodes.

However determined, a reduction of patency of affected bronchus ensues and may progress up to the complete occlusion, with the unavoidable consequence of lack of ventilation of the parenchymal area for which the interested airway is tributary. On this basis central masses, independently of their intrinsic dimensions, if occluding the lumen, are often responsible for the occurrence of important complications including atelectasis and obstructive pneumonitis.

Screening with Low-Dose CT

As concerns screening procedures, the attention is focused on the use of low-dose radiation in order to ensure a reasonable degree of safety and consequently the possibility of repeating the test either at regular time intervals or whenever needed, on the basis of individual characteristics.

Screening the general population by means of standard chest radiography does not reduce mortality from lung cancer but implies a high risk of false-positive findings. Conversely the National Lung Screening Trial (NLST) pointed out that mortality due to lung cancer may be reduced by 20% among individuals at high risk, undergoing

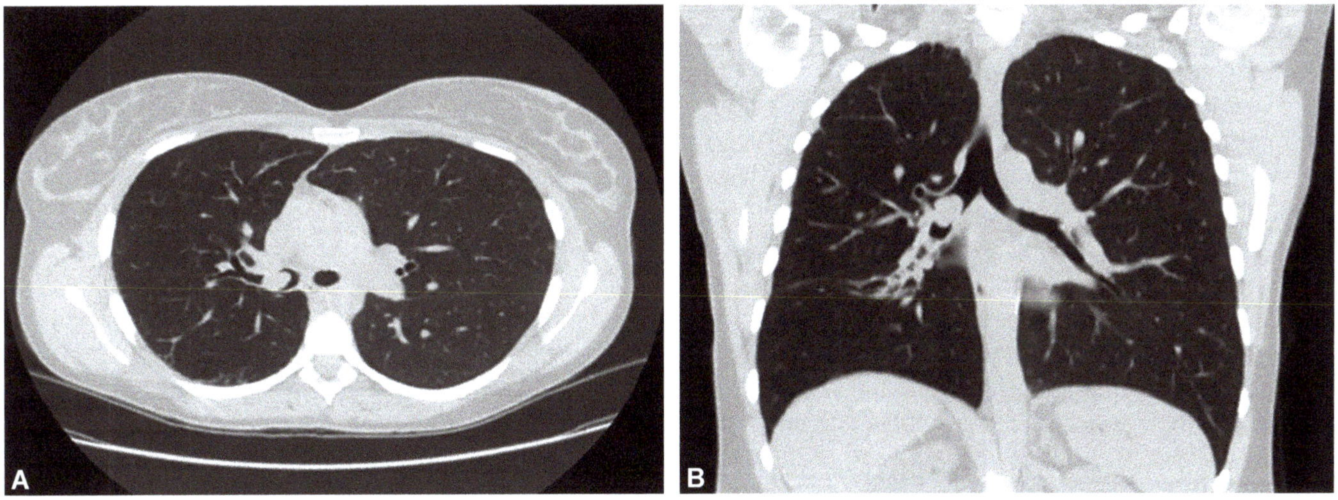

Figs. 18.10A and B: Hyperattenuating nodule within the right main bronchus. (A) Transverse plane. (B) Frontal plane. This finding suggested a lung carcinoid. Histological examination on bronchoscopic biopsy confirmed the diagnosis.

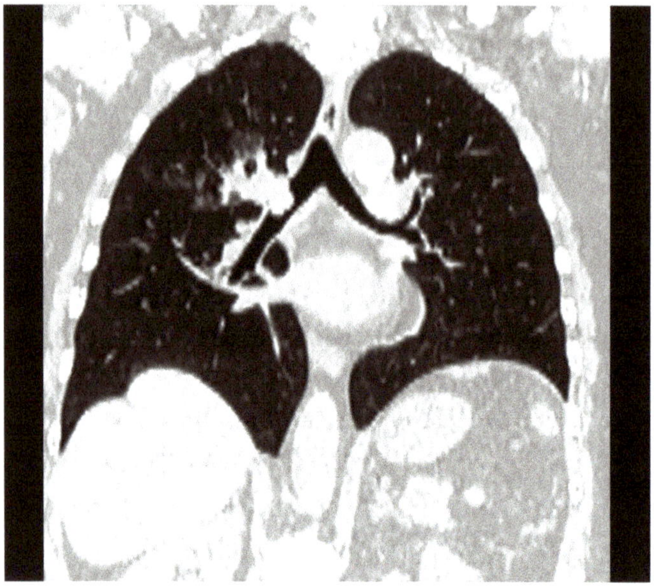

Fig. 18.11: Reconstruction of a frontal projection in a case of carcinoma of the right lung: The endoluminal growth of the tumor is made evident.

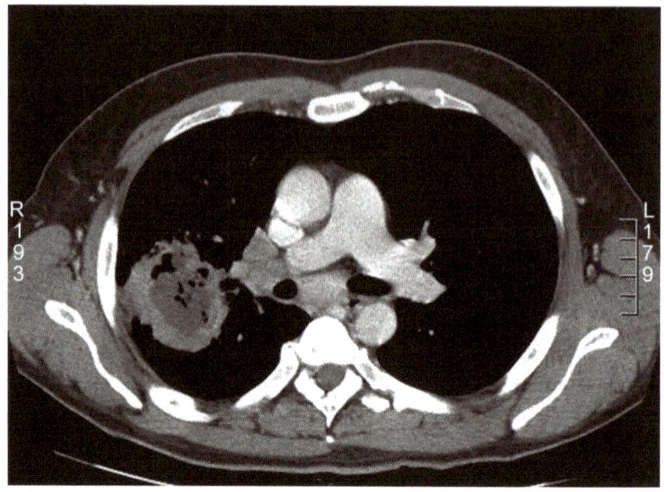

Fig. 18.12: Computed tomography shows a large neoplastic mass of the right lung. Different densities, recognizable within the structure of the mass, refer to the presence of colliquation and necrosis of neoplastic tissue.

low-dose CT. These findings represented a milestone on the way toward extensive screening programs and have been incorporated in lung cancer screening guidelines.

However, many questions remain unsolved and important studies are under the way as concerns the feasibility and cost-effectiveness of such projects for most national health services. In particular, studies are being carried out aimed at the optimization of these outcomes through the assessment of CT-derived predictors of malignancy: They include, amongst others, the size of the lesion, the spiculation of contours, the location in upper lobes, the close proximity to scarred parenchymal areas, the evidence of a necrotic area within the context (Fig. 18.12).

As a counterpart of undoubted benefits, low-dose CT screening carries a risk of adverse effects: they include false-positive results in about 20% of patients, while a portion of CT discovered nodules as high as 90% are false-positives. This implies an enormous waste of money, along with the risk connected with the application of unwarranted invasive diagnostic procedures, including repeated irradiation. On this basis the harm-benefit ratio of lung cancer screening with low-dose CT remains the object of an open debate and in particular there is still insufficient evidence to support its application in individuals with no signs or symptoms suggestive of lung cancer. Conversely evidence available so far supports low-dose CT screening only within randomized clinical trials, for people who meet the criteria for the NLST, i.e. current or former smokers, aged 55–74 years, with an adequate smoking history and no history of lung cancer.

Staging

Integrated by observations carried out after contrast enhancement, CT represents the cornerstone of the noninvasive staging procedures for lung cancer (clinical staging cTNM). The latter are aimed at confirming or excluding the resectability of the neoplasm, basing this judgment on the scalar modifications of three radiologic descriptors, namely T for the characteristics of the primary tumor mass, N for the presence of enlarged lymph nodes and M for the evidence of metastasis. A nonresectable disease is qualified by the detection of either a T4 or N3 or M1 factor. The various combinations of alterations for each TNM descriptor result in TNM subsets that, in turn, are grouped into certain stages; the latter correspond to patients who share similar prognostic and therapeutic options.

In general CT proves a very reliable tool when it is used for the assessment of the T factor of TNM classification by measuring the dimensions of the mass and the extension of area affected by atelectasis (Fig. 18.13) or by superimposed pneumonitis. Conversely diagnostic yield of CT shows definite limitations in the assessment of the involvement of chest wall and of mediastinum, as it is demonstrated by the degree of disagreement between T factor assignment based on CT (cTNM) and the result of staging after surgery (pathological TNM or pTNM).

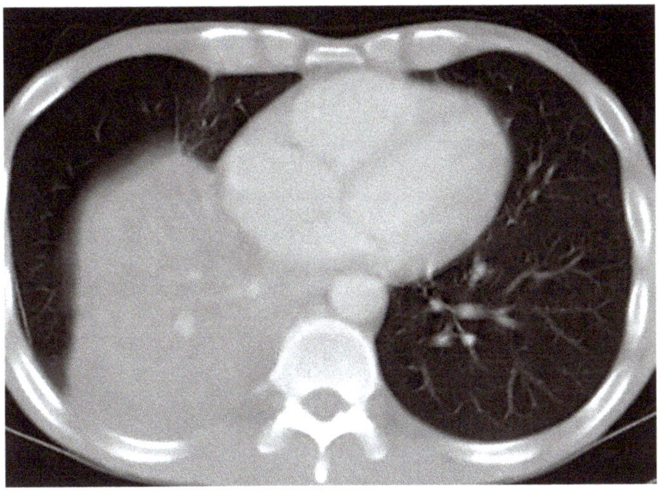

Fig. 18.13: Atelectasis of the right lower lobe.

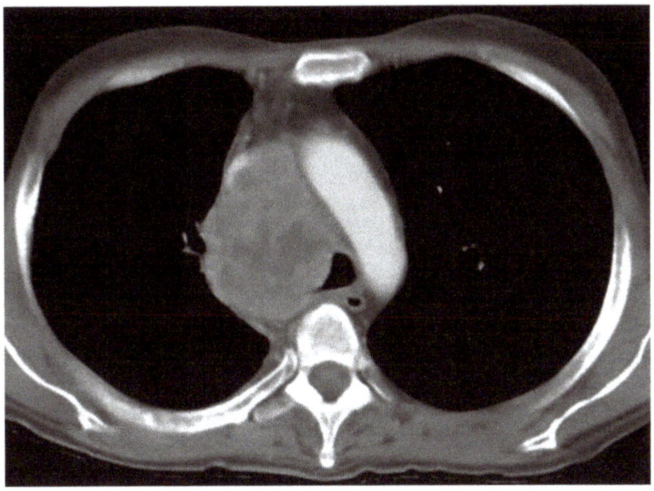

Fig. 18.14: Computed tomography picture (mediastinal window) relevant to multiple enlarged lymph nodes of mediastinum detected as a part of staging procedure in a case of pulmonary carcinoma.

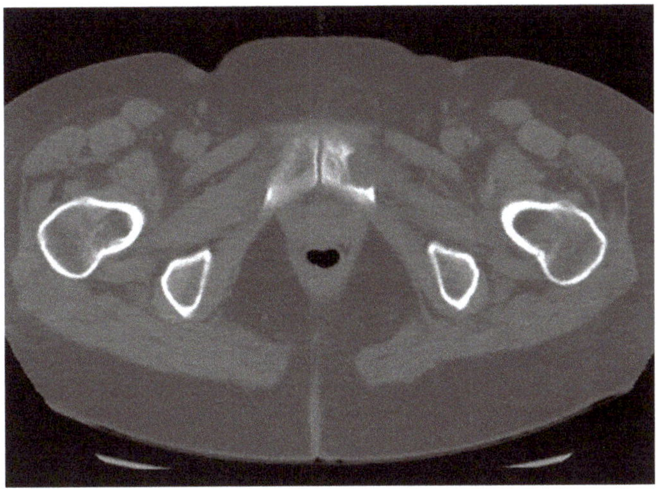

Fig. 18.15: Ischiopubic metastasis of pulmonary carcinoma.

Thoracic CT plays a pivotal role in the assessment of lymph node neoplastic involvement (N factor of TNM classification) (Fig. 18.14). This assessment is diagnosed on the basis of the assumption whereby any increase of dimensions corresponds to neoplastic involvement. Since under normal conditions the diameter of lymph node short axis is lower than 10 mm, the latter value has been assumed as a threshold to distinguish between intact and invaded nodes.

Since positive predictive power of CT slightly exceeds 50%, the finding of enlarged nodes by itself is not sufficient to establish a diagnosis of neoplastic spreading and needs confirmation by alternative procedures. Conversely, negative predictive power of CT is higher than 85%; therefore if CT research of nodes exceeding the threshold fails, it may be assumed as sound evidence in favor of negativity of N factor (cN-) with the relevant consequences upon the indication for surgery.

As far as M factor is concerned, an integrated approach is needed in all cases; CT is an important component that may be particularly useful in diagnosing the metastatic invasion of adrenal glands, pancreas, central nervous system and bones (Fig. 18.15).

In spite of the undoubted merits of CT in the staging process, a cautionary word must be said. In fact CT has important limitations, as demonstrated by the discordance between preoperative predictions based on CT and direct operative assessment in about half the cases, in the direction of both over- and under-staging.

Finally CT plays a fundamental role in the evaluation of outcome after therapy (response or stabilization or progression), according to the RECIST (Response evaluation criteria in solid tumors) criteria and in the follow-up of patient submitted to surgery with curative intent.

Solitary Pulmonary Nodule

Within the wider field of pulmonary opacities to be investigated by CT in order to confirm/exclude a malignancy, the so called *"solitary pulmonary nodule" (SPN)* is at same time a frequent and cumbersome problem. The expression SPN is used to indicate a well-circumscribed round or oval opacity of less than 3 cm in diameter (Figs. 18.16A and B).

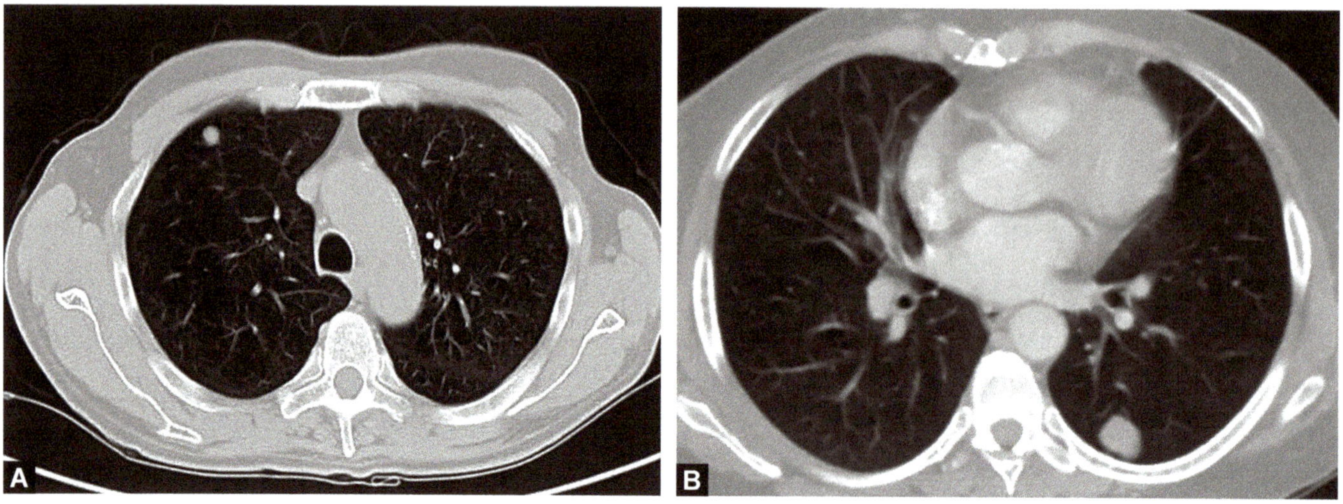

Figs. 18.16A and B: Solitary pulmonary nodule of the (A) upper right lobe and (B) lower left lobe.

To be defined as SPN the nodule must be completely surrounded by parenchyma and not accompanied by lymph node enlargement, atelectasis or pneumonia. Conversely opacities larger than 3 cm in diameter are defined as pulmonary masses and are characterized by a higher likelihood of malignancy.

Paradoxically the problem of SPN has been made more difficult by fast progress of MDCT technology: in fact the extensive use of this technique, along with the use of thin sections and maximum intensity projection reconstructions, has increased the sensitivity so much as to result in a marked increase in the number of detected nodules, at the expense of an excess of falsely positive nodules. In order to limit this risk, criteria for characterization of lung nodules have been agreed upon. Firstly, size is a central issue since increasing diameter of a lung nodule is associated with an increasing risk of cancer. At least 99% of all nodules 4 mm or smaller are benign; when the nodule is below one cm in diameter, the best strategy is surveillance. Shape and margins are also important because in general (but definitely not in all cases) smooth, regular contours increase the probability of benign characteristics, whereas lesions with spiculated margins warrant further investigations and follow-up; nevertheless irregular margins do not exclude benignity, as may be the case for focal areas of pneumonia. Calcification within the structure of nodule suggests a past inflammation healed with deposition of calcium, particularly in case of central, laminated, diffuse or popcorn calcification; conversely eccentric or amorphous calcifications are compatible with a malignant growth, superimposed over (and facilitated by) a scar. Cavitation may occur in malignant nodules as a consequence of irregular and inhomogeneous blood supply due to pathologic angiogenesis within the tumor. However evidence of necrosis by no means excludes benignity of a SPN, since alternative interpretations (infection, vasculitis, infarction) cannot be ruled out. Cavitation is not the only manifestation of irregular proliferation of vessels related to malignant growth. Another manifestation is the increase in contrast enhancement that may occur after intravenous medium injection. Lack of significant contrast enhancement is a highly sensitivity clue to a diagnosis of benign nodules.

A rare and difficult problem concerns subsolid or partly solid nodules, i.e. areas of increased attenuation at CT, that appear mixed in structure, including solid and ground-glass opacity (*see* below). This evidence raises a high suspicion of malignancy. Once defined bronchioloalveolar carcinoma, the tumor possibly underlying this picture was also referred to as pneumonia-like because of peculiar clinical and radiological presentation, mimicking an infectious pathogenesis (Figs. 18.17A and B).

The expression bronchioloalveolar carcinoma has been later abandoned and the neoplasm is now classified as adenocarcinoma in situ. The latter is characterized by a prominent or exclusive lepidic growth pattern, i.e. a growth restricted to neoplastic cells, along preexisting alveolar structures, lacking stroma, vascular or pleural invasion, with no intra-alveolar tumor cells.

Helpful hints toward a reliable differentiation of a malignant nodule from a benign one may come from

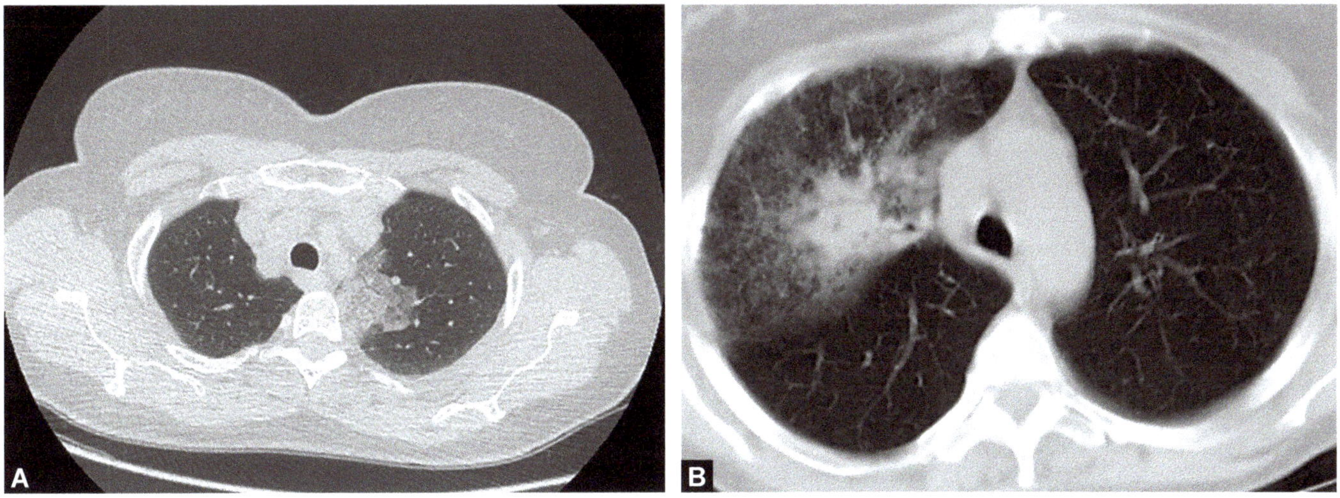

Figs. 18.17A and B: Chest CT showing two cases of adenocarcinoma in situ of (A) the left upper lobe and (B) the right lower lobe, with mixed solid and ground-glass opacity as pneumonia-like appearance.

longitudinal observation upon the dynamics of growth: the absence of any increase in dimensions over a minimum 2-year period, as determined from review of prior chest radiography or (better) of CT, is assumed as a reliable indicator of benignity.

APPLICATIONS TO DIFFUSE PARENCHYMAL LUNG DISEASES

High-resolution CT is the reference imaging method for the study of diffuse infiltrative lung diseases; it has enormously contributed to the long and cumbersome task of classifying this complex range of disorders, differing for pathogenesis and natural history but sharing the involvement of a target structure, the secondary pulmonary lobule (*see* above). In fact the availability of detailed HRCT maps of site and nature of various lesions, integrated by clinical and functional evidences, has reduced to a minimum the need for large dimension lung biopsies previously considered as unavoidable for the pathologic interpretation of chronic interstitial pneumonias. Moreover thin layer CT allows a reliable monitoring of spontaneous evolution or of response to treatment in the minority of cases in which a susceptibility to therapy, whatsoever, may be expected.

Helpful hints to interpretation may derive from the topography of the lesions within the lungs, i.e. with or without dominance in the upper or in the lower portions, in central or in peripheral parts of lung fields. In addition it must be recommended to take careful notice of additional findings, if any: evidence of cavitation, enlarged heart, fluid accumulation in the pleural space, lymphadenopathy, bronchiectasis, cutaneous or systemic involvement may lead to faster and more confident diagnostic interpretations.

Basically, approaching diffuse lung diseases the following types of lesions may be demonstrated as dominant in individual cases:

- Linear or reticular opacities
- Nodular opacities
- Increased pulmonary density (ground glass, consolidation)
- Decreased pulmonary density (emphysema, cysts).

The basic lesions listed before are organized into recognizable and recurrent architectures or patterns, as follows:

Reticular pattern: Already visible at chest radiography, a pattern of reticulation, virtually diagnostic of an interstitial lung disease, may be more clearly seen at thin-section CT. The reticular pattern is characterized by the marked prominence of the interstitial reticulum: it appears as a collection of small linear opacities that, by summation, build up a net. A twofold pathogenesis may be recognized. Firstly it may be caused by the accumulation of fluids or of fibrous tissue, or by infiltration by malignant cells, resulting in a diffuse thickening of the interlobular septa. Septal thickening may be differentiated as smooth or nodular/irregular. The former is usually seen in interstitial pulmonary edema, in lymphangitic spread of neoplasms and in the rarer occurrence of alveolar proteinosis. In the latter and in a few other conditions septal thickening is combined with ground glass opacity (*see* below) in a patchy distribution called "crazy paving" (Fig. 18.18).

Conversely a nodular or irregular thickening of interlobular septa occurs in lymphangitic neoplastic spread, as

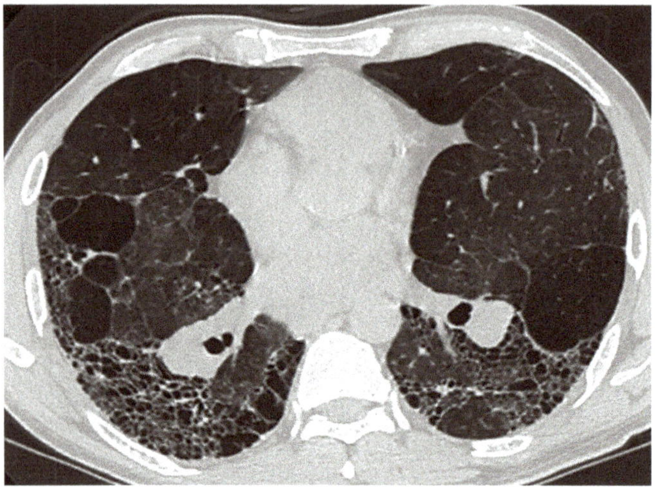

Fig. 18.18: Combination of septal thickening and ground glass opacity (crazy paving) in a case of alveolar proteinosis.

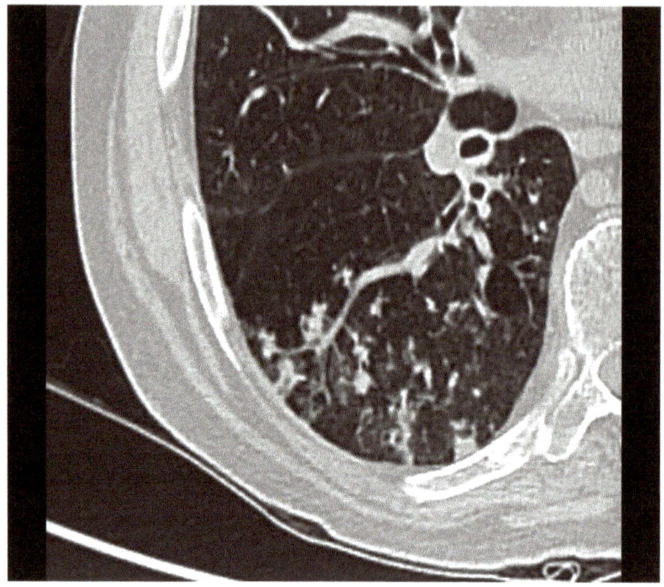

Fig. 18.19: Bronchiole filled with fluid resembling a branching tree with buds in the lower right lobe (tree-in-bud pattern).

well as in sarcoidosis and silicosis. Alternatively a reticular pattern may be the consequence of extensive fibrosis, as it may be observed in usual interstitial pneumonia and in the other diseases that share the end-stage outcome of *honeycomb lung* (*see* below).

Nodular pattern: According to the distribution of nodules over the secondary lobule, the following alternatives patterns of distribution of nodules may be differentiated.

1. *Centrilobular distribution*, i.e. predominantly toward the area located in the central part of the secondary lobule, around the small airways.

   Centrilobular nodules spare the subpleural surface, being typically at least 5–10 mm away from the pleural surfaces. Centrilobular area is usually the site of diseases that enter the lung through the airways (including hypersensitivity pneumonitis, respiratory bronchiolitis, centrilobular emphysema).

   A peculiar arrangement of centrilobular nodules, mostly evident at the periphery of the lungs, is the so-called *tree-in-bud*. This pattern is composed by an irregular and often nodular branching structure, corresponding to centrilobular bronchioles filled by mucous or purulent secretion. As such, it is usually advocated as evidence of spread of infections (e.g. tuberculosis, infected bronchiectasis) (Fig. 18.19).

2. *Perilymphatic distribution*, i.e. toward the peripheral part of the secondary lobule.

   In this case nodules are distributed with a perilymphatic predominance and are recognizable near the fissures and at subpleural level. This is usually the site of diseases that are located in the lymphatics of in the interlobular septa (such as sarcoidosis, lymphangitic carcinomatosis and pulmonary edema) (Fig. 18.20).

   These diseases usually involve also the central network of lymphatics that surround the bronchovascular bundle.

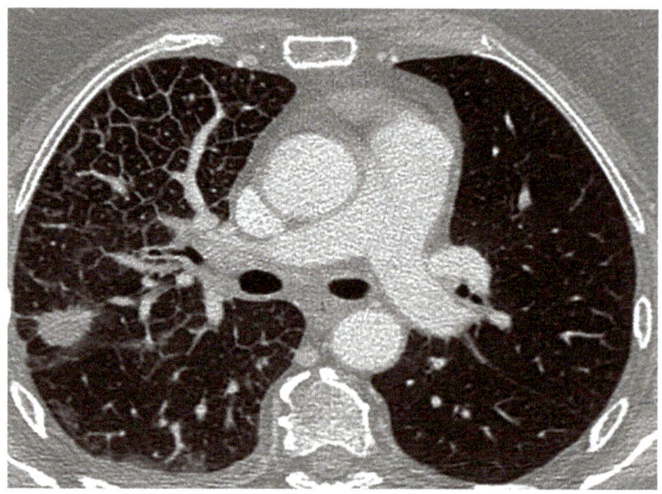

Fig. 18.20: A case of lymphangitic carcinomatosis with prevailing centrilobular distribution of nodules.

3. *Random distribution*, i.e. not showing any particular pattern of involvement with respect to the pulmonary architecture and the secondary pulmonary lobule.

   These nodules affect the fissures, the peribronchovascular structures and the center of the secondary pulmonary nodules without predominance in any of these areas. The random distribution is a result of the hematogenous spread of the offending factor, represented in the most typical cases by infections (e.g. miliary tuberculosis) or cancer (hematogenuous spread of metastases) (Fig. 18.21).

For the sake of differential diagnosis it is worthwhile to notice that sarcoidosis is typically associated with a perilymphatic distribution of nodules; however when the disease becomes very extensive, it tends to spread across the whole structure of lobule, assuming the characteristics of random distribution pattern.

HRCT Features of UIP Pattern

The radiological pattern of usual interstitial pneumonia (UIP) is one of the key features for the diagnosis of idiopathic pulmonary fibrosis (IPF). However, it is not an exclusive finding of IPF, whose diagnosis requires:

- Exclusion of all other possible causes of interstitial lung disease (iatrogenic forms, environmental exposure, connective tissues disease)
- High-resolution CT features of UIP pattern

The lack of histological or cytological data (obtained by a lung biopsy or bronchoalveolar lavage) suggestive of other diseases.

High-resolution CT features of UIP pattern include the following:

- Bilateral reticular opacities, often associated with traction bronchiectasis
- Peripheral and subpleural distribution of the alterations, mainly in the lung bases (though often patchy)
- Cystic lesions with a "honeycomb" appearance.

Absence of features not consistent with the pattern UIP, e.g. predominance of "ground glass", predominant localization to the medium-apical lung fields, numerous small nodules.

Honeycombing is manifested on HRCT as clustered cystic airspaces, typically of comparable diameters on the order of 3–10 mm but occasionally as large as 2.5 cm. It is usually subpleural and is characterized by well-defined walls. Ground glass opacities are frequent, but habitually less extensive than the reticulation. The evidence of coexistent pleural abnormalities (e.g. pleural plaques, calcifications, significant pleural effusion) suggests an alternative etiology for UIP pattern. Similarly, micronodules, air trapping, nonhoneycomb cysts, extensive ground glass opacities, consolidation or a peribronchovascular-predominant distribution should lead to consideration of an alternative diagnosis.

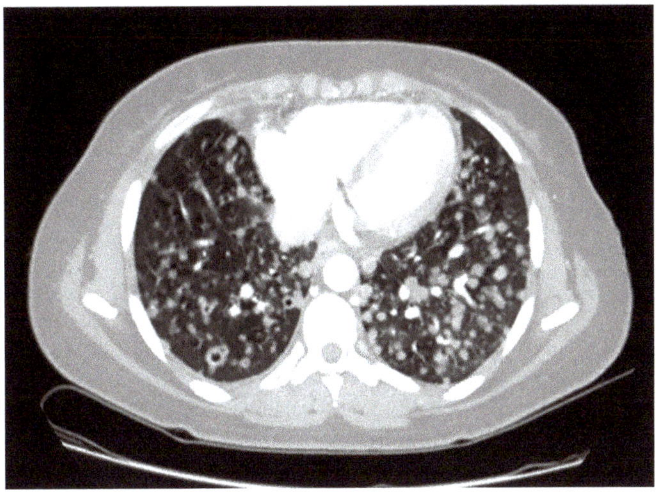

Fig. 18.21: Random distribution of nodules in a case of miliary tuberculosis. The initial cavitation of some nodules may be seen.

The most recent international guidelines on the diagnosis IPF provided radiological (HRCT) and histopathological criteria that allow to identify different levels of certainty for the UIP pattern. In particular, the HRCT criteria identify three levels of certainty: (1) UIP pattern; (2) Possible UIP pattern; (3) Inconsistent with UIP pattern (Table 18.1).

PATTERN OF INCREASED PULMONARY DENSITY

Such pattern includes opacities corresponding to parenchymal areas where a definite increased attenuation of X-rays may be pointed out; this phenomenon corresponds to the replacement of air in the alveoli by secretions, fluids, cellular infiltrates or fibrous tissue. Two different types of opacity must be distinguished, namely consolidation and ground-class opacity. In the former because of pathological filling the vascular design over the affected area is concealed; conversely in the ground-glass type of opacity, in spite of a hazy increase in density, underlying vessels are not obscured (Figs. 18.22 and 18.23). Ground glass in itself is very unspecific and there is a large overlap as concerns the etiology of ground-glass opacity and that of consolidation, with some diseases showing both abnormalities. Either isolated or combined with consolidation, ground-glass may occur in a variety of disorders including amongst others pulmonary edema and hemorrhage, infectious pneumonia, idiopathic pneumonitis and adenocarcinoma in situ. Consolidation without evidence of ground-glass may occur in a similar host of conditions in

Table 18.1: High-resolution computed tomography criteria for UIP pattern

UIP pattern (All four features)	*Possible UIP pattern (All three features)*	*Inconsistent with UIP pattern (Any of the seven features)*
Subpleural, basal predominance	Subpleural, basal predominance	Upper or mid-lung predominance
Reticular abnormality	Reticular abnormality	Peribronchovascular predominance
Honeycombing with or without traction bronchiectasis	Absence of features listed as inconsistent with UIP pattern (*see* 3rd column)	Extensive ground glass abnormality (extent > reticular abnormality)
Absence of features listed as inconsistent with UIP pattern (*see* 3rd column)		Profuse micronodules (bilateral, predominantly upper lobes)
		Discrete cysts (multiple, bilateral, away from areas of honeycombing)
		Diffuse mosaic attenuation/air-trapping (bilateral, in three or more lobes)
		Consolidation in bronchopulmonary segment(s)/lobe(s)

Source: Adapted from Raghu G, Collard HR, Egan JJ, Martinez FJ, Behr J, Brown KK, et al. An official ATS/ERS/JRS/ALAT statement: idiopathic pulmonary fibrosis: evidence-based guidelines for diagnosis and management. Am J Respir Crit Care Med. 2011;183(6):788-824.
(UIP: Usual interstitial pneumonia).

which as a result of an acute or chronic process alveoli fill up with various pathologic materials. The contrast of the patent airway appearing as full of air, superimposed over the compact area of affected parenchyma, results in the characteristic sign of air bronchogram, already visible at radiography (*see* the relevant chapter), but much better recognizable in its details at CT (Figs. 18.24A to C).

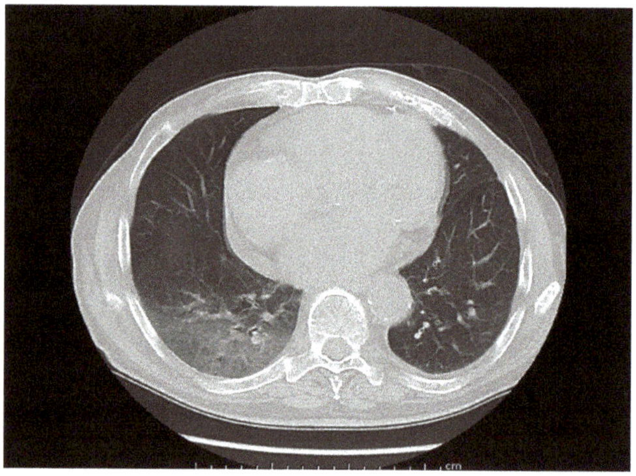

Fig. 18.22: Axial chest high-resolution CT scan showing ground glass opacity in the lower right lobe due to bleeding in patient with hemoptysis.

PATTERN OF DECREASED PULMONARY DENSITY

Under this heading we collect a group of heterogeneous disorders that share the common feature of decreased attenuation of X-rays due to increased air content: the corresponding evidence at CT is decreased pulmonary density. This pattern may occur in focal and in generalized

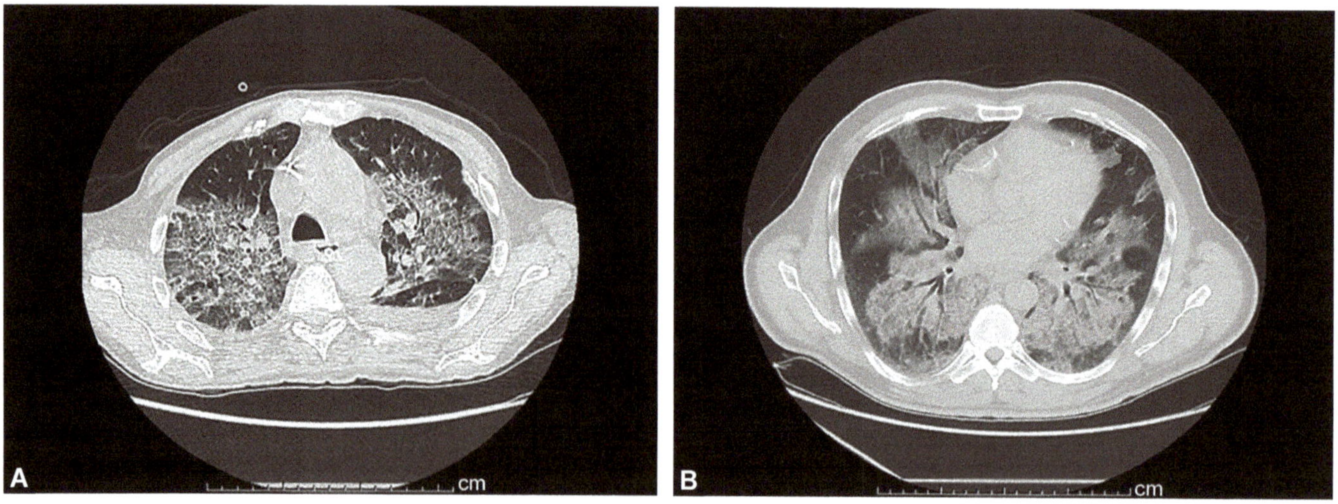

Figs. 18.23A and B: Axial chest high-resolution CT scan showing ground-glass opacities in (A) a man with adult respiratory distress syndrome (ARDS) and (B) in a man with extensive pulmonary infection by mycoplasma pneumonia.

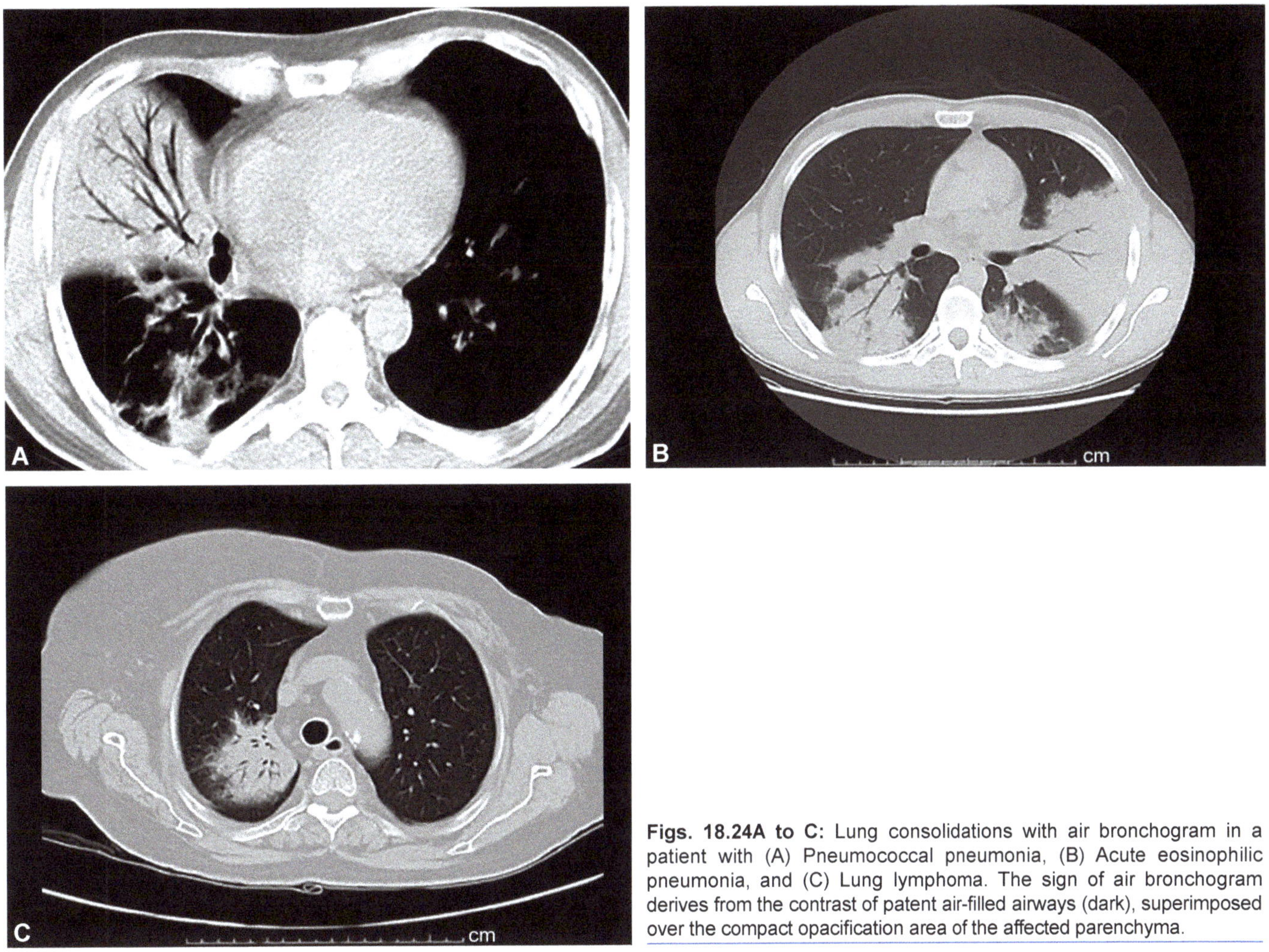

Figs. 18.24A to C: Lung consolidations with air bronchogram in a patient with (A) Pneumococcal pneumonia, (B) Acute eosinophilic pneumonia, and (C) Lung lymphoma. The sign of air bronchogram derives from the contrast of patent air-filled airways (dark), superimposed over the compact opacification area of the affected parenchyma.

diseases: among them we include disorders of common occurrence like bronchiectasis, as well as rare cystic lung diseases, like *Langerhans cell hystiocytosis* and *lymphangioleiomyomatosis* (Fig. 18.25). Cysts, i.e. radiolucent areas with a wall thickness of less than 4 mm, may also be a component of a more complex structural disorder, honeycomb lung (Fig. 18.26).

This expression is now used to refer to end-stage pulmonary fibrosis; it may be described as extensive and irregular subversion of structure with destruction and dense fibrosis, accompanied by numerous cystic airspaces, bronchiectasis and loss of acinar architecture.

Honeycombing is nonspecific in terms of etiology, since a group of different infiltrative diseases may lead to this outcome, including among others idiopathic pneumonitis, pneumoconiosis, sarcoidosis, diffuse alveolar damage.

By far the most representative and diffuse disorder where lung density is extensively reduced is pulmonary emphysema (*see* the following section of this chapter).

Emphysema

Emphysema is defined as an abnormal and permanent enlargement of distal air spaces, accompanied by destruction of alveolar walls, without overt signs of fibrosis. The definition is purely anatomical, so that until the advent of CT the diagnosis in vivo could only be presumed on a functional basis (i.e. in the presence of compatible alterations in spirometry and diffusion parameters). The scenario has been subverted by the progressive extension of applications of CT that allow a noninvasive structural diagnosis in vivo.

On anatomical/radiological basis various types of emphysema may be distinguished: the centrilobular

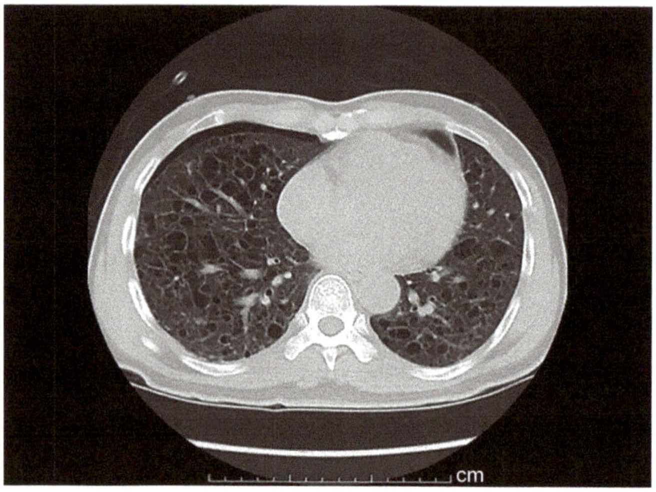

Fig. 18.25: Irregular lung cysts in a man with Langerhans cell histiocytosis (LCH). The differential diagnosis of LCH includes other cystic lung diseases, particularly lymphangioleiomyomatosis (LAM). In LCH, cysts have bizarre shapes and upper lobe predominance and may be thick walled. The cysts of LAM, in contrast, are usually round, thin walled, and diffuse in distribution. Furthermore, LAM occurs almost entirely in women.

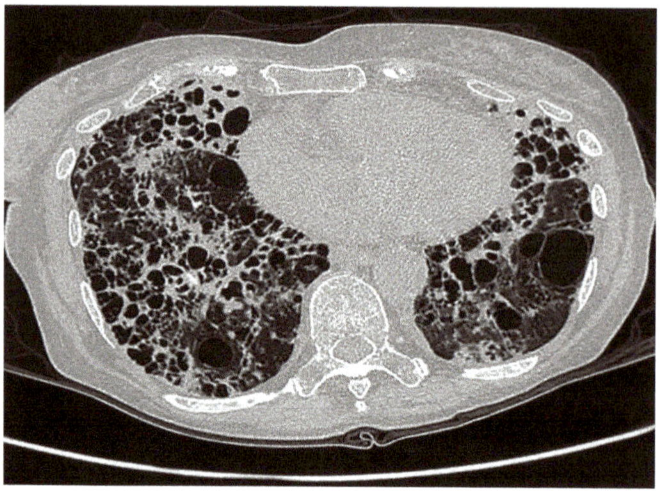

Fig. 18.26: Honeycomb lung represented by destruction and dense fibrosis of parenchyma, accompanied by numerous cystic airspaces, bronchiectasis and loss of acinar architecture.

emphysema (also referred to as proximal acinar, or centriacinar emphysema); the panlobular or panacinar emphysema and the paraseptal or distal acinar emphysema. CT allows a reliable differential diagnosis among these subtypes with the exception of the advanced forms where the extension and worsening of destructive lesions make such a differentiation more difficult.

Most often centrilobular emphysema involves the upper portion of various lobes, while as concerns the secondary pulmonary lobule the alteration is located proximally (Fig. 18.27).

Panlobular subtype is characterized by a prevalent involvement of the lower portions of the lung, although frequently it evolves toward a participation of the whole lungs. A peculiar condition very clearly demonstrated by CT is the so-called "*vanishing lung*", a rare disorder usually seen in association with centrilobular and paraseptal emphysema. It is characterized by the diffuse occurrence of very large bullae, i.e. large air-filled, thin-walled spaces in the lung consequent to widespread destruction of alveolar tissue (Fig. 18.28).

A pure form of panlobular destruction can only be found in case of emphysema due to alpha-1-protease inhibitor (*alpha-1-antitrypsin*) deficiency. At HRCT this subtype appears as large parenchymal areas with a uniformly low attenuation level and accompanied by a reduced evidence of pulmonary vessels. Alterations due to paraseptal emphysema predominantly involve the lung periphery, at subpleural level, in the form of multiple small areas located at the periphery of the secondary lobule, adjacent to interlobular septa.

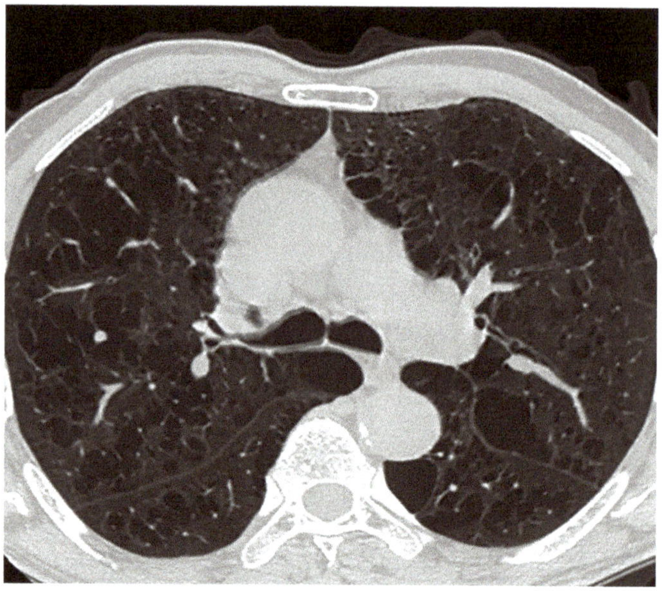

Fig. 18.27: A case of centrilobular emphysema.

The diagnostic strategy of emphysema moves from a conventional radiographic approach in two projections which may point out alterations due to hyperinflation (reduced attenuation) and to consequent adaptive modifications (e.g. lowering and flattening of diaphragm). However these findings are neither precocious nor specific and call for a closer scrutiny of the pattern of alterations as only HRCT may provide.

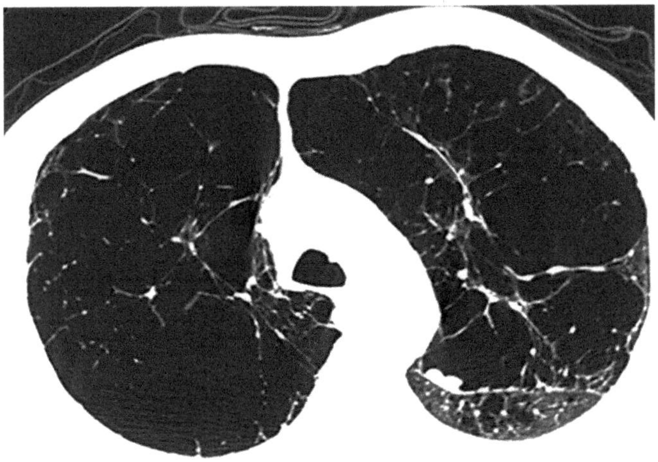

Fig. 18.28: The devastating appearance of widespread parenchymal destruction in a case of "vanishing lung".

Conventional imaging approach to such an irregularly disseminated disease was based on subjective interpretation by an expert: later, the introduction of CT opened the way to new and more reliable criteria. In the early days the progress was represented by visual scoring, i.e. the attribution of a numerical score to the subjectively evaluated lesions. Because of limitation determined by its subjective foundation this quantitative procedure tends to underestimate the lesions of milder degree and to fail in the detection of earlier stages of the diseases.

A further important progress in the field of quantification of emphysema has resulted from the introduction of densitometry, i.e. the evaluation of frequency distribution of X-rays attenuation levels. This procedure is based on the application of post-processing software that identifies and quantitates pixels placed within a determinate range of density. Areas affected by emphysema are characterized by markedly increased air content with density values ranging between –900 and – 1,000 HU.

Based on these concepts, a major technological advancement has been made by developing the "density mask", an original software allowing estimates of severity and extension of emphysema well correlated with pathology data. This software represents and quantitates *low attenuation areas (LAA)*, i.e. voxels with density lower than a predetermined threshold (e.g. –950 HU or LAA $_{-950}$). As a further evolution, two CT-based methods for determining the extent of emphysema are now available: the threshold cut-off and the percentile point analysis. The former is based on a predetermined cut-off value of attenuation to separate emphysematous from "normal" lungs. The second approach is the percentile method where a specific point on the frequency distribution curve of the X-ray attenuation values (e.g. 15th percentile) is defined and compared between subjects. Although there is no consensus on the most optimal cut-off point for this type of analysis, it is generally agreed that, for cross-sectional analysis, both the threshold and the percentile techniques are appropriate, whereas for longitudinal studies, the 15th percentile technique is preferable.

The choice of this threshold is critically important to improve the diagnostic yield in terms of sensitivity and specificity. –950 HU on HRCT (on 1 mm sections) without contrast is the value best correlated with macroscopic and microscopic findings of emphysema obtained in patients submitted to excision surgery for lung cancer or in preparation of transplantation. The selection of a suitable cut-off of density is just an aspect of the wide problem of standardization: the degree of inflation of air spaces, the type of scanner and the severity of disease are other important sources of variability of density measures. Conversely, the role of dose is controversial, although there is agreement about the need of keeping the technical parameters (including the dose) during follow-up periods.

In the interpretation of imaging studies targeted at diagnosis of emphysema, a cautious evaluation must be made in consideration of possible alternatives that can be encountered in clinical activity more often than expected. This is the case for combined pulmonary fibrosis and emphysema (CPFE), a recently defined syndrome, characterized by centrilobular and/or paraseptal emphysema in upper lung zones coexisting with pulmonary fibrosis in lower lobes. This pattern may be better interpreted in the light of a characteristic lung function profile, with unexpected subnormal static and dynamic lung volumes, contrasting with a significant reduction of carbon monoxide transfer and exercise-induced hypoxemia.

Among the disorders accompanied by a focal or diffuse decrease in attenuation, to be differentiated from emphysema, particular attention must be paid to diseases characterized by air trapping, i.e. retention of excess gas in all or part of the lung, occurring especially during expiration. This is due to functional abnormalities in patency of peripheral airways, either as a consequence of complete or partial airway obstruction or as a result of loss of stability of airway wall with consequent enhanced collapsability of the airway itself. The phenomenon may be showed through a chest CT scan performed at first in inspiration and then repeated after full expiration. Air trapping is diagnosed as less than normal increase in attenuation during expiration. The presence of air trapping may result from a variety of causes but usually suggests airway diseases, including bronchial asthma and bronchiolitis obliterans. It must be differentiated from the case of pulmonary embolism where a decreased attenuation is observed over parenchymal areas undergoing hypoperfusion secondary to locally increased pulmonary arterial resistance.

Bronchiectasis

Bronchiectasis refers to abnormal and usually irreversible dilatations of the bronchial branches, which occur in several clinical settings. *Cylindrical bronchiectasis* often produces parallel line opacities (*tram track sign*) and increased bronchoarterial ratio (*signet ring sign*), where a dilated bronchus cut in a horizontal section represents the ring, and the adjacent pulmonary artery represents the stone (*see* Fig. 18.9). The diameter of the bronchus lumen is normally 1–1.5 times that of the adjacent vessel; a diameter greater than 1.5 times that of the adjacent vessel suggests bronchiectasis. *Varicose bronchiectasis* has irregular or beaded bronchi, with alternating areas of dilatation and constriction, producing a *string of pearls* appearance. *Cystic bronchiectasis* is characterized by large cystic spaces and may have a honeycomb appearance; this contrasts with the blebs of emphysema, which have thinner walls and are not accompanied by proximal airway abnormalities (Fig. 18.29).

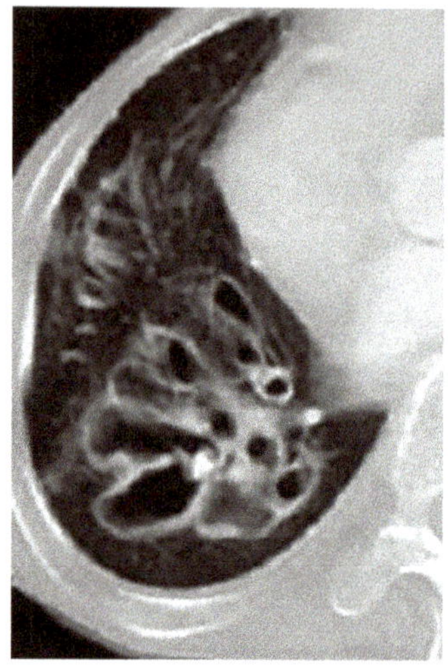

Fig. 18.29: Chest CT showing cystic bronchiectasis of the right lung.

VIRTUAL BRONCHOSCOPY

The increasingly sophisticated application of computers to the imaging techniques has caused a dramatic increase in the diffusion of "computer-aided diagnosis" (CAD) i.e. the complex of techniques of postprocessing of images aimed at increasing the diagnostic yield of CT: in particular a valuable approach is the expansion of the possibilities of the conventional axial approach to obtain 3D reconstructions.

In case of central neoplasms, because of direct and indirect effects of tumor growth on the structures of bronchial wall, the patency of lumen may be progressively limited until the complete occlusion results in obstruction atelectasis. Patency may be restored after obstruction using the approach most suitable on an individual basis, including cryosurgery, plasma coagulation, stent placement, balloon dilatation etc. In such cases fiberoptic bronchoscopy (FOB) is a mandatory step for a detailed diagnosis and for careful planning of interventions aimed at the restoration and maintenance of the ventilation of parenchymal areas. However in this perspective FOB suffers important limitations: in patients with significant stenosis of bronchial lumen, the possibility of bronchoscopic evaluation of the stenotic airway is limited to the proximal patent tract, whereas the observation of the obstructed tract and of the area placed beyond the stenosis is prevented. In addition, no clear inference can be made as to the potential participation of extraluminal pathology.

The scenario has been modified by the advent of spiral CT: the possibility of acquisition of volumetric data sets has allowed the use of axially acquired data to obtain a representation of anatomical details of large body areas in reduced time, compatible with the duration of an inspiratory apnea. By multiplanar reformatting and volume-rendering techniques axial images can be reconfigured to display the data from an endoscopic perspective (Figs. 18.30A to C).

In addition techniques of animation and of path tracking may be applied so as to represent in the most effective way the virtual exploration performed in different directions inside a hollow organ. In this way with no invasion, it is possible to provide the thoracic surgeon with anatomical data very useful for deciding the most suitable type of intervention, as well as for issuing a documented prediction as to the outcome of the procedure.

In spite of the exciting possibilities offered by virtual bronchoscopy, the diffusion of this technique in clinical practice has been hampered by some not trivial

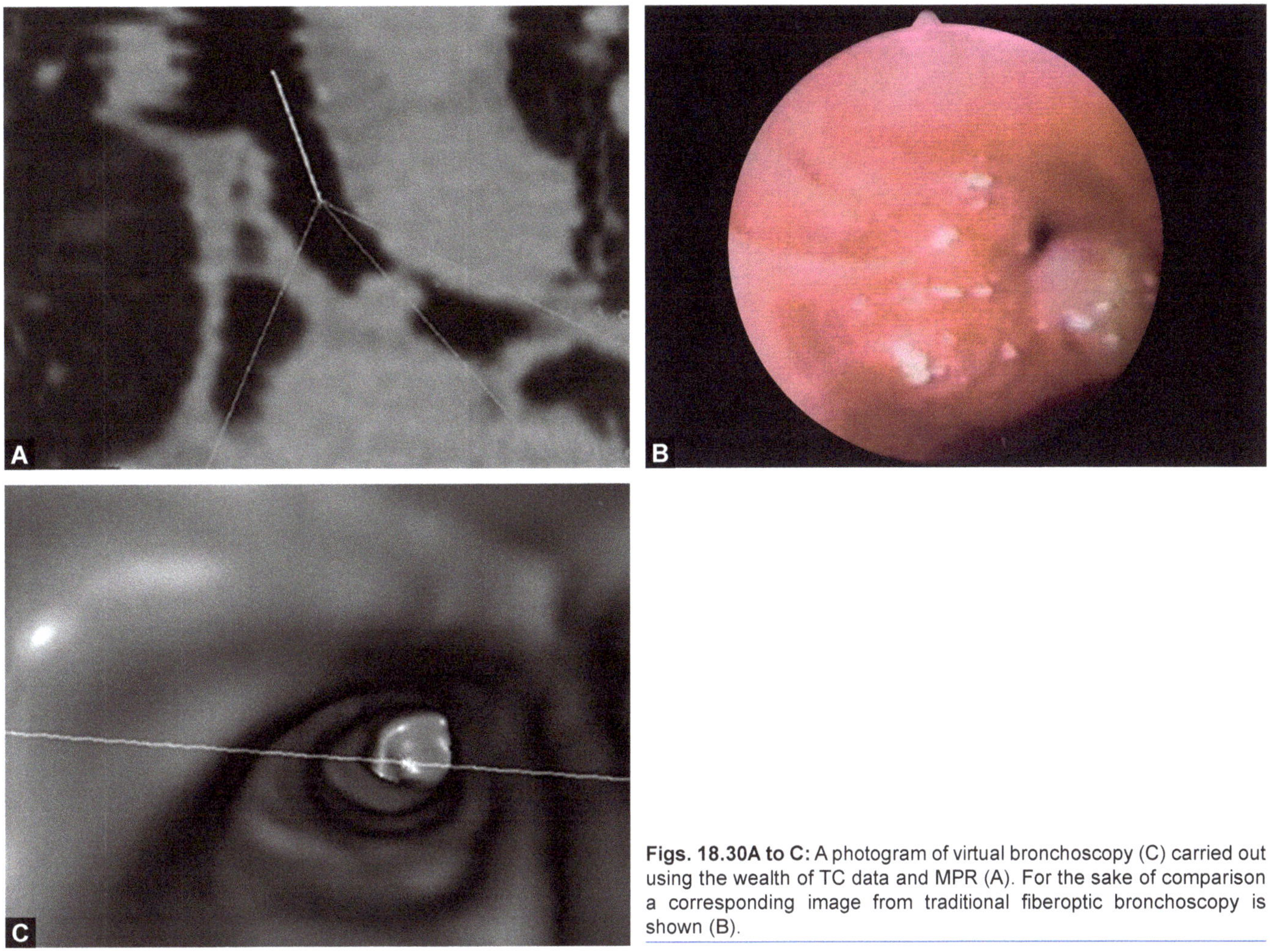

Figs. 18.30A to C: A photogram of virtual bronchoscopy (C) carried out using the wealth of TC data and MPR (A). For the sake of comparison a corresponding image from traditional fiberoptic bronchoscopy is shown (B).

limitations. The latter include: static conditions of observation, difficulty in evaluating the status of mucosa in terms of color or mobility, impossibility of performing biopsies on the sites of interest, exposure to radiation risk.

BIBLIOGRAPHY AND FURTHER READING

1. Dalal PU, Hansell DM. High-resolution computed tomography of the lungs: the borderlands of normality. Eur Radiol. 2006;16(4):771-80.
2. Gotway MB, Reddy GP, Webb WR, Elicker BM, Leung JW. High-resolution CT of the lung: patterns of disease and differential diagnoses. Radiol Clin North Am. 2005;-43(3):513-42.
3. Hansell DM, Bankier AA, MacMahon H, McLoud TC, Müller NL, Remy J. Fleischner Society: glossary of terms for thoracic imaging. Radiology. 2008;246:697-722.
4. Raghu G, Collard HR, Egan JJ, Martinez FJ, Behr J, Brown KK, et al. An Official official ATS/ERS/JRS/ALAT statement: idiopathic pulmonary fibrosis: evidence-based guidelines for diagnosis and management. Am J Respir Crit Care Med. 2011;183(6):788-824.
5. Verma N, Chung JH, Mohammed TL. Tree-in-bud sign. J Thorac Imaging. 2012;27:W27.
6. Walker CM, Abbott GF, Greene RE, Shepard JA, Vummidi D, Digumarthy SR. Imaging pulmonary infection: classic signs and patterns. AJR Am J Roentgenol. 2014;202:479-92.
7. Whiting P, Singatullina N, Rosser JH. Computed tomography of the chest: I. Basic principles. BJA Educ. 2015;15(6):299-304

Chapter

19 High-Resolution Computed Tomography for the Evaluation of Airways Distensibility

Alida Benfante, Robert H Brown, Claudio Sorino, Nicola Scichilone

AIRWAY DISTENSION AND DEEP INSPIRATIONS

Our airways are constantly subjected to a cycling process of distention and recoil resulting from our breathing function, which appears to play a major role in maintaining airway patency. This is most probably because, during the inspiratory phase of breathing, a stretch is imposed on airway tissue and particularly on the airway smooth muscle, thus altering its contractile state toward a condition of relaxation. The magnitude of the stretch is even more important: full lung inflations through deep inspirations provide a powerful mechanism for airway protection from subsequent bronchospastic stimuli. In healthy subjects, a deep inspiratory maneuver also acts as a *bronchodilator*, that is, it distends constricted airways. The bronchoprotective effect of deep inspiration has been found to be lost in individuals with airway hyperresponsiveness, suggesting a mechanistic association between the two components. On the other hand, the bronchodilatory effect of deep inspirations has been shown to decrease with increasing severity of asthma, and to be severely impaired in individuals suffering from chronic obstructive diseases [chronic obstructive pulmonary disease (COPD)]. Taken together, these findings suggest that the impairment of the ability of deep inspirations to dilate constricted airways affects and modulates the occurrence of chronic respiratory symptoms.

It has been postulated that the beneficial effect of deep inspirations is mediated by airway distension. A deep inspiration exerts its stretching effect on the airways by virtue of airway to parenchyma interdependence that is sustained by a network of connective fibers. Therefore, with the deep inspiratory maneuver, radial traction is applied to the airway wall, resulting in bronchial distension. It is postulated that structural changes of the airways (thickening) and the parenchyma (loss of alveolar attachments) induced by the inflammatory processes may affect the beneficial effect of deep inspirations by attenuating the tethering forces between the airways and the surrounding parenchyma. Computed tomography (CT) has been used to assess airway wall thickness and luminal area, and to quantify the parenchymal alterations associated with lung diseases. In addition, by looking at the airway caliber at different lung volumes, the magnitude of airway distensibility can be estimated. Therefore, this technique can provide a tool to investigate the relation between structural changes of the lung and functional impairment in subjects with chronic lung diseases. This approach could also provide novel information on the mechanisms underlying the bronchodilatory effect of deep inspirations and its relationship with the clinical characteristics of subjects with asthma and COPD. This chapter will describe the clinical applicability of high-resolution computed tomography (HRCT) in the assessment of the "dynamic" changes of the airways in COPD.

BENEFICIAL EFFECTS OF LUNG INFLATION

Airways in healthy individuals are distended with each inspiration. This cyclic process is even more pronounced during sighing and deep inspirations to full lung inflation. This physiological function of the respiratory system is essential in repeatedly distending airway smooth muscle and maintaining airway patency. The above-described phenomenon has been largely explored, and several

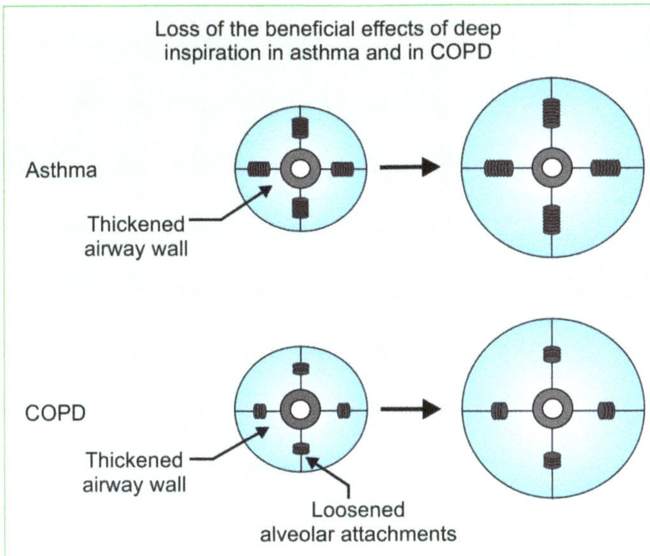

Fig. 19.1: Schematic of the mechanisms involved in the impairment of airway distensibility in asthma and in chronic obstructive pulmonary disease (COPD). The stretching effect of lung inflation is limited by the thickened airway wall that opposes the distending effect, and by the loss of alveolar attachments that reduces the distending forces.

human studies have demonstrated that a deep inspiratory maneuver in healthy subjects acts as a *bronchodilator*. The bronchodilatory effect of deep inspirations has been shown to be as effective in mild asthmatics, but to decrease with increasing severity of disease. In addition, studies have shown that the bronchodilatory effect of deep inspirations is severely blunted in individuals with COPD, and significantly impaired in healthy elderly subjects. These observations lend support to the notion that the impairment of the ability of deep inspirations to dilate constricted airways contributes to the occurrence and the degree of respiratory symptoms.

It has been argued that the extent of the airway stretch is important to activate the beneficial properties of deep inspirations. Assuming that this is true, then any factor affecting the airway to parenchyma interdependence should influence the effectiveness of deep inspiration to distend constricted airways. Thickened airway walls, which are seen in individuals with the most severe forms of asthma, could reasonably be responsible for the lack of the beneficial effect of deep inspiration, counteracting the distending forces of lung inflations. In addition, loosened alveolar attachments observed in lungs of individuals with emphysema may also account for the loss of the beneficial effect of lung inflation in this pathological condition due to the lack of the tethering forces (Fig. 19.1).

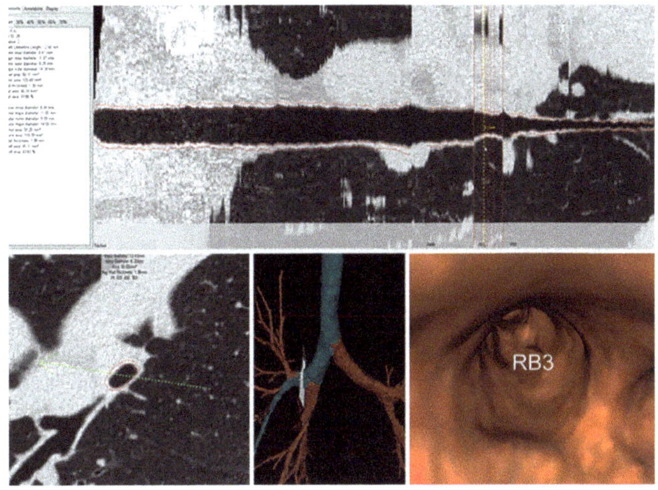

Fig. 19.2: High-resolution CT images of the airway for analysis of wall thickness.
Vida software package.

One of the only methods to measure changes in airway size in vivo is HRCT. HRCT is a repeatable, direct and noninvasive radiological technique that can be used for qualitative and quantitative parenchymal and airway measurements in vivo. Indeed, HRCT is capable of excellent spatial resolution and provides anatomic detail of pulmonary structures. Total lung volume and parenchymal density can also be measured on the HRCT scans, the latter as an estimate of parenchymal damage. Parenchymal density can be expressed by lung attenuation parameters, such as mean lung density (Mean HU), the percent of the lung with a low attenuation area at total lung capacity (TLC) below -950 HU (LAA_{-950}) as an estimate of the degree of emphysema, and the percent of the lung with low attenuation area at functional residual capacity (FRC) below -856 (RA_{-856}) as an estimate of the degree of air trapping. HRCT can assess airway diameter and airway wall thickness in multiple airways (2nd to 8th generation airways) in nonobstructed and obstructive subjects (Fig. 19.2).

High-resolution CT is uniquely capable of addressing questions about airway responsiveness in vivo that are not answerable by other techniques. Previous studies using HRCT in animal models have confirmed and validated the ability to measure airway constrictor responses and to monitor the effect of lung inflation. For example, HRCT can be used to measure the same airway before and after a bronchodilator to assess the presences and degree of airway tone. Most important, by assessing the caliber of the same airway measured at two different lung volumes, i.e. FRC and TLC, the magnitude of the increase of the

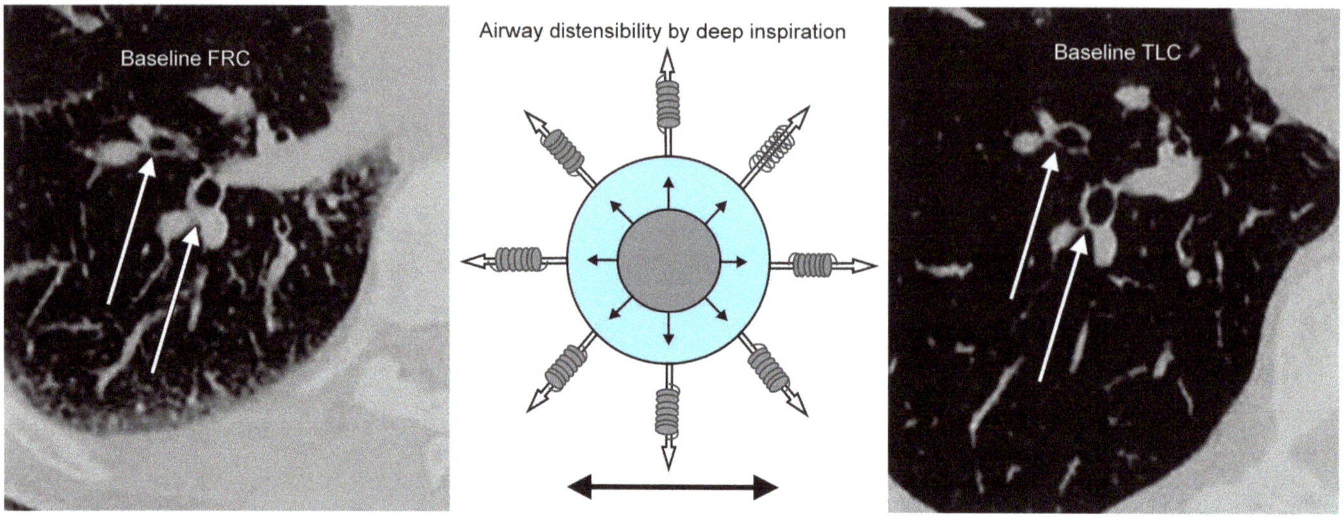

Fig. 19.3: High-resolution CT scans obtained at functional residual capacity (FRC) and total lung capacity (TLC) to assess the degree of distensibility of the same airway.

airway lumenal area represents the airway distensibility (Fig. 19.3). This response to lung inflation (or the lack of it), is associated with the clinical phenotype of chronic respiratory patients, and could be proposed as a tool to monitor lung function in these patients.

FACTORS AFFECTING THE BENEFICIAL EFFECTS OF LUNG INFLATION

In the context of the asthmatic phenotype, Brown and collaborators previously showed that deep inspirations stretch the airways of mild asthmatic individuals whose disease was stable at the time to the same degree as the airways of healthy individuals. This is in contrast with the hypothesis that lung inflation is impaired in all asthmatics. However, the same group showed that deep inspiration-induced bronchodilation was impaired with increasing severity of asthma, leading the authors to hypothesize that this phenomenon is severity related. In that study, the more severe asthmatic subjects were the ones who lacked the bronchodilatory effect of deep inspiration and showed the lowest airway distensibility by HRCT. Although no direct histological demonstration of airway remodeling could be demonstrated, it is plausible that the airways of the most severe asthmatics presented with features of remodeling. Indeed, a large body of evidence has shown that airway remodeling is significant in severe asthma. Other investigators have attempted to examine airway wall thickening as a measure of severity with the use of HRCT; however, the data are inconclusive.

A possible mechanism for limited airway distention could lie in the structural, non-reversible changes of the airway wall. The airway mucosa is incompressible, so as airway smooth muscle contracts, the mucosa buckles and folds. Histological studies of the airways have assumed that the epithelial basement membrane is not distensible, thus representing a limiting structure for airway distention. More recently, James et al. showed an increase in the extracellular matrix in both fatal and nonfatal asthma cases. The increased extracellular matrix may be a factor in decreased airway distension in asthma. Another component of the airway wall is the airway smooth muscle. Increases in the amount of airway smooth muscle, as a result of either hypertrophy or hyperplasia, may lead not only to increased contractility, but also to decreased distensibility. Studies in dogs, sheep and in humans showed that when the airways had tone, not only was their baseline size reduced, but their distensibility was also depressed. Using HRCT, Brown and colleagues measured the change in airway size after complete airway smooth muscle relaxation. The authors observed an inverse correlation between the chronic airflow obstruction and the beta-adrenergic-responsive airway smooth muscle. The asthmatic subjects with the greatest airflow obstruction showed the lowest response to beta-adrenergic bronchodilation. Since the airways in asthmatics did not bronchodilate to the same degree, factors other than airway smooth muscle tone must be involved in the chronic airway obstruction observed in moderate and severe asthma.

One of the factors that could oppose airway distension is edema in the airway wall or in the peribronchial space, which could decrease the interdependence between the airway and the parenchyma, resulting in decreased radial forces acting on the smooth muscle with lung inflation. Brown and coworkers demonstrated in dogs and sheep that substantial airway wall edema, up to a 50% increase in airway wall area, did not affect airway distensibility. Therefore, it is less likely that airway edema is a primary cause of decreased airway distensibility.

Of course, remodeling changes in the airways, such as those observed in asthma and COPD, can stiffen the airways, thus opposing the distending forces of a deep inspiratory maneuver. However, recent findings showed that, even though the airway walls of subjects suffering from asthma and COPD of comparable degree of airway obstruction are thicker, this increased thickness does not appear to impede airway distensibility. The authors inferred that the remodeling processes leading to increased airway wall thickness did not appear to change the basic passive force-tension dynamics in vivo, and therefore did not appear to make airways more resistant to imposed stretch by deep inspiration.

An alternative (or complementary) mechanism that is implicated in the impairment of the beneficial effect of lung inflations is the reduction in the distending forces. Permutt demonstrated that, in healthy humans, lung elastic recoil becomes significantly depressed with increasing age. This explains why a series of lung inflation maneuvers immediately after experimentally induced bronchoconstriction was only partially able to reinstate airway patency in healthy elderly subjects. In individuals with COPD, lung elastic recoil diminished as a function of the degree of emphysema, primarily because of the disruption of the alveolar attachments that were responsible for the "stretching effect". For stretch to be exerted on the airway wall, the anatomic and functional interdependence between the lung parenchyma and the airways needs to be intact. In COPD, alveolar attachments on airway walls are progressively destroyed and this is expected to impact the ability of lung inflation by deep inspiration to stretch the airways. In this respect, Scichilone and colleagues found a clear correlation between the amount of destroyed alveolar attachments and the magnitude of the reduction in the beneficial effects of deep inspiration. In addition, a significant inverse relationship between airway distensibility and features of hyperinflation were demonstrated, suggesting that the increase in lung volume could be one of the factors that limits this process. This is of great importance in COPD, where lung hyperinflation is a pivotal functional abnormality resulting from the loss of elastic recoil and emphysematous damage to the lung parenchyma. Recently, Diaz and colleagues demonstrated that airway distensibility by lung inflation was largely attenuated in subjects with an emphysema-predominant phenotype as opposed to those with airway-predominant alterations. On the basis of these observations, it is plausible to hypothesize that, in subjects with COPD, the impaired ability of deep inspiration to dilate the airways contributes to the occurrence and/or the severity of chronic respiratory symptoms.

An interesting aspect of the airway distensibility is the relationship with the magnitude of lung inflations. To examine the effects on subsequent airway caliber of varying transpulmonary pressure during the deep inspiratory maneuver, changes in airway size following lung inflations of increasing magnitude taken immediately after infusion of bronchoconstrictor agent were measured by HRCT in anesthetized and ventilated dogs. The results showed that the magnitude of the transpulmonary pressure was associated with a qualitative change in the airway response. Furthermore, the duration of the deep inpiration also affected the subsequent airway caliber.

ROLE OF HRCT IN ASSESSING AIRWAY DISTENSIBILITY

To further explore the factors that affect the magnitude of deep inspiration-induced airway distensibility with HRCT, Benfante et al. tested the degree of distensibility in subjects with asthma and COPD with comparable degree of bronchial obstruction, as previously discussed. Airway wall thickness and lung density were measured to evaluate which radiological abnormalities could potentially affect the main outcome, and a total of 701 airways were analyzed in 12 asthmatics and 8 subjects with COPD. No significant differences between the two groups were detected when airway distensibility was calculated for either all airways (Fig. 19.4) or by airway size for the small ($p = 0.27$), the medium ($p = 0.94$), and the large ($p = 0.40$) airways. These results suggest that the lack of airway distensibility is the main cause of persistent airflow limitation, regardless of the obstructive lung disease etiology. However, the major determinants of airway distensibility were different for the two groups. In the asthmatic group, the dynamic ability to alter lung volume was the main factor that affected airway distensibility, while, in the subjects with COPD, the static lung volumes influenced the degree of airway distensibility.

Taken together, these observations confirm that the HRCT-assessed dynamic behavior of the respiratory system can provide unique information. The increased thickness

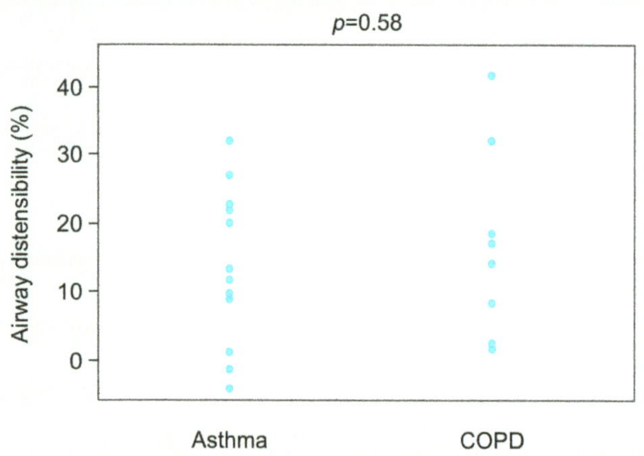

Fig. 19.4: Comparison of airway distensibility between asthmatics and chronic obstructive pulmonary disease (COPD) individuals of same degree of airway obstruction.

of the airway wall, such as that observed in the more severe stages of asthma, or the loss of alveolar attachments, such as that documented in the emphysematous lungs, can impair the ability to distend airways. Both in asthma and in COPD, the severity of the disease, as assessed by lung function impairment, is associated with the decreasing bronchodilatory ability of deep inspirations as assessed by HRCT.

In conclusion, it is postulated that in asthma and COPD functional alterations can be defined not only by the degree of bronchial obstruction, but also by the change in the magnitude of the distensibility of the airways following deep inspirations. Functional imaging of airway distensibility can contribute to an understanding of the mechanisms of action of deep inspirations and, consequently, to the understanding of the disease processes in asthma and COPD. Future studies could explore the role of functional imaging in the monitoring of the severity of the disease and the response to treatment. A body of evidence supports the notion that lung inflation is a major modulatory mechanism of airway patency in healthy humans. Disturbances of the effects of lung inflation are associated with airway dysfunction, and studying this process by HRCT may provide insight into the pathophysiology, progression of disease and response to therapy in asthmatic patients.

BIBLIOGRAPHY AND FURTHER READING

1. Amirav I, Kramer SS, Grunstein MM, Hoffman EA. Assessment of methacholine-induced airway constriction by ultrafast high-resolution computed tomography. J Appl Physiol. 1993;75(5):2239-50.
2. Baldi S, Miniati M, Bellina CR, Battolla L, Catapano G, Begliomini E, et al. Relationship between extent of pulmonary emphysema by high-resolution computed tomography and lung elastic recoil in patients with chronic obstructive pulmonary disease. Am J Respir Crit Care Med. 2001;164(4):585-9.
3. Benfante A, Bellia M, Scichilone N, Canizzaro F, Midiri M, Brown RH, et al. Airway distensibility by HRCT in asthmatics and COPD with comparable airway obstruction. COPD. 2013;10:560-6.
4. Brightling CE, Gupta S, Gonem S, Siddiqui S. Lung damage and airway remodelling in severe asthma. Clin Exp Allergy. 2012;42:638-49.
5. Broide DH. Immunologic and inflammatory mechanisms that drive asthma progression to remodeling. J Allergy Clin Immunol. 2008;121(3):560-72.
6. Brown RH, Herold CJ, Hirshman CA, Zerhouni EA, Mitzner W. In vivo measurements of airway reactivity using high-resolution computed tomography. The American review of respiratory disease. 1991;144(1):208-12.
7. Brown RH, Herold CJ, Hirshman CA, Zerhouni EA, Mitzner W. Individual airway constrictor response heterogeneity to histamine assessed by high-resolution computed tomography. J Appl Physiol. 1993;74(6):2615-20.
8. Brown RH, Mitzner W, Bulut Y, Wagner EM. Effect of lung inflation in vivo on airways with smooth muscle tone or edema. J Appl Physiol. 1997;82(2):491-9.
9. Brown RH, Mitzner W, Wagner EM. Interaction between airway edema and lung inflation on responsiveness of individual airways in vivo. J Appl Physiol. 1997;83(2):366-70.
10. Brown RH, Mitzner W. Duration of deep inspiration and subsequent airway constriction in vivo. The Journal of asthma: official journal of the Association for the Care of Asthma. 2003;40(2):119-24.
11. Brown RH, Mitzner W. Effect of lung inflation and airway muscle tone on airway diameter in vivo. J Appl Physiol. 1996;80(5):1581-8.
12. Brown RH, Pearse DB, Pyrgos G, Liu MC, Togias A, Permutt S. The structural basis of airways hyperresponsiveness in asthma. J Appl Physiol. 2006;101:30-9.
13. Brown RH, Scichilone N, Mudge B, Diemer FB, Permutt S, Togias A. High-resolution computed tomographic evaluation of airway distensibility and the effects of lung inflation on airway caliber in healthy subjects and individuals with asthma. Am J Respir Crit Care Med. 2001;163(4):994-1001.
14. Brown RH, Zerhouni EA, Mitzner W. Airway edema potentiates airway reactivity. J Appl Physiol. 1995;79(4):1242-8.
15. Brown RH, Zerhouni EA, Mitzner W. Visualization of airway obstruction in vivo during pulmonary vascular engorgement and edema. J Appl Physiol. 1995;78(3):1070-8.
16. Brusasco V, Crimi E, Barisione G, Spanevello A, Rodarte JR, Pelligrino R. Airway responsiveness to methacholine: effects of deep inhalations and airway inflammation. J Appl Physiol. 1999;87:567-73.
17. Corsico A, Milanese M, Baraldo S, Casoni GL, Papi A, Riccio AM, et al. Small airway morphology and lung

function in the transition from normality to chronic airway obstruction. J Appl Physiol. 2003;95:441-7.
18. Crimi E, Pelligrino R, Milanese M, Brusasco V. Deep breaths, methacholine, and airway narrowing in healthy and mild asthmatic subjects. J Appl Physiol. 2002;93:1384-90.
19. Diaz AA, Come CE, Ross JC, San Jose Estepar R, Han MK, Loring SH, et al. Association between airway caliber changes with lung inflation and emphysema assessed by volumetric CT scan in subjects with COPD. Chest. 2012;141(3):736-44.
20. Fish JE, Ankin MG, Kelly JF, Peterman VI. Regulation of bronchomotor tone by lung inflation in asthmatic and non-asthmatic subjects. J Appl Physiol. 1981;50:1079-86.
21. Fredberg JJ. Frozen objects: small airways, big breaths, and asthma. J Allergy Clin Immunol. 2000;106:615-24.
22. James AL, Elliot JG, Jones RL, Carroll ML, Mauad T, Bai TR, et al. Airway smooth muscle hypertrophy and hyperplasia in asthma. Am J Respir Crit Care Med. 2012;185(10):1058-64.
23. James AL, Hogg JC, Dunn LA, Pare PD. The use of the internal perimeter to compare airway size and to calculate smooth muscle shortening. The American review of respiratory disease. 1988;138(1):136-9.
24. Jensen A, Atileh H, Suki B, Ingenito EP, Lutchen KR. Selected contribution: airway caliber in healthy and asthmatic subjects: effects of bronchial challenge and deep inspirations. J Appl Physiol. 2001;91:506-15.
25. Kapsali T, Permutt S, Laube B, Scichilone N, Togias A. The potent bronchoprotective effects of deep inspiration and its absence in asthma. J Appl Physiol. 2000;89:711-20.
26. Lai-Fook SJ, Beck KC, Sutcliffe AM, Donaldson JT. Effect of edema and height on bronchial diameter and shape in excised dog lung. Respiration Physiology. 1984;55(2):223-37.
27. Lambert RK, Codd SL, Alley MR, Pack RJ. Physical determinants of bronchial mucosal folding. J Appl Physiol. 1994;77(3):1206-16.
28. Little SA, Sproule MW, Cowan MD, Macleod KJ, Robertson M, Love JG, et al. High resolution computed tomographic assessment of airway wall thickness in chronic asthma: reproducibility and relationship with lung function and severity. Thorax. 2002;57(3):247-53.
29. Macklem PT. Mechanical factors determining maximum bronchoconstriction. Eur Respir J Suppl. 1989;6:516-9.
30. Niimi A, Matsumoto H, Amitani R, Nakano Y, Mishima M, Minakuchi M, et al. Airway wall thickness in asthma assessed by computed tomography. Relation to clinical indices. Am J Respir Crit Care Med. 2000;162(4 Pt 1):1518-23.
31. Niimi A, Matsumoto H, Takemura M, Ueda T, Chin K, Mishima M. Relationship of airway wall thickness to airway sensitivity and airway reactivity in asthma. American journal of respiratory and critical care medicine. 2003;168(8):983-8.
32. Permutt S, Martin HB. Static pressure-volume characteristics of lungs in normal males. J Appl Physiol. 1960;15:819-25.
33. Pyrgos G, Scichilone N, Togias A, Brown RH. Bronchodilation response to deep inspirations in asthma is dependent on airway distensibility and air trapping. J Appl Physiol. 2011;110: 472-9.
34. Scichilone N, Bruno A, Marchese R, Vignola AM, Togias A, Bellia V. Association between reduced bronchodilatory effect of deep inspiration and loss of alveolar attachments. Respir Res. 2005;6:55.
35. Scichilone N, La Sala A, Bellia M, Fallano K, Togias A, Brown RH, et al. The airway response to deep inspirations decreases with COPD severity and is associated with airway distensibility assessed by computed tomography. J Appl Physiol. 2008;105:832-8.
36. Scichilone N, Marchese R, Catalano F, Togias A, Vignola AM, Bellia V. Bronchodilatory effect of deep inspiration diminishes with aging. Respir Med. 2004;98:838-43.
37. Scichilone N, Marchese R, Catalano F, Vignola AM, Togias A, Bellia V. Bronchodilatory effect of deep inspiration is absent in subjects with mild COPD. Chest. 2004;125:2029-35.
38. Scichilone N, Marchese R, Soresi S, Interrante A, Togias A, Bellia V. Deep inspiration-induced changes in lung volume decrease with severity of asthma. Respir Med. 2007;101:-951-6.
39. Silvers GW, Petty TL, Stanford RE. Elastic recoil changes in early emphysema. Thorax. 1980;35(7):490-5.
40. Skloot G, Permutt S, Togias A. Airway hyperresponsiveness in asthma: a problem of limited smooth muscle relaxation with inspiration. J Clin Invest. 1995;96(5):2393-403.
41. Sundblad BM, Larsson K. Effect of deep inhalations after a bronchial methacholine provocation in asthmatic and non-asthmatic subjects. Respir Med. 2002;96:477-81.
42. Wheatley JR, Pare PD, Engel LA. Reversibility of induced bronchoconstriction by deep inspiration in asthmatic and normal subjects. Eur Respir J. 1989;2:331-9.
43. Wood SA, Zerhouni EA, Hoford JD, Hoffman EA, Mitzner W. Measurement of three-dimensional lung tree structures by using computed tomography. J Appl Physiol. 1995;79(5):-1687-97.

Chapter

20 Computed Tomographic Pulmonary Angiography

Johannes Gossner, Claudio Sorino

OVERVIEW ON COMPUTED TOMOGRAPHIC PULMONARY ANGIOGRAPHY

Computed tomographic pulmonary angiography (CTPA) is a noninvasive diagnostic technique that employs computed tomography and a contrast agent to obtain an image of the pulmonary arteries.

Since the first description of imaging pulmonary embolism (PE) with computed tomography (CT) in three cases in 1980, CTPA has evolved into one of the most useful test in diagnosing PE. The introduction of spiral-CT into clinical practice in the early 90s offered the possibility to acquire image of the whole thorax during one breath hold and made CTPA possible. In one of the first studies examining the pulmonary arteries with a single slice spiral-CT, Remy-Jardin et al. reported perfect agreement with the findings of pulmonary angiography. Studies with 1- or 4-slice scanners reported sensitivities between 91% and 100% compared to the "gold standard" pulmonary angiography. Using different scanners in a miulticenter study the PIOPED II investigators found sensitivity of CTPA of 83% compared to an often criticized composite reference standard (positive findings on pulmonary angiography, ventilation-perfusion scintigraphy or venous ultrasound). In this study additional CT-venography improved sensitivity to 90%. Interestingly, comparing 4- and 64-slice CT scanners no difference in the overall prevalence of PE was found, but more subsegmental emboli were found using the 64-slice scanner. Actually CTPA has become itself a "gold standard" for newer tests like magnetic resonance pulmonary angiography. CTPA is now central part of most clinical guidelines in the diagnosis of PE, for example the guideline of the European Society of Cardiology. There several advantages of CTPA in patient management. Compared to scintigraphy CT is widely available and most radiology departments offer a round the clock CT service. It has been shown that correct interpretation of CTPA is reliable also in radiology residents at the early stage of training, which are often the first-line interpreters in out of office hour scans. CTPA is fast and can also be performed in critical ill patients. And in a large number of patients (more than 40%) alternative diagnosis are found, which is of high clinical impact for the choice of further treatment.

INDICATIONS AND CONTRAINDICATIONS

Computed tomographic pulmonary angiography is now the central investigation in suspected PE. The guidelines of the British Thoracic Society already stated in 2003 that "CTPA is now the recommended initial lung imaging". The actual guidelines of the European Society of Cardiology advocates CTPA immediately in patients with suspected PE and signs of shock or hypotension or in compensated patients with high clinical probability of PE. In patients with low or intermediate probability and elevated D-Dimer levels CTPA is also advocated. These guidelines have been widely adopted in Europe. A modified algorithm for the use of CTPA is shown in Flowchart 20.1.

The indication for CTPA in the pregnant patient is under discussion. In this scenario applied radiation dose is a concern. The imaging of choice depends on the initial chest radiography. If normal, scintigraphy is preferred over CTPA because of the lower radiation burden of scintigraphy. CTPA should only be performed in patients with abnormal chest radiography, in which the sensitivity of scintigraphy is significantly lowered. Alternative imaging

Flowchart 20.1: Modified algorithm for the diagnosis of pulmonary embolism. Indications for CTPA and simplified algorithm for pulmonary embolism.

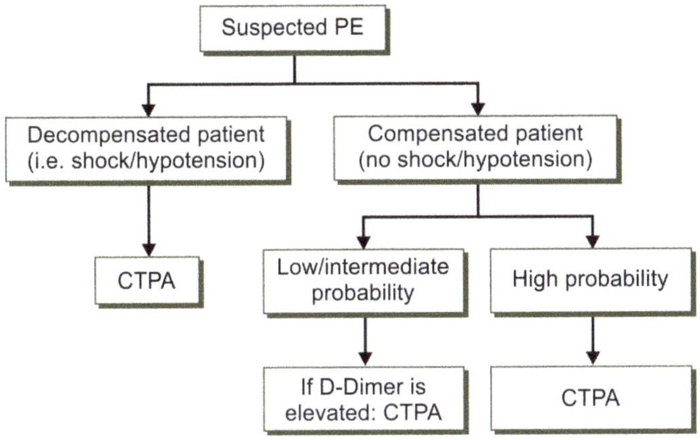

Source: Adapted from the guidelines of the European Society of Cardiology (2008).
(CTPA: Computed tomographic pulmonary angiography).

approaches like compression ultrasound of the legs and echocardiography to rule out deep venous thromboembolism or right heart dysfunction as an indirect sign of PE are also used. Another group of patients in which radiation risks deserve special attention are children. It has been estimated that in 1800 CT scans result in 1 excess cancer in children compared to children without CT exposition. Venous thromboembolism and PE are a seldom occurrence in children and occur most often in patients with underlying disease. In the pediatric patient chest radiography and D-Dimer testing should be the initial tests in cases of suspect PE. It has been shown that alternative explanations of dyspnea found on chest radiography are common and in such cases PE is very unlikely. CTPA should be reserved in children for patients with unremarkable chest radiography, elevated D-Dimer and not otherwise explainable dyspnea.

Contraindications for CTPA are largely contraindications for iodinated contrast media. Iodinated contrast media may impair renal function [contrast-induced nephropathy (CIN)]. The frequency of CIN and relevance of CIN is under debate. It has to be considered that the definition of CIN is quite weak (rise in serum creatinine of 25% after application of contrast media) and only a very small part of patients with CIN require hemodialysis. In patients with chronic kidney disease as well in patients under peritoneal dialysis with residual kidney function no persistent decline of renal function was found after administration of iodinated contrast media. It has been shown that serum creatinine changes comparable to the criteria of CIN are also occurring in hospitalized patients without application of contrast media and in a recent randomized study with matching of patients undergoing imaging with or without iodinated contrast media no significant difference in rise in serum creatinine was found. Despite this discussion and the possible overestimation of CIN in the past actual guidelines should be followed (for example the ESGUR guideline). Reduction of the applied amount of contrast media and adequate hydration are most important in patient at risk for CIN. But CTPA sometimes is an indispensable test in critically ill patient and needs to be performed also in patients with severely diminished renal function, eventually in these circumstances dialysis is required to restore renal function. Another contraindication is hyperthyroidism. The risk of developing hyperthyroidism in unselected patients is about 0.3%. If available, thyroid laboratory markers should be considered. In patients with latent hyperthyroidism contrast media can be given if the iodine uptake into the thyroid is blocked with perchlorate and eventually carbimazole. Because iodine is only slowly leaving its binding with plasma proteins initiation of thyrostatic therapy is also possible several hours after application of iodinated contrast media. In patients with manifest hyperthyroidism CTPA with iodinated contrast media should only be performed if other tests like scintigraphy are not performable, for example in patients with shock and suspected PE. Thyrostatic medication is mandatory in this scenario. Another possibility is the use of gadolinium as contrast media. The feasibility of this approach has been described. But from our own experience obtaining sufficient contrast is complicated, because only a small amount of gadolinium-based contrast media can be applied and the subsequent small bolus length. Other contraindications are related to the patient clinical state and habitus. Patients, who cannot lay down for 1 or 2 minutes are usually not examinable. Adipose patients may be too heavy for the scanner or may be too large for the gantry.

HOW THE TEST IS PERFORMED?

Technical Aspects of CTPA

The positioning of the patient is not different from other body CT examinations. Patients are positioned supine on the examination table. If possible the arms should be positioned above the head, this is reducing streak artifacts with subsequent better image quality. There are two important factors for optimal image quality. First there should no or minimal motion artifacts and second optimal opacification with contrast media of the pulmonary arteries is crucial for the detection PE. To minimize motion artifacts several strategies have been proposed. Technical advance has diminished examination times. With the introduction of single-slice CT scanners into practice examination during one breath hold got feasible. But even with the 16-slice scanner in our department imaging of the whole chest means a breath hold of about 15 seconds, this is often not possible in the ill patient. Newer scanners (64-, 128-, and 256-slice) have further diminished examination times. To minimize motion artifacts due to breathing we are scanning in caudocranial direction. There is less movement of the upper lung if breath hold cannot be performed anymore and embolism is usually more pronounced in the basal part of the lung. With slower scanners reduction of scan field, with sparring of the lung apices as well as the costophrenic angles, does not diminish sensitivity in the diagnosis of PE. Especially in younger patients this may be an approach to reduce radiation. Usually we are advocating a scan of the whole lung and not to miss pathology of the parenchyma. Minor motion artifacts of the heart, aortic root and main pulmonary trunk are often visible. These can be diminished by using ECG-gated scans. But ECG gating is not widely available and until now there is no data showing improvement in accuracy of PE detection with ECG-gated scans. To visualize PE a contrast difference between the emboli and the opacified blood must be present. In a study a minimum contrast enhancement of pulmonary arterial blood of 93 hounsfield units (HU) to detect all acute emboli was proposed, given the calculations by Wittram a double threshold should be reached. Some researchers are claiming higher density values for acute embolism and it is known that chronic embolism has also higher density. Therefore enhancement of an examinable vessel should exceed 200 HU (Fig. 20.1). After CTPA the radiologist or the technician has quickly to decide if vascular opacification is satisfying. A density measurement of all relevant arteries is not practicable. A single measurement of the density of the main pulmonary trunk may give impression of the obtained contrast. In a recent study all CTPA minimum density of 211 HU in the main pulmonary trunk were diagnostic. As a practical rule radiographers should measure central density in patients with CTPA. If density of the main pulmonary trunk exceeds 200 HU the examination may be classified as diagnostic and the patient can leave the department. If this level is not reached the patient should remain on the examination table. A density lower than 200 HU in the main pulmonary trunk does not mean that the examination is not diagnostic, but examination of the whole data set should be performed to decide if an additional scan with repeated administration of contrast media is necessary.

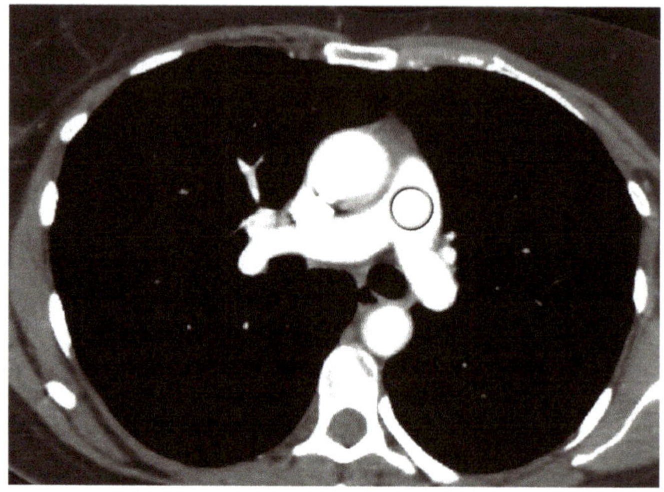

Fig. 20.1: Detail of a CTPA in a 43-year-old women. Using 60 mL of iodinated contrast media perfect opacification of the pulmonary vessels is achieved. Density measurement in the main pulmonary trunk revealed 340 HU.

To optimize arterial enhancement, high flow rates of contrast media are usually recommended. For example the usage of large bore (18 G) and proximally placed intravenous cannula (antecubital fossa) with a flow rate of 4 mL/s. In daily practice these high flow rates can often not be achieved because of poor peripheral venous status or fine bore central venous access. We have shown that even with a low injection flow rate of 2.0 mL/s enhancement of the central pulmonary arteries in most patients is also of diagnostic quality. This finding is important for everyday patient care. In patients with poor peripheral venous status the use of small bore cannulas may be adequate. Transistory fine bore central venous devices as well as port catheters may also be used. It has to be kept in mind that only a few port catheter systems do not have an approval for power injectors. However, "off- label" use of these devices is frequently performed and this is supported by data from an in vitro study, showing that tested port catheters (none had an approval for power injectors) tolerated an injection rate of 2.0 mL/s. The optimal dose and concentration of contrast media has also been debated. With higher iodine concentration the opacification of the vessel increases. On the other hand the total amount of contrast media is diminished, that is followed by a more complex timing of the scan. There have been no differences in diagnostic confidence using 75 mL or 125 mL of contrast media. Even with the use of 30 mL contrast media in a small study sufficient contrast was found in all but one patient. Several departments regularly use 60 mL of iodinated contrast media with a concentration of 350 mg iodine/mL.

An interesting option to enhance contrast is the reduction of peak tube voltage. It has bee n shown that compared to standard settings (120 kV) a reduced tube voltage of 80 kV resulted in significantly higher density values in the pulmonary arteries. However, these differences may not be clinically relevant as subjective impression of image quality does not differ between different kV values. But reduced kV setting does also result in lower radiation burden, this may be of interest in imaging younger patients. Especially with low volume of contrast media and high iodine concentrations bolus tracking is essential for optimal vessel opacification. Bolus tracking is adopting the scan to individual circulation times. A region of interest is positioned in the main pulmonary artery and after a chosen threshold for contrast media density is achieved the scan is started. This threshold varies considerably due to the used scanner and the amount of contrast media used. With a 16-slice CT scanner and 60 mL of iodinated contrast media (350 mg iodine/mL) we use a threshold of 90 HU with good results. The region of interest for bolus tracking is positioned in the main pulmonary trunk. In different studies the reconstructed slice thicknesses considerable varied, we use a reconstructed slice thickness of 1 mm. This also facilitates judgment of the lung parenchyma. But even with slice thicknesses of 2.5 mm in early studies a high sensitivity of CTPA was found. A common problem in CTPA is the so-called transient interruption of contrast media, which can be found in up to 37% of CTPA scans and may result in nondiagnostic scans. A recent study found this phenomenon in 12% of scans and 2% of the scans were nondiagnostic. Transient interruption of contrast media is thought to be connected to elevated intrathoracic pressure during deep inspiration. With deep inspiration some patients perform a valsalva maneuver, this leads to reduced inflow of contrast media from the upper extremity and increased inflow of noncontrasted blood from the abdominal cavity causing interruption of contrast. Several strategies have been proposed. Imaging in expiration leads to increased density of the pulmonary vasculature, but the diagnostic imaging of the lung parenchyma is impaired. The use of a second scan in expiration after insufficient CTPA has been proposed. Using "breath holding at ease" seems to improve pulmonary vasculature enhancement. The coaching of patients prior to CTPA (not to inhale deeply) did not reduce the number of inappropriate scans. Because of the visibility of the lung parenchyma we are using standard imaging with breath hold in deep inspiration for CTPA scans. If significant interruption of contrast occurs we are adding a second central scan with further 30 mL of contrast media and a fixed delay of 15 seconds in expiration or without breathing instructions (Figs. 20.2A and B). In the rare case of CTPA during pregnancy imaging should always be performed in expiration, because of physiologically increased abdominal blood flow severe interruption of contrast media with deep inspiration is common.

Imaging Findings of Pulmonary Embolism

We recommend examination on the primary axial slices using an adjusted soft tissue window setting. With using standard soft-tissue settings and strong opacification small emboli may be missed. The opacified vessel brightness should be diminished until the wall of the large pulmonary arteries can be clearly depicted (Figs. 20.3A and B). Secondary reconstructions (for example, maximum intensity projections) may give a global impression but may not show small emboli. In contrast to other modalities one of the main advantages of CTPA is the direct visualization of PE. Emboli are hypodense and can be differentiated from the opacified blood (Fig. 20.4). Computer-assisted detection (CAD) has been applied in several studies. In general, sensitivity is increased, especially in the inexperienced reader. Usually small subsegmental emboli are additionally detected by CAD. But high numbers of false-positive findings are interfering with efficient use in everyday clinical work. CAD for detection of embolism is commercially available and may be CAD will be a valuable second reader of CTPA in the future. With direct visualization of embolism an estimation of the clot burden is possible and different semiquantitative scores have been proposed. Extensive clot burden has been correlated to adverse outcomes. The modified Miller score was initially developed for pulmonary angiography and has been adopted for CTPA. Each of the segmental vessels which are partly or totally occluded by embolism is given 1 point. If the proximal vessel is occluded the following vessels are also scored that means MMS ranges from 0 to 16 (all lobar arteries or saddle embolus) (Figs. 20.5A and B). It has been shown that with higher scores signs of right heart dysfunction develop. Patients with a MMS of 12 or more are more likely to develop

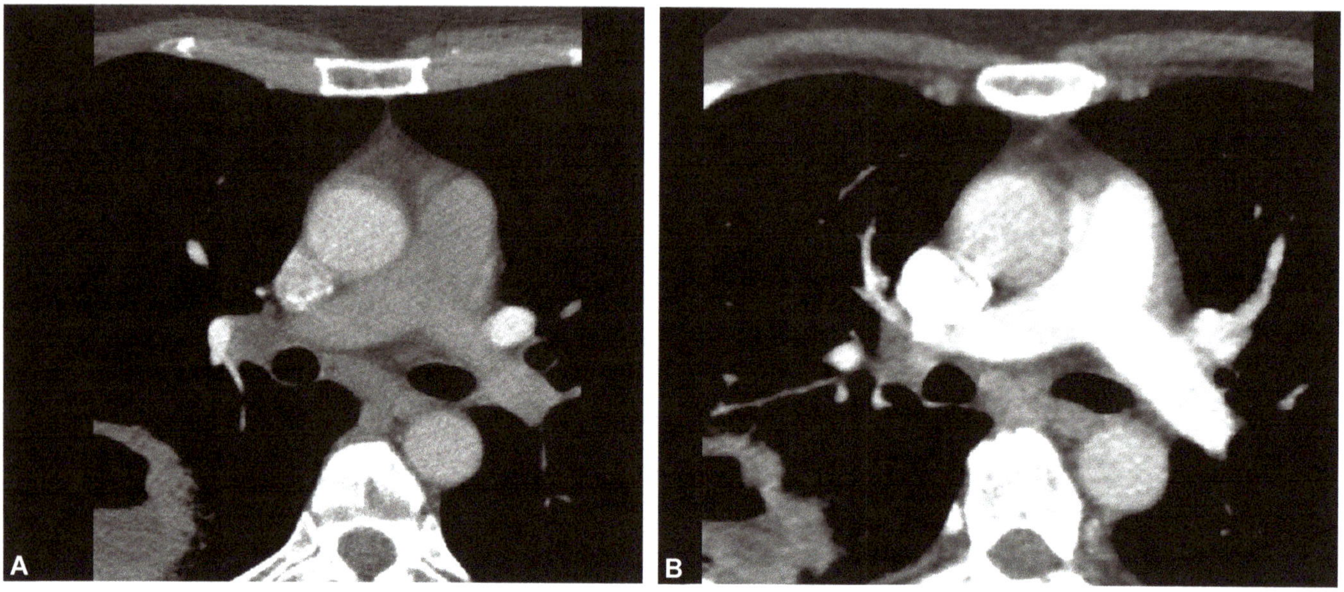

Figs. 20.2A and B: CTPA in a 44-year-old woman. With deep inspiration there is severe interruption of contrast media and the scan is non-diagnostic (A). A second scan with another 30 mL of contrast media and in expiration now shows a diagnostic opacification of the pulmonary arteries (B). Note the large necrotizing tumor of the left lung.

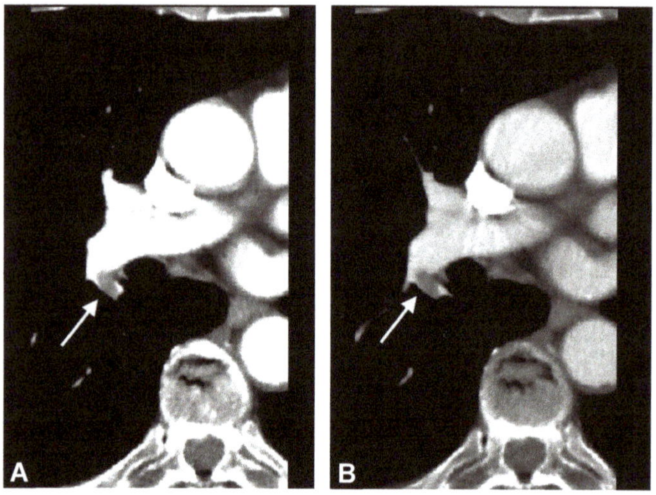

Figs. 20.3A and B: CTPA in a standard soft tissue window setting (A) and in an adjusted soft tissue window setting (B). The adjusted settings give a more detailed and better impression of the small pulmonary embolus (arrow). Small PE is sometimes difficult to see using a standard soft tissue window setting.

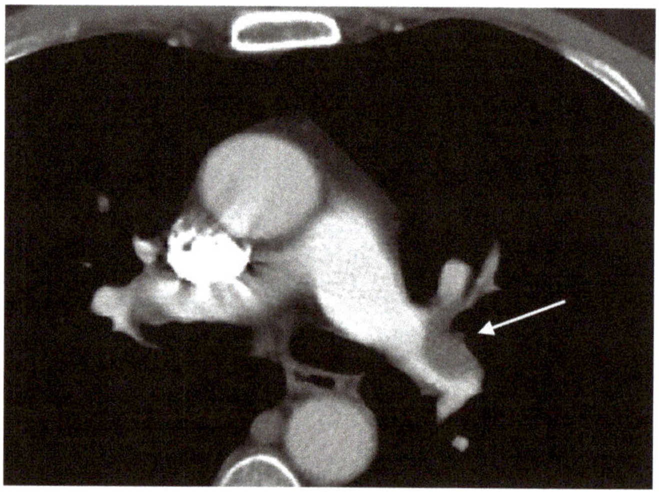

Fig. 20.4: CTPA showing pulmonary embolism at left lower and upper lung artery (arrow).

right heart decompensation (a MMS score of 12 has been described as a "tipping point" for right heart dysfunction). Right heart dysfunction is the crucial part of PE prognosis. Patients with PE usually die because of right ventricular failure. In patients with signs of shock or hypotension therefore thrombolysis or even surgical thrombectomy is indicated. But there are also patients with clinical compensated aspect, who also showing signs of right heart dysfunction. Treatment of these patients is under discussion. It has been shown that early thrombolysis in patients with signs of right heart dysfunction may improve prognosis, the influence on long-term outcome is addressed in the ongoing Pulmonary embolism thrombolysis study (PEITHO) trial. With CTPA signs of right heart dysfunction can be seen. The most useful sign is the reversal of diameters of the ventricles. Normally the short axis of the left ventricle is larger than the diameter of the right ventricle. With right heart dysfunction this reverses and a straightening

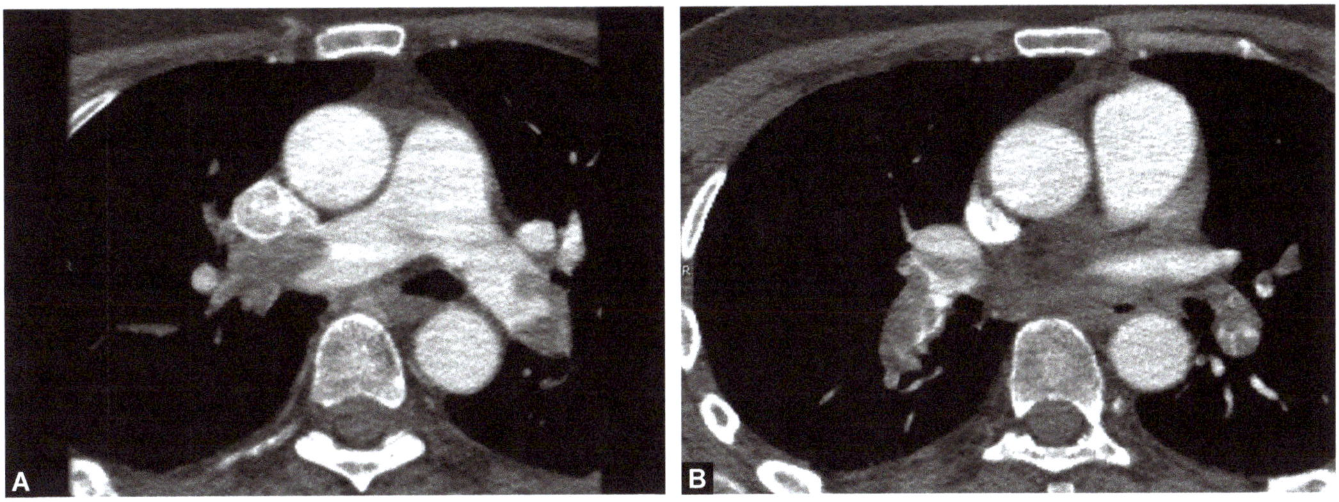

Figs. 20.5A and B: Massive bilateral pulmonary embolism on CTPA. Central (A) as well as peripheral embolism (B) is present. The high thrombus load corresponds to a modified Miller score of 16.

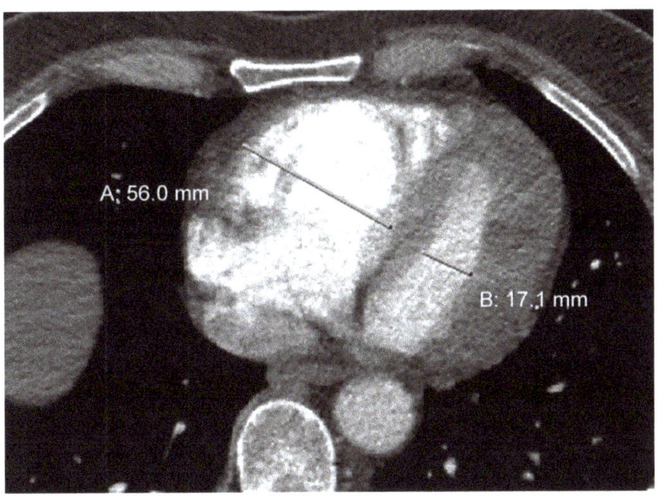

Fig. 20.6: Signs of right heart dysfunction in a patient with massive pulmonary embolism. (A) The diameter of the right ventricle is larger than (B) the diameter of the left ventricle. The interventricular septum is straightened and slightly moved into the left ventricle.

of the septum or bowing to the left ventricle can be found (Fig. 20.6). The reversal of diameters has been repeatedly linked to higher short-term mortality. Measurements on standard axial planes are reliable, reconstructions like the four-chamber views are not necessary. The signs of right heart dysfunction on CTPA correlate well with echocardiography.

Reporting of Findings

If CTPA is performed it should be read quickly. It has been shown that delayed communication of positive findings is not only associated with a longer time until the start of therapy, but also with increased mortality within 30 days. Radiologistsshouldreportroutinelyonthefollowingaspects if there is evidence of PE on the obtained CTPA: technical adequacy, localization of the embolism, clot burden and signs of right heart dysfunction. Despite all technical evolutions radiologists are usually a describing all the findings in a prose text. The introduction of elements of structured reporting in CTPA reports may improve the transferability into treatment decisions, like it has been shown with CT coronary angiography.

Diagnostic Yield

Like described at the beginning of this chapter CT has a high sensitivity in diagnosing PE, in some studies being 100% compared to the former gold-standard pulmonary angiography. In retrospective analysis of the Prospective investigation of pulmonary embolism diagnosis study (PIOPED)II data it has also been shown that some subsegmental emboli where detected by CTPA, but missed by pulmonary angiography. It has now become the imaging of choice in ruling out PE. The value of a negative CTPA has been studied extensively. The negative predictive value of CTPA has been shown to range between 94% and 100%. Several investigators have shown that withholding anticoagulation after negative CTPA is safe. Recently two issues have been discussed: the overutilization of CTPA and the overdiagnosis of PE with CTPA. The issue of overutilization arises from the low incidence of positive findings on request CTPA, in most studies around 10% of CTPA only

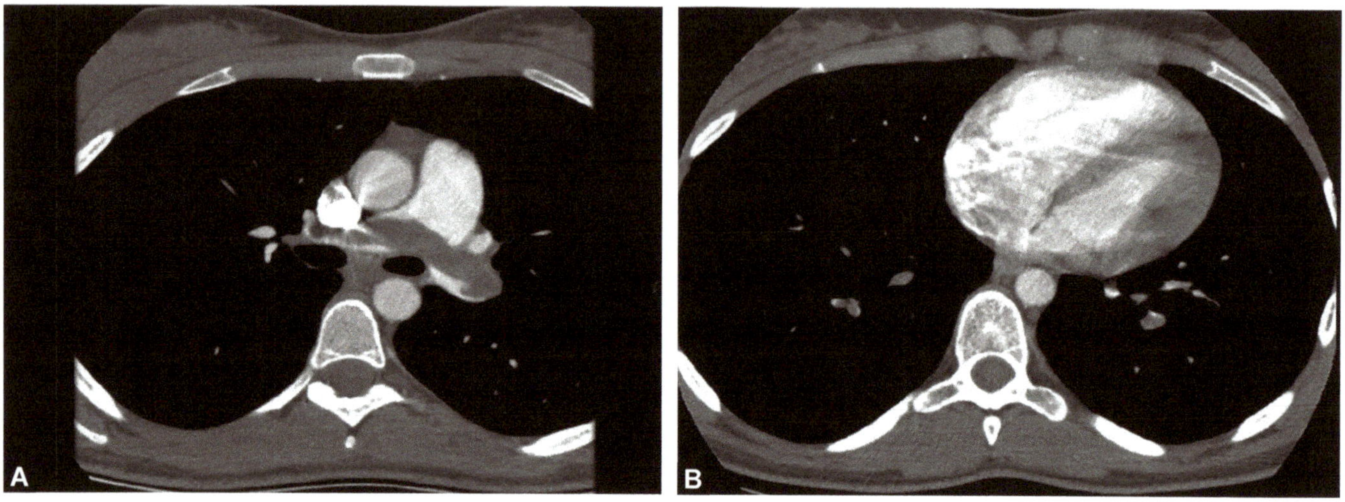

Figs. 20.7A and B: Computed tomographic pulmonary angiography (CTPA) in a 20-year-old women showing massive bilateral embolism with high thrombus load and signs of right heart dysfunction. Based on CT findings lysis was started immediately and patient recovered with no signs of persistent right heart dysfunction.

showed PE. This may be explained by nonspecific symptoms (dyspnea, thoracic pain) and the nonspecific finding of an elevated D-Dimer level. It has been shown that there are also individual factors in requiring CTPA, i.e. with a more defensive style of medicine CTPA will be requested more often. Clinical judgment and the use of established scoring systems like the Wells score are crucial for correct patient selection for CTPA. The implementation of age-adjusted D-Dimer levels also reduces the number of negative CTPA examinations. Worry because of probable overdiagnosis arises from studies showing an increase in the diagnosis of PE with no obvious changes in mortality. It has to be noted that incidental PE can be found in up to 6% of inpatients undergoing imaging of the chest with CT. These incidental PEs are usually found on the subsegmental level. More frequently with a rise in CTPA utilization less severe PE are detected and these more frequently detected. The clinical significance of subsegmental is unclear and under debate. While reviews are suggesting limited relevance, this has been challenged by newer findings. It seems that a differentiation of incidental found subsegmental emboli and symptomatic emboli is warranted. In symptomatic subsegmental PE outcome may not to differ significantly from more proximal located embolism. In contrast, currently available data suggests that without treatment, mortality is not elevated in incidental found subsegmental PE. Some authors even argue that the lung acts as a filter, and the clearance of small emboli is a physiological process.

In conclusion, CTPA is the imaging of choice in suspected PE and central part of established guidelines. PE is still frequently not clinically suspected and therefore not diagnosed, but on the other hand with increased use of CTPA overdiagnosis may occur. In the proper clinical context CTPA reliable detects or excludes PE. In the case of PE the estimation of clot burden and judgment of right heart dysfunction from the CTPA may rapidly guide further treatment (Figs. 20.7A and B).

BIBLIOGRAPHY AND FURTHER READING

1. Arnold RW, Janitz E, Boulton TB, Bacic J, Frush DP. CT pulmonary angiography to evaluate for pulmonary embolism in children visiting adult- centered community hospitals. AJR. 2011;196:W823-30.
2. Aymard T, Kadner A, Widmer A, Basciani R, Tevaearai H, Weber A, et al. Massive pulmonary embolism: surgical embolectomy versus thrombolytic therapy—should surgical indication be revisited? Eur J Cardiothor Surg. 2013;43:90-4.
3. Bernabé-García JM, García-Espasa C, Arenas-Jiménez J, Sánchez-Payá J, de la Hoz-Rosa J, Carreres-Polo JO. Has "respiratory coaching" before deep inspiration an impact on the incidence of transient contrast interruption during pulmonary CT angiography? Insights Imaging. 2012;3:505-11.
4. British Thoracic Society Standards of commitee pulmonary embolism guideline development group. British Thoracic Society guidelines for the managment of suspected acute pulmonary embolism. Thorax. 2003;58:470-84.
5. Carrier M, Rhighini M, Wells PS, Perrier A, Anderson DR, Rodger MA, et al. Subsegmental pulmonary embolism diagnosed by computed tomography: incidence and clinical implications. A systematic review and meta- analysis of the management outcome tudies. J Thromb Haemost. 2010; 8:1716-22.
6. Cervini P, Bell CM, Roberts HC, Provost YL, Chung TB, Paul NS. Radiology resident interpretation of on- call pulmonary angiogramms. Acad Radiol. 2008;15:556-62.

7. Chen YH, Velayudhan V, Weltman DI, Balsam D, Patel N, Draves KA, et al. Waiting to exhale: salvaging the nondiagnostic CT pulmonary angiogram by using expiratory imaging to improve contrast dynamics. Emerg Radiol. 2008;15:161-9.
8. Cobelli R, Zompatori M, De Luca G, Chiari G, Bresciani P, Marcato C. Clincal usefulness of computed tomography study without contrast injection in the evaluation of acute pulmonary embolism. J Comput Assist Tomogr. 2005;29:6-12.
9. Cok G, Tasbakan MS, Ceylan N, Bayraktaroglu S, Duman S. Can we use CT pulmonary angiography as an alternative to echocardiography in determining right ventricular dysfunction and its severity in patients with acute pulmonary thromboembolism? Jpn J Radiol. 2013;31:172-8.
10. Costa AF, Basseri H, Sheikh A, Stiell I, Dennie C. The yield of CT pulmonary angiograms to exclude acute pulmonary embolism. Emerg Radiol. 2014;21:133-41.
11. Den Exter PL, van Es J, Klok FA, Kroft LJ, Kruip MJ, Kamphuisen PW, et al. Risk profile and clinical outcome of symptomatic subsegmental acute pulmonary embolism. Blood. 2013;122:1144-9.
12. Desai R. Unsuspected pulmonary embolism on CT scanning: yet another headache for clinicians? Thorax. 2007;62:470-2.
13. Dittrich E, Puttinger H, Schillinger M, Lang I, Stefenelli T, Hörl WH, et al. Effect of radio contrast media on residual renal function in peritoneal dialysis patients- a prospective study. Nephrol Dial Transplant. 2006;21:1334-9.
14. Douma RA, Hofstee HM, Schaefer-Prokop C, van Waesberghe JH, Lely RJ, Kamphuisen PW, et al. Comparison of 4- and 64-slice CT scanning in the diagnosis of pulmonary embolism. Throm Haemost. 2010;103:242-6.
15. Gebauer B, Teichgräber UK, Hothan T, Felix R, Wagner HJ. Contrast media pressure injection using a portal catheter system- results of an *in vitro* study. Rofo. 2005;177:1417-23.
16. Ghoshhajra BB, Lee AM, Ferencik M, Elmariah S, Margey RJ, Onuma O, et al. Interpreting the interpretations: the use of structured reporting improves reffering clinicians' comprehension of coronary CT angiography reports. J Am Coll Radiol. 2013;10(6):432-8.
17. Godwin JD, Webb WR, Gamsu G, Ovenfors OV. Computed tomography of pulmonary embolism. AJR. 1980;135:691-5.
18. Gossner J. Feasibility of computed tomographic angiography with low flow rates. J Clin Imag Sci. 2012;2:57.
19. Guilabert JP, Manzur DN, Tarrasa MJ, Llorens ML, Braun P, Arques MP. Can multislice CT alone rule out reliably pulmonary embolism? A prospective study. Eur J Radiol. 2007;62:220-6.
20. Gurney JW. No fooling around: direct visualization of pulmonary embolism. Radiology. 1993;188:618-9.
21. Hintze G, Blombach O, Fink H, Burkhardt U, Köbberling J. Risk of iodine induced thyreotoxicosis after coronary angiography: an investigation in 788 unselected subjects. Eur J Endocrin. 1999;140:264-7.
22. Hunsacker AR, Oliva IB, Cai T, Trotman-Dickenson B, Gill RR, Hatabu H, et al. Contrast opacification using a reduced volume of iodinated contrast material and low peak kilovoltage in pulmonary CT angiography: objective and subjective evaluation. AJR. 2010;195:W118-24.
23. Hunsaker AR, Lu MT, Goldhaber SZ, Rybicki FJ. Imaging in acute pulmonary embolism with spezial clinical scenarios. Cir Cardiovasc imaging. 2010;3:491-500.
24. Kalva SP, Jagannathan JP, Hahn PF, Wicky ST. Venous thromboembolism: indirect CT venography during CT pulmonary angiography- should the pelvis be imaged. Radiology. 2008;246:605-11.
25. Karabulut N. Inferior caval blood flow affects quality of CTPA during pregnancy. Eur Radiol. 2009;19:1693.
26. Kim IY, Lee SB, Lee DW, Song SH, Seong EY, Kwak IS. Long- term effect of radiocontrast- enhanced computed tomography on the renal function of chronic kidney disease patient. Clin Exp Nephrol. 2012;16: 755-9.
27. Konstandinides S, Geibel A, Heusel G, Heinrich F, Kasper W; Management Strategies and Prognosis of Pulmonary Embolism-3 Trial Investigators. Heparin plus alteplase compared with heparine alone in patients with submassive pulmonary embolism. N Engl J Med. 2002;347:1143-50.
28. Kumamaru KK, Hunsaker AR, Kumamaru H, George E, Bedayat A, Rybicki FJ. Correlation between early direct communication of positive pulmonary angiography findings and improved clinical outcome. Chest. 2013;144:1546-54.
29. Kurcz J, Garacek J, Guzinski M, Czarnecka A, S⊠siadek MJ. Multislice computed tomography angiography as an imaging modality of choice in patients with suspicion of pulmonary embolism—own experiences and modern imaging techniques. Adv Clin Exp Med. 2013;22:705-13.
30. Kuzo RS, Pooley RA, Crook JE, Heckman MG, Gerber TC. Measurement of caval blood flow with MRI during respiratory maneuvers: implications for vascular contrast opacification on pulmonary CT angiographic studies. AJR. 2007;188:839-42.
31. Leung AN, Bull TM, Jaeschke R, Lockwood CJ, Boiselle PM, Hurwitz LM, et al. An official American Thoracic Society/Society of Thoracic Imaging clinical practice guideline: evaluation of suspected pulmonary embolism in pregnancy. Am J Resp Crit Care Med. 2011;184:1200-8.
32. Li YK, Lau KK, Ardley N, Lau T. Effiacy of 'breath holding at ease' during CT pulmonary angiography in the improvement of contrast enhancement in pulmonary arteries. J Med Imaging Radiat Oncol. 2013;57:415-22.
33. Lloyd S, Sahu A, Riordan R. Diagnosis of pulmonary embolism by computed tomographic pulmonary angiography with and without optimal contrast enhancement: a prospective single centre audit. Hong Kong J Radiol. 2012;15:162-9.
34. Lu MT, Demehri S, Cai T, Parast L, Hunsaker AR, Goldhaber SZ, et al. Axial and reformatted four-chamber right ventricle-to-left ventricle diameter ratios on pulmonary angiography as predictors of death after acute pulmonary embolism. AJR. 2012;198:1353-60.
35. Mathews JD, Forsythe AV, Brady Z, Butler MW, Goergen SK, Byrnes GB, et al. Cancer risk in 680000 people exposed to computed tomographiy scans in childhood or adolescence: data linkage study of 11 million Australians. BMJ. 2013;346:f2360.
36. McDonald RJ, McDonald JS, Bida JP, Carter RE, Fleming CJ, Misra S, et al. Intravenous contrast material- induced

nephropathy: causal or coincident phenomenon? Radiology. 2013;267:106-8.

37. Meanley TF, Raudikivi U, McIntyre WJ, Gallagher JH, Haaga JR, Havrilla TR, et al. Detection of low-contrast in computed body tomography: an experimental study of simulated lesions. Radiology 1980;134:149-54.
38. Mortimer AM, Singh RK, Hughes J, Greenwood R, Hamilton MC. Use of exspiratory CT pulmonary angiography to reduce inspiration and breath-hold artefact: contrast dynamics and implication for scan protocol. Clin Radiol. 2011;66:1159-66.
39. Newhouse JH, Kho D, Rao QA, Starren J. Frequency of serum creatinine changes in the absence of iodinated contrast material: implications for studies of contrast nephrotoxicity. AJR. 2008;191:376-82.
40. Pérez de Llano LA, Veres Racamonde A, Ortiz Piquer M, López Díaz MJ, Janeiro Amela M, Méndez Maroto L, et al. Safety of withholding anticoagulant therapy in patients who have clinically suspected pulmonary embolism and negative results on helical computed tomography. Respiration. 2006;73:514-9.
41. Remy-Jardin M, Remy J, Deschildre F, Artaud D, Beregi JP, Hossein-Foucher C, et al. Diagnosis of pulmonary embolism with spiral CT: comparison with pulmonary angiography and scintigraphy. Radiology. 1996;200:699-706.
42. Remy-Jardin M, Remy J, Wattine L, Giraud F. Central pulmonary thromboembolism: diagnosi with spiral volumetric CT with single breath-hold technique- comparison with pulmonary angiography. Radiology. 1992;185:381-7.
43. Rendl J, Saller B. Schilddrüse und Röntgenkontrastmittel. Dt Ärztebl. 2001;98:A402-6.
44. Righini M, van Es J, Den Exter PL, Roy PM, Verschuren F, Ghuysen A, et al. Age-adjusted D-Dimer cutoff levels to rule out pulmonary embolism: ADJUST-PE study. JAMA. 2014;311:1117-24.
45. Ritchie G, McGurk S, McCreath C, Graham C, Murchison JT. Prospective evaluation of unsuspected pulmonary embolism on contrast enhanced multidetector CT (MDCT) scanning. Thorax. 2007;62:536-40.
46. Schafer-Prokop C, Bankier A, Janata K, et al. Complete CTA versus limited range CTA for the diagnosis of PE: what do we miss? Abstract presented at the European Congress of Radiology (ECR). 2005; Eur Radiol Suppl; B-595.
47. Schellhaass A, Walther A, Konstantinides S, Böttiger BW. The diagnosis and treatment of acute pulmonary embolism. Dtsch Arztebl Int. 2010;107:589-95.
48. Schissler AJ, Rozensthtein A, Kulon ME, Pearson GD, Green RA, Stetson PD, CT pulmonary angiography: increasingly diagnosing less severe pulmonary emboli. PLoS One. 2013;12:e65669.
49. Shuman WP, Leipsic JA, Busey JM, Green DE, Pipavath SN, Hague CJ, et al. Prospective ECG gated CT pulmonary angiography versus helical ungated CT pulmonary angiography: impact on cardiac related motion artifacts and patient radiation dose. Eur J Radiol. 2012;81:2444-9.
50. Singh T, Lam KV, Murray C. Low volume contrast CTPA in patients with renal dysfunction. J Med Imaging Radiat Oncol. 2011;55:143-8.
51. Smadja L, Remy-Jardin M, Dupuis P, Deken-Delannoy V, Devos P, Duhamel A, et al. Gadolinium-enhanced thoracic CTA: retropsective analysis of image quality and tolerability in 45 patients evaluated prior to the description of nephrogenic systemic fibrosis. J Radiol. 2009;90:287-98.
52. Stacul F, van der Molen AJ, Reimer P, Webb JA, Thomsen HS, Morcos SK, et al. Contrast induced nephropathy: updated ESUR contrast media safety committee guidelines. Eur Rad. 2011;21:2527-41.
53. Stein PD, Fowler SE, Goodman LR, Gottschalk A, Hales CA, Hull RD, et al. Multidetector computed tomography for acute pulmonary embolism. N Engl J Med. 2006;354: 2317-27.
54. Swensen SJ, Sheedy PF, Ryu JH, Pickett DD, Schleck CD, Ilstrup DM, et al. Outcomes after withholding anticoagulation from patients with suspected acute pulmonary embolism and negative computed tomographic findings: a cohort study. Mayo Clin Proc. 2002;77:130-8.
55. Szucs- Farkas Z, Christe A, Megyeri B, Rohacek M, Vock P, Nagy EV, et al. Diagnostic accuracy of computed tomography pulmonary angiography with reduced radiation and contrast material dose: a prospective randomized clinical trial. Invest Radiol. 2014;49:201-8.
56. Toprak O, Cirit M. Risk factors for contrast-induced nephropathy. Kidney Blood Press Res. 2006;29:84-93.
57. Torbicki A, Perrier A, Konstantinides S, Agnelli G, Galiè N, Pruszczyk P, et al. Gudeline on the diagnosis and managment of acute pulmonary embolism. The task force for the diagnosis and amangment of acute pulmonary embolism of the European Society of Cardiology (ESC). Europ Heart J. 2008;29:2276-315.
58. van der Meer RW1, Pattynama PM, van Strijen MJ, van den Berg-Huijsmans AA, Hartmann IJ, Putter H, et al. Right ventricular dysfunction and pulmonary obstruction index at helical CT: prediction of clinical outcome dusring 3- month follow- up in patients with acute pulmonary embolism. Radiology. 2005;235:798-803.
59. Wiener RS, Schwartz LM, Woloshin S. Time trends in pulmonary embolism in the United States: evidence of overdiagnosis. Arch Intern Med. 2011;171:831-7.
60. Winer- Muram HT, Rydberg J, Johnson MS, Tarver RD, Williams MD, Shah H, et al. Suspected pulmonary embolism: evaluation with multi-detector CT versus digital substraction pulmonary angiography. Radiology. 2004;233:806-15.
61. Wittenberg R, Peters JF, Sonnemans JJ, Prokop M, Schaefer-Prokop CM. Computer assisted detection of pulmonary embolism: evaluation of of CT pulmonary angiograms performed in an on-call setting. Eur Radiol. 2010;20:801-6.

62. Wittram C, Waltman AC, Shepard AJ, Halpern E, Goodman LR. Discordance between CT and angiography in the PIOPED II study. Radiology. 2007;244:883-9.
63. Wittram C. How I do it: CT pulmonary angiography. AJR Am J Roentgenol. 2007;188:1255-61.
64. Wong LF, Akram AR, McGurk S, Van Beek EJ, Reid JH, Murchison JT. Thrombus load and acute right ventricul failure in pulmonary embolism: correlation and demonstration of a "tipping point" on CT pulmonary angiography. Br J Radiol. 2012;85:1471-6.
65. Yilmaz Ö, Üstün ED, Kayan M, Kayan F, Akta⊠ AR, Unlü EN, et al. Diagnostic quality of CT pulmonary angiography in pulmonary thromboembolism: a comparison of three different kV values. Med Sci Monit. 2013;19:908-15.

Chapter 21

Conventional Pulmonary Angiography

Filippo Russo, Claudio Sorino, Mario Galli

OVERVIEW OF PULMONARY ANGIOGRAPHY

Catheter-directed pulmonary angiography (PA) is a well-established, safe and quite accurate invasive method of evaluating main and branch pulmonary arteries by use of contrast agent and X-rays.

Over the last two decades alternative noninvasive technologies with higher sensitivity for capturing pulmonary vascular images have also evolved, including computed tomography (CT) and magnetic resonance imaging (MRI), so that diagnostic PA is performed in less cases.

However, PA remains an important tool in catheterization laboratory since more therapeutic options are catheter guided; moreover it is an important tool to obtain diagnostic information when noninvasive techniques are insufficient.

First PA was reported by Robb and Steinberg in 1938 and through subsequent decades the procedure became faster, simpler and safer thanks to technology evolution including different catheters and guidewires availability, iodinated contrast safety and radiographic image resolution.

INDICATIONS

Pulmonary angiography indications are well established and summarized in the last revised guidelines for performance of arteriography by the *American College of Radiology (ACR)*, the *Society of Interventional Radiology (SIR)*, and the *Society of Pediatric Radiology (SPR)*.

Guidelines highly recommend to determine the relative benefit and risk of diagnostic arteriography compared with alternative noninvasive diagnostic techniques for each patient, suggesting that PA should be used as an adjunction when other diagnostic tests are inconclusive or discordant with clinical data or when it is preparatory to interventional procedures on pulmonary circulation.

Main PA indications are:

- Suspected acute pulmonary embolism
- Suspected chronic pulmonary embolism
- Suspected other pulmonary vascular abnormalities, congenital or acquired, such as aneurysm, arteriovenous fistula, stenosis, neoplasm, foreign bodies.

Acute Pulmonary Embolism

Pulmonary embolus angiographic images include abrupt intraluminal defect, tapered peripheral vessels, and avascular lung regions. Nowadays the most common PA indication is the diagnosis and treatment of acute pulmonary embolism in particular clinical settings such as high risk acute pulmonary embolism (Table 21.1).

Although in literature only some case series are available, *catheter directed thrombectomy* is considered a feasible, safe and effective life-saving therapeutic option; it is indicated by the *European Society of Cardiology (ESC)*

Table 21.1: Features useful in identifying patient with high mortality risk from pulmonary embolism and consequent approach suggested.

Risk	*Low*	*Intermediate*	*High*
Clinical features	NO Right ventricle disfunction NO myocardial injury NO shock or hypotension	Right ventricle disfunction AND/OR Myocardial injury NO shock or hypotension	Shock or hypotension
Possible approach	Early discharge or home treatment	Hospital admission	Thrombolysis or embolectomy

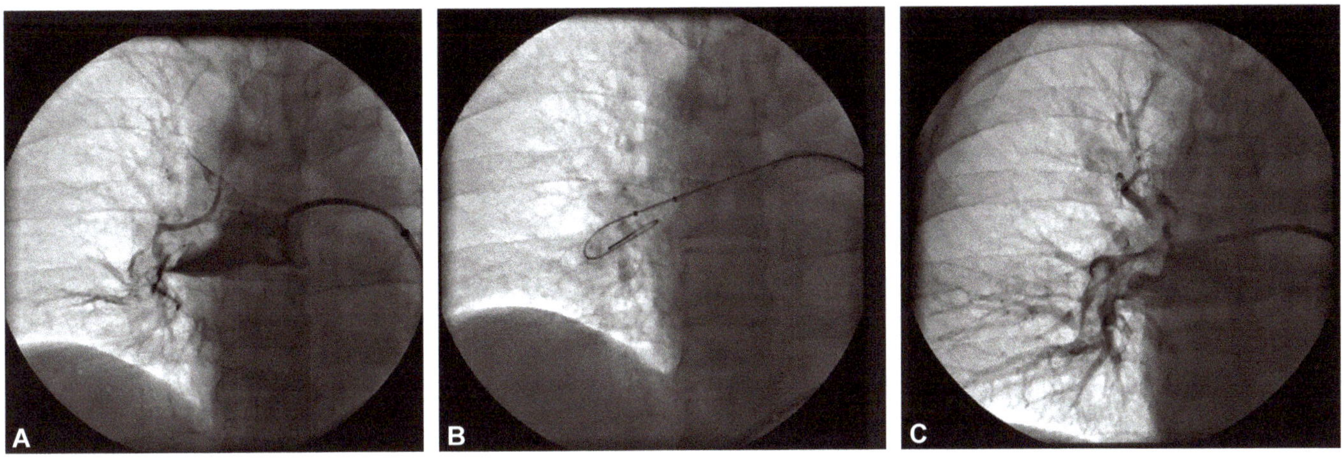

Figs. 21.1A to C: Pulmonary angiogram of acute right pulmonary embolism in 75-year-old patient treated by *rheolytic thrombectomy*. (A) Basal right pulmonary artery angiogram showing intraluminal massive obstructive thrombosis. (B) Catheter-guided rheolytic thrombectomy by use of *Xpeedior Angiojet catheter*. (C) Final angiographic result after treatment showing perfusion improvement.

guidelines (IIa class recommendation) in case of thrombolytic absolute contraindications or failure, or as an alternative to surgery if immediate access to cardiopulmonary bypass is unavailable. Catheter-guided thrombectomy provides significant blood flow improvement and is associated with hemodynamic restoring even if only modest angiographic changes appear to the operating physician (Figs. 21.1A to C).

Preliminary pulmonary imaging, in particular CT, is highly recommended in order to access thrombectomy technical feasibility and to guide physicians to a specific lung segment, allowing the less time consuming examination.

European Society of Cardiology guidelines also recommend that catheter technique should only be used when the main pulmonary artery branches are involved. Indeed, no benefit is expected from embolus fragmentation in smaller branches, whereas it is often associated with high risk of artery perforation.

The Greenfield suction embolectomy catheter introduced in 1969 remains the only device approved by the *Food and Drug Administration (FDA)*; over the last two decades a variety of different catheters has been introduced, including specific designed pulmonary catheters and rheolytic catheters. More recently, devices which can be introduced via sheath ranging from 6 to 11F have been developed, so that procedures are associated with less vascular access site complications.

Chronic Pulmonary Embolism

Pulmonary angiography in chronic pulmonary embolism is rarely performed because of its inability to fully described the disease location and extension, which is necessary for surgical thrombendoarterectomy planning.

Some other well established technologies have a higher sensitivity and specificity than PA for obtaining pulmonary angiographic images, such as CT and MRI.

In literature a some reports describe good clinical outcomes after surgical endarterectomy in patients affected by pulmonary hypertension secondary to chronic thromboembolism.

Pulmonary Vascular Abnormalities

Pulmonary angiography is sometimes performed after other noninvasive diagnostic screening when vascular abnormalities a better definition or catheter-guided treatment is required.

Pulmonary artery aneurysm is a quite rare vascular abnormality, defined as an increase in diameter vessel by 50% over normal diameter.

Aneurysms could be fusiform or saccular, focal or multiple, located in the main branches of pulmonary arteries or in peripheral vessels.

In most case they are acquired and mainly secondary to acute or chronic pulmonary infections (tuberculosis, syphilis, septic emboli), chronic pulmonary hypertension, inflammatory disease (vasculitis) and surgical repair of congenital heart disease; congenital aneurysm are unusual and may be seen in Bechet's disease, Marfan and Hughes-Stovin syndromes.

Pseudoaneurysms are usually of iatrogenic nature, secondary to wall trauma during pulmonary arteries catheterization.

Percutaneous repair of a pulmonary artery aneurysm is feasible, safe and effective, mainly by coils embolization; aneurysm rupture usually leads to fatal hemorrhage.

Systemic to pulmonary circulation communication are unusually described; they may be congenital, due to an embryologic defect in terminal capillary loop (e.g. Osler-Weber-Rendu syndrome), or acquired, secondary to trauma, infections (e.g. aspergillosis, tuberculosis, schistosomiasis), or hepatogenic angiodysplasia (Figs. 21.2 to 21.5).

Pulmonary arteriovenous fistula (PAVF) screening should be done only by noninvasive imaging techniques such as echocardiography, spiral CT and MRI; PA should be considered only if percutaneous treatment is required.

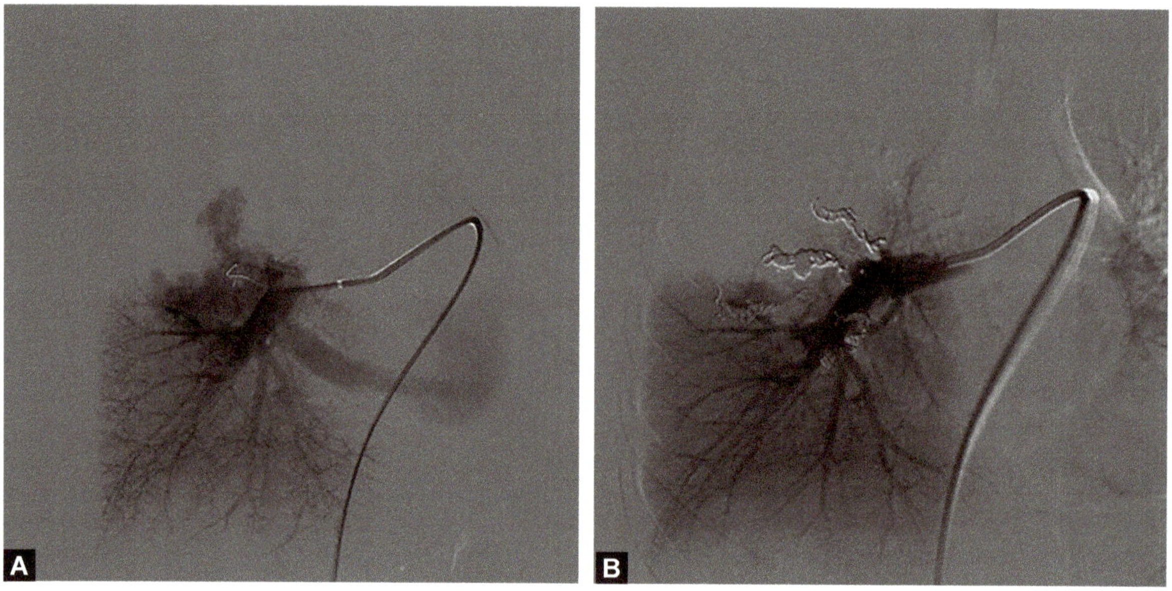

Figs. 21.2A and B: (A) A symptomatic pediatric case with *Osler-Weber-Rendu syndrome*. Right pulmonary digital subtraction angiography showing a complex right *pulmonary arteriovenous malformation (PAVM)*. (B) Right pulmonary arteriography showing complete exclusion of the feeding vessels of the PAVM, using large volume detachable coils and an *Amplatzer occluder*.

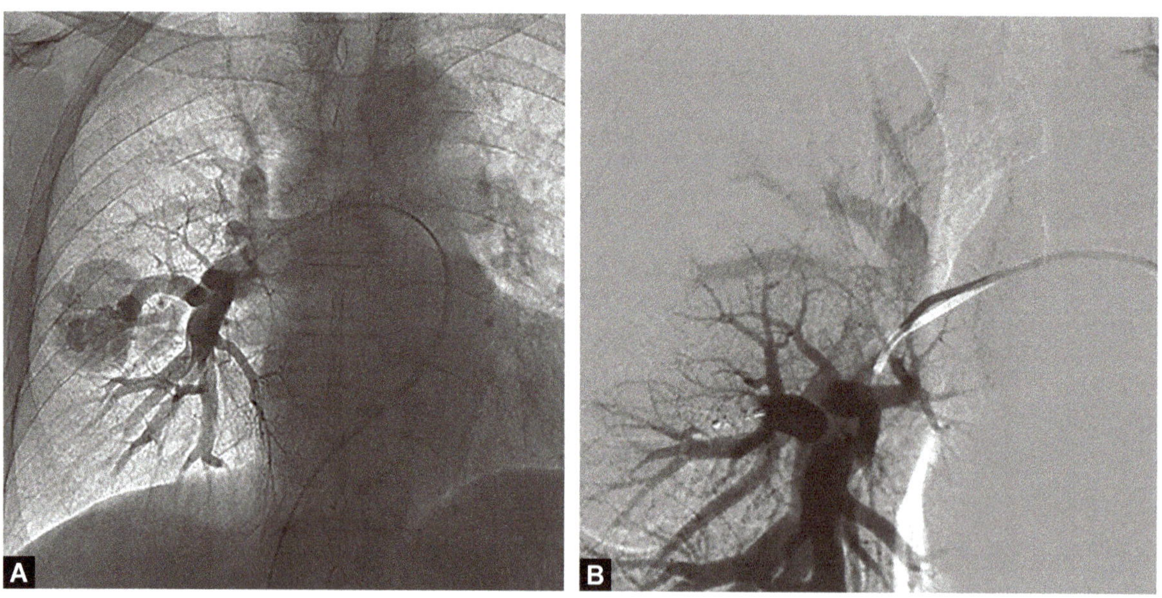

Figs. 21.3A and B: (A) Massive right *pulmonary arteriovenous malformation* in a patient affected by *Osler-Weber-Rendu syndrome*. (B) Right pulmonary angiography confirming occlusion of the right pulmonary arteriovenous malformation by use of *Amplatzer occluder*.

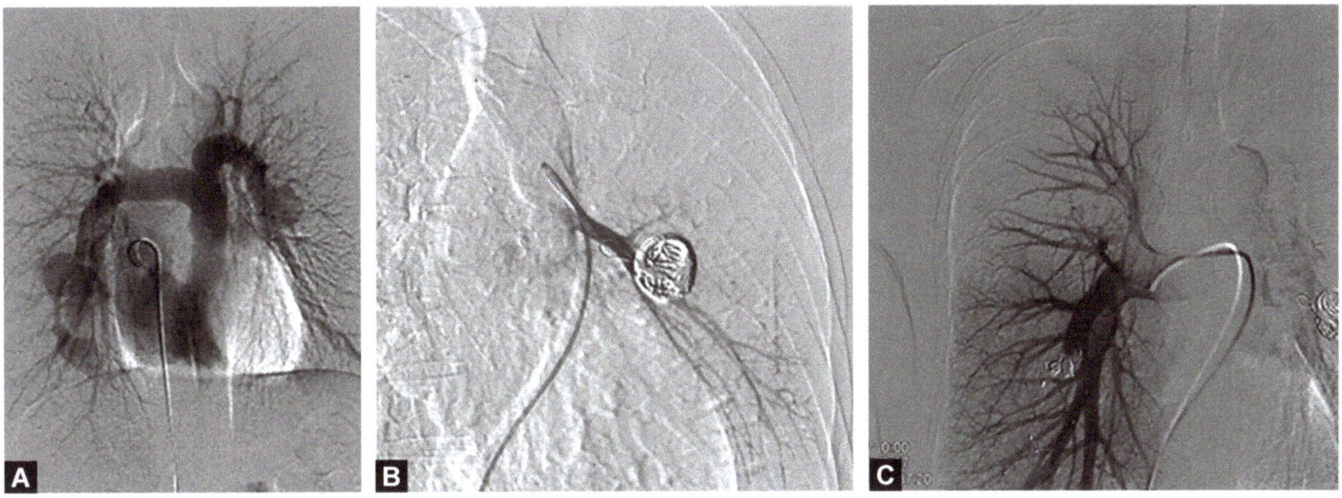

Figs. 21.4A to C: (A) Bilateral pulmonary angiogram demonstrating voluminous bilateral pulmonary arteriovenous malformations in a patient with *Osler-Weber-Rendu syndrome*. (B) Embolization of the left pulmonary arteriovenous malformation with large volume detachable coils. (C) Occlusion of the right pulmonary arteriovenous malformations with multiple *Amplatzer occluders* and several large volume detachable coils.

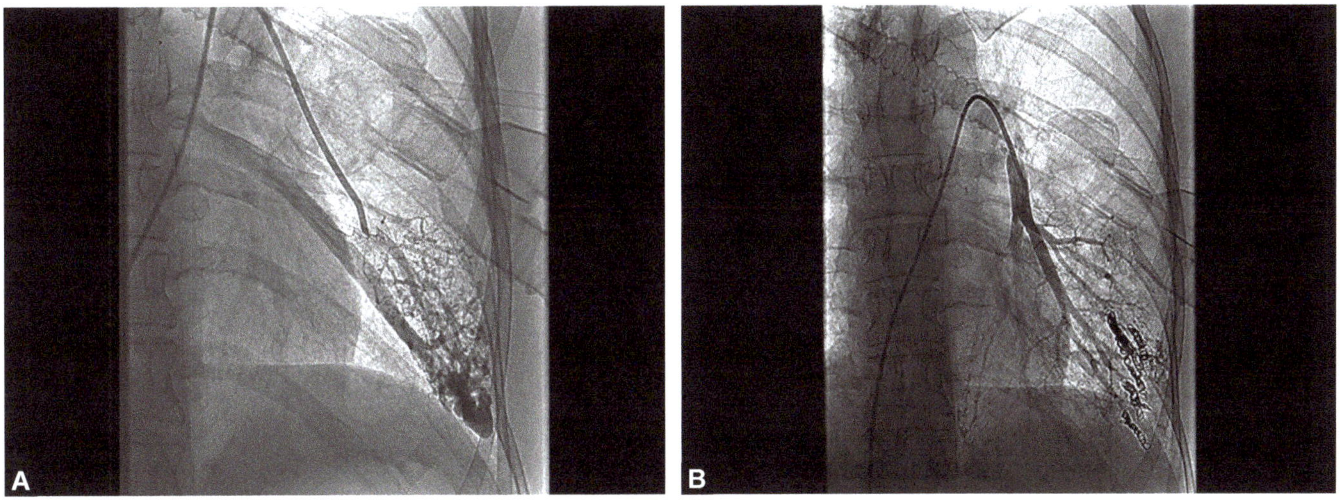

Figs. 21.5A and B: (A) Right basal pulmonary angiogram representing arteriovenous fistulas in a patient affected by *Osler-Weber-Rendu syndrome*. (B) Right pulmonary arteriography indicating good exclusion of the pulmonary arteriovenous fistulas (PAVFs).

When major symptoms are present, repair should be considered and percutaneous embolization by use of coils and detachable balloons is feasible, safe, and effective.

Pulmonary artery stenoses are uncommon and may be congenital or acquired. Congenital stenosis may be present without cardiac abnormalities or associated with some of them, such as aortic stenosis, tetralogy of Fallot, truncus arteriosus and ventricular septal defects.

Pulmonary artery stenosis may be secondary to chronic infections (e.g. histoplasmosis, schistosomiasis), associated with idiopathic hypercalcemia or following pulmonary artery shunts banding. When a pulmonary artery stenosis is found, it should be evaluated functionally by pressure gradient measurement across it; percutaneous treatment by angioplasty and stent implantation is described mainly in congenital stenosis and appears associated with good immediate and mid-term results; only few case reports are reported in literature about acquired stenosis treatment.

Pulmonary vascular neoplasms are very rare and mainly observed in leiomyosarcoma. They appear as irregular masses usually located in pulmonary main branches which may cause obstruction, encasement or displacement.

Pulmonary angiography is also necessary when the *removal of foreign bodies*, especially medical devices such as stents, catheters and filter, is required.

CONTRAINDICATIONS

No absolute contraindications to PA exist.

In according with the *ACR-SIR-SPR guidelines* for arteriography performance, only relative contraindications should be considered and every effort should be made for their correction, if feasible.

Relative contraindications include:

- Left bundle branch block because of the risk of complete heart block developing during right heart catheterization
- Systemic or pulmonary severe hypertension
- Uncorrectable coagulopathy or thrombocytopenia
- Clinical significant sensitivity to iodinated contrast material
- Renal failure based on the estimated glomerular filtration rate (eGFR)
- Congestive heart failure
- Certain connective tissue disorders because of reported complications at the puncture site.

Table 21.2: Indicators and thresholds for complications in diagnostic arteriography.

Department indicators	*Reported rates*	*Major adverse event threshold*
Puncture site complications		
Hematoma (requiring trasfusion, surgery or delayed discharge)	0.0% to 0.68%	0.5%
Occlusion	0.0% to 0.76%	0.2%
Pseudoaneurysm or arteriovenous fistula	0.04% to 0.3%	0.2%
Catheter-induced complications in the aorta or principal branches (other than puncture site)		
Distal emboli	0.0% to 0.10%	0.2%
Arterial dissection/subintimal passage	0.43%	0.5%
Subintimal injection of contrast media	0.0% to 0.44%	0.5%
Other procedure-related complications		
Major contrast media reactions	0.0% to 3.58%	0.5%
Contrast-media-induced Nephrotoxicity requiring renal replacement therapy (such as dialysis)	0.2% to 3.0%	0.2%
Overall procedure threshold for major complications	0.1%	

RISKS AND POSSIBLE COMPLICATIONS

Pulmonary angiography, as an invasive procedure, may be associated with some possible, but uncommon, complications which can be classified as major and minor complications (Table 21.2).

Major complications are defined as those that are life-threatening, do not promptly respond to medical therapy or require invasive treatment, unplanned increase in patient's level of care and prolonged hospitalization (e.g. cardiopulmonary resuscitation, endotracheal intubation, blood transfusion, dialysis, percutaneous or surgical vascular access repair).

Minor complications are those that result in no long-term morbidity, spontaneously regress or require nominal medical therapy.

According with the ACR-SIR-SPR guidelines for performance of arteriography, complications may be classified into three groups: puncture site, systemic and catheter induced.

Puncture site complications include arterial hematoma, thrombosis, spasm, dissection, pseudoaneurysm, arteriovenous fistula. Most puncture site complications occur in small size patients (e.g. infants and children) because of their small size vessels relative to sheaths' and catheters' size.

Hematoma is the most common puncture site complication with very low incidence of major hematoma requiring repair, transfusion or prolonged hospitalization, and variable incidence of minor hematoma (between 5% and 10%), depending on the puncture site chosen (femoral or axillary vein).

Other puncture site complications are rare, occurring in less than 1% of puncture.

Infections at puncture site with bacteriemia is rare, mainly interesting high risk patient (e.g. immunocompromised, diabetics) or in case of repeated puncture at same access site over a short period, long procedures, long-term sheath access; in those cases antibiotic prophylaxis should be considered.

Systemic complications include vaso-vagal symptoms, usually with mild intensity that pass in few minutes without requiring medical therapy (nausea, vomiting, bradicardia, syncope), contrast related reactions that require hospitalization in less than 1% (urticaria, periorbital edema, wheezing), and contrast induced nephropathy (CIN).

Contrast induced nephropathy is usually defined as a relative (>25%) or absolute (>0,5 mg/dL; 44 mcmol/L) increase of serum creatinine from preintervention value; CIN physiopathology is multifactorial but still incompletely understood. Risk factors of CIN development are pre-existing renal insufficiency, diabetes, dehydration, large contrast volume. Digital subtraction arteriographic systems, low-osmolar contrast medium and preprocedural hydration allow lower acute kidney injury incidence, especially among high risk patients.

All systemic complications occur in less than 5%.

Complications related to catheter manipulation include dissection and emboli due to subintimal sheath, guidewire or catheter passage or contrast medium injection; their incidence is less than 0.5%.

The overall procedure threshold for major complications is determined by the following formula:

Number of patients with major complications =

$$\frac{\text{Undergoing diagnostic arteriography only} \times 100}{\text{Total number of patients undergoing arteriography only}}$$

TECHNIQUE

Pulmonary angiography procedure is usually performed by interventional cardiologist or radiologist together with properly trained support personnel (nurses and radiologic technologist) and requires a catheterization laboratory provided with some technical equipment in order to ensure a safe and successful examination.

A high resolution flat-panel detector or image intensifier and television chain with arteriographic filming capabilities is required; digital angiographic is preferred in order to reduce examination time, fluoroscopy time exposure and contrast media volume.

Adequate angiographic supplies include different needles, sheaths, guidewires, catheters, an adequate contrast media injector, capable of varying injection volumes and rates.

Appropriate equipment to allow patient's vital sign monitoring is also required.

Emergency facilities such as intravenous pump, respirators, anesthesia equipment and defibrillator should be present in catheterization laboratory as well.

Preprocedural Care: Patient Preparation and Premedication

Pulmonary angiography procedure requires both "emotional" and "clinical" patient preparation.

Patient should receive complete explanation about procedural indications, alternatives, possible risks and complications in order to give truly written informed consent in compliance with state laws.

Clinically significant history, including indication, physical examination and vital signs should be documented and recorded on patient's chart.

Laboratory examination including hemoglobin, creatinine, electrolytes and coagulation should be available. If pre-existing renal failure or other CIN risk factors are present, pre-procedural patient hydration should be done. INR less than 2.0 and no heparin administered for 6 hours are associated with low vascular access site and catheter related complications, although in some urgent settings, such as acute pulmonary embolism treatment, anticoagulants or thrombolytic therapy may have been previously administered.

Patient should be fast except for oral medication since the day before.

Patient vascular access site should be carefully prepared: an area approximately 20 cm in diameter surrounding access site point should be carefully shaved and disinfected.

Antibiotic prophylaxis is not mandatory for PA but it should be considered in high risk patient such as diabetics and immunocompromised.

Premedication before the patient is sent to catheterization laboratory and sedation once the patient is in catheterization laboratory is up to single operator's and center's decision but should be considered in specific case (low-compliant patient, long diagnostic and interventional procedures).

Vascular Access

Right or left common veins are the preferred access site thanks to the straight course to inferior vena cava and right heart chambers; right jugular vein is also considered a good access site especially if inferior vena cava filter is present or iliac or inferior vena cava thrombosis is present.

After careful access site preparation, puncture should be done by Seldinger technique and single wall puncture is recommended in order to avoid access site complications, especially in patients taking anticoagulant drugs.

Sheath, Catheters, and Guidewires

A 6F to 8F sheath may be placed, after vascular access site appropriate dilatation; in case of long interventional procedures requiring multiple catheter exchanges, long sheath placement may be considered.

Although many different catheters with various configurations and shapes are available to perform diagnostic PA, pigtail and balloon-tipped catheters are most frequently used. Pigtail catheter facilitates right heart and main pulmonary artery passage and pulmonary artery branches good selection; balloon-tipped catheter is also used thanks to its property to be passively carried by heart flow till pulmonary circulation.

J wire is generally used but also floppy tip or straight wires may be adopted although careful manipulation under fluoroscopy is recommended in order to avoid possible perforations.

Image Acquisition

During contrast media injection, patient should stop breathing for few seconds after taking a full inspiration in order to obtain a good diagnostic pulmonary angiogram with minimal motion artifact.

In most studies it is recommended to obtain 3-4 images per second for the first 5 seconds and then 1-2 images per seconds.

Usually two views of each lung are performed; in particular a frontal and 45° oblique view has been validated in large clinical trials on pulmonary embolism.

Procedural Care

All patients should have vital parameters monitoring during the procedure (systemic arterial pressure, heart rate, pulse oximetry).

All patients should have a peripheral venous access as well in order to permit drug administration if needed.

All vitals parameters, drugs and contrast media administered, fluoroscopy time exposure and total procedural time should be recorded.

Any possible procedural complication should be adequately treated and recorded.

Postprocedural Care

At the end of the procedure, sheath removal should be performed by qualified personnel and adequate hemostasis of puncture site should be ensured prior to patient transfer from catheterization laboratory to postprocedural care area.

According to local practice a procedure note should be written in patient's chart summarizing major PA findings and possible complications occurred during the procedure; an official interpretation should be available immediately later or within few hours.

All patients should remain at rest during initial post-procedural period and qualified personnel should be available in order to access patient's clinical condition and vascular access site stability, especially if any interventional procedure following diagnostic PA has been performed.

All patients' vital sign should be monitored and his initial ambulation should be supervised.

Test Interpretation

Pulmonary angiography must be performed under supervision and interpretation by qualified physicians according to state law and international guidelines.

A successful PA is considered when the arteriogram is complete, including gaining access to the artery, obtaining complete image set, adequate to support full interpretation and further medical decision; a successful PA does not necessarily imply it is complication free.

Physician performing PA must completely appreciate procedural indications, contraindications, benefits, alternatives, potential risks and complications; a complete understanding of pulmonary vascular anatomy including potential congenital variants and common collateral pathways is mandatory.

BIBLIOGRAPHY AND FURTHER READING

1. ACR-SIR-SPR Practice Guideline for Performance of Arteriography; Revised 2012 (Resolution 5)
2. Brady AJ, Crake T, Oakley CM. Percutaneous catheter fragmentation and distal dispersion of proximal pulmonary embolus. Lancet. 1991;338:1186-19.
3. Chechi T, Vecchio S, Spaziani G, Giuliani G, Giannotti F, Arcangeli C, et al. Rheolytic thrombectomy in patients with massive and submassive acute pulmonary embolism. Catheter Cardiovasc Interv. 2009;73(4):506-13.
4. Corr P. Pulmonary artery aneurysm as a cause of massive hemoptysis: diagnosis and management. Case Rep Radiol. 2011;2011:141563.
5. Greenfield LJ, Kimmel GO, McCurdy WC. Transvenous removal of pulmonary emboli by vacuum cup catheter technique. J Surg Res. 1969;9:347-52.
6. Guidelines on the diagnosis and management of acute pulmonary embolism: the Task Force for the Diagnosis and Management of Acute Pulmonary Embolism of the European Society of Cardiology (ESC). Eur Heart J. 2014;35:3033-3080.
7. Ing FF, Khan A, Kobayashi D, Hagler DJ, Forbes TJ. Pulmonary artery stents in the recent era: Immediate and intermediate follow-up. Catheter cardiovasc Interv. 2014;84(7):1123-30.

8. Kucher N, Goldhaber SZ. Pulmonary angiography. In: Baim DS. Grossman's cardiac catheterization, angiography and intervention, 7th edition. Philadelphia: Lippincott Williams and Wilkins, 2006. pp. 234-51.
9. Mayer E, Jenkins D, Lindner J, D'Armini A, Kloek J, Meyns B, et al. Surgical management and outcome of patients with chronic thromboembolic pulmonary hypertension: results from an international prospective registry. J Thorac Cardiovasc Surg. 2011;141(3):702-10.
10. McCullogh PA, Sandberg KR. Epidemiology of contrast-induced nephropathy. Rev Cardiovasc Med. 2003;4(Suppl 5): S3-9.
11. Morsolini M, Nicolardi S, Milanesi E, Sarchi E, Mattiucci C, et al. Evolving surgical techniques for pulmonary endoarterectomyaccording to the changing features of chronic thromboembolic pulmonary hypertension patients during 17-year single center experience. J Thorac Cardiovasc Surg. 2012;144(1):100-7.
12. Murphy SW, Barret BJ, Parfrey PS. Contrast nephropathy. J Am Soc Nephrol. 2000;11(1):177-82.
13. Ray CE, Kaufmann JA, Geller SC, Rivitz SM, Kanarek DJ, Waltman AC. Embolization of pulmonary catheter-induced pulmonary artery pseudoaneurysm. Chest. 1996;110:1370-3.
14. Robb GP, Steinberg I. A pratical method of visualization of the chambers of the heart, the pulmonary circulation and the great blood vessels in man. J Clin Invest. 1938;17:507.
15. Schoept UJ, Costello P. CT angiography for diagnosis of pulmonary embolism: state of the art. Radiology. 2004;-230:329-37.
16. Seldinger SI. Catheter replacement of the needle in percutaneous arteriography; a new technique. Acta radiol. 1953;39(5):368-76.
17. Silvetti S, Pappalardo F, Melisurgo G, Nisi T, Latib A, Figini F, et al. Ultrasound accelerated thrombolysis and extracorporeal membrane oxigenation in a patient with massive pulmonary embolism and cardiac arrest. Circ Cardiovasc Interv. 2013;6(3):e34-6.
18. Stein PD, Athanasoulis C, Alavi A. Complications and validity of pulmonary angiography in acute pulmonary embolism. Circulation. 1992;85:462-8.
19. Timsit JF, Reynaud P, Meyer G, Sors H. Pulmonary embolectomy by catheter device in massive pulmonary embolism. Chest. 1991;100:655-8.
20. Vawdrey DB, Fitzsimmons F, Veldtman GR, Carpenter JP. Therapeutic pulmonary artery stenting for metastatic bronchial carcinoid. BMJ Case Rep. 2013.
21. White I, Pollak JS, Wirth JA. Pulmonary arteriovenous malformations: diagnosis and transcatheter embolotherapy. J Vac Interv radiol. 1996;7:787-804.
22. Wittram C, Waltman AC, Shepard JA, Halpern E, Goodman LR. Discordance between CT and angiography in the PIOPED II study. Radiology. 2007;244(3):883-9.

Chapter 22

Role of Magnetic Resonance Imaging in the Evaluation of Respiratory Diseases

Miranda Kirby, Harvey O Coxson, Claudio Sorino, Grace Parraga

OVERVIEW AND HISTORY

Since the first image of the human body, using magnetic resonance imaging (MRI)—an axial image of the chest showing the heart, lungs and chest wall—was produced in 1977 by Damadian and colleagues, the field has grown to the point where now MRI is recognized as the imaging modality of choice for many clinical indications. In contrast to X-ray-based methods that identify structures based on differences in X-ray attenuation, MRI takes advantage of the fact that our bodies are composed primarily of proton (^1H) atoms in fat and water. ^1H atoms, along with several other nuclei, possess a quantum mechanical property called "spin" that allows these atoms to produce a signal that can be detected by the MRI hardware.

Over the last 30 years, MRI has demonstrated that it has important advantages over other imaging methods. In contrast to X-ray based imaging methods, MRI does not involve the use of ionizing radiation and yet still provides very high spatial resolution images of soft tissue and bone. The fact that MRI does not use ionizing radiation is an advantage for imaging children because they are more radiosensitive than adults and therefore are more susceptible to radiation-induced cancers. For example, it was recently reported that the use of computed tomography (CT) in children may nearly triple their risk of developing leukemia and brain cancer depending on the radiation dose.

Magnetic resonance imaging has also become the imaging modality of choice for many diseases and organ systems because the excellent soft tissue contrast produces exquisite images of the spinal cord and brain, as well as the musculoskeletal system. As a result, imaging of the brain using MRI is the clinical standard for neurological diseases.

Another reason that MRI may be preferred to X-ray-based imaging is for serial studies. Intensive serial investigations and longitudinal studies may provide a way to better understand disease pathogenesis and progression, and for the development and assessment of therapeutic interventions.

However, MRI has not become the clinical standard for the routine evaluation of respiratory disease. In this Chapter, we will begin by discussing some of the technical challenges for MRI of the lung that has thus far prevented its use in respiratory disease evaluation. We will then discuss how these challenges are being overcome with the development of novel MRI approaches for lung evaluation, and identify some potential applications where MRI of the lung may become the imaging modality of choice.

LUNG PARENCHYMA: THE BLACK HOLE OF MRI

During normal inspiration, air passes through the conducting airways to the respiratory zone. There are more than 20 generations or branches of airways between the trachea and the alveolar ducts and sacs, and yet the airways and the blood vessels constitute only 10% of the lung volume while the alveoli ducts and sacs account for the remaining 90%. Although these numerous small alveoli air sacs, of which there are estimated to be approximately 480 million in the human lungs, are essential for the exchange of oxygen to the pulmonary capillaries, they pose a serious challenge for MRI of the lung.

First, MRI of the lung is challenging due to its inherently low ^1H density. Because the respiratory region of the lung is predominately air-filled, there is very little tissue and consequently very little signal that can be detected

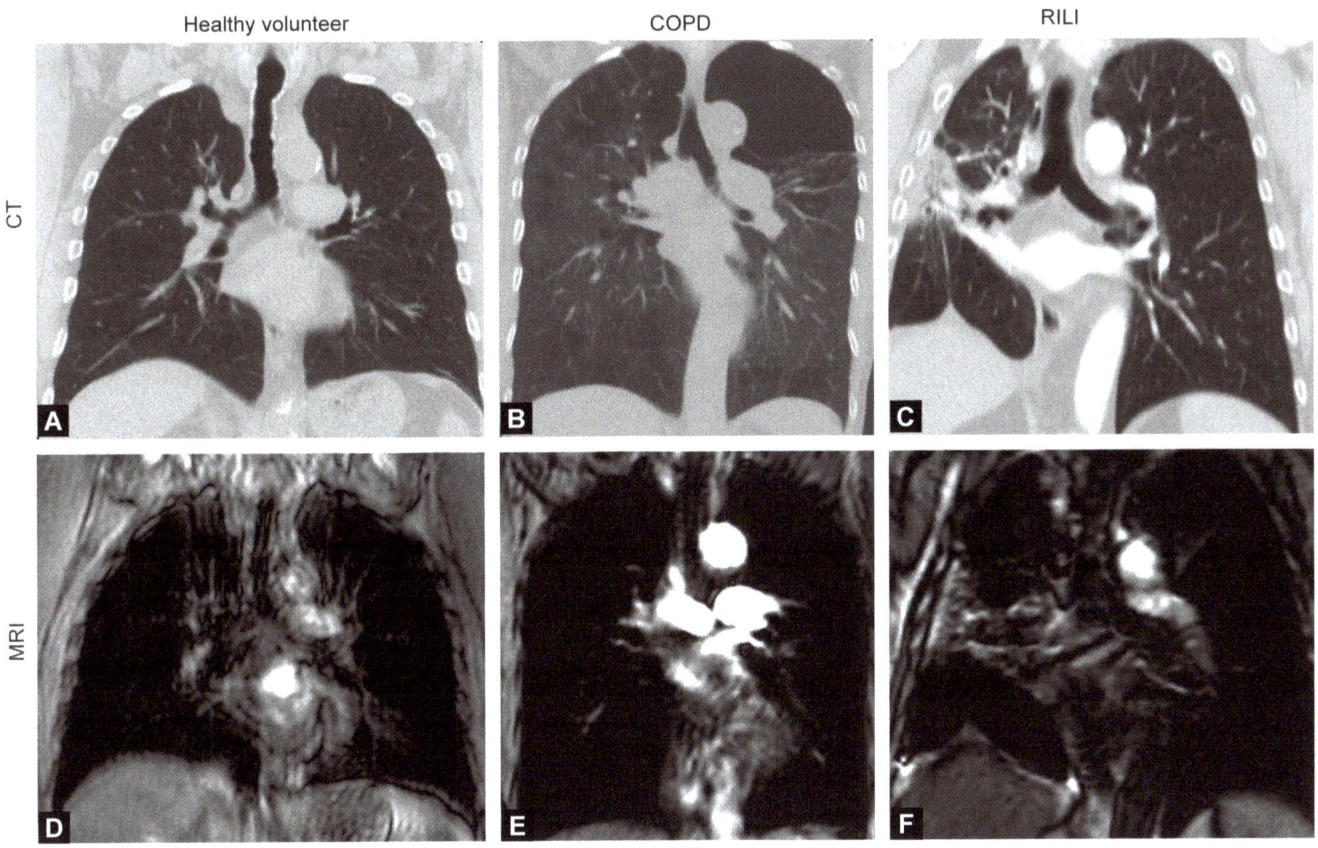

Figs. 22.1A to F: Computed tomography (CT) and conventional ^{1}H MRI for a healthy volunteer and a subject with chronic obstructive pulmonary disease (COPD) and radiation-induced lung injury (RILI). The center slice coronal CT image with the corresponding ^{1}H MRI image shown below for a healthy volunteer, and a subject with COPD and RILI.

from the lung parenchyma. The lung parenchyma also has a short *transverse magnetization relaxation time*, known as T2, resulting in a much faster signal decay for the lung parenchyma compared to other tissues. In addition to the short T2, another problem for MRI of the lung relates to the fact that air and tissue have very different magnetic susceptibilities. At air-tissue interfaces, such as those at the alveolar membrane, the difference in magnetic susceptibilities results in magnetic field gradients that may further degrade the ^{1}H signal and distort the image. Therefore, with on average approximately 480 million alveoli in the human lungs, there are substantial magnetic susceptibility effects. Moreover, MRI signal and image quality is also degraded by respiratory motion as well as the heart pulsation during image acquisition. Therefore, the combined effect of magnetic susceptibility at air-tissue interfaces and respiratory and cardiac motion during image acquisition, with the already intrinsically low ^{1}H density in the lung and short T2 of the lung parenchyma does not bode well for the use of conventional ^{1}H MRI for pulmonary evaluations.

Figures 22.1A to F shows a conventional ^{1}H MRI image and a CT image of the lung in the coronal view for a volunteer with normal pulmonary function as well as a subject with *radiation-induced lung injury (RILI)* and *chronic obstructive pulmonary disease (COPD)*. Despite the fact that conventional ^{1}H MRI can identify important image features, such as increased signal intensity in regions of radiation pneumonitis as shown for the subject with RILI, in comparison to CT, MRI of the lung parenchyma appears as a black hole with very little signal visible. This leads to the inability to distinguish lung parenchyma in general and the complete loss of structural information, such as emphysema and bullae, when compared to CT lung imaging.

Despite these challenges, there is still interest in MRI of the lung, particularly as concern about radiation exposure from CT continues to grow. The following sections will introduce several new and emerging MRI methodologies and show how these approaches may be useful for the quantitative evaluation of respiratory disease.

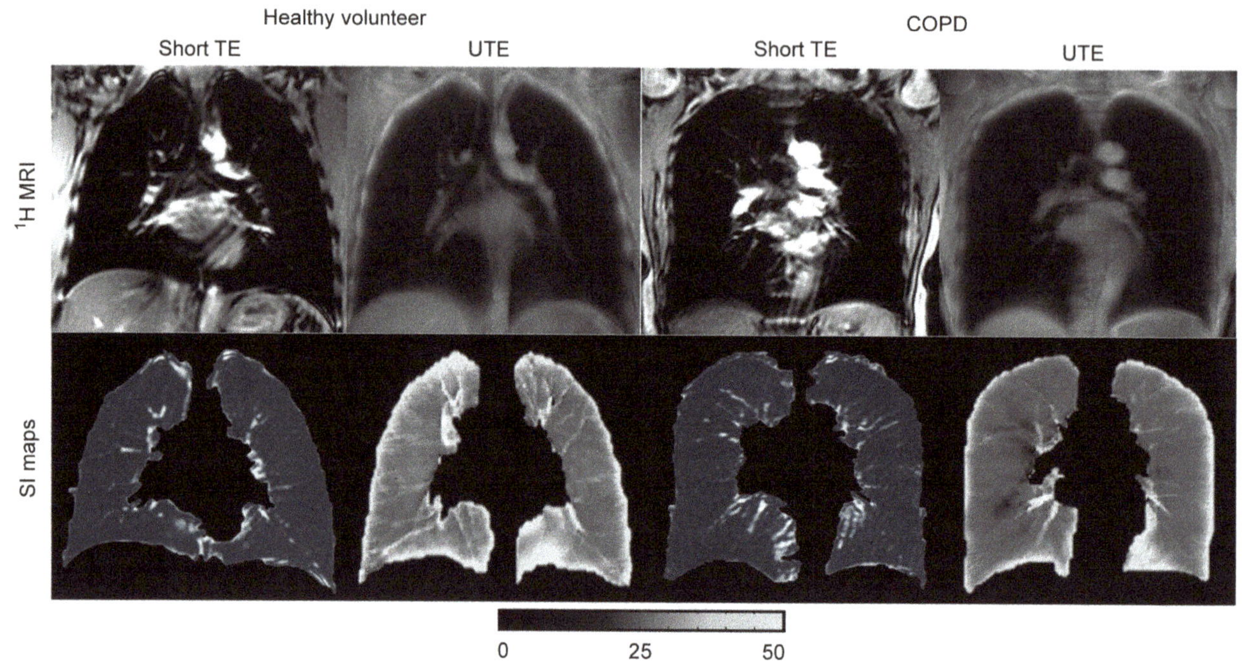

Fig. 22.2: Short TE and UTE MR images of a healthy volunteer and subject with chronic obstructive pulmonary disease (COPD). The ^{1}H MRIs acquired using a short TE and UTE sequence with the corresponding signal intensity (SI) maps shown below for healthy volunteer and subject with COPD.
Source: Khadija Sheikh, Robarts Research Institute, London, ON, Canada.

IS THERE ADDED-VALUE OF MRI FOR PATIENT ASSESSMENT?

Short Echo Time and Ultra Short Echo Time MRI

While little can be done to overcome many of the limitations of ^{1}H MRI described above, investigators have discovered that some improvement in image quality can be achieved by altering how the images are acquired. By acquiring the images very quickly using *short echo times (TE)*, defined as the delay time between the end of radiofrequency excitation and the beginning of data collection, signal loss from the lung parenchyma can be minimized.

Early investigations using short TE pulmonary ^{1}H MRI showed very promising results in comparison to more standard TE. Mayo and colleagues demonstrated that the signal intensity from the lung parenchyma was statistically significantly greater using a TE of 7 ms compared with 20 ms. They also provided evidence that MRI using a TE of 7 ms may differentiate normal lung from emphysematous lung in COPD patients better than a TE of 20 ms, and in patients with lung transplants, the extent of diffuse infiltrate may also be more easily differentiated.

Several investigators have also demonstrated that MR images with short TE may be comparable to CT for identifying pathological changes in several pulmonary applications. MRI has been shown to be useful in describing diffuse lung disease and cancer staging, both of which are dominated by CT and/or positron-emission tomography (PET) imaging. An early study by Lutterbey and colleagues compared MRI and CT for identifying pathological changes in diffuse lung disease patients and found that MRI could detect 93% of the same pathological changes that were detected by CT. A study comparing MRI with fluorodeoxyglucose (FDG) PET/CT demonstrated that MRI measurements of mediastinal and hilar lymph node metastases were more sensitive and accurate than those derived from FDG combined PET/CT.

While short TE MRI demonstrated improved image quality over conventional MRI, even greater improvements in image quality with the improved visualization of fine lung structures can be achieved with *ultra short TE (UTE)* MRI. Figure 22.2 shows a coronal MRI of a healthy volunteer and a COPD subject acquired using short TE MRI and UTE MRI, with the corresponding signal intensity maps below. As shown in the MRI signal intensity maps in Figure 22.2, increased signal intensity can be observed with UTE MRI compared to short TE MRI sequences. Moreover, it has been demonstrated that measurements derived from UTE MRI can differentiate smokers without COPD from smokers with very mild airflow limitation, i.e. with forced expiratory volume in 1 second greater than or equal to 80%, corresponding to COPD at stage I according to the Global Initiative for Chronic Obstructive Lung Disease (GOLD). Similarly, it can differentiate between subjects with COPD at stage I and stage III/IV according to the GOLD. MRI-derived measurements have also been shown to have moderate correlations with spirometric measurements of airflow limitation and the diffusing capacity of the lung for carbon monoxide (DL_{CO}), as well as with CT measures of emphysema and airway disease. In another investigation, UTE MRI measurements were shown to differentiate patients with interstitial lung disease from healthy volunteers, and measurements correlated significantly with pulmonary function measurements and CT disease severity scoring.

More recently, it has been suggested that developing three-dimensional (3D) UTE MRI approaches, in contrast to 2D approaches, may provide further improvements in image quality allowing isotropic spatial resolution and full chest coverage. Although, 3D UTE MRI is not practical to perform in a single breath-hold and therefore involves the added challenges of motion correction and respiratory gating, preliminary work provides evidence that 3D UTE is feasible in patients, and similar patterns of fibrosis have been visualized using 3D UTE MRI and CT in patients with interstitial pulmonary fibrosis.

While MRI cannot provide a way visualize some of the finer anatomical structures and more physiological validation is required, these studies certainly demonstrate that the field is rapidly advancing to improve image quality of magnetic resonance (MR) technique. As demonstrated by many of the studies discussed, MRI does add value to the clinical assessment of a number of pulmonary pathologies, and in some cases may even perform better than the more standard imaging modalities used for disease diagnosis and assessment. Although ^{1}H MRI may never replace CT for many pulmonary evaluations, it may be possible to use MRI for follow-up evaluations in patients with respiratory disease in order to reduce the number of CT examinations required.

Fourier Decomposition MRI

Another method for extracting MRI pulmonary information, referred to as Fourier decomposition MRI, has been recently developed and pioneered by Bauman and colleagues. This technique acquires images during free breathing and measures the changes in MR signal intensity on a voxel-by-voxel basis. Each voxel in the MR image will change in signal intensity during free breathing due to the increase or decrease in tissue volume during inspiration and expiration, as well as the changes in blood flow during the systolic and diastolic phase of the cardiac cycle. Interestingly, the MRI signal modifications from these two physiological processes can be decomposed to yield ventilation-weighted and perfusion-weighted MR images.

To develop this technique, investigators have used a large animal model to compare Fourier decomposition MRI with traditional ventilation and perfusion measurements derived from single photon emission computed tomography (SPECT)/CT. In this study the authors demonstrated that there was a significant correlation between measurements obtained using Fourier decomposition MRI and SPECT/CT, and that the imaging findings were qualitatively consistent between both methods. To determine whether abnormal lung function can be measured with this technique, another large animal study was performed that aimed to compared Fourier decomposition MRI with well-established hyperpolarized ^{3}He MRI and dynamic contrast-enhanced MRI. In this study, the investigators simulated atelectasis and gas trapping by occluding a bronchus with a balloon catheter. These studies showed that regions of gas trapping and atelectasis were visualized as ventilation defects using both Fourier decomposition MRI and ^{3}He MRI, and the corresponding perfusion changes could be identified by both Fourier decomposition MRI and dynamic contrast enhanced MRI (Figs. 22.3A to D). Although clinical studies using Fourier decomposition MRI are still limited, Bauman and colleagues found very good agreement between perfusion defects identified using Fourier decomposition MRI and dynamic contrast enhance MRI in patients with cystic fibrosis.

A limitation of Fourier decomposition MRI is that image quality is very dependent on the changes in signal intensity caused by the respiratory and cardiac cycle during image acquisition. Although very high reproducibility of this technique has been reported in healthy volunteers, any irregularities in the respiratory and cardiac cycle may reduce image quality and therefore future studies should aim to evaluate the reproducibility of this technique in younger patients and patients with respiratory disease. Despite these limitations, a very important advantage of Fourier decomposition MRI is that it can be easily implemented on standard and clinically available MRI systems

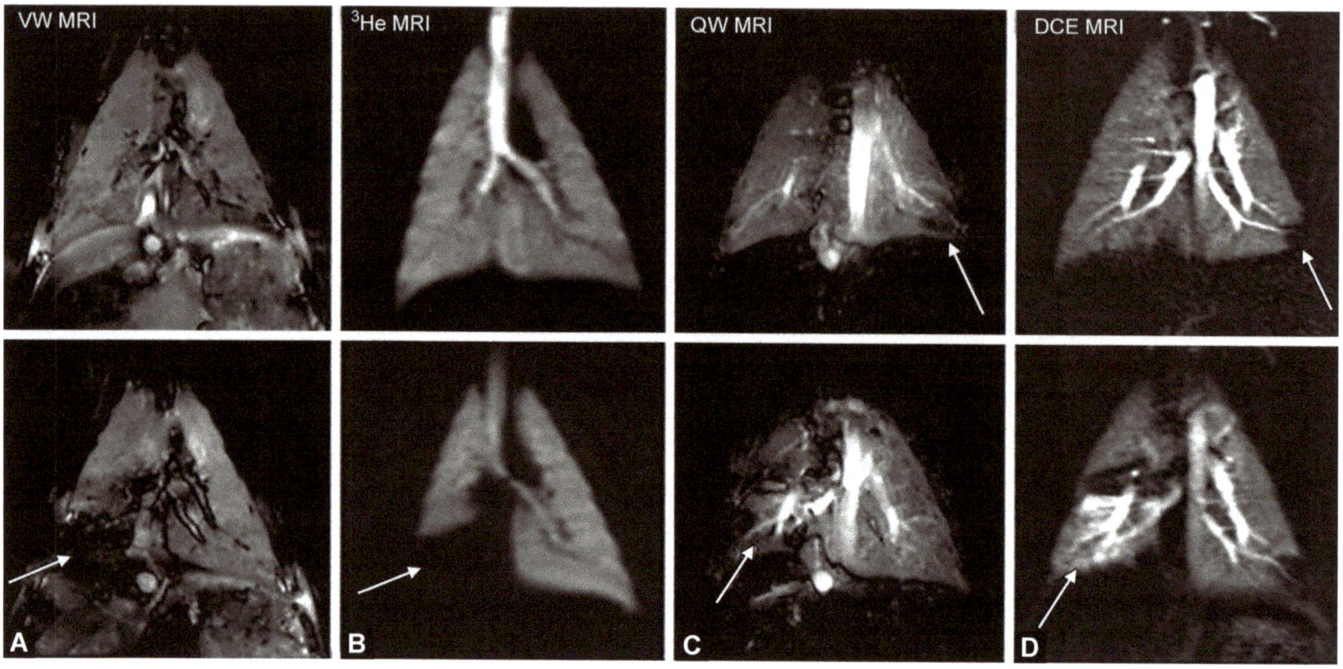

Figs. 22.3A to D: Ventilation-weighted (VW) Fourier decomposition MRI, ^{3}He MRI, perfusion-weighted Fourier decomposition MRI and dynamic Contrast-enhanced (DCE) MRI of porcine lungs following obstruction of a segmental bronchus. (A) The VW FD MRI. (B) ^{3}He MRI. (C) QW FD MRI. (D) DCE MRI of porcine lungs following induction of pulmonary embolism is shown in the top row. The bottom row shows images acquired after obstruction of a segmental bronchus. Regional lung atelectasis can be visualized in the right lower lobe in VW FD MRI and ^{3}He MRI as indicated by the white arrows. Heterogeneous perfusion can also be visualized in the atelectatic lung region using QW MRI and DCE MRI.
Source: Reprinted with permission of John Wiley and Sons.
Bauman G, Scholz A, Rivoire J, Terekhov M, Friedrich J, de Oliveira A, et al. Lung ventilation- and perfusion-weighted Fourier decomposition magnetic resonance imaging: in vivo validation with hyperpolarized ^{3}He and dynamic contrast-enhanced MRI. Magn Reson Med. 2013;69(1):229-37.

without additional contrast agents, which are contraindicated for some patients. Although Fourier decomposition MRI is still in the early stages of development, these first investigations and preliminary work in cystic fibrosis (CF) patients suggest that it is a promising method for evaluating respiratory disease.

Gas Contrast Enhanced MRI

Although the new proton-based MRI approaches, described above, have overcome many of the limitations and shortcomings of conventional MRI, other methods have been developed that utilize inhaled contrast agents in order to further improve the lung signal.

Oxygen-Enhanced MRI

The primary function of the lung is to deliver oxygen to the blood and remove carbon dioxide from the body. Once oxygen has diffused across the barrier into the pulmonary capillary blood, it primarily binds to hemoglobin or dissolves as molecular oxygen to be carried away to the body tissues for cellular respiration. Oxygen-enhanced MRI takes advantage of this process. Molecular oxygen is weakly paramagnetic which means that it is attracted to magnetic fields and as a result, will shorten the T1 times of the lung tissue. In other words, the presence of molecular oxygen in the blood leads to more rapid decay of the MR signal intensity for the surrounding lung parenchyma. Therefore, since the concentration of oxygen is increased for inhalation of 100% oxygen inhalation compared to room air, the extent of T1 shortening is also greater for 100% oxygen inhalation. Subtraction of MR images acquired by inhaling room-air from images acquired by inhaling 100% oxygen yields functional MR images depicting a combination of regional ventilation as well as oxygen transfer.

Edelman and colleagues first used oxygen-enhanced MRI in 1996 to demonstrate that 100% oxygen inhalation reduced the T1 values of the lung compared to room-air, and that pathological changes could be identified as functional defects in the oxygen-enhanced MR images. Since then, many of the studies performed to-date using oxygen-enhanced MRI have been for the evaluation of

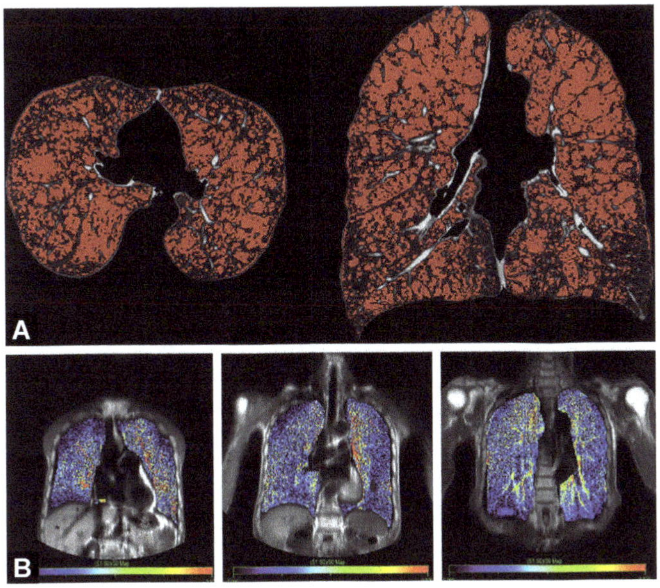

Figs. 22.4A and B: Computed tomography density mask and oxygen-enhanced MRI for a severe chronic obstructive pulmonary disease (COPD) Subject. (A) The CT density mask in the axial and coronal view highlighting emphysematous regions, (B) with the relative enhancement maps derived from oxygen-enhanced MRI for three central coronal slices of a 69-year-old subject with very severe COPD.
Source: Reprinted with permission of the American Thoracic Society. Copyright © 2014 American Thoracic Society.
Ohno Y, Iwasawa T, Seo JB, Koyama H, Takahashi H, Oh YM, et al. Oxygen-enhanced magnetic resonance imaging versus computed tomography: multicenter study for clinical stage classification of smoking-related chronic obstructive pulmonary disease. Am J Respir Crit Care Med. 2008;177(10):1095-102.

COPD patients. Similar to density masks highlighting emphysematous regions in CT, Figures 22.4A and B shows that oxygen-enhanced MRI depicts markedly abnormal and heterogeneous signal enhancement in severe COPD patients. In a clinical study, Ohno and colleagues investigated the relationship between oxygen-enhanced MRI and the diffusing capacity of the lung (DL_{CO}). They showed the lungs of subjects with emphysema had a significantly reduced mean relative enhancement ratio (ratio of the difference in signal intensity between the images acquired during 100% oxygen breathing and room-air breathing to the signal intensity of the images acquired at room air breathing), and showed greater heterogeneity in signal enhancement in comparison to healthy volunteers. They also demonstrated that the mean relative enhancement ratio was strongly and significantly correlated with DL_{CO}, suggesting that the reduced and heterogeneous signal intensity in pulmonary emphysema patients may reflect reduced diffusion of oxygen to the capillary bed. Another study that evaluated COPD patients demonstrated that oxygen-enhanced MRI could differentiate between smokers with different stages of disease severity. Moreover, it was shown that the strength of the correlation between pulmonary function parameters for oxygen-enhanced MRI and CT were very comparable in COPD subjects.

Oxygen-enhanced MRI has also been used in patients with interstitial lung disease. Investigators demonstrated that both CT- and MRI-derived measures could differentiate patients with interstitial lung disease from healthy volunteers. It was also demonstrated that there was no significant differences in diagnostic performance between oxygen-enhanced MRI and CT for sensitivity, specificity or accuracy.

One limitation of oxygen-enhanced MRI is the fact that images must be acquired over several respiratory cycles for sufficient signal-to-noise and this has to the potential to introduce motion artifacts. Breathing motion may result in misplaced pulmonary vessels, chest wall and diaphragm leading to signal variability in the subtraction images. However, recent reports demonstrated that non-rigid registration of the images can overcome this limitation and result in improved image quality and reduced signal variability. Another limitation is related to the fact that inhalation of oxygen in patients with pulmonary diseases may alter or modify existing pulmonary pathophysiology by reversing hypoxic vasoconstriction. Clearly, this may lead to an underestimation in the measurement of the extent of functional abnormalities in patients with respiratory disease when assessed using oxygen-enhanced MRI. While oxygen-enhanced MRI has vast potential in the clinical setting because it is inexpensive and easy to implement, further improvements in image quality and postprocessing of these images are required. Moreover, further comparisons between oxygen-enhanced MRI with other functional imaging methods, such as ^{3}He or ^{129}Xe MRI for comparison of ventilation abnormalities and nuclear medicine approaches for comparison of perfusion abnormalities, in patients with pathological changes may provide improved understanding of these measurements and their potential for assessing respiratory disease.

Hyperpolarized Noble Gas MRI

The use of hyperpolarized noble gases as contrast agents for MRI lung imaging was first recognized by Albert and colleagues in 1994. For hyperpolarized noble gas MRI, the MRI system is tuned to the resonance frequency of the gaseous contrast agent, instead of resonance frequency of ^{1}H, and therefore when the contrast agent is inhaled

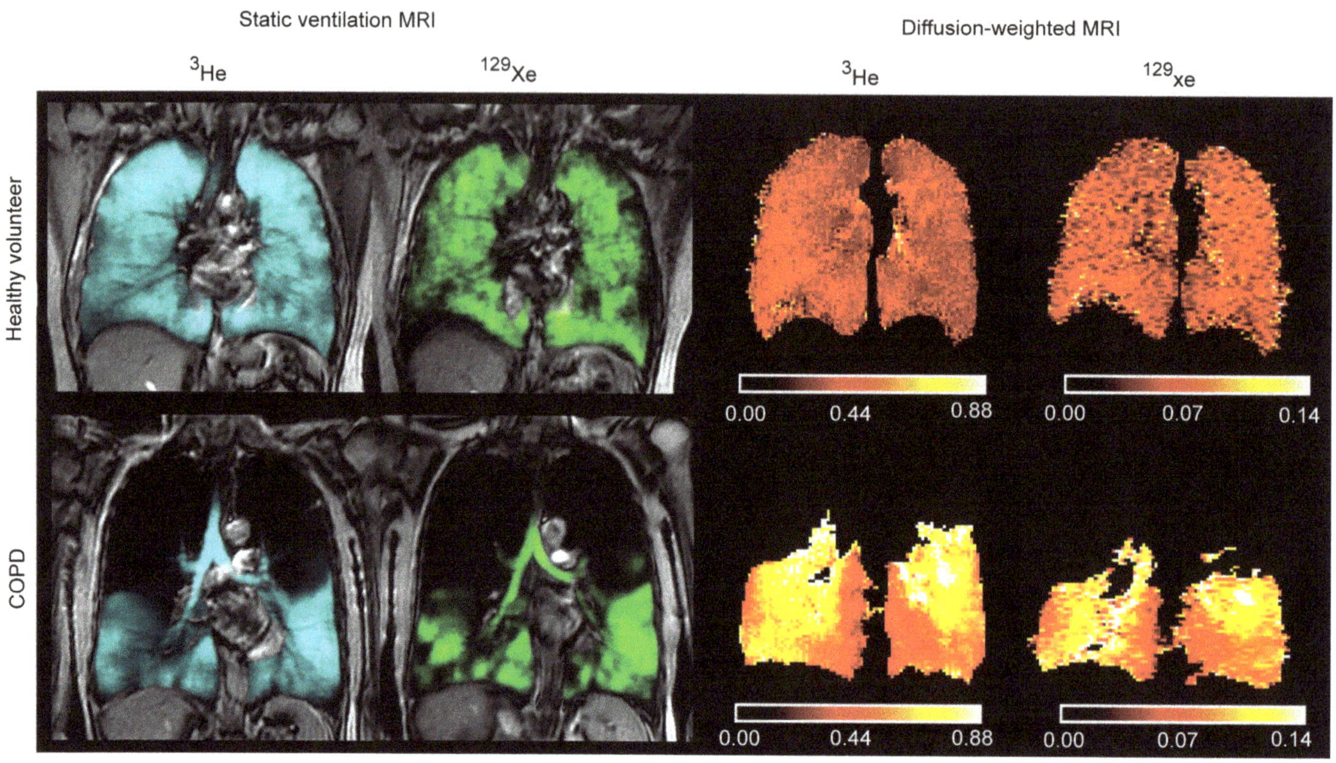

Fig. 22.5: Hyperpolarized ^{3}He MRI and ^{129}Xe MRI of a healthy volunteer and subject with chronic obstructive pulmonary disease (COPD). For static ventilation MRI, the center slice coronal ^{3}He MR image (in blue) and the ^{129}Xe MR image (in green) coregistered to conventional ^{1}H MR image is shown for a healthy volunteer and subject with COPD. For diffusion-weighted MRI, the center slice coronal ^{3}He and ^{129}Xe ADC map is also shown for the same healthy volunteer and COPD subject.

by the subject while inside the MRI scanner, the distribution of the gas during breath-hold imaging can be directly visualized.

An important advantage of hyperpolarized gas MRI is that a number of pulmonary structural/functional measurements may be obtained. Figure 22.5 shows hyperpolarized ^{3}He and ^{129}Xe MRI for a healthy volunteer and subject with emphysema. In contrast to the homogenous signal intensity within the lungs of healthy volunteers, static ventilation imaging in subjects with respiratory disease allows for regions with local hypoventilation or nonventilated regions of the lung, known as ventilation defects, to be directly visualized and quantified. Importantly, these ventilation defects correspond to signal voids in ^{133}Xe ventilation scintigraphy images, and correlate significantly with airflow limitation assessed using spirometry.

Structural lung information regarding the size of the pulmonary airspaces can also be obtained using diffusion-weighted MRI. Hyperpolarized gas diffusion-weighted MRI is sensitive to the self-diffusion of the gas within the lung microstructure. When a healthy volunteer inhales the hyperpolarized gas and it reaches the alveoli, the diffusion of the gas is restricted by the alveolar walls. In contrast, emphysematous destruction of the lung parenchyma creates enlarged airspaces and therefore allows greater displacement of the hyperpolarized gas during the breath-hold. This is illustrated in the apparent diffusion coefficient (ADC) maps shown in Figure 22.5; the healthy volunteer has relatively homogeneous and reduced ADC values as a result of the restricted displacement of the hyperpolarized gas within the lung microstructure. The COPD subject, on the other hand, has significant emphysema or bullae which results in greater gas displacement and greater ADC values as shown in the ADC map. Studies investigating diffusion-weighted MRI have demonstrated the ADC correlates significantly with age, CT emphysema measurements and histology.

Other less commonly used measurements, such as those obtained using dynamic imaging for visualizing gas flow and measurements of oxygen uptake with the longitudinal relaxation time (T1) may also be performed using hyperpolarized noble gases. Finally, ^{129}Xe gas is soluble in

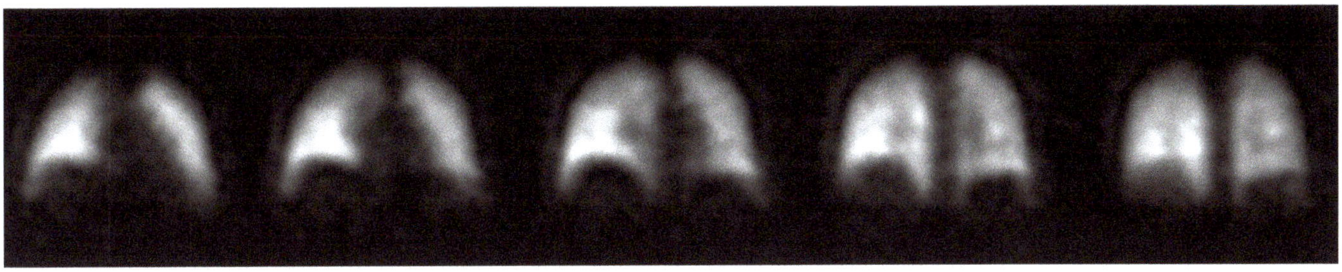

Fig. 22.6: Coronal ^{19}F MR images of a healthy volunteer. Coronal ^{19}F MR images acquired during continuous breathing of ^{19}F gas mixture show homogeneous gas distribution through the lung for a healthy volunteer.
Source: Marcus Couch, Thunder Bay Regional Research Institute, Thunder Bay, ON, Canada.
Couch MJ, Ball IK, Li T, Fox MS, Littlefield SL, Biman B, et al. Pulmonary ultrashort echo time 19F MR imaging with inhaled fluorinated gas mixtures in healthy volunteers: feasibility. Radiology. 2013;269(3):903-9.

tissue and, unlike ^{3}He, will diffuse across the alveoli-capillary membrane. In tissues, ^{129}Xe resonates at a different frequency than in the gas phase, offering new opportunities to measure ventilation and perfusion simultaneously and at high resolution.

Hyperpolarized noble gas MRI provides a way to generate measurements never-before available. Specialized polarization equipment, coils and physics expertise is required. Furthermore, until now, the limited supply of ^{3}He gas globally has restricting the clinical translation of this technique. Fortunately, ^{129}Xe gas is a substantially more abundant noble gas, and recent commercialization of polarizer equipment enables more wide-spread use.

^{19}F MRI

Another type of gas-contrast MRI that has been gaining interest very recently is MRI of inhaled fluorinated gases [e.g. sulfur hexafluoride (SF_6), hexafluoroethane (C_2F_6), and tetrafluoromethane (CF_4)]. ^{19}F MRI does not require specialized polarization equipment due to the high gyromagnetic ratio of ^{19}F (^{19}F = 40.1 MHz/T), and the fact that the signal per mole of gas is proportional to the number of ^{19}F atoms per molecule. The longitudinal relaxation time (T1) of ^{19}F is also very short (on the order of milliseconds) and therefore SNR can be enhanced by obtaining multiple snapshots during a breath-hold. In contrast to ^{3}He gas, only slight reductions in signal intensity occur when ^{19}F gas is mixed with oxygen and therefore image acquisition during continuous breathing of oxygen and fluorinated gas mixtures is possible.

The first ^{19}F MRI pulmonary images were reported by Kuethe and colleagues in 1998. They demonstrated that gas distribution images of rat lungs could be acquired using an 80:20 mixture of C_2F_6 and oxygen. Other early studies demonstrated that wash-in and wash-out kinetics of the fluorinated gases could be measured in rat lung and, in ex-vivo human lungs it was demonstrated that the ADC could distinguish between healthy and emphysematous lung tissue.

Very recently, Soher and colleagues reported the first ^{19}F MR images in a single healthy volunteer. Although this study demonstrated that in vivo ^{19}F MRI is feasible in humans, it was clear that improvements in image quality for ^{19}F MRI were required for the evaluation of respiratory disease. In another study Albert and colleagues aimed to improve image quality by directly comparing two breathing protocols; one in which images were acquired during a single breath-hold and another where images were acquired during continuous breathing of the ^{19}F gas mixture. The advantage of acquiring images during continuous breathing is that there is a greater density of ^{19}F nuclei in the lungs and therefore greater signal, which is exactly what these investigators found; signal-to-noise-ratio was significantly greater in images acquired during continuous compared to breath-hold imaging. Figure 22.6 shows ^{19}F MR images acquired using the continuous breathing protocol for a healthy volunteer that was evaluated in this study.

Another important step in demonstrating the utility of ^{19}F MRI for pulmonary imaging is to demonstrate that pathological changes can be measured. Halaweish and colleagues evaluated subjects with a range of pulmonary conditions, including subjects with COPD, asthma and those that had undergone lung transplant. In contrast to healthy volunteers that demonstrated homogenous gas distribution, the subjects with lung disease demonstrated more heterogeneous signal intensity with observable ventilation defects.

Although these studies have shown that ^{19}F MRI is feasible in humans and that pathological changes can be observed, further improvements in image quality are required. Moreover, once image quality is improved and ventilation abnormities can be quantified, future studies should aim to evaluate the relationship between ^{19}F MRI ventilation defects with physiological measurements. It would also be of interest to investigate how ^{19}F MRI gas distribution compares to hyperpolarized ^{3}He and ^{129}Xe MRI in healthy volunteers and subjects with respiratory disease. Although ^{19}F MRI is still in the very early stages of development, the lack of polarization equipment required, the low cost and high abundance of ^{19}F gas, and the fact that it is inert make this emerging technique a very promising candidate for imaging pulmonary structure and function.

WHEN IS PULMONARY MRI THE MODALITY OF CHOICE?

Longitudinal and Serial Studies

Magnetic resonance imaging of the lung does not involve the use of ionizing radiation and therefore it is an ideal imaging modality for the longitudinal evaluation of respiratory diseases, as well as for serial assessment following treatment or other interventions. However, despite the potential of MRI to be the imaging modality of choice, more serial studies demonstrating that MRI can detect change are required for this to be realized, and to-date these studies are limited. Of these emerging techniques, hyperpolarized ^{3}He MRI has been the most frequently used for longitudinal and serial studies.

Serial studies to assess ^{3}He MRI short-term reproducibility have demonstrated that ^{3}He MRI ventilation defects are highly reproducible in older never-smokers. Similar to the older never-smokers, ventilation defects have been shown to be reproducible in subjects with COPD, while greater variability is seen in asthmatics and CF subjects (Figs. 22.7A to C) that likely reflects the day-to-day physiological changes in airway patency.

In a longitudinal ^{3}He MRI study that evaluated COPD subjects over 2 years, statistically significantly greater ventilation defects and ADC measurements (reflective of emphysema) were reported at the 2 year follow-up compared to baseline, irrespective of changes in standard spirometry measurements which was suggestive of anatomic disease progression. These ventilation defects, as shown in Figures 22.7A to C, were visually larger and the ventilation distribution was more heterogeneous in the MR static ventilation images at the 2-year follow-up in comparison to baseline. RILI subjects have also been monitored longitudinally using ^{3}He MRI. Figures 22.7A to C shows that significant changes can be observed in the contralateral lung 35 weeks following radiation therapy, suggesting that ^{3}He MRI may be detecting functional compensatory changes in the contralateral lung due to ipsilateral lung radiation-induced injury.

Serial studies have also demonstrated that ^{3}He MRI can sensitively detect significant improvements in ^{3}He gas distribution within the lung following inhalation of a bronchodilator in COPD subjects as well as following airway bypass stenting for severe emphysema, and these changes were detected despite minimal change in airflow limitation measured using spirometry. In adult asthmatic patients, ^{3}He ventilation defects have been reported to increase in number and extent following an exercise challenge and methacholine provocation (Figs. 22.7A to C), and persist or recur in the same locations over time. Importantly, ^{3}He ventilation defects in asthmatics have also been reported to resolve following bronchodilator therapy, demonstrating that treatment efficacy can be evaluated with ^{3}He MRI.

For the other emerging imaging techniques, the technical reproducibility as well as the variability introduced by quantitative evaluation of the images must be established before longitudinal and serial studies should be performed. In this regard, very recently the reproducibility of oxygen-enhanced MRI and Fourier decomposition MRI has been demonstrated to be high, and therefore these methods have potential to be used for longitudinal monitoring of respiratory disease.

MRI of Pediatric Lung Disease

Although CT provides very high resolution anatomical images and plays a key role in the detection and evaluation of many lung diseases, for children, MRI can also provide high resolution structural *and functional* information that does not require ionizing radiation. Therefore there is considerable interest in the development and implementation of these techniques for pediatric lung disease evaluation. Two pulmonary diseases in particular where MRI has shown promise is for the evaluation of asthma and CF.

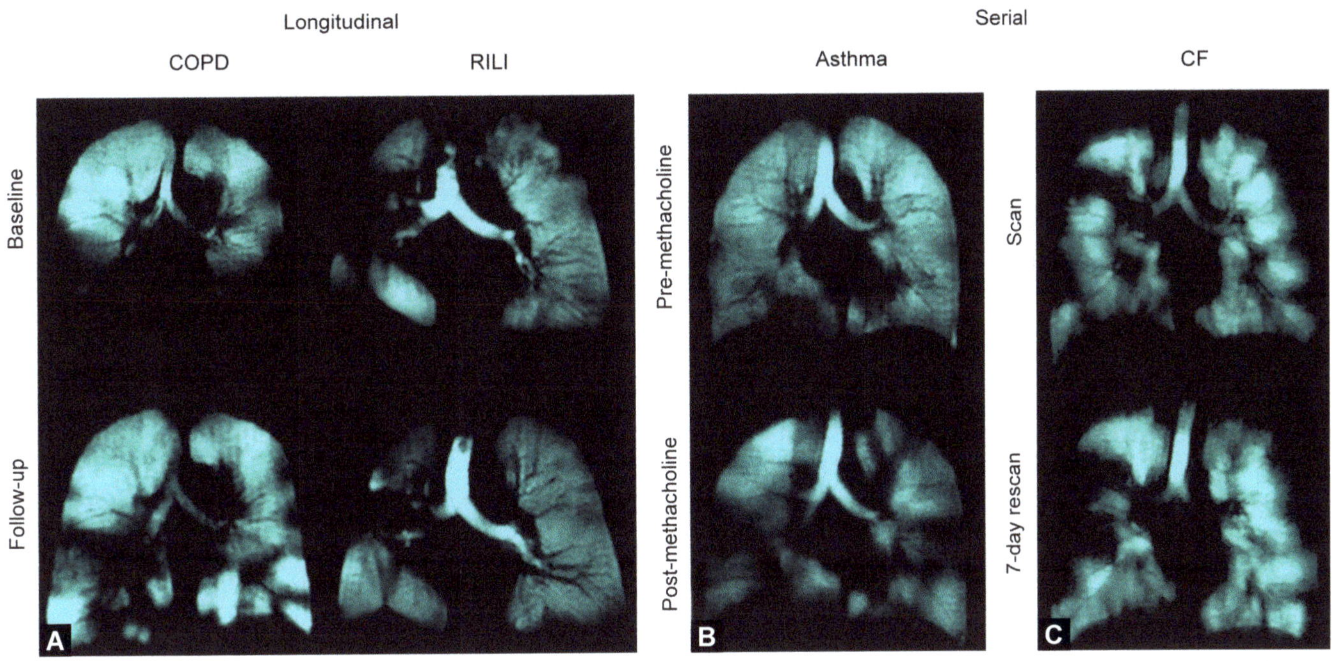

Figs. 22.7A to C: ^{3}He MRI static ventilation images of longitudinal and serial studies in subjects with chronic obstructive pulmonary disease (COPD), radiation-induced lung injury (RILI), asthma and cystic fibrosis (CF). Longitudinal studies show a COPD subject at baseline and 2 years following and a RILI subject at baseline and 35 weeks following radiation therapy. Serial studies show an asthma subject pre- and post-methacholine administration and a CF subject at scan and 7-day rescan.

Asthma

Asthma is a complex, chronic inflammatory disease associated with abnormal remodeling of the airways. In children, asthma is currently the most common chronic disease, affecting 16% of children between 4 and 11 years of age. In addition, asthma is a major cause of emergency visits and hospitalizations for children. The development of novel treatments and therapies to improve asthma symptoms and control are required in order to prevent hospitalizations. Toward this end, in order to evaluate these novel treatments, techniques capable of detecting regional improvements in pulmonary function are required.

Recently, one of the first investigations of childhood asthma was performed using hyperpolarized ^{3}He MRI in a small group of children aged 9–10 years with a current diagnosis of mild-to-moderate asthma. In comparison to a group of aged-matched children without asthma, asthmatic children demonstrated visually obvious and significantly greater ventilation defects as well as abnormal ^{3}He structural ADC measurements. This important study demonstrates that ^{3}He MRI may provide sensitive biomarkers of small airway dysfunction in asthma. Long-term follow-up of these subjects will be important to determine whether ^{3}He MRI measurements of early disease can predict long-term changes in disease progression and treatment response.

These emerging MR imaging techniques may also be used for evaluating new treatments to improve asthma control and reduced symptoms, such as bronchial thermoplasty—an approved airway treatment for severe asthma. Some preliminary studies have suggested that ^{3}He MRI may be useful to evaluate improvements in regional gas distribution following thermoplasty, as well as use ^{3}He MRI to guide treatment to regions with the most significant airflow obstruction. Although bronchial thermoplasty may not be used as an asthma treatment for children, these studies certainly demonstrate that there may be a role for MRI in guiding airway treatment or for evaluating the efficacy of treatments over time in asthmatics.

Cystic Fibrosis

Among all fatal genetic diseases affecting children, CF is the most common and currently there is no cure. CF is a multisystem disease, affecting mainly the digestive and respiratory system. Although therapies have improved leading to an increase in survival of CF patients, the improvements in therapies directed at addressing the severe lung problems are limited and therefore most CF deaths are due to respiratory complications. Biomarkers capable of predicting disease progression and exacerbations as well as evaluating the efficacy of new therapies are urgently needed in CF children, and some investigators have recommended that CT be used as part of a multimodality approach for monitoring CF lung disease. However, the radiation burden associated with serial CT imaging is not insignificant and, therefore, this remains a controversial technique.

Because ^{3}He MRI involves no ionizing radiation and is well tolerated in children, several studies have investigated the role of ^{3}He MRI for evaluating treatments in CF. It has been demonstrated in children that regional changes in ^{3}He MRI gas distribution can be visualized following chest physiotherapy, following inhalation of a bronchodilator and after mechanical airway clearance treatment. Moreover, the first investigation to use hyperpolarized ^{3}He MRI to assess an investigational CF drug was recently performed; ^{3}He MRI showed dramatic improvements in gas distribution in children with CF following treatment with Ivacaftor, demonstrating that ^{3}He MRI can provide a way to evaluate regional improvements in airflow obstruction.

Lung Growth and Abnormal Lung Development

Another area where MRI may be the imaging modality of choice is for the study of lung growth (alveolarization) as well as normal and abnormal lung development. Although CT may be used to investigate changes in lung weight, gas volume as well as changes in airway and parenchymal structure during the growth period, the radiation exposure due to CT limits longitudinal evaluation. Diffusion-weighted MRI can provide structural pulmonary information at the alveolar level without ionizing radiation and therefore this technique provides the opportunity to investigate the normal age-related changes that occur in the lung in individuals over time.

Although some ex-vivo studies suggest that alveolarization ceases in early life (~8 years), without in vivo longitudinal studies that can directly investigate alveolarization we do not have a definitive answer, and this knowledge may have very important implications. For example, the timing of pneumonectomy may be very important. Although pneumonectomy in children is rare, if pneumonectomy were to be performed during a period of time when the patient's lungs are still undergoing alveolarization, better outcomes may be possible. An important hyperpolarized ^{3}He MRI study recently provided evidence that alveolar growth continues throughout childhood and adolescence—much later than previously thought. Interestingly, another study recently demonstrated evidence of alveolarization using diffusion-weighted MRI in an adult women following pneumonectomy.

In addition, there is very little known about the impact of respiratory disease or illness that occurs early in life on subsequent lung growth and development. These novel MRI techniques may provide a very important opportunity to investigate lung growth and development longitudinally, especially in infants and children.

SUMMARY AND FUTURE DIRECTIONS

Conventional ^{1}H MRI of the lung suffers from the inherently low proton density and short T2 of the lung parenchyma, as well as magnetic susceptibility artifacts and respiratory and cardiac motion. Because of these limitations, several novel MRI approaches for the lung have emerged. The development of short TE and UTE MRI has greatly improved the lung ^{1}H signal and, as a result, has led to visualization of pathological lung changes. Other proton-based techniques, such as Fourier Decomposition MRI have also been introduced and provide ventilation- and perfusion-weighted information that is comparable to other established imaging approaches. The introduction of gas-contrast MRI has also led to improvements in both the quality and quantity of pulmonary information that can be obtained, and very promising results in patients with respiratory disease using oxygen-enhanced and hyperpolarized noble gas MRI have been demonstrated. Although ^{19}F MRI is one of the newer MRI techniques, the fact that gas-contrast images can be obtained using clinically available MRI systems without requiring expensive polarization equipment suggests that this technique has great promise for the evaluation of respiratory disease.

While many of these novel MRI methodologies are still under development and there are currently very few clinical studies, these techniques are well on their way to demonstrating that MRI may be the imaging modality of choice for providing pulmonary structural and functional information in patients with respiratory disease. The greatest potential of MRI of the lung may be for evaluating respiratory disease in infants and children, as well as for longitudinal or serial studies as a complement to other standard approaches.

BIBLIOGRAPHY AND FURTHER READING

1. Ajay S, Robert T, James K, David SG, Jaime T, Tammy K, et al. Ventilation defects with hyperpolarized Helium MRI in severe asthma before and after bronchial thermoplasty. D29 Use of Emerging Imaging Techniques as Biomarkers of Lung Disease. American Thoracic Society International Conference Abstracts: American Thoracic Society; 2013. p. A5443-A.

2. Albert MS, Cates GD, Driehuys B, Happer W, Saam B, Springer CS, et al. Biological magnetic resonance imaging using laser-polarized 129Xe. Nature. 1994;370(6486):199-201.
3. Aliverti A, Kayser B, Macklem PT. A human model of the pathophysiology of chronic obstructive pulmonary disease. Respirology. 2007;12(4):478-85.
4. Altes, TA, Johnson, M, Mugler, JP, Froh, D, Flors, L, Wilson Miller G, Mata JH, Salinas, CL, Tustison, N, Lee, P-S, Song, T, Yen, K, deLange EE and Botfield MC. Hyperpolarised helium-3 MRI detects the effects of a CFTR potentiator (ivacaftor) therapy in subjects with cystic fibrosis and the G551D mutation. Abstract 1359 International Society for Magnetic Resonance in Medicine 20th Annual Meeting Melbourne Australia May 8 2012.
5. Altes TA, Mata J, de Lange EE, Brookeman JR, Mugler JP, Assessment of lung development using hyperpolarized helium-3 diffusion MR imaging. J Magn Reson Imaging. 2006;24(6):1277-83.
6. Altes TA, Powers PL, Knight-Scott J, Rakes G, Platts-Mills TA, de Lange EE, et al. Hyperpolarized 3He MR lung ventilation imaging in asthmatics: preliminary findings. J Magn Reson Imaging. 2001;13(3):378-84.
7. Altes TA, Rehm PK, Harrell F, Salerno M, Daniel TM, de Lange EE. Ventilation imaging of the lung: comparison of hyperpolarized helium-3 MR imaging with Xe-133 scintigraphy. AcadRadiol. 2004;11(7):729-34.
8. Bannier E, Cieslar K, Mosbah K, Aubert F, Duboeuf F, Salhi Z, et al. Hyperpolarized 3He MR for sensitive imaging of ventilation function and treatment efficiency in young cystic fibrosis patients with normal lung function. Radiology. 2010;255(1):225-32.
9. Bauman G, Lutzen U, Ullrich M, Gaass T, Dinkel J, Elke G, et al. Pulmonary functional imaging: qualitative comparison of Fourier decomposition MR imaging with SPECT/CT in porcine lung. Radiology. 2011;260(2):551-9.
10. Bauman G, Puderbach M, Deimling M, Jellus V, Chefd'hotel C, Dinkel J, et al. Non-contrast-enhanced perfusion and ventilation assessment of the human lung by means of fourier decomposition in proton MRI. Magn Reson Med. 2009;62(3):656-64.
11. Bauman G, Puderbach M, Heimann T, Kopp-Schneider A, Fritzsching E, et al. Validation of Fourier decomposition MRI with dynamic contrast-enhanced MRI using visual and automated scoring of pulmonary perfusion in young cystic fibrosis patients. European journal of radiology. 2013;82(12):2371-7.
12. Bauman G, Scholz A, Rivoire J, Terekhov M, Friedrich J, de Oliveira A, et al. Lung ventilation- and perfusion-weighted Fourier decomposition magnetic resonance imaging: in vivo validation with hyperpolarized 3He and dynamic contrast-enhanced MRI. Magn Reson Med. 2013;69(1): 229-37.
13. Bergin CJ, Pauly JM, Macovski A. Lung parenchyma: projection reconstruction MR imaging. Radiology. 1991; 179(3):777-81.
14. Butler JP, Loring SH, Patz S, Tsuda A, Yablonskiy DA, Mentzer SJ. Evidence for adult lung growth in humans. N Engl JMed. 2012;367(3):244-7.
15. Cadman RV, Lemanske RF, Evans MD, Jackson DJ, Gern JE, Sorkness RL, et al. Pulmonary 3He magnetic resonance imaging of childhood asthma. J Allergy Clin Immunol. 2013;131(2):369-76.e1-5.
16. Canada CF. Canadian Cystic Fibrosis Registry 2011 Annual Report. Toronto, ON; 2011.
17. Cleveland ZI, Cofer GP, Metz G, Beaver D, Nouls J, Kaushik SS, et al. Hyperpolarized Xe MR imaging of alveolar gas uptake in humans. PLoSOne. 2010;5(8):e12192.
18. Couch MJ, Ball IK, Li T, Fox MS, Littlefield SL, Biman B, et al. Pulmonary ultrashort echo time 19F MR imaging with inhaled fluorinated gas mixtures in healthy volunteers: feasibility. Radiology. 2013;269(3):903-9.
19. Damadian R, Goldsmith M, Minkoff L. NMR in cancer: XVI. FONAR image of the live human body. Physiol Chem Phys. 1977;9(1):97-100, 108.
20. Deimling M, Jellus V, Geiger B, Chefd'hotel C. Time Resolved Lung Ventilation Imaging by Fourier Decomposition. Proceedings of the 16th Annual Meeting of ISMRM, Toronto, Canada. 2008;2639.
21. de Jong PA, Long FR, Wong JC, Merkus PJ, Tiddens HA, Hogg JC, et al. Computed tomographic estimation of lung dimensions throughout the growth period. The European respiratory journal. 2006;27(2):261-7.
22. de Jong PA, Mayo JR, Golmohammadi K, Nakano Y, Lequin MH, Tiddens HA, et al. Estimation of cancer mortality associated with repetitive computed tomography scanning. Am J Respir Crit Care Med. 2006;173(2):199-203.
23. de Jong PA, Nakano Y, Lequin MH, Merkus PJ, Tiddens HA, Hogg JC, et al. Estimation of lung growth using computed tomography. Eur Respir J. 2003;22(2):235-8.
24. de Lange EE, Altes TA, Patrie JT, Battiston JJ, Juersivich AP, Mugler JP, et al. Changes in regional airflow obstruction over time in the lungs of patients with asthma: evaluation with 3He MR imaging. Radiology. 2009;250(2):567-75.
25. de Lange EE, Altes TA, Patrie JT, Parmar J, Brookeman JR, Mugler JP, et al. The variability of regional airflow obstruction within the lungs of patients with asthma: assessment with hyperpolarized helium-3 magnetic resonance imaging. JAllergy ClinImmunol. 2007;119(5):1072-8.
26. de Lange EE, Mugler JP, Brookeman JR, Knight-Scott J, Truwit JD, Teates CD, et al. Lung air spaces: MR imaging evaluation with hyperpolarized 3He gas. Radiology. 1999; 210(3):851-7.
27. Deninger AJ, Eberle B, Bermuth J, Escat B, Markstaller K, Schmiedeskamp J, et al. Assessment of a single-acquisition imaging sequence for oxygen-sensitive (3)He-MRI. Magnetic resonance in medicine : official journal of the Society of Magnetic Resonance in Medicine/Society of Magnetic Resonance in Medicine. 2002;47(1):105-14.
28. Deninger AJ, Eberle B, Ebert M, Grossmann T, Heil W, Kauczor H, et al. Quantification of regional intrapulmonary oxygen partial pressure evolution during apnea by (3)He MRI. Journal of magnetic resonance. 1999;141(2):207-16.

29. Diaz S, Casselbrant I, Piitulainen E, Magnusson P, Peterson B, Wollmer P, et al. Validity of apparent diffusion coefficient hyperpolarized 3He-MRI using MSCT and pulmonary function tests as references. Eur J Radiol. 2009;71(2):257-63.
30. Diaz S, Casselbrant I, Piitulainen E, Pettersson G, Magnusson P, Peterson B, et al. Hyperpolarized 3He apparent diffusion coefficient MRI of the lung: reproducibility and volume dependency in healthy volunteers and patients with emphysema. JMagn Reson Imaging. 2008;27(4):763-70.
31. Donnelly LF, MacFall JR, McAdams HP, Majure JM, Smith J, Frush DP, et al. Cystic fibrosis: combined hyperpolarized 3He-enhanced and conventional proton MR imaging in the lung-preliminary observations. Radiology. 1999;212(3): 885-9.
32. Dregely I, Mugler JP, Ruset IC, Altes TA, Mata JF, Miller GW, et al. Hyperpolarized Xenon-129 gas-exchange imaging of lung microstructure: first case studies in subjects with obstructive lung disease. J Magn Reson Imaging. 2011; 33(5):1052-62.
33. Dregely I, Ruset IC, Mata JF, Ketel J, Ketel S, Distelbrink J, et al. Multiple-exchange-time xenon polarization transfer contrast (MXTC) MRI: initial results in animals and healthy volunteers. Magn Reson Med. 2012;67(4):943-53.
34. Driehuys B, Cofer GP, Pollaro J, Mackel JB, Hedlund LW, Johnson GA. Imaging alveolar-capillary gas transfer using hyperpolarized 129Xe MRI. Proc Natl Acad Sci USA. 2006;103(48):18278-83.
35. Driehuys B, Martinez-Jimenez S, Cleveland ZI, Metz GM, Beaver DM, Nouls JC, et al. Chronic obstructive pulmonary disease: safety and tolerability of hyperpolarized 129Xe MR imaging in healthy volunteers and patients. Radiology. 2012;262(1):279-89.
36. Dunnill MS. The problem of lung growth. Thorax. 1982;-37(8):561-3.
37. Edelman RR, Hatabu H, Tadamura E, Li W, Prasad PV. Noninvasive assessment of regional ventilation in the human lung using oxygen-enhanced magnetic resonance imaging. Nat Med. 1996;2(11):1236-9.
38. Fain SB, Altes TA, Panth SR, Evans MD, Waters B, Mugler JP, et al. Detection of age-dependent changes in healthy adult lungs with diffusion-weighted 3He MRI. Acad Radiol. 2005;12(11):1385-93.
39. Fain SB, Gonzalez-Fernandez G, Peterson ET, Evans MD, Sorkness RL, Jarjour NN, et al. Evaluation of structure-function relationships in asthma using multidetector CT and hyperpolarized He-3 MRI. Acad Radiol. 2008;15(6): 753-62.
40. Fain SB, Panth SR, Evans MD, Wentland AL, Holmes JH, Korosec FR, et al. Early emphysematous changes in asymptomatic smokers: detection with 3He MR imaging. Radiology. 2006;239(3):875-83.
41. Fischer MC, Spector ZZ, Ishii M, Yu J, Emami K, Itkin M, et al. Single-acquisition sequence for the measurement of oxygen partial pressure by hyperpolarized gas MRI. Magnetic resonance in medicine: official journal of the Society of Magnetic Resonance in Medicine/Society of Magnetic Resonance in Medicine. 2004;52(4):766-73.
42. Halaweish AF, Moon RE, Foster WM, Soher BJ, McAdams HP, MacFall JR, et al. Perfluoropropane gas as a magnetic resonance lung imaging contrast agent in humans. Chest. 2013;144(4):1300-10.
43. Hatabu H, Gaa J, Tadamura E, Edinburgh KJ, Stock KW, Garpestad E, et al. MR imaging of pulmonary parenchyma with a half-Fourier single-shot turbo spin-echo (HASTE) sequence. Eur J Radiol. 1999;29(2):152-9.
44. Holmes JH, O'Halloran RL, Brodsky EK, Bley TA, Francois CJ, Velikina JV, et al. Three-dimensional imaging of ventilation dynamics in asthmatics using multiecho projection acquisition with constrained reconstruction. Magn Reson Med. 2009;62(6):1543-56.
45. Holmes JH, O'Halloran RL, Brodsky EK, Jung Y, Block WF, Fain SB. 3D hyperpolarized He-3 MRI of ventilation using a multi-echo projection acquisition. Magn Reson Med. 2008;59(5):1062-71.
46. Jacob RE, Chang YV, Choong CK, Bierhals A, Zheng Hu D, Zheng J, et al. 19F MR imaging of ventilation and diffusion in excised lungs. Magn Reson Med. 2005;54(3):577-85.
47. Johnson KM, Fain SB, Schiebler ML, Nagle S. Optimized 3D ultrashort echo time pulmonary MRI. Magn Reson Med. 2013;70(5):1241-50.
48. Kauczor HU, Ebert M, Kreitner KF, Nilgens H, Surkau R, Heil W, et al. Imaging of the lungs using 3He MRI: preliminary clinical experience in 18 patients with and without lung disease. J Magn Reson Imaging. 1997;7(3):538-43.
49. Kaushik SS, Cleveland ZI, Cofer GP, Metz G, Beaver D, Nouls J, et al. Diffusion-weighted hyperpolarized 129Xe MRI in healthy volunteers and subjects with chronic obstructive pulmonary disease. Magn Reson Med. 2011;65(4):1154-65.
50. Kirby M, Heydarian M, Svenningsen S, Wheatley A, McCormack DG, Etemad-Rezai R, et al. Hyperpolarized 3He magnetic resonance functional imaging semiautomated segmentation. Acad Radiol. 2012;19(2):141-52.
51. Kirby M, Mathew L, Heydarian M, Etemad-Rezai R, McCormack DG, Parraga G. Chronic obstructive pulmonary disease: quantification of bronchodilator effects by using hyperpolarized 3He MR imaging. Radiology. 2011;261(1): 283-92.
52. Kirby M, Mathew L, Wheatley A, Santyr GE, McCormack DG, Parraga G. Chronic obstructive pulmonary disease: longitudinal hyperpolarized 3He MR imaging. Radiology. 2010;256(1):280-9.
53. Kirby M, Svenningsen S, Ahmed H, Wheatley A, Etemad-Rezai R, Paterson NA, et al. Quantitative evaluation of hyperpolarized helium-3 magnetic resonance imaging of lung function variability in cystic fibrosis. Acad Radiol. 2011;18(8):1006-13.
54. Kirby M, Svenningsen S, Owrangi A, Wheatley A, Farag A, Ouriadov A, et al. Hyperpolarized 3He and 129Xe MR Imaging in Healthy Volunteers and Patients with Chronic Obstructive Pulmonary Disease. Radiology. 2012;265(2): 600-10.
55. Koumellis P, van Beek EJ, Woodhouse N, Fichele S, Swift AJ, Paley MN, et al. Quantitative analysis of regional airways obstruction using dynamic hyperpolarized 3He

MRI-preliminary results in children with cystic fibrosis. J Magn Reson Imaging. 2005;22(3):420-6.
56. Kuethe DO, Caprihan A, Fukushima E, Waggoner RA. Imaging lungs using inert fluorinated gases. Magn Reson Med. 1998;39(1):85-8.
57. Lederlin M, Bauman G, Eichinger M, Dinkel J, Brault M, Biederer J, et al. Functional MRI using Fourier decomposition of lung signal: reproducibility of ventilation- and perfusion-weighted imaging in healthy volunteers. Eur J Radiol. 2013;82(6):1015-22.
58. Lutterbey G, Gieseke J, von Falkenhausen M, Morakkabati N, Schild H. Lung MRI at 3.0 T: a comparison of helical CT and high-field MRI in the detection of diffuse lung disease. European radiology. 2005;15(2):324-8.
59. Mathew L, Evans A, Ouriadov A, Etemad-Rezai R, Fogel R, Santyr G, et al. Hyperpolarized 3He magnetic resonance imaging of chronic obstructive pulmonary disease: reproducibility at 3.0 tesla. Acad Radiol. 2008;15(10):1298-311.
60. Mathew L, Gaede S, Wheatley A, Etemad-Rezai R, Rodrigues GB, Parraga G. Detection of longitudinal lung structural and functional changes after diagnosis of radiation-induced lung injury using hyperpolarized 3He magnetic resonance imaging. Med Phys. 2010;37(1):22-31.
61. Mathew L, Kirby M, Etemad-Rezai R, Wheatley A, McCormack DG, Parraga G. Hyperpolarized 3He magnetic resonance imaging: preliminary evaluation of phenotyping potential in chronic obstructive pulmonary disease. EurJ Radiol. 2011;79(1):140-6.
62. Mathew L, Kirby M, Farquhar D, Licskai C, Santyr G, Etemad-Rezai R, et al. Hyperpolarized 3He functional magnetic resonance imaging of bronchoscopic airway bypass in chronic obstructive pulmonary disease. Can Respir J. 2012;19(1):41-3.
63. Mayo JR, MacKay A, Muller NL. MR imaging of the lungs: value of short TE spin-echo pulse sequences. AJR AmJ Roentgenol. 1992;159(5):951-6.
64. Mentore K, Froh DK, de Lange EE, Brookeman JR, Paget-Brown AO, Altes TA. Hyperpolarized HHe 3 MRI of the lung in cystic fibrosis: assessment at baseline and after bronchodilator and airway clearance treatment. AcadRadiol. 2005;12(11):1423-9.
65. Miller GW, Mugler JP, Altes TA, Cai J, Mata JF, de Lange EE, et al. A short-breath-hold technique for lung pO2 mapping with 3He MRI. Magn Reson Med. 2010;63(1):127-36.
66. Molinari F, Bauman G, Paolantonio G, Geisler T, Geiger B, Bonomo L, et al. Improvement of multislice oxygen-enhanced MRI of the lung by fully automatic non-rigid image registration. Eur J Radiol. 2012;81(10):2900-6.
67. Morbach AE, Gast KK, Schmiedeskamp J, Dahmen A, Herweling A, Heussel CP, et al. Diffusion-weighted MRI of the lung with hyperpolarized helium-3: a study of reproducibility. J Magn Reson Imaging. 2005;21(6):765-74.
68. Mugler JP, Altes TA, Ruset IC, Dregely IM, Mata JF, Miller GW, et al. Simultaneous magnetic resonance imaging of ventilation distribution and gas uptake in the human lung using hyperpolarized xenon-129. Proc Natl Acad Sci USA. 2010;107(50):21707-12.
69. Mugler JP, Mata JF, Wang HTJ, Tobias WA, Cates GD, Christopher JM, et al. The apparent diffusion coefficient of 129-Xe in the lung: preliminary human results. Proceedings of the 12th Annual Meeting of ISMRM, Kyoto, Japan. 2004:769.
70. Narayanan M, Owers-Bradley J, Beardsmore CS, Mada M, Ball I, Garipov R, et al. Alveolarization continues during childhood and adolescence: new evidence from helium-3 magnetic resonance. Am J Respir Crit Care Med. 2012;185(2):186-91.
71. Niles DJ, Kruger SJ, Dardzinski BJ, Harman A, Jarjour NN, Ruddy M, et al. Exercise-induced bronchoconstriction: reproducibility of hyperpolarized 3He MR imaging. Radiology. 2013;266(2):618-25.
72. Ochs M, Nyengaard JR, Jung A, Knudsen L, Voigt M, Wahlers T, et al. The number of alveoli in the human lung. AmJ Respir Crit Care Med. 2004;169(1):120-4.
73. Ohno Y, Hatabu H, Takenaka D, Van CM, Fujii M, Sugimura K. Dynamic oxygen-enhanced MRI reflects diffusing capacity of the lung. Magn Reson Med. 2002;47(6):1139-44.
74. Ohno Y, Iwasawa T, Seo JB, Koyama H, Takahashi H, Oh YM, et al. Oxygen-enhanced magnetic resonance imaging versus computed tomography: multicenter study for clinical stage classification of smoking-related chronic obstructive pulmonary disease. AmJ Respir Crit Care Med. 2008;177(10):1095-102.
75. Ohno Y, Koyama H, Yoshikawa T, Matsumoto K, Aoyama N, Onishi Y, et al. Comparison of capability of dynamic O(2)-enhanced MRI and quantitative thin-section MDCT to assess COPD in smokers. EurJRadiol. 2012;81(5):1068-75.
76. Ohno Y, Koyama H, Yoshikawa T, Matsumoto K, Takahashi M, Van Cauteren M, et al. T2* measurements of 3-T MRI with ultrashort TEs: capabilities of pulmonary function assessment and clinical stage classification in smokers. AJR Am J Roentgenol.. 2011;197(2):W279-85.
77. Ohno Y, Koyama H, Yoshikawa T, Nishio M, Aoyama N, Onishi Y, et al. N stage disease in patients with non-small cell lung cancer: efficacy of quantitative and qualitative assessment with STIR turbo spin-echo imaging, diffusion-weighted MR imaging, and fluorodeoxyglucose PET/CT. Radiology. 2011;261(2):605-15.
78. Ohno Y, Nishio M, Koyama H, Takenaka D, Takahashi M, Yoshikawa T, et al. Pulmonary MR imaging with ultra-short TEs: utility for disease severity assessment of connective tissue disease patients. Eur J Radiol. 2013;82(8):1359-65.
79. Ohno Y, Nishio M, Koyama H, Yoshikawa T, Matsumoto S, Seki S, et al. Oxygen-enhanced MRI for patients with connective tissue diseases: Comparison with thin-section CT of capability for pulmonary functional and disease severity assessment. Eur J Radiol. 2014;83(2):391-7.
80. O'Connell OJ, McWilliams S, McGarrigle A, O'Connor OJ, Shanahan F, Mullane D, et al. Radiologic imaging in cystic fibrosis: cumulative effective dose and changing trends over 2 decades. Chest. 2012;141(6):1575-83.
81. Parraga G, Mathew L, Etemad-Rezai R, McCormack DG, Santyr GE. Hyperpolarized 3He magnetic resonance imaging of ventilation defects in healthy elderly volunteers: initial findings at 3.0 Tesla. AcadRadiol. 2008;15(6):776-85.

82. Patz S, Hersman FW, Muradian I, Hrovat MI, Ruset IC, Ketel S, et al. Hyperpolarized (129)Xe MRI: a viable functional lung imaging modality? Eur J Radiol. 2007;64(3):335-44.
83. Patz S, Muradian I, Hrovat MI, Ruset IC, Topulos G, Covrig SD, et al. Human pulmonary imaging and spectroscopy with hyperpolarized 129Xe at 0.2T. Acad Radiol. 2008;15(6): 713-27.
84. Pearce MS, Salotti JA, Little MP, McHugh K, Lee C, Kim KP, et al. Radiation exposure from CT scans in childhood and subsequent risk of leukaemia and brain tumours: a retrospective cohort study. Lancet. 2012;380(9840):499-505.
85. Renne J, Lauermann P, Hinrichs J, Schonfeld C, Sorrentino S, Gutberlet M, et al. Clinical use of oxygen-enhanced T mapping MRI of the lung: Reproducibility and impact of closed versus loose fit oxygen delivery system. Journal of magnetic resonance imaging: J Magn Reson Imaging. 2015;41(1):60-6.
86. Rizi RR, Baumgardner JE, Ishii M, Spector ZZ, Edvinsson JM, Jalali A, et al. Determination of regional VA/Q by hyperpolarized 3He MRI. Magn Reson Med. 2004;52(1): 65-72.
87. Saam BT, Yablonskiy DA, Kodibagkar VD, Leawoods JC, Gierada DS, Cooper JD, et al. MR imaging of diffusion of (3)He gas in healthy and diseased lungs. Magn Reson Med. 2000;44(2):174-9.
88. Salerno M, Altes TA, Brookeman JR, de Lange EE, Mugler JP. Dynamic spiral MRI of pulmonary gas flow using hyperpolarized (3)He: preliminary studies in healthy and diseased lungs. Magn Reson Med. 2001;46(4):667-77.
89. Salerno M, de Lange EE, Altes TA, Truwit JD, Brookeman JR, Mugler JP. Emphysema: hyperpolarized helium 3 diffusion MR imaging of the lungs compared with spirometric indexes--initial experience. Radiology. 2002;222(1):252-60.
90. Sarah S, Miranda K, Stephen C, Andrew W, David GM, Grace P. Temporal-Spatial maps of asthma ventilation to identify therapy targets. A19 understanding ventilation distribution in airways disease. American Thoracic Society International Conference Abstracts: American Thoracic Society; 2013. p. A1049-A.
91. Schreiber WG, Eberle B, Laukemper-Ostendorf S, Markstaller K, Weiler N, Scholz A, et al. Dynamic (19) F-MRI of pulmonary ventilation using sulfur hexafluoride (SF(6)) gas. Magn Reson Med. 2001;45(4):605-13.
92. Sindile A, Muradian I, Hrovat M, Johnson DC, Hersman FW, Patz S. Human pulmonary diffusion weighted imaging at 0.2T with hyperpolarizd 129Xe. Proceedings of the 15th Annual Meeting of ISMRM, Berlin, Germany. 2007:1290.
93. Soher BJ AM, MacFall J, Hashoian R, Charles HC, (Eds). Lung Imaging in Humans at 3T using Perfluorinated Gases as MR Contrast Agents. Proc Intl Soc Mag Reson Med. 2010.
94. Svenningsen S, Kirby M, Starr D, Leary D, Wheatley A, Maksym GN, et al. Hyperpolarized (3) He and (129) Xe MRI: Differences in asthma before bronchodilation. Journal of magnetic resonance imaging: J Magn Reson Imaging. 2013 Dec;38(6):1521-30.
95. Swift AJ, Wild JM, Fichele S, Woodhouse N, Fleming S, Waterhouse J, et al. Emphysematous changes and normal variation in smokers and COPD patients using diffusion 3He MRI. EurJ Radiol. 2005;54(3):352-8.
96. Tadamura E, Hatabu H, Li W, Prasad PV, Edelman RR. Effect of oxygen inhalation on relaxation times in various tissues. J Magn Reson Imaging. 1997;7(1):220-5.
97. Takahashi M, Togao O, Obara M, van Cauteren M, Ohno Y, Doi S, et al. Ultra-short echo time (UTE) MR imaging of the lung: comparison between normal and emphysematous lungs in mutant mice. J Magn Reson Imaging. 2010;32(2):326-33.
98. Tiddens HA, Stick SM, Davis S. Multi-modality monitoring of cystic fibrosis lung disease: The role of chest computed tomography. Paediatric respiratory reviews. Paediatr Respir Rev. 2014;15(1):92-7.
99. Togao O, Tsuji R, Ohno Y, Dimitrov I, Takahashi M. Ultrashort echo time (UTE) MRI of the lung: assessment of tissue density in the lung parenchyma. Magnetic resonance in medicine. Magn Reson Med. 2010;64(5):1491-8.
100. Tustison NJ, Avants BB, Flors L, Altes TA, de Lange EE, Mugler JP, et al. Ventilation-based segmentation of the lungs using hyperpolarized (3)He MRI. J Magn ResonImaging. 2011;34(4):831-41.
101. Weibel ER, Gomez DM. Architecture of the human lung. Use of quantitative methods establishes fundamental relations between size and number of lung structures. Science. 1962;137(3530):577-85.
102. Wild JM, Paley MN, Kasuboski L, Swift A, Fichele S, Woodhouse N, et al. Dynamic radial projection MRI of inhaled hyperpolarized 3He gas. Magn Reson Med. 2003;49(6):991-7.
103. Woodhouse N, Wild JM, Paley MN, Fichele S, Said Z, Swift AJ, et al. Combined helium-3/proton magnetic resonance imaging measurement of ventilated lung volumes in smokers compared to never-smokers. J Magn Reson Imaging. 2005;21(4):365-9.
104. Woodhouse N, Wild JM, van Beek EJ, Hoggard N, Barker N, Taylor CJ. Assessment of hyperpolarized 3He lung MRI for regional evaluation of interventional therapy: a pilot study in pediatric cystic fibrosis. J Magn Reson Imaging. 2009;30(5):981-8.
105. Woods JC, Choong CK, Yablonskiy DA, Bentley J, Wong J, Pierce JA, et al. Hyperpolarized 3He diffusion MRI and histology in pulmonary emphysema. Magn Reson Med. 2006;56(6):1293-300.

Chapter 23

Lung Ultrasonography

Riccardo Inchingolo, Andrew S Liteplo, Claudio Sorino

OVERVIEW OF LUNG ULTRASOUND

Transthoracic ultrasound (US) of the lungs is a useful diagnostic tool for pulmonologists, emergency and critical care physicians, or anyone interested in the evaluation of the lungs. It allows for rapid, immediate, noninvasive assessment at the patient's bedside. Ultrasound is clearly useful in the diagnosis and characterization of pleural diseases like pneumothorax (PTX) and pleural effusion. It is also critical in improving the safety of pleural interventions. Moreover, it is useful in detecting other lung pathologies that reach the pleura such as pulmonary edema, consolidation, pulmonary infarction, pulmonary contusion, acute respiratory distress syndrome (ARDS) and even malignancy.

BASIC KNOWLEDGE OF LUNG ULTRASONOGRAPHY TECHNIQUE

Lung ultrasonography is a noninvasive clinical imaging technique that uses sound waves to evaluate thoracic structures. It is performed at the patient's bedside allowing for real-time integration of findings with the physical examination and clinical history. A methodological approach can help with decision-making about the optimal use of other imaging techniques, like radiography or computed tomography (CT) scan. Finally, this technique does not use ionizing radiation, making it a safe option for radiation reduction for all patients, and especially in the ones in whom radiation exposure is particularly concerning such as children and pregnant patients.

Sound waves in the 2.5–20 MHz frequency range are used for imaging the chest by detecting the intensity of the echo reflected and displaying this reflected intensity as a gray-scale image. Each chest structure has its own acoustic impedance, due to intrinsic tissue properties, and the difference in the acoustic impedance of contiguous structures creates a series of interfaces. At these interfaces, sound waves are reflected, refracted, and reverberated. Lungs, being air-filled organs will scatter ultrasound waves and under normal circumstances no meaningful image of the lungs is generated.

However, an interface of very large differences of acoustic impedances exists between tissue and air at the level of the pleural line. This generates particular artifacts which can be observed and interpreted in the right clinical context to give the clinician an understanding of the lung tissue underlying the probe. Thus, the science of lung ultrasound is really the interpretation of normal or abnormal artifact.

ULTRASOUND EQUIPMENT AND PROBES

A comprehensive ultrasound evaluation of the lungs is best performed using one of three types of probe: (1) a convex low frequency probe, with a frequency range between 2.5 MHz and 5 MHz, suitable for the general overview of tissues of interest, the characterization of pleural effusion and pleural thickening and the study of diaphragmatic kinetics, (2) a high frequency linear probe, with a frequency range between 7 MHz and 12 MHz, best used for the study of the chest wall, pleural line and for a detailed characterization of the pleuroparenchymal interface; and, finally, (3) a sector phased array probe can also be used, in similar fashion as the convex probe, and is the ideal probe for echocardiographic ultrasound which is often performed

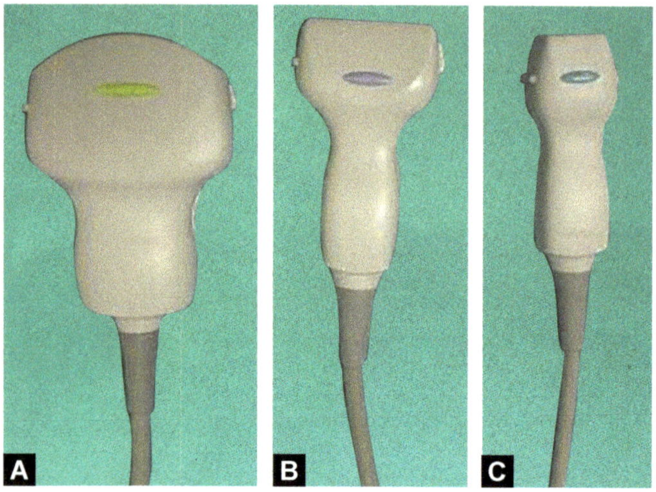

Figs. 23.1A to C: (A) The convex probe with frequency range between 2.5 MHz and 5 MHz. (B) The linear probe with frequency range between 7 MHz and 12 MHz. (C) The sector probe to perform echocardiography.

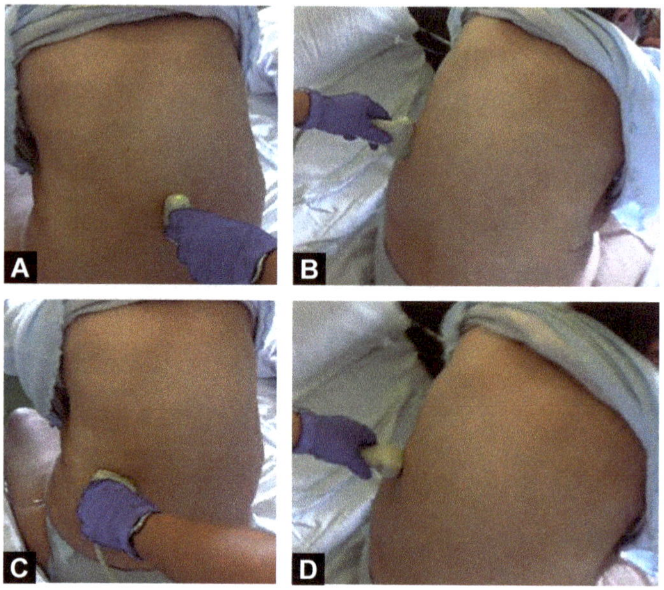

Figs. 23.2A to D: (A) Longitudinal scan along the paravertebral line with convex probe. (B) Longitudinal scan along posterior axillary line with convex probe. (C and D) Transverse scan along posterior axillary line with convex probe.

in conjunction with lung ultrasound (Figs. 23.1A to C). Using both convex and linear probes is ideal in order to combine the evaluation of deeper structures (convex probe), with the details arising from the higher spatial resolution power of the linear probe.

Before proceeding with the lung ultrasound examination, it is important to have a general understanding of the machine being used. Nowadays, there are three common types of machines: small "hand-held" devices, medium-sized portable devices and large devices equipped with more complex diagnostic imaging modalities and functions. However, usually these machines do not have a specific lung preset. Therefore, the operator should use the abdominal preset for the convex probe and the vascular preset for the linear probe. Moreover, the operator chooses the mode with which to perform the examination: "B-mode" (modulation of the "brightness", that creates a bright dot for each reflected echo creating the typical image ones sees using ultrasound) or "M-Mode" (visualization of the "Movement" of the tissue structures positioned along a single line in the ultrasound beam over time, creating a graph of motion over time). Finally, it is important to properly adjust depth and gain to generate the optimal image of the structure(s) of interest.

IMAGING OF THE CHEST WALL

The ultrasonographer begins by placing a generous layer of gel on the probe to eliminate any air between the probe and the skin, which could act as a barrier to ultrasound wave penetration. The operator then places the probe on the selected area of interest. Whenever possible, it is better to perform the examination in a sitting position. In this way, the operator can place the probe longitudinally or transversely (by rotating the probe 90 degrees) on the posterior axillary line/paravertebral line and move around the chest to the parasternal line, and thus investigate all lung fields. It should be noted that by convention the cephalad structures of the area examined should appear on the left of the screen. Often in critical settings the patient cannot be placed in a sitting position, and thus the examination proceeds similarly with the patient in the supine position scanning the ventrolateral fields (from parasternal to midaxillary line) (Figs. 23.2A to D).

Normally, an ultrasound examination of the chest will generate a particular image different from most ultrasonography since an air-filled organ lies underneath the probe. The first structures to appear in the near field or top of the screen will be skin and subcutaneous tissue, followed by a layer of muscle and fascia. Deep to these structures one should first begin by identifying the hyperechoic immobile surface of the bones of the rib cage. The bright lines of each rib can be easily recognized by the shadowing of the image they create just below, since the bone absorbs and reflects all ultrasound beams back to the probe. Finally, and most importantly, a couple of centimeters below, in between each rib, one should be

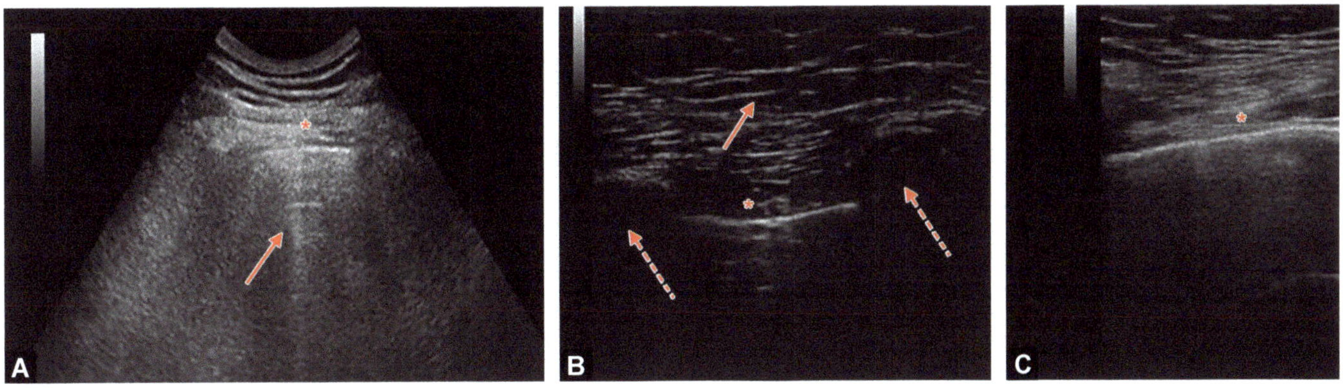

Figs. 23.3A to C: (A) A transverse scan with convex probe on the posterior axillary line. It is visible the pleural line (star) and underlying artifactual pleural-parenchymal field (arrow) due to "mirror effect" (arrow). (B) A longitudinal scan with linear probe with 10 MHz frequency on emiclavear line. It is possible to appreciate the details of the chest wall (arrow), the shadowing effect of the contiguous ribs (dashed arrow) and underlying pleural line (circle). (C) The pleural line (star) evaluated by a transverse scan with linear probe.

able to identify a bright white shimmering line representing the pleural line. In normal well-aerated lungs, the ultrasound beams should then be scattered and no recognizable image generated below.

Whenever there are structures with acoustic impedance similar to that of nonaerated tissues, the ultrasound beam can pass through them permitting the visualization of both them and adjacent structures. The *pleural line*, due to the interface between chest wall and aerated lung, moves with the act of breathing, giving the shimmering appearance of ants marching along a straight white line. This property of the normal pleural line is referred to as the *sliding sign* or *lung sliding*. It is due to movement of the visceral and the parietal layers of the pleura over each other. This sign, best seen with linear probe in B-mode real-time imaging, demonstrates the contact of the visceral and parietal pleura and, therefore, excludes the presence of PTX at that location (*see* below). The operator can improve the visualization of this sign, through the reduction of gain and depth, especially when ventral and cephalad lung fields are scanned in supine and sitting position, respectively.

The contiguity of structures with acoustic impedance that are different from each other creates a very important acoustic interface, in this case at the *pleural line*: the hyper-reflective line lying beyond the tissues of the chest wall which should not allow for real anatomical image generation of what lies beyond. This phenomenon is similar to the effect of a "mirror" (Figs. 23.3A to C). At this interface, however, one will find recognizable artifacts through the image below, known as A-Lines and B-Lines, both of which are be used to interpret the physiology of the lung below.

Thus, ultrasound imaging of the lung per se implies analysis of artifacts and dynamic estimates (*artifactual analysis*) rather than an analysis of the shape or structures (*morphological analysis*). In fact, chest ultrasound is basically a morphological study of the chest wall until the *pleural line* and is then an "artifactual" study of the pleural dynamics and artifacts created at the pleural-parenchymal field interface.

A LINES AND B LINES

The normal subpleural lung field (i.e. what that lies beneath the pleural line) generates the so-called *A Lines*. These are normal artifacts that appear as parallel and equidistant lines below the pleural line. They are horizontal artifacts and represent reverberations of the acoustic interfaces situated above (the above-mentioned "mirror effect") (Fig. 23.4).

Another kind of artifact, recognizable in the subpleural lung field, is the so-called *B Line*. B Lines are defined as discrete laser-like vertical hyperechoic artifacts that arise from the pleural line and extend deep into the lung, to the bottom of the screen without fading, moving synchronously with lung sliding (Fig. 23.5). When such artifacts appear on the screen but are small and do not penetrate deep into the tissue, they are commonly referred to simply as "comet tails". However, their genesis is not completely clear.

As of yet, there is poor understanding of the anatomic and physical genesis of B Lines. They are thought of as a reflection of the variations of density of the initial subpleural layer of the lung parenchyma. In fact, any parenchymal lung disease that increases lung density—through

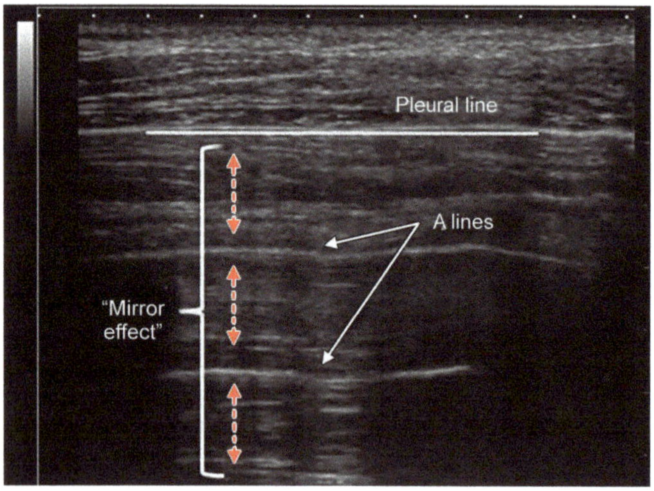

Fig. 23.4: Mirror effect.

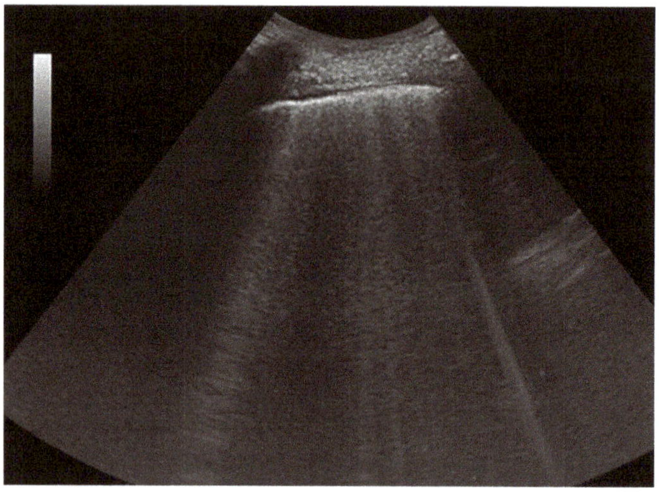

Fig. 23.5: B Lines.

the reduction of air content and/or the increase of solid (water/tissue) content - generates B Lines. Normal lung ultrasound could produce sporadic B lines, particularly at lung fissures. The presence of B Lines in relation to disease exists along a continuum, where the more diseased a lung (or the more the loss of normal, aerated lung) the more B Lines.

Another important site of transition from an "artifactual" analysis to a "morphological" one takes place during the movement of supradiaphragmatic pulmonary segments down in the costophrenic recesses. As the diaphragm moves inferiorly with inspiration so does the lung which scatters the ultrasound beams and thus image below. The appearance is similar to that of a curtain which obscures the hypochondriac organs (liver and spleen) as it move caudally (*curtain sign*) (Fig. 23.6).

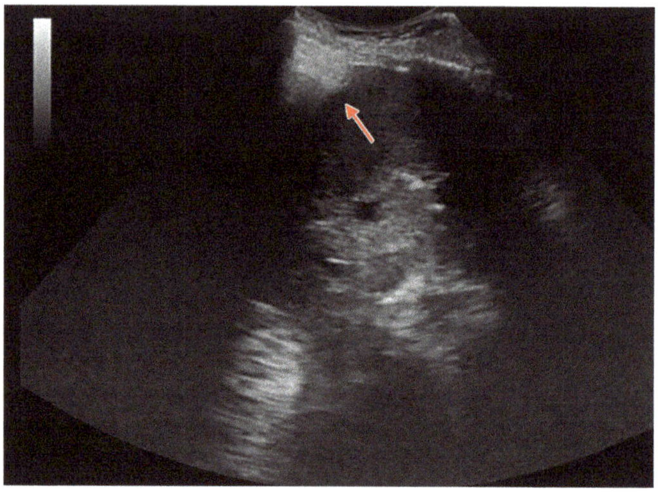

Fig. 23.6: Curtain sign on the liver. The inspiratory movement of supra diaphragmatic pulmonary segments down in the right costophrenic recess, similar to a curtain, obscures the diaphragmatic limit and the liver.

Whenever there is a supradiaphragmatic acoustic window (like in pleural effusion, atelectasis, lung consolidation) it is possible to obtain an image of the diaphragm through the transthoracic views. The images generated through the transthoracic diaphragmatic region are different from that obtained by transabdominal scanning since the hypochondriac organs (liver and spleen) act as acoustic windows and allow identification of the bright echoes of the diaphragm. The analysis of the supradiaphragmatic region is particularly relevant because it is the area most sensitive for pleural effusions (*see* below). Moreover, the presence of the curtain sign allows one to assess the costophrenic recesses as well as diaphragmatic kinetics.

EVALUATION OF PLEURAL DISEASE

Under normal conditions, lung ultrasound cannot physically distinguish the visceral from parietal pleural surfaces. In fact, as previously discussed, the pleural line is an acoustic interface, and not a morphologic structure. Therefore, it is only when there is pathologic involvement of the pleura and/or of the pleural space that it is possible to distinguish the two layers of the pleurae. This is what happens in the case of pleural effusions, PTX and pleural thickening.

A *pleural effusion* is a fluid-filled space localized above the diaphragm and bordered by the parietal pleural layer at the surface (near field on ultrasound) and by the visceral layer at its depth (far field). It is typically completely or predominantly anechoic, however, the cause and chronicity of the pleural effusion influence its sonographic appearance. The echographic aspect of pleural effusions depends on the physical characteristics of the fluid. Based on internal echogenicity, pleural effusions are usually classified into

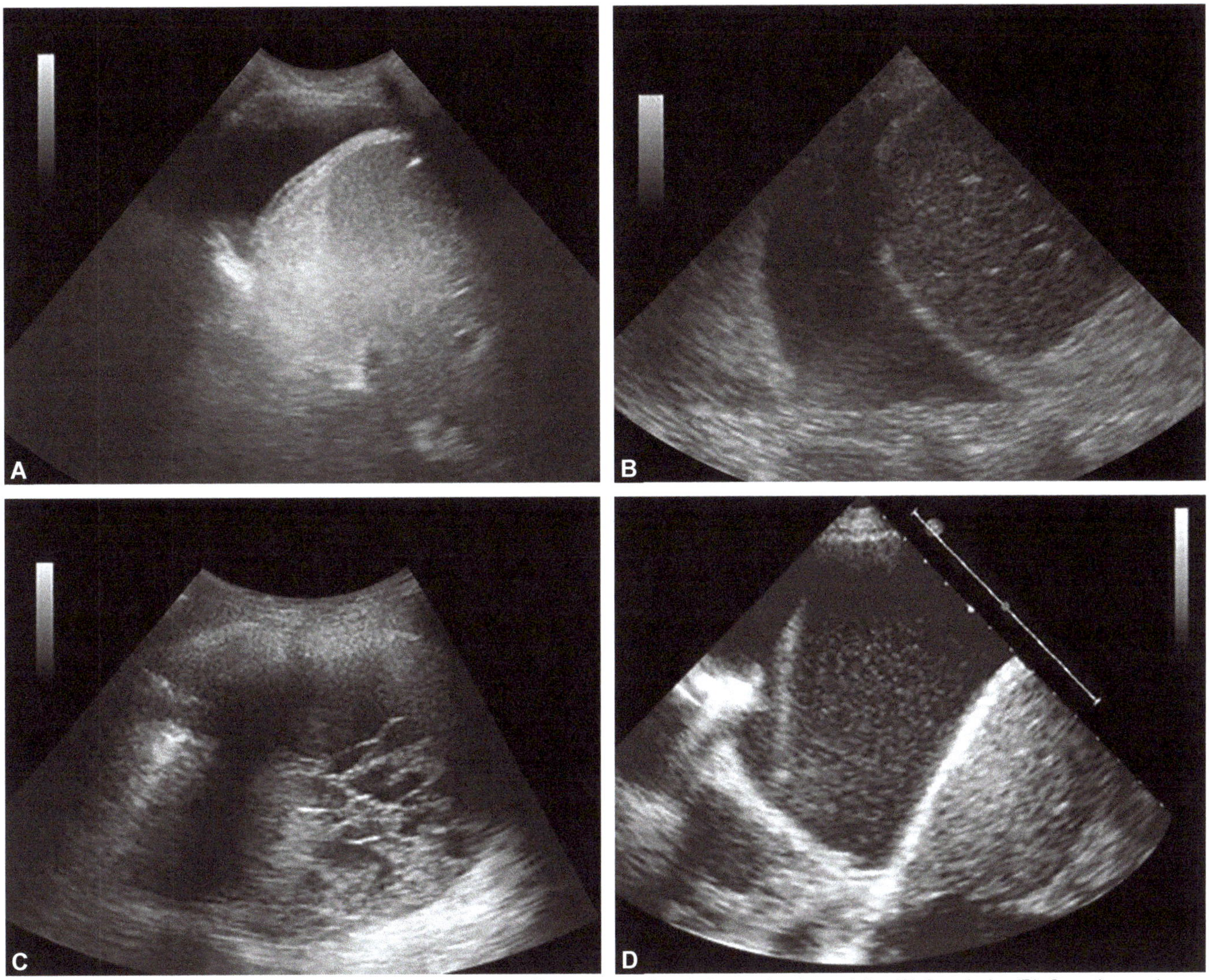

Figs. 23.7A to D: Ultrasonographic classification of pleural effusion according to internal echogenicity. (A) Anechoic. (B) Complex and non-septated (containing floating corpuscular material of variable density). (C) Complex and septated (composed of fibrin strands or septae in a lattice-like pattern). (D) Homogeneously hyperechogenic (densely corpusculated).

four sonographic patterns: (1) anechoic, (2) complex and nonseptated (containing floating corpuscular material of variable density), (3) complex and septated (composed of fibrin strands or septae in a lattice-like pattern), and (4) homogeneously hyperechoic (densely corpusculated) (Figs. 23.7A to D).

Effusions are defined as loculated when they are fixed and limited to a restricted area by a wall of a fibrinous tissue. The identification of a pleural effusion can be easily performed using the convex probe in a craniocaudal direction, proceeding with longitudinal scans from the base up to the cephalad zone of the lung in sitting position. The use of a linear probe can be used to better visualize small pleural effusions.

The operator should characterize the pleural effusion in terms of its localization, sonographic pattern and "functional" impact on the lung. The known thoracic vertical lines as well as intercostal spaces allows one to delineate the extent of a pleural effusion longitudinally and transversely (Figs. 23.8A and B).

The "functional" impact of pleural effusion on the lung depends essentially on the volume of the effusion. Its "quantitative" assessment is crucial to select the appropriate diagnostic and therapeutic approach. Different techniques have been proposed to estimate the volume of effusions. One such technique illustrated in Figures 23.9A to F uses a grading system to classify pleural effusions using the following ultrasonographic landmarks: the level of

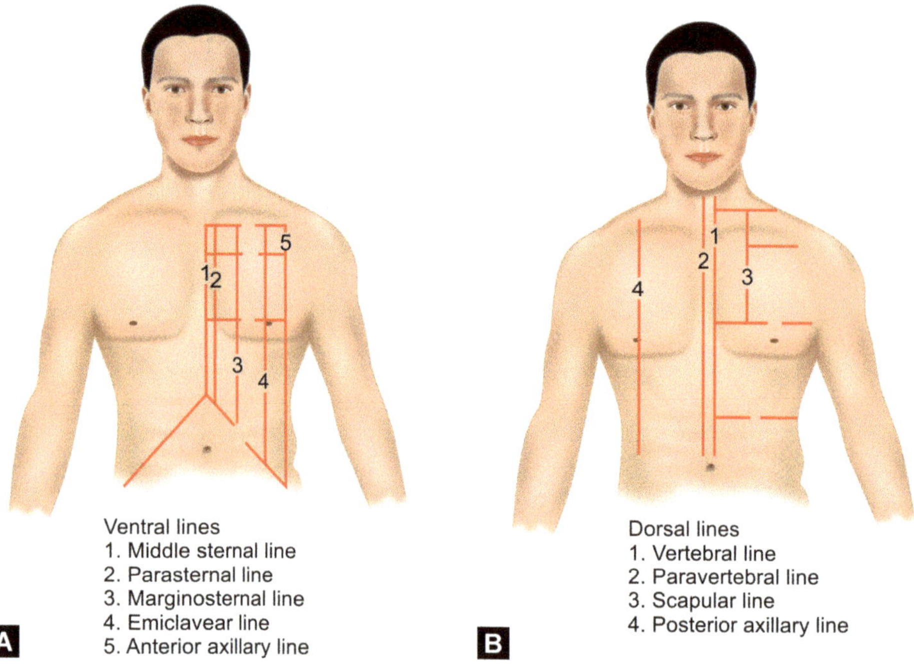

Figs. 23.8A and B: Ventral and dorsal thoracic vertical lines.

compression/atelectasis of the lobes, the visualization of the diaphragmatic dome and the pulmonary hilum, as well as the number of intercostal spaces through which fluid is visualized in caudal-cranial direction (Figs. 23.9A to F).

The first application of ultrasonography for the identification of PTX dates back to 1986, when the veterinarian Rantanen diagnosed PTX in a horse by the absence of the typically "sliding sign" artifact of normal moving pleurae. Appreciation of the presence or absence of the normal artifacts of the pleural-parenchymal field is crucial for ultrasonographic diagnosis of PTX. The combination of four ultrasonographic signs allows one to identify PTX. These signs are: (1) presence of lung point(s), (2) absence of lung sliding, (3) absence of B Lines, and (4) absence of lung pulse.

The *lung point* is an artifact that identifies the transition from a zone with no sliding to one with clear evidence of sliding of the pleural line. This point is the physical limit of PTX, the actual spot where the lung is touching the chest wall. It is important to note, however, that with full collapse of the lung, no lung point will be identified. The absence of both the sliding sign and B Lines is caused by the separation of visceral and parietal pleura due to the interposition of air.

In certain patients, however, the sliding sign can be difficult to appreciate (such as in patients with hyperinflated lungs). In such cases, the identification of another artifact known as the the *lung pulse* can be helpful to exclude PTX at that location. The *lung pulse* refers to the subtle rhythmic sliding of the visceral pleura along the parietal pleura with cardiac oscillations and can only occur if both pleurae are in contact. This essentially means that any pleural movement assures that there is no air in between the pleura and thereby excludes a PTX at that location.

Finally, M mode can be used to confirm movement of the pleural. By placing the cursor in an intercostal space directly over the pleura, one can see in the near field parallel horizontal lines generated by soft tissue above the pleura and a grainy image in the far field below representing normal aerated lung, often referred to as the *seashore sign*. In the setting of a PTX, the grainy image in the far field is replaced by lines like those above the pleura, creating an image of only vertical lines, referred to as the *barcode sign* (Figs. 23.10 to 23.12).

In order to identify a PTX in the supine patient, it is crucial to first explore areas least gravitationally dependent (i.e. anterior chest wall around the second or third intercostal space). If lung sliding is not seen, the probe should be moved laterally in search of a lung point, which definitively confirms a PTX and provides clues regarding its size. This method has a very high sensitivity and specificity. It is often suggested to use the linear probe as the high

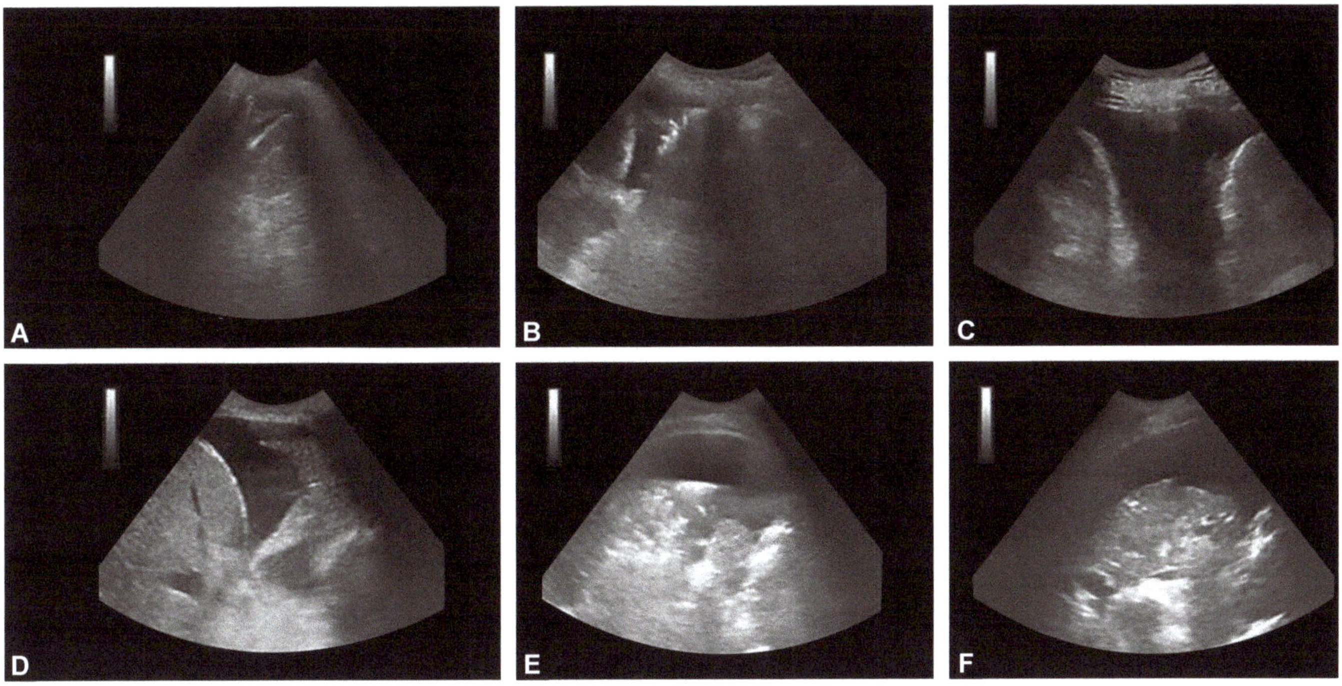

Figs. 23.9A to F: Standardized grading method for free pleural effusions. (A) Grade 1: limited to costophrenic sinus with diaphragmatic dome partially evident. (B) Grade 2: lower lung lobe partially involved with diaphragmatic dome completely evident. (C) Grade 3: lower lung lobe partially atelectasic with pulmonary hilum not visible. (D) Grade 4: atelectasis of the lower lung lobe and pulmonary hilum visible. (E) Grade 5: atelectasis of the lower lung and upper lung lobe partially atelectasic. (F) Grade 6: atelectasis of the whole lung and hilum completely visible. *Source:* Modified by bibliography 72 Copyright © 2013 Karger Publishers, Basel, Switzerland.

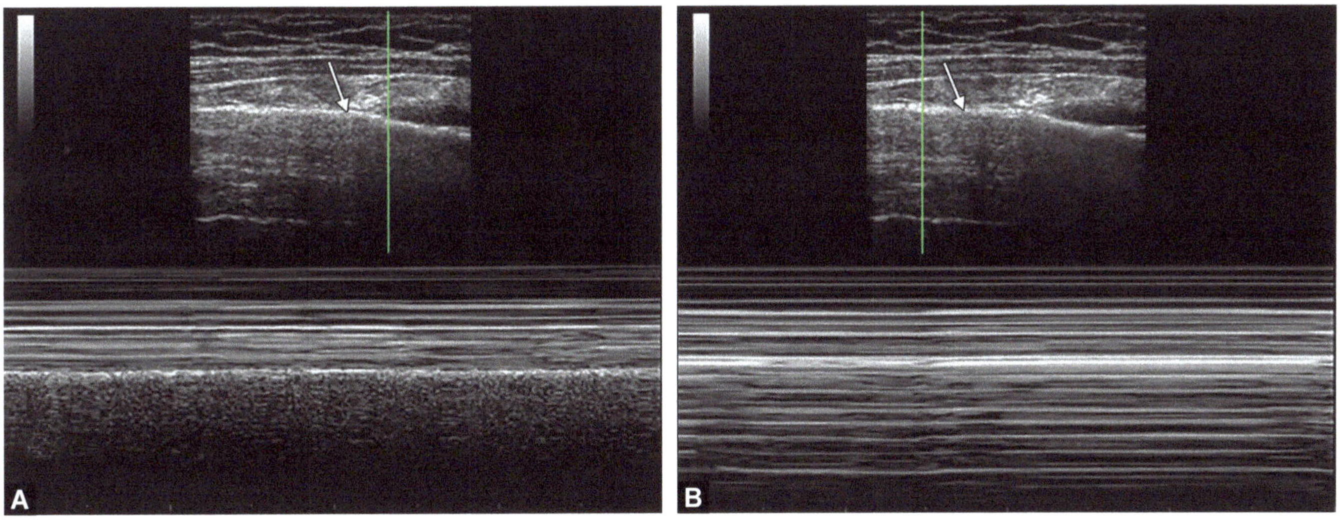

Figs. 23.10A and B: M-mode for the ultrasonographic diagnosis of pneumothorax (PTX). (A) Healthy lung with fine echogenicity below the pleural line (*seashore sign*). (B) Pneumothorax: the normal grainy image in the far field is replaced by lines like those above the pleural line, creating an image of only horizontal lines, referred to as the *barcode sign*. The white arrow indicates the lung point.

frequency range typically provides increased details of the pleural interface. This is crucial in case of "radio-occult" PTX for which chest ultrasound has sensitivity similar to CT. Finally, the use of chest ultrasound to rule out PTX is of paramount importance in critical situations like cardiac arrest and unstable patients requiring ventilatory support.

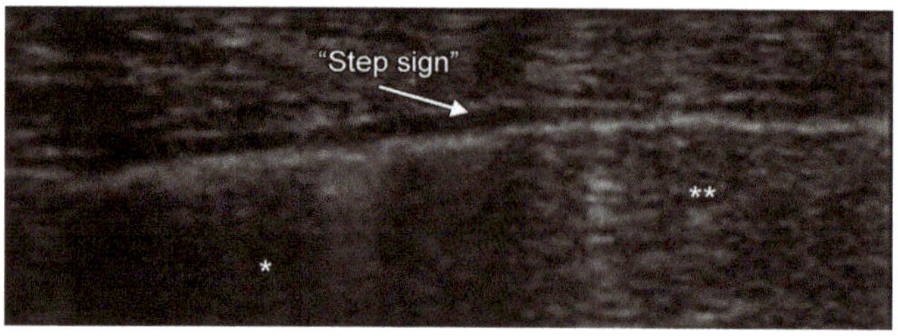

Fig. 23.11: Step sign in case of pneumothorax: the minimum difference in level of the pleural line at the zone of the lung point for which the true pleural line appears slightly deeper.
*Artifacts of pleural-parenchymal field,
**Pneumothorax (PTX).

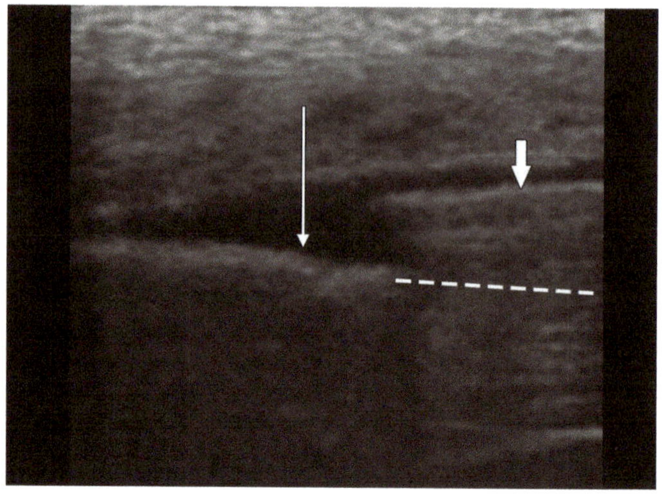

Fig. 23.12: Curtain sign in case of hydropneumothorax: the large arrows indicate the air, the small arrows indicate the plane effusion, while the dashed line indicates the position of the pleural line behind artifacts from air.

STUDY OF DIAPHRAGMATIC KINETICS

Different approaches can be used to study the movement of diaphragm. Some authors describe the visualization of diaphragmatic movement with a transhepatic approach using M-mode, by directing the ultrasound beam perpendicular to the diaphragmatic dome. With this approach, the diaphragm appears as a thick hyperechoic line, representing the interface between abdominal organ and ventilated lung. Using M-mode, the operator can visualize the movement of structures positioned along a line in the ultrasound beam. The diaphragmatic interface will appear in M-mode as an echogenic line with a sinusoidal form. During inspiration, the diaphragm descends, moving closer to the probe; during expiration, it rises, moving away from the probe, and thus the image generated shows a bright line which descends with expiration and rises with inspiration. In this way, it is possible to measure both resting diaphragmatic excursion during spontaneous breathing and maximal diaphragmatic excursion during forced inspiratory and expiratory maneuvers (Figs. 23.14A to D).

Mean diaphragmatic excursion ranges from 42 ± 16 to 79 ± 13 mm during forced maneuver and from 11 ± 4 to 21 ± 6 mm during spontaneous breathing. It is also possible to measure muscle thickness with linear probe in a longitudinal position at the level of the 8th–9th intercostal space on the midaxillary line, i.e. the so-called zones of apposition where the diaphragm is apposed to the rib cage.

EVALUATION OF PULMONARY DISEASE

Pulmonary parenchymal patterns detectable with chest ultrasound include preconsolidating states and lung consolidations. The first are known as *sonographic interstitial syndromes* and range from multiple vertical artifacts — multiple B Lines — to a full coalescence of those lines to form what is known as a *white lung*. This is seen when multiple B Lines are so close together that they become indistinguishable from one another and have the appearance of a white curtain. When infection or inflammation fills the alveoli, the lung behaves more like a solid organ than an airy one, and *consolidation* can be seen (Figs. 23.13A to D).

From a pathophysiological point of view, it is useful to consider four mechanisms of alteration of the normal artifacts generated at pleural line:

- Single or multiple interlobular and/or intralobular septal thickening
- Increase of lung parenchymal water content
- Increase of "tissue" content of the lung parenchyma
- Diminution of ventilation and porosity.

All of these mechanisms can generate B Lines, and though the genesis of B Lines is not yet fully understood, the study of these vertical artifacts is crucial to identify different pathological conditions.

Sonographic interstitial syndromes can be classified as: focal or diffuse. Focal sonographic interstitial syndrome can be identified in focal interstitial pneumonias, areas of pulmonary infarction or contusion, or areas of impaired ventilation. Diffuse interstitial syndromes, characterized by multiple, diffuse and bilateral B Lines, can be due to pulmonary edema of various causes, interstitial pneumonia or pneumonitis and diffuse parenchymal lung disease (pulmonary fibrosis). These etiologies are not mutually exclusive, and as such B lines can be present in any one of these conditions, or a combination thereof.

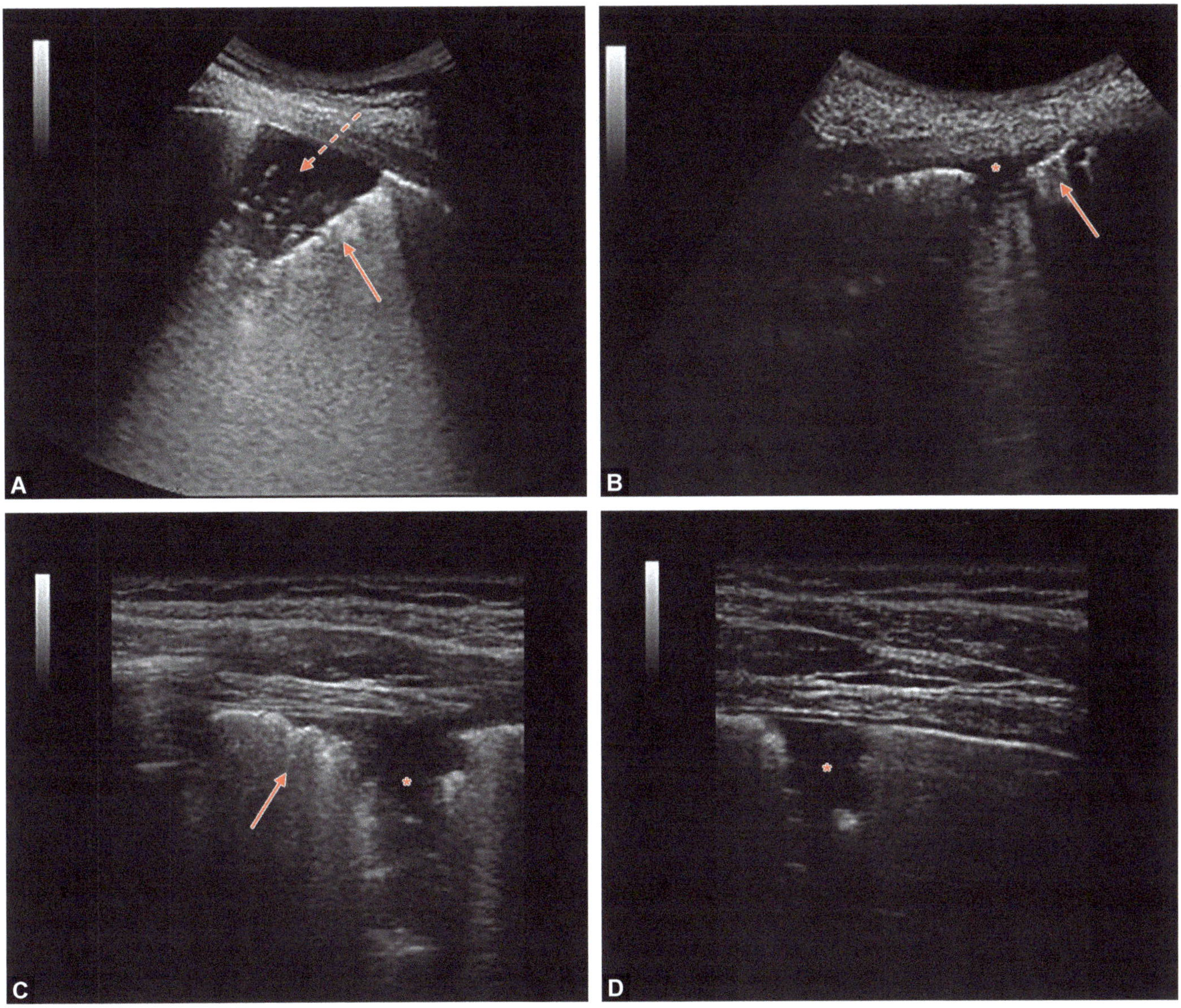

Figs. 23.13A to D: Lung consolidations. Four examples of lung consolidations evaluated by convex probe (top) and linear probe (bottom). It is evident the characteristic aspect of a region with tissue like echotexture in image A (red dotted arrow) and three sub pleural echo-poor regions in images B, C and D (red stars) with perilesional focal interstitial syndrome (red arrows).

The operator should also consider the appearance of the pleural line: smooth, thin, and regular versus thickened, coarse, and irregular. Thus considering both the B Line and pleural characteristics, it is possible to distinguish two principal diffuse patterns: (1) diffuse homogeneous sonographic interstitial syndrome, with a smooth, thin, regular pleural line, and (2) diffuse heterogeneous sonographic interstitial syndrome, with a thickened, coarse, irregular pleural line.

Additionally, the operator should pay attention to the gradient of concentration of B Lines in the cranial-caudal or ventral-dorsal sense, in sitting and supine position, respectively. The identification of diffuse bilateral homogeneous sonographic interstitial syndrome, with a smooth, thin and regular pleural line involving mostly the caudal and dorsal regions, that is gravitationally dependent, is highly suggestive of cardiogenic pulmonary edema in the right clinical setting (Figs. 23.15A and B). On the other hand, if the operator finds a diffuse heterogeneous sonographic interstitial syndrome, with a thickened, coarse and irregular pleural line, without a clear cranial-caudal or ventral-dorsal gradient, the diagnosis of noncardiogenic

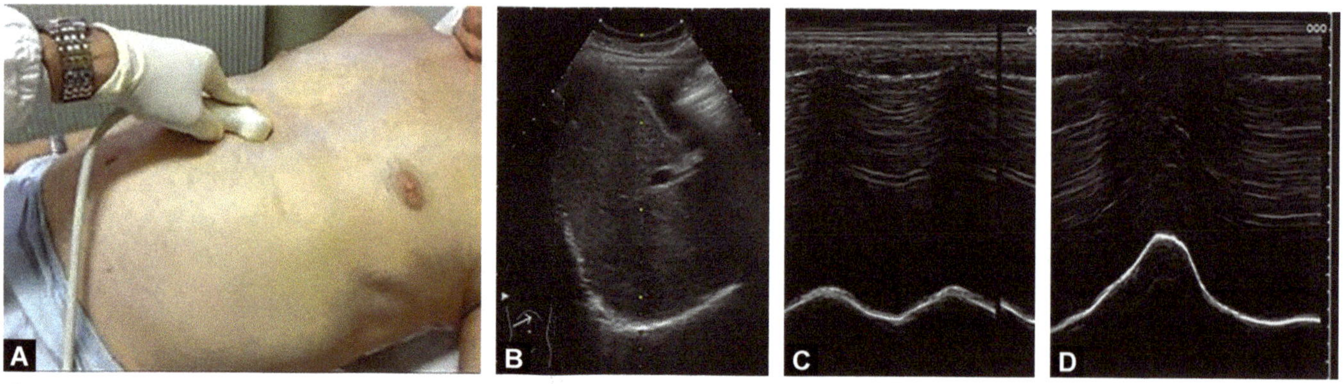

Figs. 23.14A to D: (A) Trans hepatic scan using convex probe. (B) B-mode visualization of diaphragmatic dome (the diaphragm appears as a thick hyperechoic line, i.e. the interface between liver and right lung). (C) M-mode visualization of the ultrasound beam perpendicular to the diaphragmatic dome. During spontaneous breathing, diaphragmatic excursions create a sinusoidal form in time. (D) During forced inspiration, the diaphragm descends, moving closer to the probe.

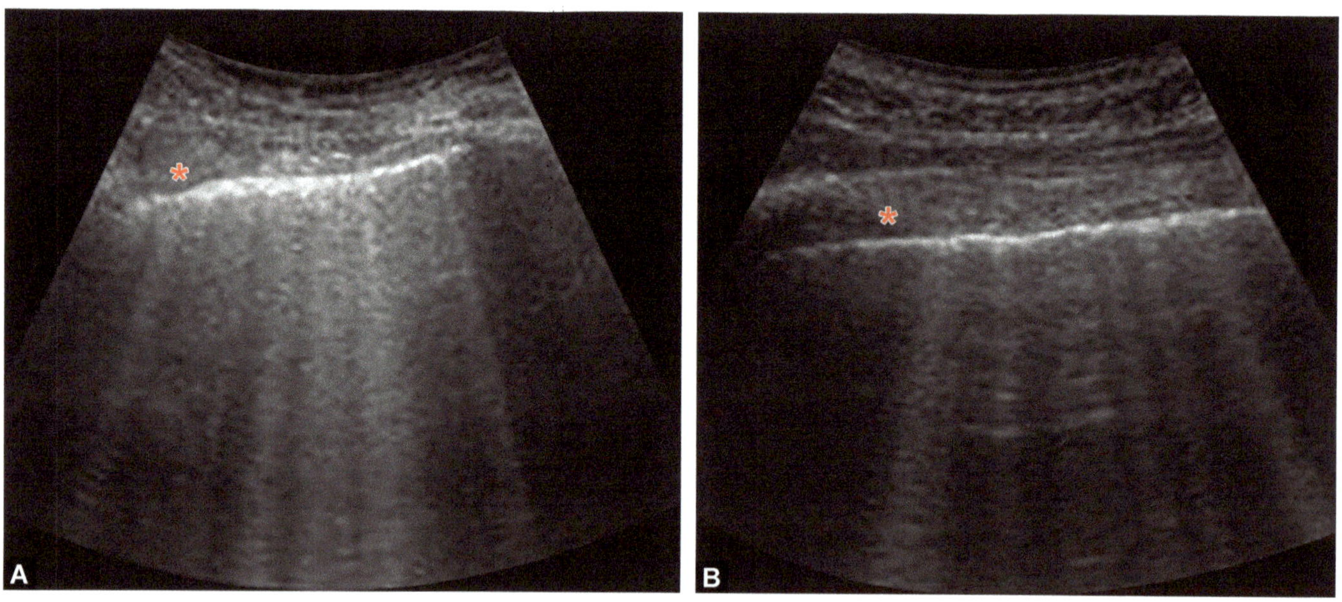

Figs. 23.15A and B: Acute cardiogenic pulmonary oedema. (A) Diffuse bilateral homogeneous sonographic interstitial syndrome with multiple B Lines and smooth, thin and regular pleural line (star) (transverse scan with convex probe on posterior axillary line in sitting position). (B) The reduction of "density" of B Lines in the same patient in sitting position with transverse scan of lung apices with convex probe.

pulmonary edema is highly likely, especially if there are also multiple subpleural consolidations and/or areas of normal clear lung (Figs. 23.16A to C).

In critical settings, differentiating between acute cardiogenic pulmonary edema and ARDS is difficult. Ultrasound can be a useful tool in this setting. Both syndromes are characterized by bilateral B Lines, however, the distribution and the density of B Lines and the appearance of the pleural line are different. In ARDS, the pulmonary heterogeneous impairment of alveolar capillary membrane and the consequent heterogeneous alveolar flooding result in a range of ultrasonographic findings consistent with multiple bilateral B Lines with a heterogeneous distribution pattern, subpleural consolidations and areas of "sparing" with normal parenchyma. Moreover, patients with ARDS will usually have pleural line abnormalities such as reduced lung sliding, irregular/fragmented pleura and subpleural consolidations.

Patients with acute cardiogenic pulmonary edema will typically have ultrasound findings of bilateral, diffuse and homogeneous B Lines, ranging from multiple B Lines to bilateral *white lung*, without areas of "sparing", typically

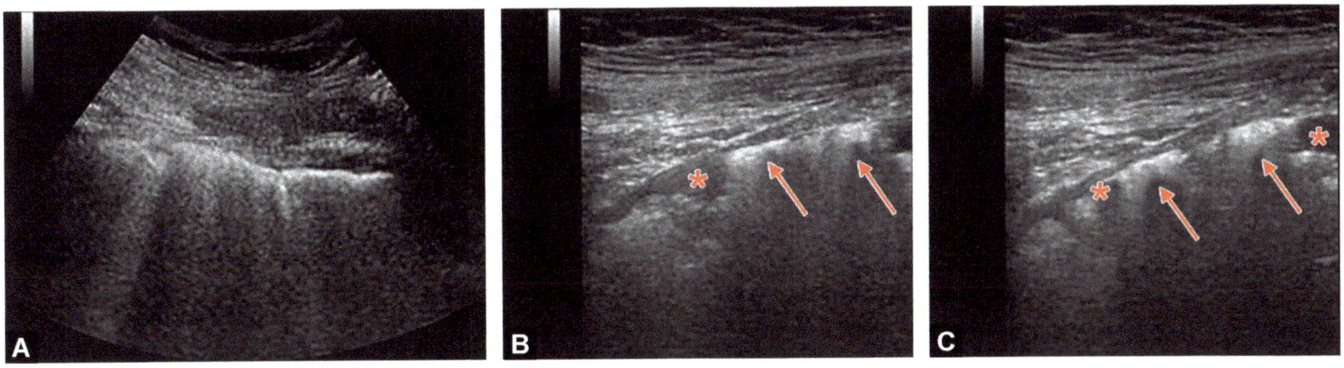

Figs. 23.16A to C: Acute noncardiogenic pulmonary oedema. (A) Diffuse bilateral dishomogeneous sonographic interstitial syndrome (transverse scan with convex probe on mid-axillary line in supine position). (B and C) The same area scanned with linear probe to better appreciate the signs of interstitial syndrome (red arrows) with thickened, coarse and irregular pleural line and sub pleural micro consolidations (stars).

decreasing in number as one scans from gravitationally dependent to less dependent areas. Also, there are often associated pleural effusions. The development of B Lines is a dynamic process and can be observed in real time. When properly integrated with physical examination it can lead to the earlier identification of pulmonary edema as well as help to directly monitor the effects resulting from treatment.

Lung ultrasound is also a useful diagnostic tool in the setting of diffuse parenchymal lung disease (DPLD). Reissig A and Kroegel C studied the pleural and parenchymal ultrasonographic alterations in patients with DPLD and they found a characteristic pattern of diffuse interstitial syndrome with multiple vertical artifacts associated with an irregular and fragmented pleural line. Typically, the abnormalities were detected in both lungs, more frequently visible in the lower segments, reflecting the diffuse fibrosing process and corresponding well to typical findings seen on high-resolution computed tomography (HRCT) scan. Delle Sedie A et al. evaluated the use of the linear probe for the study of vertical artifacts (B Lines) in systemic sclerosis and found a good correlation with HRCT findings. Again, in addition to its utility in the diagnosis of diffuse parenchymal lung disease, chest ultrasound can be very useful in monitoring and evaluating treatment response, allowing for a reduction in radiation exposure of recurrent radiography and CT scans.

Lung consolidation, when imaged by ultrasound is seen as a subpleural echo-rich region, one with tissue-like echotexture. Different pathologies can generate lung consolidations: pulmonary infection, pulmonary embolism, lung cancer and metastasis, compression atelectasis, obstructive atelectasis and lung contusion. Independent from the etiology, the consolidation of the lung is characterized by a loss of alveolar air and an increase in fluid content. This is responsible for the disappearance of the "normal" artifactual A-Lines below the pleural line and the genesis of a discernable image of the lung resulting from a given pathologic process. The consolidated region is visualized as a tissue-like image depending on the various degrees of air loss and fluid accumulation.

In the case of pneumonia, the echo texture of the consolidated lung is similar to that of the liver and hence is referred to as *lung hepatization*. In this setting, it is also possible to find a dynamic tree-shaped *air bronchogram* and irregular and serrated margins of the consolidated lung. The *air bronchogram* sign sonographically appears as hyperechoic foci and spots within linear structures within the consolidated lung. If the bright foci move with respirations, they are considered to be *dynamic air bronchograms*, and if not then they are *static air bronchograms*. In cases of post-obstructive pneumonia, where bronchi may be filled with fluid rather than air, it is possible to find the *fluid bronchogram* sign, so called for the presence of tubular structures with hypo- or anechoic content. These lack any Doppler flow and hence are distinguishable from blood vessels.

Other variations of consolidation can be seen in patients with pulmonary embolism, where one can occasionally view small pleural-based echo-poor consolidations with wedge-shaped margins and without central vascularization. Also, peripheral lung carcinomas and metastases can appear as hypoechoic or moderately echogenic heterogeneous structures on ultrasound. Their shape is quite variable: rounded, oval, or polycystic. Compression atelectasis is caused by large pleural effusion, and

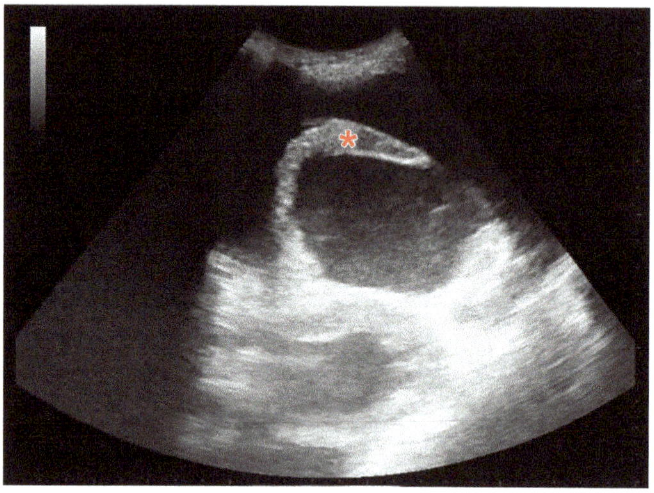

Fig. 23.17: Compression atelectasis caused by large pleural effusion. The involved pulmonary parenchyma (star) floats in the effusion like "a waving hand".

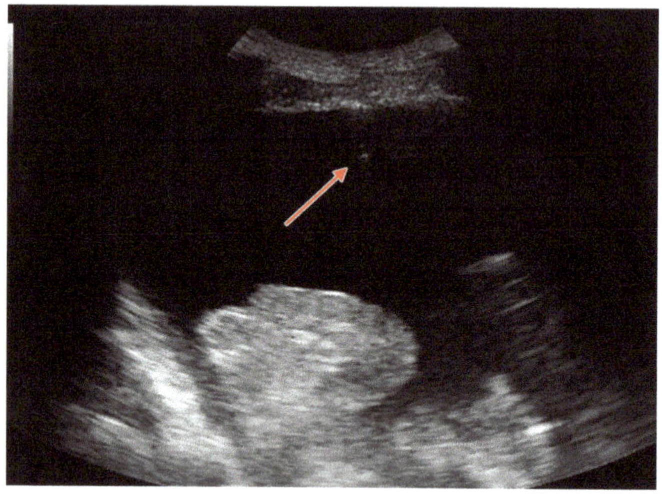

Fig. 23.18: Ultrasound-guided thoracentesis with a 15-gauge Veres needle (arrow).

in this situation, the involved pulmonary parenchyma has a triangular shape and floats in the effusion like *a waving hand* (Fig. 23.17). Using color Doppler, compression atelectasis shows increased branch-like vessel visualization, in distinction to the typical liver pattern. The definitive confirmation of compressive atelectasis is its resolution after thoracentesis. In contrast, obstructive atelectasis may generate an image of *hepatization* of the lung similar to that of pneumonia but with significantly fewer air bronchograms. The distinctive feature of obstructive atelectasis is the fluid bronchogram sign previously described. It is sometimes also possible to see a *lung pulse* as described above. Differentiating compressive and obstructive atelectasis is important because the latter is a clear indication for bronchoscopy. Finally, in cases of blunt chest trauma, the area of pulmonary contusion is usually visualized as hypoechoic, plate-like or complex consolidation with adjacent focal interstitial syndrome.

It is crucial to understand that one of the major limitations of chest ultrasonography for the detection of lung consolidations is that the consolidations must reach the lung surface to be visualized. Fortunately, this is frequently the case. That being said, the ultrasound can be a highly useful tool for the pulmonologist to rapidly and easily distinguish various types of lung consolidations in mechanically ventilated patients. Moreover, the use of lung ultrasound significantly reduces the number of chest radiographs and CT scans and limits the need for transportation of patients out of the monitored and controlled critical care setting of an intensive care unit.

ULTRASOUND-GUIDED INTERVENTIONAL PROCEDURES

Ultrasound can be used as a guide for interventional procedures, particularly for thoracentesis and chest tube insertion. The details of these invasive diagnostic procedures are covered in detail elsewhere in the book.

One of the main advantages of the use of lung ultrasound for performing thoracentesis and/or insertion of chest drainage tubes is the identification of the best site for the procedure, taking into account the need for sufficient depth of pleural fluid and the absence of adjacent lung parenchyma. The assessment should be carried out, in all phases of the respiratory cycle as diaphragmatic movement may change the position of the fluid and its relationship to nearby structures (Fig. 23.18). The use of lung ultrasound as a guide for procedural interventions is particularly useful in critical care conditions, as in patients on mechanical ventilation. The main advantage of lung ultrasound-guided thoracentesis is the reduction of rate of PTX. Moreover, in case of "difficult-to-manage" multiloculated pleural effusion, the ultrasonographic approach allows drainage of the more voluminous loculation and determination of the ideal needle position, thereby optimizing likelihood of success.

BIBLIOGRAPHY AND FURTHER READING

1. Agricola E, Bove T, Opizzi M, Marino G, Zangrillo A, Margonato A, et al. "Ultrasound comet tail images": a marker of pulmonary edema: a comparative study with

wedge pressure and extravascular lung water. Chest. 2005;127:1690-5.

2. Akhan O, Ozkan O, Akinci D, Hassan A, Ozmen M. Image-guided catheter drainage of infected pleural effusions. Diagn Interv Radiol. 2007;13(4):204-9.
3. Ayoub J, Metge L, Dauzat M, Lemerre C, Pourcelot L, Prefaut C, et al. Diaphragm kinetics coupled with spirometry: Mmode ultrasonographic and fluoroscopic study; preliminary results. J Radiol. 1997;78:563-8.
4. Baldi G, Gargani L, Abramo A, D'Errico L, Caramella D, Picano E, et al. Lung water assessment by lung ultrasonography in intensive care: a pilot study. Intensive Care Med. 2013;39(1):74-84.
5. Balik M, Plasil P, Waldauf P, Pazout J, Fric M, Otahal M, et al. Ultrasound estimation of volume of pleural fluid in mechanically ventilated patients. Intensive Care Med. 2006;32(2):318-21.
6. Ball CG, Kirkpatrick AW, Feliciano DV. The occult pneumothorax: what have we learned? Can J Surg. 2009;-52:E173-9.
7. Ball CG, Kirkpatrick AW, Laupland KB, Fox DL, Litvinchuk S, Dyer DM, et al. Factors related to the failure of radiographic recognition of occult posttraumatic pneumothoraces. Am J Surg. 2005;189:541-6.
8. Beckh S, Bolcskei PL, Lessnau KD. Real-time chest ultrasonography: a comprehensive review for the pulmonologist. Chest. 2002;122:1759-73.
9. Blaivas M, Lyon M, Duggal S. A prospective comparison of supine chest radiography and bedside ultrasound for the diagnosis of traumatic pneumothorax. Acad Emerg Med. 2005;12:844-9.
10. Bolliger CT, Mathur PN, Beamis JF, Becker HD, Cavaliere S, Colt H, et al. ERS/ATS statement on interventional pulmonology. European Respiratory Society/American Thoracic Society. Eur Respir J. 2002;19(2):356-73.
11. Bouhemad B, Brisson H, Le-Guen M, Arbelot C, Lu Q, Rouby JJ. Bedside ultrasound assessment of positive end-expiratory pressure-induced lung recruitment. Am J Respir Crit Care Med. 2011;183:341-7.
12. Boussuges A, Gole Y, Blanc P. Diaphragmatic motion studied by M-mode ultrasonography: Methods, reproducibility, and normal values. Chest. 2009;135:391-400.
13. Breitkreutz R, Price S, Steiger HV, Seeger FH, Ilper H, Ackermann H, et al. Focused echocardiographic evaluation in life support and peri-resuscitation of emergency patients: a prospective trial. Resuscitation. 2010;81:1527-33.
14. Chen HJ, Tu CY, Ling SJ, Chen W, Chiu KL, Hsia TC, et al. Sonographic appearances in transudative pleural effusions: not always an anechoic pattern. Ultrasound Med Biol. 2008;34(3):362-9.
15. Chian CF, Su WL, Soh LH, Yan HC, Perng WC, Wu CP. Echogenic swirling pattern as a predictor of malignant pleural effusions in patients with malignancies. Chest. 2004;126(1):129-34.
16. Cohen E, Mier A, Heywood P, Murphy K, Boultbee J, Guz A. Excursion-volume relation of the right hemidiaphragm measured by ultrasonography and respiratory airflow measurements. Thorax. 1994;49:885-9.
17. Copetti R, Soldati G, Copetti P. Chest sonography: a useful tool to differentiate acute cardiogenic pulmonary edema from acute respiratory distress syndrome. Cardiovasc Ultrasound. 2008;29;6:16.
18. Delle Sedie A, Doveri M, Frassi F, Gargani L, D'Errico G, Pepe P, et al. Ultrasound lung comets in systemic sclerosis: a useful tool to detect lung interstitial fibrosis. Clin Exp Rheumatol. 2010;28:S54.
19. Eibenberger KL, Dock WI, Ammann ME, Dorffner R, Hörmann MF, et al. Quantification of pleural effusions: sonography versus radiography. Radiology. 1994;191:681-4.
20. Epelman M, Navarro OM, Daneman A, Miller SF. M-mode sonography of diaphragmatic motion: Description of technique and experience in 278 pediatric patients. Pediatr Radiol. 2005;35:661-7.
21. Gargani L, Doveri M, D'Errico L, Frassi F, Bazzichi ML, Delle Sedie A, et al. Ultrasound lung comets in systemic sclerosis: a chest sonography hallmark of pulmonary interstitial fibrosis. Rheumatology (Oxford). 2009;48:1382-7.
22. Gehmacher O, Mathis G, Kopf A, Scheier M. Ultrasound imaging of pneumonia. Ultrasound Med Biol. 1995;21:-1119-22.
23. Gerscovich EO, Cronan M, McGahan JP, Jain K, Jones CD, McDonald C. Ultrasonographic evaluation of diaphragmatic motion. J Ultrasound Med. 2001;20:597-604.
24. Gillman LM, Alkadi A, Kirkpatrick AW. The "pseudo-lung point" sign: all focal respiratory coupled alternating pleural patterns are not diagnostic of a pneumothorax. J Trauma. 2009;67:672-3.
25. Gordon CE, Feller-Kopman D, Balk EM, Smetana GW. Pneumothorax following thoracentesis: a systematic review and meta-analysis. Arch Intern Med. 2010;170(4):332-9.
26. Haber K, Asher M, Freimanis AK. Ultrasonographic evaluation of diaphragmatic motion in intra-abdominal diseases. Radiology. 1975;114:141-4.
27. Hamilton DR, Sargsyan AE, Kirkpatrick AW, Nicolaou S, Campbell M, Dawson DL, Melton SL, et al. Sonographic detection of pneumothorax and hemothorax in microgravity. Aviat Space Environ Med. 2004;75:272-7.
28. Harris RS, Giovannetti M, Kim BK. Normal ventilatory movement of the right hemidiaphragm studied by ultrasonography and pneumotachography. Radiology. 1983;146:141-4.
29. Houston JG, Angus RM, Cowan MD, McMillan NC, Thomson NC. Ultrasound assessment of normal hemidiaphragmatic movement: Relation to inspiratory volume. Thorax. 1994;49:500-3.
30. Islam S, Tonn H. Thoracic Ultrasound Overview. In: Bolliger CT, Herth FJF, Mayo PH, Miyazawa T, Beamis JF (Eds). Clinical Chest Ultrasound: From the ICU to the Bronchoscopy Suite. Prog in Respir Res. Switzerland: Karger; 2009; vol 37, pp 11-20.
31. Jiang JRm Tsai TH, Jerng JS, Yu CJ, Wu HD, Yang PC. Ultrasonographic evaluation of liver/spleen movements and estubation outcome. Chest. 2004;126:179-85.

32. Kantarci F, Mihmanli I, Demirel MK, Harmanci K, Akman C, Aydogan F, et al. Normal diaphragmatic motion and the effects of body composition: Determination with M-mode sonography. J Ultrasound Med. 2004;23:255-60.
33. Kirkpatrick AW, Sirois M, Laupland KB, Liu D, Rowan K, Ball CG, et al. Hand-held thoracic sonography for detecting post-traumatic pneumothoraces: the Extended Focused Assessment with Sonography for Trauma (EFAST). J Trauma. 2004;57:288-95.
34. Kocijancic I, Kocijancic K, Cufer T. Imaging of pleural fluid in healthy individuals Clin Radiol. 2004;59:826-9.
35. Koegelenberg CF, Diacon AH, Bolliger CT. Transthoracic Ultrasound for Chest Wall, Pleura, and the Peripheral Lung. In: Bolliger CT, Herth FJF, Mayo PH, Miyazawa T, Beamis JF (Eds). Clinical Chest Ultrasound: From the ICU to the Bronchoscopy Suite. Prog in Respir Res. Switzerland: Karger; 2009; vol 37, pp. 22-33.
36. Koegelenberg CF, von Groote-Bidlingmaier F, Bolliger CT. Transthoracic ultrasonography for the respiratory physician. Respiration. 2012;84(4):337-50.
37. Koenig SJ, Narasimhan M, Mayo PH. Thoracic ultrasonography for the pulmonary specialist. Chest. 2011;-140(5):1332-41.
38. Lichtenstein D, Lascols N, Mezière G, Gepner A. Ultrasound diagnosis of alveolar consolidation in the critically ill. Intensive Care Med. 2004;30:276-81.
39. Lichtenstein D, Meziere G, Seitz J. The dynamic air bronchogram. A lung ultrasound sign of alveolar consolidation ruling out atelectasis. Chest. 2009;135:1421-5.
40. Lichtenstein DA, Lascols N, Meziere G, Gepner A. Ultrasound diagnosis of alveolar consolidation in the critically ill. Intensive Care Med. 2004;30:276-81.
41. Lichtenstein DA, Lascols N, Prin S, Meziere G. The "lung pulse": an early ultrasound sign of complete atelectasis. Intensive Care Med. 2003;29:2187-92.
42. Lichtenstein DA, Lascols N, Prin S, Mezière G. The "lung pulse": an early ultrasound sign of complete atelectasis. Intensive Care Med. 2003;29(12):2187-92.
43. Lichtenstein DA, Menu Y. A bedside ultrasound sign ruling out pneumothorax in the critically ill. Lung sliding. Chest. 1995;108(5):1345-8.
44. Lichtenstein DA, Meziere G, Biderman P, Gepner A. The "lung point": an ultrasound sign specific to pneumothorax. Intensive Care Med. 2000;26:1434-40.
45. Lichtenstein DA, Meziere G, Lascols N, Biderman P, Courret JP, Gepner A, et al. Ultrasound diagnosis of occult pneumothorax. Crit Care Med. 2005;33(6):1231-8.
46. Lichtenstein DA, Meziere G, Lascols N, Biderman P, Courret JP, Gepner A, Goldstein I, et al. Ultrasound diagnosis of occult pneumothorax. Crit Care Med. 2005;33:1231-8.
47. Lichtenstein DA, Meziere GA. Relevance of lung ultrasound in the diagnosis of acute respiratory failure: the BLUE protocol. Chest. 2008;134:117-25.
48. Lichtenstein DA. Lung ultrasound in the critically ill. Ann Intensive Care. 2014;4(1):1.
49. Lichtenstein DA. Whole Body Ultrasonography in the Critically Ill. Berlin, Germany; Springer; 2010. pp. 117-208.
50. Lomas DJ, Padley SG, Flower CD. The sonographic appearances of pleural fluid. Br J Radiol. 1993;66(787):619-24.
51. Lowe SA. Diagnostic radiography in pregnancy: risks and reality. Aust N Z J Obstet Gynaecol. 2004;44(3):191-6.
52. Maslove DM, Chen BT, Wang H, Kuschner WG. The diagnosis and management of pleural effusions in the ICU. J Intensive Care Med. 2013;28(1):24-36.
53. Mathis G, Blank W, Reissig A, Lechleitner P, Reuss J, Schuler A, et al. Thoracic ultrasound for diagnosing pulmonary embolism: a prospective multicenter study of 352 patients. Chest. 2005;128:1531-8.
54. Mathis G, Dirschmid K. Pulmonary infarction: sonographic appearance with pathologic correlation. Eur J Radiol. 1993;17:170-4.
55. Mathis G, Metzler J, Fussenegger D, Sutterlutti G, Feurstein M, Fritzsche H. Sonographic observation of pulmonary infarction and early infarctions by pulmonary embolism. Eur Heart J. 1993;14:804-8.
56. Mathis G. Thorax sonography – Part II: Peripheral pulmonary consolidation. Ultrasound Med Biol. 1997;23:1141-53.
57. Miglioranza MH, Gargani L, Sant'Anna RT, Rover MM, Martins VM, Mantovani A, et al. Lung ultrasound for the evaluation of pulmonary congestion in outpatients: a comparison with clinical assessment, natriuretic peptides, and echocardiography. JACC Cardiovasc Imaging. 2013; 6(11):1141-51.
58. Parlamento S, Copetti R, Di Bartolomeo S. Evaluation of lung ultrasound for the diagnosis of pneumonia in the ED. Am J Emerg Med. 2009;27:379-84.
59. Peris A, Tutino L, Zagli G, Batacchi S, Cianchi G, Spina R, et al. The use of point-of-care bedside lung ultrasound significantly reduces the number of radiographs and computed tomography scans in critically ill patients. Anesth Analg. 2010;111:687-92.
60. Rantanen NW. Disease of the thorax. Vet Clin North Am Equine Pract. 1986;2:49-66.
61. Reissig A, Copetti R, Mathis G, Mempel C, Schuler A, Zechner P, et al. Lung ultrasound in the diagnosis and follow-up of community-acquired pneumonia: a prospective, multicenter, diagnostic accuracy study. Chest. 2012;142(4):965-72.
62. Reissig A, Görg C, Mathis G. Transthoracic sonography in the diagnosis of pulmonary diseases: a systematic approach. Ultraschall Med. 2009;30(5):438-54.
63. Reissig A, Kroegel C. Accuracy of transthoracic sonography in excluding postinterventional pneumothorax and hydropneumothorax. Comparison to chest radiography. Eur J Radiol. 2005;53(3):463-70.
64. Reissig A, Kroegel C. Transthoracic sonography of diffuse parenchymal lung disease: the role of comet tail artifacts. J Ultrasound Med. 2003;22:173-80.
65. Reuter KL, Bogdan A. Physics of diagnostic ultrasound: creating the image. In: Bolliger CT, Herth FJF, Mayo PH, Miyazawa T, Beamis JF (Eds). Clinical Chest Ultrasound: From the ICU to the Bronchoscopy Suite. Prog in Respir Res. Switzerland: Karger; 2009; vol 37, pp. 2-10.

66. Roch A, Bojan M, Michelet P, Romain F, Bregeon F, Papazian L, et al. Usefulness of ultrasonography in predicting pleural effusions >500ml in patients receiving mechanical ventilation. Chest. 2005;127: 224-32.
67. Rowan KR, Kirkpatrick AW, Liu D, Forkheim KE, Mayo JR, Nicolaou S. Traumatic pneumothorax detection with thoracic US: correlation with chest radiography and CT - initial experience. Radiology. 2002;225:210-4.
68. Sargsyan AE, Hamilton DR, Nicolaou S, Kirkpatrick AW, Campbell MR, Billica RD, et al. Ultrasound evaluation of the magnitude of pneumothorax: a new concept. Am Surg. 2001;67:232-5; discussion 235-6.
69. Sartori S, Tombesi P. Emerging roles for transthoracic ultrasonography in pulmonary diseases. World J Radiol. 2010;2(6):203-14.
70. Scott S, Fuld JP, Carter R, McEntegart M, MacFarlane NG. Diaphragm ultrasonography as an alternative to whole-body plethysmography in pulmonary function testing. J Ultrasound Med. 2006;25:225-32.
71. Smargiassi A, Inchingolo R, Soldati G, Copetti R, Marchetti G, Zanforlin A, et al. The role of chest ultrasonography in the management of respiratory diseases: document II. Multidiscip Respir Med. 2013;8(1):55.
72. Smargiassi A, Inchingolo R, Zanforlin A, Valente S, Soldati G, Corbo GM. Description of free-flowing pleural effusions in medical reports after echographic assessment. Respiration. 2013;85(5):439-41.
73. Soldati G, Inchingolo R, Smargiassi A, Sher S, Nenna R, Inchingolo CD, et al. Ex vivo lung sonography: morphologic-ultrasound relationship. Ultrasound Med Biol. 2012;-38(7):1169-79.
74. Soldati G, Sher S, Copetti R. If you see the contusion, there is no pneumothorax. Am J Emerg Med. 2010;28(1):106-7.
75. Soldati G, Smargiassi A, Inchingolo R, Sher S, Valente S, Corbo GM. Ultrasound-guided pleural puncture in supine or recumbent lateral position - feasibility study. Multidiscip Respir Med. 2013;8(1):18.
76. Soldati G, Testa A, Sher S, Pignataro G, La Sala M, Silveri NG. Occult traumatic pneumothorax: diagnostic accuracy of lung ultrasonography in the emergency department. Chest. 2008;133(1):204-11.
77. Soldati G, Testa A, Silva FR, Carbone L, Portale G, Silveri NG. Chest ultrasonography in lung contusion. Chest. 2006;130(2):533-8.
78. Sperandeo M, Filabozzi P, Varriale A, Carnevale V, Piattelli ML, Sperandeo G, et al. Role of thoracic ultrasound in the assessment of pleural and pulmonary diseases. J Ultrasound. 2008;11:39-46.
79. Targhetta R, Chavagneux R, Ayoub J, Lemerre C, Prefaut C, Bourgeois JM, et al. Right diaphragmatic kinetics measured by TM-mode ultrasonography with concomitant spirometry in normal subjects and asthmatic patients: Preliminary results. Rev Med Interne. 1995;16:819-26.
80. Testa A, Soldati G, Giannuzzi R, Berardi S, Portale G, Gentiloni Silveri N. Ultrasound M-mode assessment of diaphragmatic kinetics by anterior transverse scanning in healthy subjects. Ultrasound Med Biol. 2011;37(1):44-52.
81. Testa A, Soldati G, Giannuzzi R, Berardi S, Portale G, Gentiloni Silveri N. Ultrasound M-mode assessment of diaphragmatic kinetics by anterior transverse scanning in healthy subjects. Ultrasound Med Biol. 2011;37:44-52.
82. Tomà P, Owens CM. Chest ultrasound in children: critical appraisal. Pediatr Radiol. 2013;43(11):1427-34.
83. Tu CY, Hsu WH, Hsia TC, Chen HJ, Tsai KD, Hung CW, et al. Pleural effusions in febrile medical ICU patients: chest ultrasound study. Chest. 2004;126(4):1274-80.
84. Vignon P, Chastagner C, Berkane V, Chardac E, François B, Normand S, et al. Quantitative assessment of pleural effusion in critically ill patients by means of ultrasonography. Crit Care Med. 2005;33:1757-63.
85. Vitturi N, Soattin M, Allemand E, Simoni F, Realdi G. Thoracic ultrasonography: A new method for the work-up of patients with dyspnea. J Ultrasound. 2011;14(3):147-51.
86. Vivier E, Mekontso Dessap A, Dimassi S, Vargas F, Lyazidi A, Thille AW, et al. Diaphragm ultrasonography to estimate the work of breathing during non-invasive ventilation. Intensive Care Med. 2012;38(5):796-803.
87. Volpicelli G, Caramello V, Cardinale L, Mussa A, Bar F, Frascisco MF. Bedside ultrasound of the lung for the monitoring of acute decompensated heart failure. Am J Emerg Med. 2008;26:585-91.
88. Volpicelli G, Elbarbary M, Blaivas M, Lichtenstein DA, Mathis G, Kirkpatrick AW, et al. International evidence-based recommendations for point-of-care lung ultrasound. Intensive Care Med. 2012;38(4):577-91.
89. Volpicelli G, Melniker LA, Cardinale L, Lamorte A, Frascisco MF. Lung ultrasound in diagnosing and monitoring pulmonary interstitial fluid. Radiol Med. 2013;118(2):196-205.
90. Volpicelli G, Mussa A, Garofalo G, Cardinale L, Casoli G, Perotto F, et al. Bedside lung ultrasound in the assessment of alveolar-interstitial syndrome. Am J Emerg Med. 2006;-24(6):689-96.
91. Volpicelli G, Silva F, Radeos M. Real-time lung ultrasound for the diagnosis of alveolar consolidation and interstitial syndrome in the emergency department. Eur J Emerg Med. 2010;17:63-72.
92. Volpicelli G. Sonographic diagnosis of pneumothorax. Intensive Care Med. 2011;37(2):224-32.
93. Volpicelli G. The double lung point. Am J Emerg Med. 2011;29(7):832-3.
94. Volpicelli G. Usefulness of emergency ultrasound in non-traumatic cardiac arrest. Am J Emerg Med. 2011;29:216-23.
95. Wustner A, Gehmacher O, Hammerle S, Schenkenbach C, Hafele H, Mathis G. Ultrasound diagnosis in blunt thoracic trauma. Ultraschall Med. 2005;26:285-90.
96. Zanforlin A, Giannuzzi R, Nardini S, Testa A, Soldati G, Copetti R, et al. The role of chest ultrasonography in the management of respiratory diseases: document I. Multidiscip Respir Med. 2013;8(1):54.
97. Zhang M, Liu ZH, Yang JX, Gan JX, Xu SW, You XD, et al. Rapid detection of pneumothorax by ultrasonography in patients with multiple trauma. Crit Care. 2006;10:R112.

Chapter 24

Single Photon Emission Computed Tomography in the Evaluation of Lung Diseases

Marika Bajc, Claudio Sorino

OVERVIEW OF VENTILATION/PERFUSION SPECT

Ventilation/perfusion single photon emission computed tomography (V/P SPECT) is the recommended scintigraphic technique for the diagnosis of *pulmonary embolism (PE)* and many other disorders that affect lung function. Moreover, according to *European Association of Nuclear Medicine* guidelines, it should be the preferred modality whenever possible for the diagnosis of PE because it has the highest sensitivity and accuracy and neither contraindications nor complications. It produces very few nondiagnostic reports, and radiation doses are very low. This is particularly important for women in the reproductive period and during pregnancy.

To take full advantage of the V/P SPECT potential, it is crucial to apply an optimal protocol for a single session imaging of both ventilation and perfusion using low nuclide activities.

Furthermore, full use should be made of display options, which are integrated in modern camera systems. Holistic interpretation is the most important strategy for V/P SPECT, giving a clear report with respect to PE, its extension as well as other diagnoses based on V/P patterns typical for various diseases. Interpretation is based upon all relevant clinical information about the patient and all V/P patterns. PE is diagnosed when there is more than one subsegment showing a V/P mismatch representing an anatomic lung unit.

The above mentioned advantages of V/P SPECT for studying PE imply that it may be the most suitable technique both for follow-up in patients with PE as well as for research regarding its treatment and pathophysiology.

Recent studies showed that for the ventilation *Technegas* particles show advantages of over radiolabeled liquid aerosols and are not restricted to the presence of obstructive lung disease. Radiolabeled macroaggregated human albumin is the imaging agent of choice for perfusion scintigraphy. An optimal combination of nuclide activities and acquisition times for ventilation and perfusion, collimators, and imaging matrix yields an adequate ventilation/perfusion (V/Q) SPECT study in approximately 20 minutes of imaging time. The recommended protocol based on the patient remaining in an unchanged position during the initial ventilation study and the perfusion study allows presentation of matching ventilation and perfusion slices in all projections as well as in rotating volume images based upon maximum intensity projections (MIPs).

Apart from PE, other pathologies should be identified and reported, such as broncho-obstructive disease, left heart failure (LHF), pneumonia and suspicion of other parenchymal process like tumors. Pitfalls exist both with respect to imaging technique and scan interpretation.

V/P SPECT AND PULMONARY EMBOLISM

Pulmonary embolism is a common disease with about 250,000 patients diagnosed each year in the American population. In spite of advanced technology, it remains a big diagnostic challenge because the clinical symptoms and signs which are frequently observed in PE, are also a feature of other conditions. Accordingly, the initial clinical suspicion needs to be confirmed or negated using a conclusive imaging test. Routinely multidetector computed tomography (MDCT) is suggested as the initial imaging study. However, the latest evidence shows that the optimal test is V/P SPECT interpreted with holistic principles according to European guideline. Before performing imaging tests, it is recommended to estimate the clinical probability for PE. Usually Wells score is applied. Although a more precise predictive model developed by Miniati et al. is recommended. Easy-to-use softwares are also available for computation (palm computer) (e.g. http://www.ifc.cnr.it/pisamodel).

The measurement of *D-dimer*—a breakdown product of cross-linked fibrin clot—is widely used in the investigative workup of patients with suspected venous thromboembolism. However, D-dimer has a low specificity (about 40%) because a number of conditions, other than venous thromboembolism, may cause its increase, e.g. acute myocardial infarction, stroke, inflammation, active cancer, and pregnancy. The specificity declines even further with age and, in the elderly, may reach only 10%. Due to the low predictive value, a positive quantitative D-dimer test does not modify the pretest probability. A negative quantitative D-dimer test combined with a low clinical probability is associated with a low risk of thromboembolic disease. At moderate to high pretest clinical probability, D-dimer has no incremental value.

BASIC PRINCIPLES OF PULMONARY EMBOLISM DIAGNOSIS WITH V/P SPECT

The lung circulation has a distinct architecture where each bronchopulmonary segment and subsegment is supplied by a single end-artery. Emboli are usually multiple, occluding the arteries causing segmental or subsegmental perfusion defects within still ventilated regions, causing the so-called mismatch (Fig. 24.1). PE is often a recurring process giving rise to multiple emboli in various stages of resolution (Fig. 24.2).

In clinical practice, it is essential to have a procedure that is both fast and conclusive to avoid the risks associated with untreated disease. Therefore, it is recommended that imaging tests for PE diagnosis should be carried out as soon as possible, preferably within 24 hours of the onset of symptoms.

IMAGING PROTOCOLS

V/P SPECT Acquisition

Administration of ventilation and perfusion agents should be performed with patients in the same position (usually supine) to be able to compare the studies. Different position of administration will cause different distribution of activity due to different gravitational gradients. During inhalation, activity over the lungs should be monitored to ensure adequacy of pulmonary deposition. The procedure starts with ventilation scintigraphy which is usually based upon inhalation of a radioaerosol (Table 24.1).

Large particles (> 2 μm) are deposited mainly by impaction in large airways. Very fine particles, less than

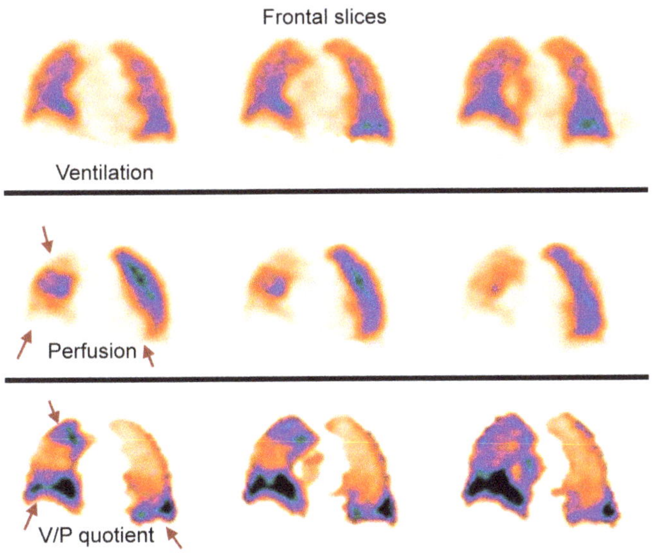

Fig. 24.1: Patient with pulmonary embolism (PE). Frontal slices; ventilation with corresponding perfusion images and quotient images. Multiple areas with absent perfusion (arrows) and preserved ventilation, clearly visible as mismatch on ventilation/perfusion quotient (V/P quotient) (arrows) images.

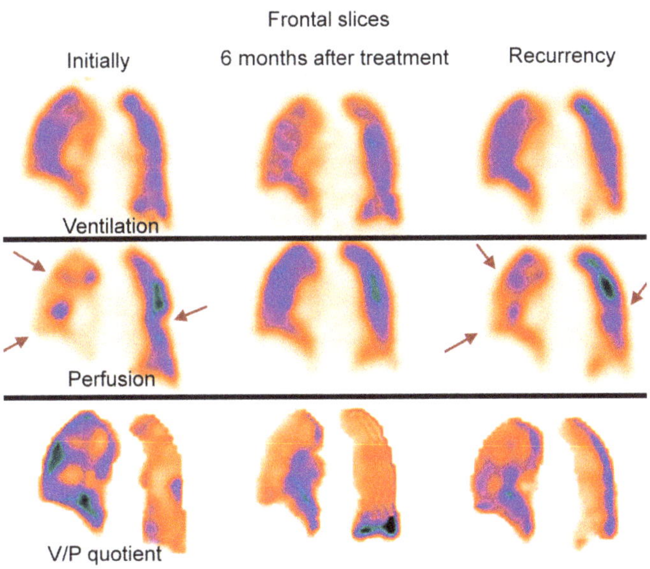

Fig. 24.2: Patient with PE; initially follow-up 6 months after treatment and recurrence. Frontal and ventilation with corresponding perfusion images and V/P quotient images. Areas with PE; absent perfusion (arrows) and preserved ventilation. (PE: Pulmonary embolism).

Table 24.1: Ventilation/perfusion protocol for lung tomography (V/P SPECT). Patient preparation is not needed. Patient is in the supine position during inhalation, intravenous (IV) injection and during the acquisition.

	Ventilation	*Perfusion*
Administration	Inhalation	IV injection
Radiopharmaceutical and administered activity	Technegas® 25–30 MBq to reach the lung	^{99m}Tc-MAA 120–160 MBq
Particle size	0.09 µm	15–100 µm
Time of imaging	about 11 minutes	about 5 minutes
Acquisition protocol	General purpose collimator: 64 × 64 matrix, 60–64 steps for each head, 10 s/step	General purpose collimator: 64 × 64 matrix, 60–64 steps for each head, 5 s/step
Reconstruction	Iterative reconstruction— 8 subsets and 4 iterations	Iterative reconstruction— 8 subsets and 4 iterations

1 µm, are mainly deposited in alveoli by diffusion. In comparison with liquid aerosols, *Technegas* showed significantly reduced problems of central airway deposition and peripheral hotspot formation in patients with obstructive lung disease. Therefore, the use of *Technegas* is recommended in chronic obstructive pulmonary disease (COPD).

Perfusion tomography follows immediately after ventilation SPECT without changing the patient position. The nearly universally used agent for perfusion scintigraphy is technetium labeled particles of macroaggregates of human albumin (^{99m}Tc-MAA). After intravenous (IV) injection, the particles of size 15–100 µm are lodged in the pulmonary capillaries and in the precapillary arterioles in proportion to perfusion.

To achieve adequate imaging quality, with low radiation exposure, in a short time, relationships between activities, acquisition times, collimators and matrices for SPECT imaging must be optimized. This problem was systematically analyzed by Palmer et al. in the context of a dual-head gamma camera. Doses of 25–30 megabecqueral (MBq) for ventilation studies and 120–160 MBq for perfusion studies were found optimal by using a general purpose collimator, and 64 × 64 matrix. A total acquisition time is about 20 minutes. If a matrix of 128 × 128 is used, than a higher doses and/or longer acquisition time is required. This is not promoted as it did not yield images of significantly higher quality.

Many centers are using much higher doses. To follow a good medical practice, radiation exposure should be minimized to the lowest level consistent with satisfactory image quality. For V/P SPECT, it is essential to use iterative reconstruction. Recommended is *ordered-subset expectation maximization (OSEM)* with 4 iterations and 8 subsets. Standard software can be used for image presentation in frontal, sagittal and transversal projections as well as for presentation of rotating three-dimensional (3D) images. Johan Palmer et al, have developed a way of calculating and displaying V/P quotient images. This is based upon acquisition as described above. Ventilation is normalized to perfusion counts, and then the V/P quotient images are calculated. V/P quotient images facilitate diagnosis and quantification of PE extension. Using this protocol, attenuation correction is not needed.

For quality control and fast orientation, an overview of ventilation and perfusion in frontal and sagittal slices is useful. It is important to present the images so that ventilation and perfusion are carefully aligned to each other (Fig. 24.3). This is greatly facilitated by the one session protocol with the patient in unchanged position. The option to triangulate between frontal (coronal), sagittal and transverse slices is valuable for identification of matching and nonmatching ventilation and perfusion changes. Proper alignment is also a prerequisite for V/P quotient images. These facilitate the interpretation and quantification of PE extension and all ventilation and perfusion defects. However, quotient images are not prerequisite for high-quality V/P SPECT.

REPORTING FINDINGS

Ventilation-Perfusion Patterns

For V/P SPECT, interpretation criteria are as important as the imaging technique itself. According to European guidelines, all patterns of ventilation and perfusion as well as numbers of defects are described and clinical probability is taken into account. This holistic principle for reporting,

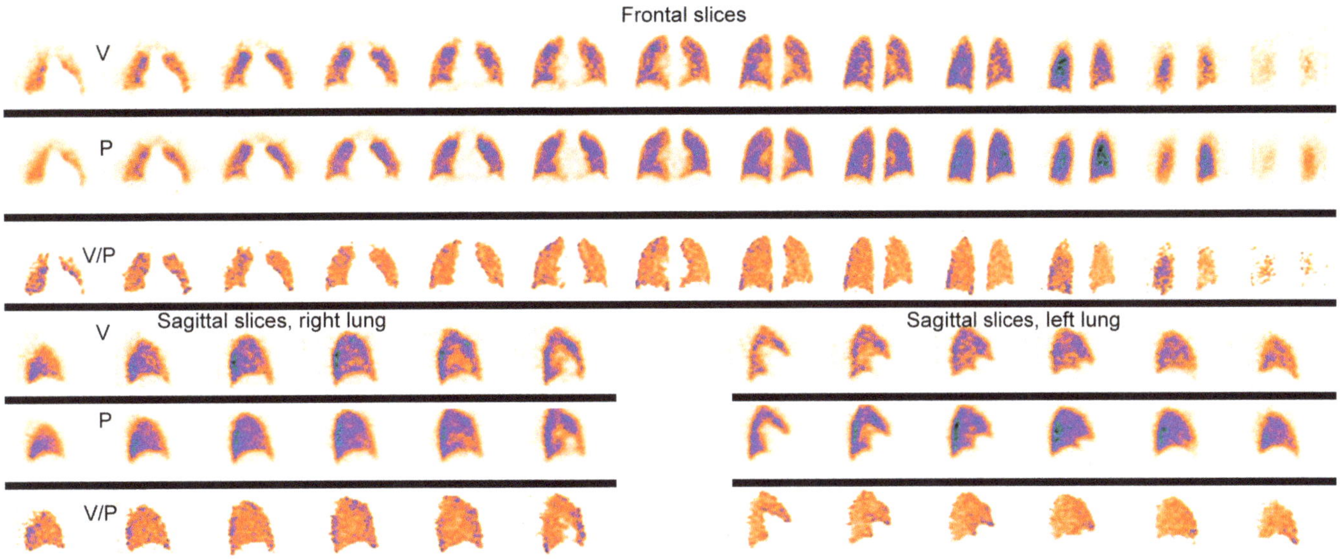

Fig. 24.3: Overview image of ventilation and perfusion in frontal and sagittal slices. Ventilation and perfusion are carefully aligned to each other.

give also a clear answer; yes or no for PE. This goal was not achieved with previous probabilistic reporting methods according to the Prospective Investigation of Pulmonary Embolism Diagnosis (PIOPED) study or modified PIOPED. Large V/P SPECT studies have shown that interpretation of all patterns representing ventilation together with perfusion achieves this result. Conclusive reports were given in 97–99% of cases.

Criteria for Acute Pulmonary Embolism

Recommended criteria for reading V/P SPECT with respect to acute PE are the following:

- *Pulmonary embolism* is reported if there is V/P mismatch of at least one segment or two subsegments that conforms to the pulmonary vascular anatomy.
- *No PE* is reported if there is: (1) normal perfusion pattern conforming to the anatomic boundaries of the lungs matched or reversed mismatch V/P defects of any size, shape or number in the absence of mismatch; (2) mismatch that does not have a lobar, segmental or subsegmental pattern.
- *Nondiagnostic for PE* is reported if there are multiple V/P abnormalities not typical of specific diseases.

It is important to report that with PE, a mismatch has its base along the pleura and conforms to known subsegmental and segmental vascular anatomy as stressed in the Prospective Investigative Study of Acute Pulmonary Embolism Diagnosis (PISAPED) study. Applying these principles of interpretation, recent V/P SPECT studies amounting to over 5,000 cases report a negative predictive value of 97–99%, sensitivities of 9699%, and specificities of 91–98% for PE diagnosis and rates of nondiagnostic findings were 1–3%.

An important step in the diagnostic procedure is to quantify the extent of embolism. V/P SPECT is particularly suitable for this because of its greater sensitivity compared to alternative planar scintigraphy and MDCT. The number of segments and subsegments indicating PE typical mismatch are counted and expressed in percentage of the total lung parenchyma. Furthermore, areas with ventilation abnormalities were recognized and this allowed the degree of total lung malfunction to be estimated. The study showed that patients with up 40% PE could be safely treated at home if ventilation abnormalities engaged not more that 20% of the lung. Outpatient management in hemodynamically stable patients with PE is safe provided that the embolic burden, quantified using V/P SPECT is included in the treatment decision algorithm. In Lund University the home treatment based on V/P SPECT has been implemented in 2004 and Elf at all has recently published that the treatment based on this setting is safe.

Chronic Pulmonary Embolism

Chronic PE is a progressive disease that develops in about 1–5% after an acute episode of PE, even in treated patients. It might lead to pulmonary hypertension, right heart failure and arrhythmia, which are frequent causes of death. The value of V/Q scintigraphy in this situation is well established. This has been confirmed in a head-to-head comparison between MDCT and planar scintigraphy with pulmonary angiography as reference. Among patients with pulmonary hypertension, scintigraphy had a sensitivity of 96–97% and specificity of 90%, whereas MDCT had a sensitivity of 51%. The conclusion was that V/Q scintigraphy "has a higher sensitivity than MDCT as well as very good specificity in detecting chronic pulmonary thromboembolic disease as a potentially curable cause of pulmonary hypertension". Scintigraphic features of chronic PE vary. Figure 24.4 illustrates one case of a typical pattern for chronic PE. MDCT was normal. In some patients, mismatch without clear segmental or subsegmental pattern is observed.

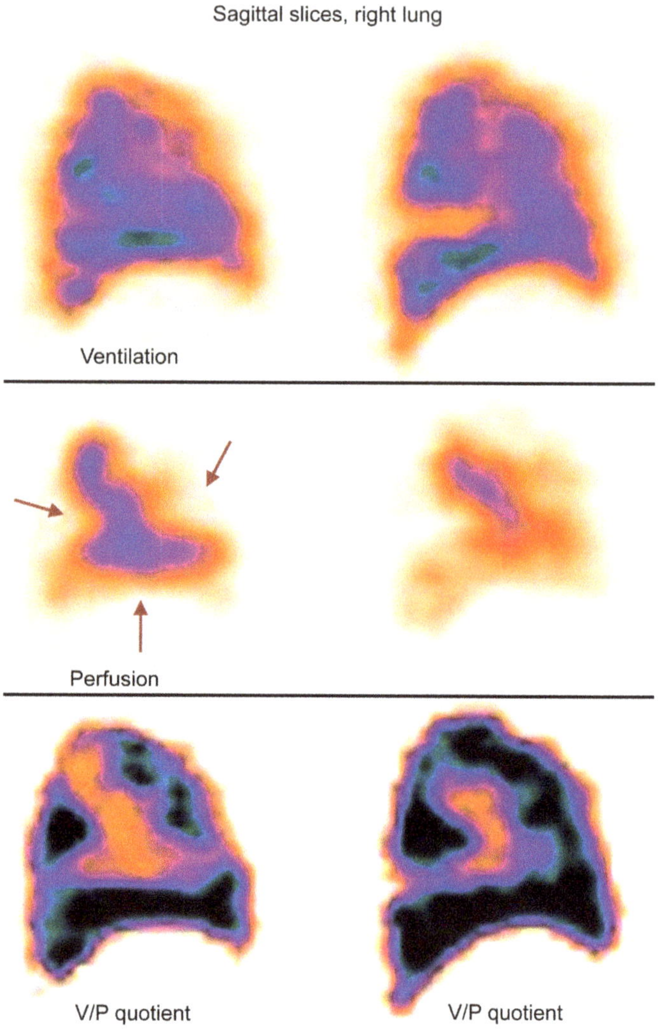

Fig. 24.4: Patient with chronic pulmonary embolism. Sagittal slices; uneven ventilation. The corresponding perfusion images show perfusion only in the central part of the lung. Perfusion defects (arrows) around the lung, clearly visible on V/P quotient images.

ROLE OF VENTILATION SPECT IN DIAGNOSIS OF OTHER LUNG DISEASES

Chronic Obstructive Pulmonary Disease

A common alternative or additional diagnosis is COPD. The characteristic is a general unevenness of ventilation. Focal deposition may be observed in central or peripheral airways even when using *Technegas*. A very important fact is that COPD patients are at high risk of PE. The rate of PE in patients hospitalized for acute exacerbations of COPD may be as high as 25%. Different from PIOPED study with V/P SPECT PE can be diagnosed even in the presence of COPD. PE accounts for up to 10% of deaths in stable COPD patients. The degree of unevenness of aerosol distribution correlated with lung function tests. Significantly, as there are no contraindications to V/P SPECT, even very sick and breathless patients can be studied. Figure 24.5 shows frontal slices in a patient with severe COPD and emphysema. Figure 24.6 shows frontal slices in a patient with COPD and PE. Furthermore, a grading of obstruction has been standardized (Fig. 24.7), with a strong correlation with spirometric stratification of the Global Initiative for Chronic Obstructive Lung Disease (GOLD). Moreover, V/P SPECT has a high sensitivity, and experimentally able to show an obstructive pattern in many apparently healthy smokers.

The method gives the possibility for physiological phenotyping having ability to localize ventilation and perfusion impairment and also estimate the total lung function.

Pneumonia

Pneumonia is also frequent in patients investigated for suspected PE. A typical finding is a ventilation defect in an area usually with better preserved perfusion, known as reverse mismatch. One of the typical patterns, which strongly support the diagnosis of pneumonia, is the "stripe sign". This refers to maintained perfusion along the pleural surface, peripheral to a central matched defect as seen in Figure 24.8. Moreover, the patient has also a PE in the middle lobe.

Left Heart Failure

Left heart failure is another diagnosis that is often observed among patients suspected of PE. The typical pattern is antigravitational redistribution of perfusion. In consecutive patients with suspected PE, V/P SPECT showed antigravitational redistribution of perfusion from posterior to anterior region in 15% of the cases indicating

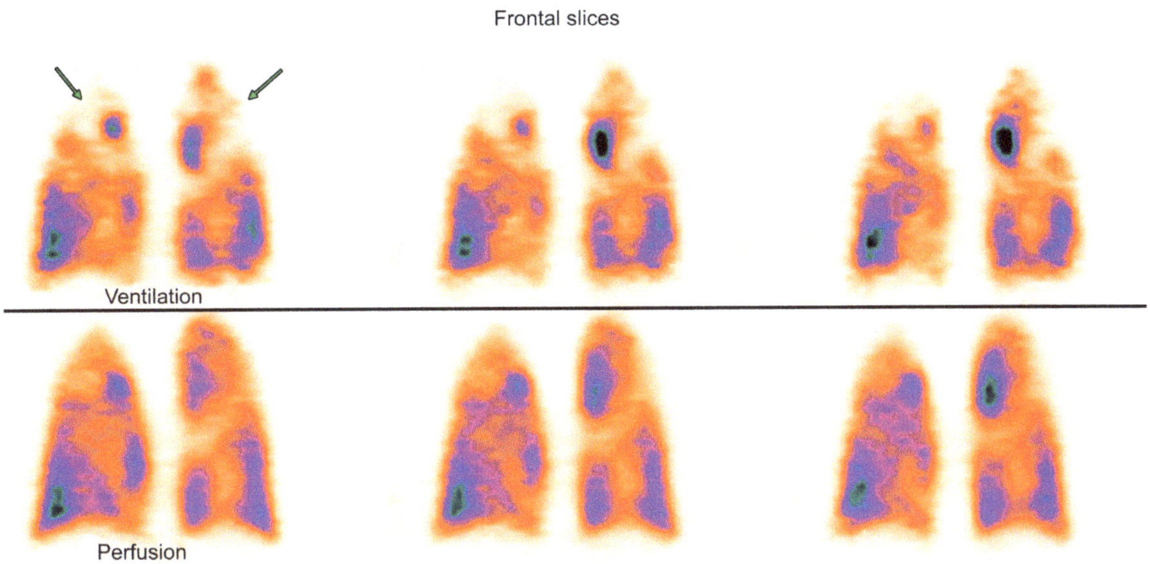

Fig. 24.5: Patient with severe chronic obstructive pulmonary disease and emphysema. Frontal slices; very uneven distribution of ventilation with deposition of aerosols in small airways (upper row) and reduced/absent ventilation in the upper lobes bilaterally (arrows). Perfusion is better preserved.

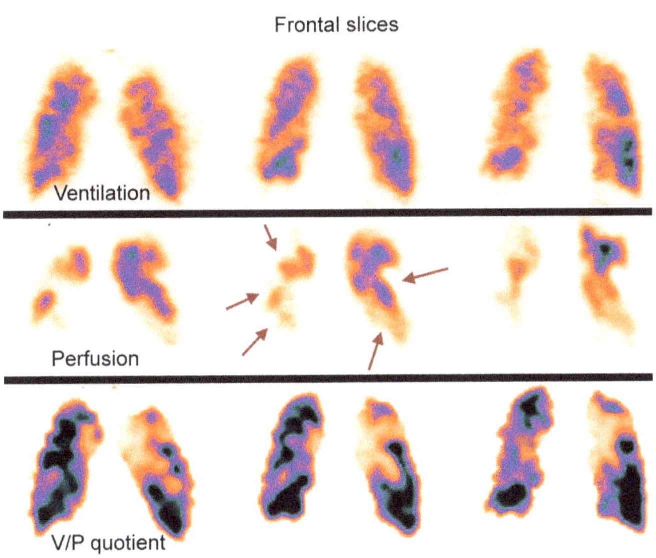

Fig. 24.6: Patient with severe chronic obstructive pulmonary disease and pulmonary embolism. Frontal slices; uneven distribution of ventilation with deposition of aerosols in small airways (upper row). Corresponding perfusion images (middle row) show multiple segmental perfusion defects (arrows) in the ventilated areas, nicely delineated on V/P quotient images.

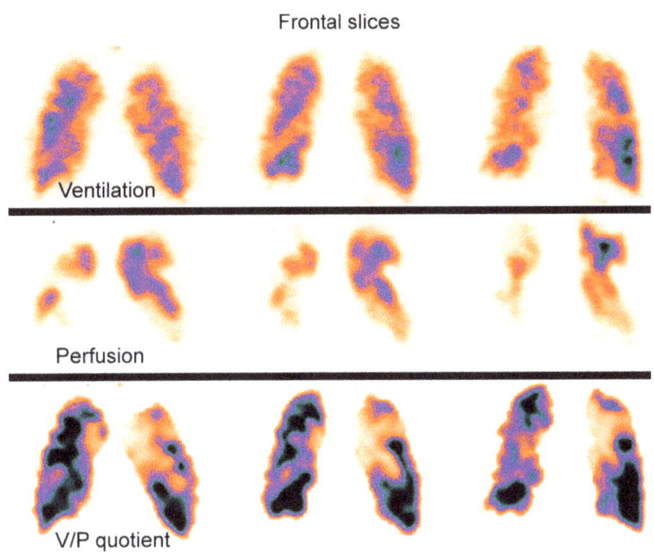

Fig. 24.7: Degree of obstruction. Frontal slices; ventilation and corresponding perfusion images; normal pattern, mild, moderate and severe chronic obstructive pulmonary disease.

LHF. The positive predictive value for heart failure in the study published by Jogi et al. was at least 88%. As ventilation is usually less redistributed than perfusion, V/P mismatch may be observed in dorsal regions. This VP mismatch has a nonsegmental pattern (does not conform pulmonary vascular architecture) and should not be misinterpreted as PE (Fig. 24.9).

V/P SPECT VERSUS MDCT

Diagnosis of Pulmonary Embolism

Multidetector computed tomography is often recommended as the first-line test for PE diagnosis. However, the principal study evaluating the use of MDCT as an imaging tool for PE diagnosis shows that sensitivity is not more than 78% and that there are a high number of false positive

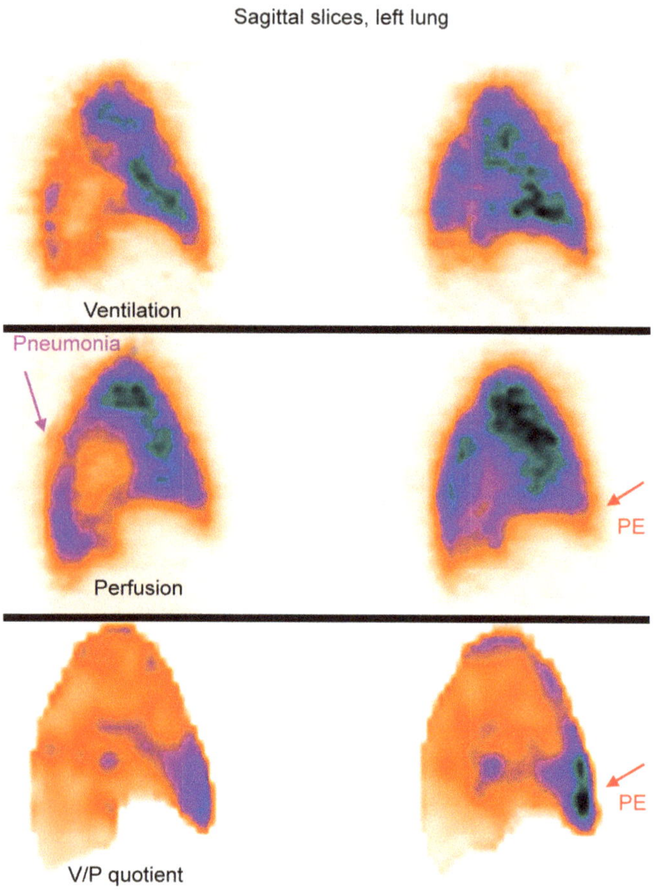

Fig. 24.8: Patient with pneumonia and pulmonary embolism in the right lung. Sagittal slices; reduced/absent ventilation posteriorly with reduced perfusion in the same area. Preserved perfusion adjacent to the pleura—stripe sign—arrow. In the middle lobe perfusion defect is seen (arrow) in the ventilated area.

results when clinical probability is not high. In the prospective study, PIOPED 2, the positive predictive value for a PE within a lobar pulmonary artery was 97% but fell to 68% and 25% in segmental and subsegmental pulmonary vessels respectively.

Advocates for MDCT stress that this method has the advantage over V/P SPECT by allowing also alternative diagnoses. Nevertheless, V/P SPECT provides evidence about alternative diagnoses as well. Actually, a properly performed V/P SPECT interpreted on the basis of all patterns of ventilation and perfusion, frequently allows diagnosis of other pulmonary disease with or without PE and a comprehensive understanding of the patient's symptoms. This added value of V/P SPECT appears at least as high as for additional diagnosis with MDCT. Further studies are needed in order to demonstrate the clinical impact of alternative diagnoses obtained by both methods.

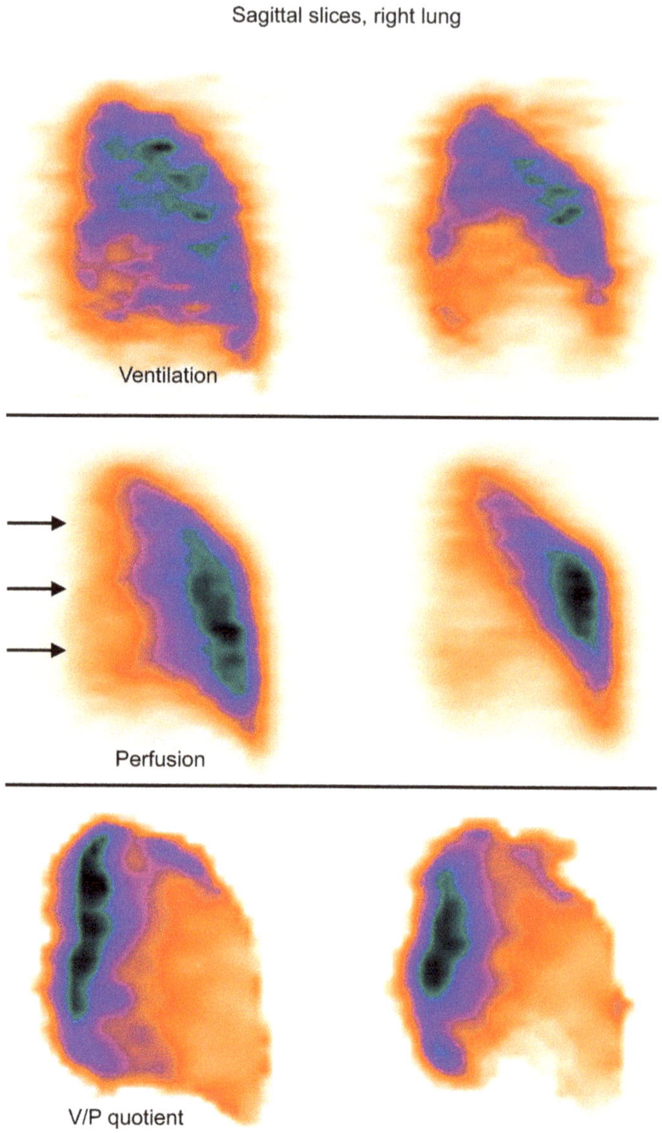

Fig. 24.9: Patient with left heart failure. Sagittal slices; antigravitational distribution of ventilation and more so of perfusion, causing nonsegmental V/P mismatch in dorsal regions (arrows).

The lack of a satisfactory gold standard for PE diagnosis poses difficulties for the assessment of sensitivity, specificity, and accuracy of all diagnostic methods for PE. The best available point of reference is an adequate follow-up of the patients to identify a recurrence of PE or alternative diagnoses as seen in Figures 24.2 and 24.5, respectively.

According to the most recent evidences, PE occurs in 1.4% of patients after a negative single slice CT, in 1.6% after a negative pulmonary angiography study and in 1.5% after a negative MDCT.

Bajc et al, showed in a large study that after a negative V/P scintigraphy, occurrence of PE during follow-up was 0.4%. Further prospective comparisons between up to date V/P SPECT and MDCT are needed. Moreover, results illustrate well the limited clinical utility of computed tomography pulmonary angiography (CTPA) because of kidney failure, critical illness, recent myocardial infarction, ventilator support and allergy to the contrast agent. By contrast, V/P SPECT has no contraindications and suboptimal studies are very rare.

Radiation Doses

Based upon data from the International Commission on Radiation Protection (ICRP) reports, the effective dose for V/P SPECT with the recommended protocol is about 35-40% of the dose from MDCT. The absorbed dose to the female breast for V/P SPECT is only 4% of the dose from MDCT with full-dose saving means according to Hurwitz. This may have particular importance in pregnant women with proliferating breast tissue and in the whole generative period. During the first trimester of pregnancy, the fetal dose of MDCT is greater than or equivalent to that of V/P SPECT. The advantage of V/P SPECT increases after the first trimester.

Follow-up

Follow-up of PE using imaging is essential to assess: (1) the effect of therapy, (2) to be able to differentiate between new and old PE where there is a suspicion of PE recurrence, and (3) explain physical incapacity after PE. Figure 24.2 shows that there were the rest of perfusion defects when terminated therapy and PE recurrence on same locations.

These demands for follow-up are only met with V/P SPECT. Obviously, the same method should be used for diagnosis and for follow-up.

Research

The suitability of an imaging technique for research into PE and its treatment and clinical follow-up are in principle the same. However, in research, there are even stronger, ethical, grounds for the use of nontraumatic procedures associated with lowest possible risks.

CLINICAL USE OF HYBRID V/P SPECT/CT

The hybrid SPECT/CT system is a dual imaging modality technique whose clinical application is particularly relevant in oncological diseases as it leads to improved sensitivity and specificity, combining coregistration of anatomical and functional data. It may lead to improved staging and treatment monitoring. As nuclear medicine procedures have the ability to visualize early functional changes much sooner than structural changes occur, additional CT procedure may improve correction for photon attenuation and allow coregistration of morphology and function. However, SPECT/CT acquisition of the chest constitutes a challenge due to respiratory movements, which can cause image artifacts and thus decrease diagnostic accuracy. A system which combines dual-head gamma camera with a Brilliance 16 slice CT can be a useful option.

Table 24.2: V/P SPECT/CT protocol.

	CT overview image			
	Tube potential	*Tube current*	*Collimation/slice width*	*Pitch*
Low dose CT	120 kV	20 mAs	16 × 1.5 – 0.5 s (second) rotation	0.813

The procedure starts with CT overview image and continues with diagnostic low-dose CT (120 kV, 20 mAs/slice, 16 × 1.5 collimator, 0.5 second rotation time and pitch of 0.813) not used for attenuation correction but to exactly colocalize the morphological and functional changes visualized in either of the two modalities (Table 24.2). Thereafter, follows the protocol for V/P SPECT as described above and according to the European guideline. Low-dose CT delivers approximately 1 mSv when used for alignment and attenuation correction. However, as a diagnostic tool in this hybrid system, it delivers 2-3 mSv and V/P SPECT 2.1-2.4 mSv.

Some authors have recently recommended V/P SPECT low-dose CT as a first-line procedure in patients with suspected PE. They showed 97% sensitivity and 88% specificity when only V/P SPECT was used. However, adding low-dose CT the sensitivity was unchanged but specificity increased to 100%.

Many departments in most developed countries use V/P SPECT as a primary tool in patients with suspected PE. Current evidence does not support the use of hybrid V/P SPECT/CT as a first-line procedure for all patients with suspected PE. It is not ethical to advocate higher radiation dose (2-3 mSv) for every patient with suspected PE where prevalence of PE might be as low as 10%. Following the good clinical practice recommendation to use hybrid system for PE diagnosis appears to be premature.

CT utilization has increased dramatically in the evaluation of patients with suspected PE, without improving rate of PE or other clinically significant diagnoses. Moreover, the patients are exposed at risks of radiation. Therefore, it is important to validate the V/P SPECT/CT system and not to adopt it too quickly, without fully assessing the benefits and risks.

The dual modality, however, will have impact in some group of patients. SPECT/CT may provide a significant contribution to COPD patients where architecture of the lung is changed and remodeled. COPD patients are usually also more prone to complications such as PE, pneumonia, LHF. Moreover, many of these patients have a tendency to develop tumors. These tumors are usually small and could only be visualized with CT. Correlation of perfusion defects on perfusion slices with specific pulmonary arterial branches seen on CT slices and heterogeneous defects on ventilation slices caused by airways changes could be easier to understand and interpret when applying both modalities. Figure 24.10 shows V/P SPECT images in patient with COPD. Uneven distribution of ventilation and corresponding perfusion images, typical for COPD are seen. On CT—transversal slice, small tumor is delineated in the left upper lobe. Tumor caused decreased/absent perfusion that is clear first when aligning both modalities (Fig. 24.10). Furthermore, V/P SPECT show LHF not visible on low-dose CT (Figs. 24.11A to C). Increased knowledge will improve future interpretation.

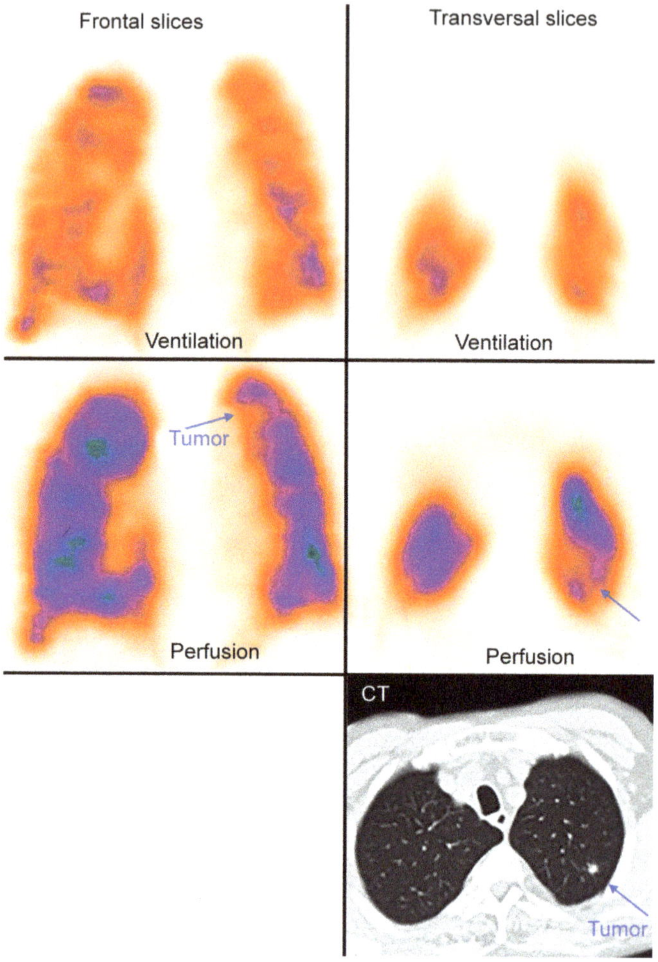

Fig. 24.10: Patient with chronic obstructive pulmonary disease; left column; frontal slices; the upper image displays uneven distribution of ventilation with deposition of Technegas. Corresponding perfusion image presenting similar pattern. Right column, transversal slices of ventilation SPECT upper row, with corresponding perfusion SPECT in the middle row. On CT image in lower row small tumor (1 cm) is visualized. Aligning both modalities small perfusion defect is observed in this area (arrow).

CONCLUSION

The V/P SPECT should be used as a primary tool for the diagnosis of PE because it has the highest sensitivity and accuracy and neither contraindications nor complications. In addition, it produces very few nondiagnostic reports. Furthermore, radiation doses are very low. This is particularly important for women in the reproductive period and during pregnancy.

To take full advantage of the V/P SPECT potential, it is crucial to apply an optimal protocol for a single session imaging of both ventilation and perfusion using low nuclide activities. Furthermore, full use should be made of display options, which are integrated in modern camera systems. Most important of all is holistic interpretation, giving a clear report with respect to PE, its extension as well as other diagnoses based on V/P patterns typical for various diseases.

The above mentioned advantages of V/P SPECT for studying PE imply that it may be the most suitable technique both for follow-up in patients with PE as well as for research regarding its treatment and pathophysiology.

BIBLIOGRAPHY AND FURTHER READING

1. Bajc M, Jonson B. Ventilation/perfusion SPECT for diagnosis of pulmonary embolism and other diseases. Int J Mol Imaging. 2011;2011:682949.
2. Bajc M, Maffioli L, Miniati M. Good clinical practice in pulmonary embolism diagnosis: where do we stand today? Eur J Nucl Med Mol Imaging. 2014;41(2):333-6.

Sagittal slices

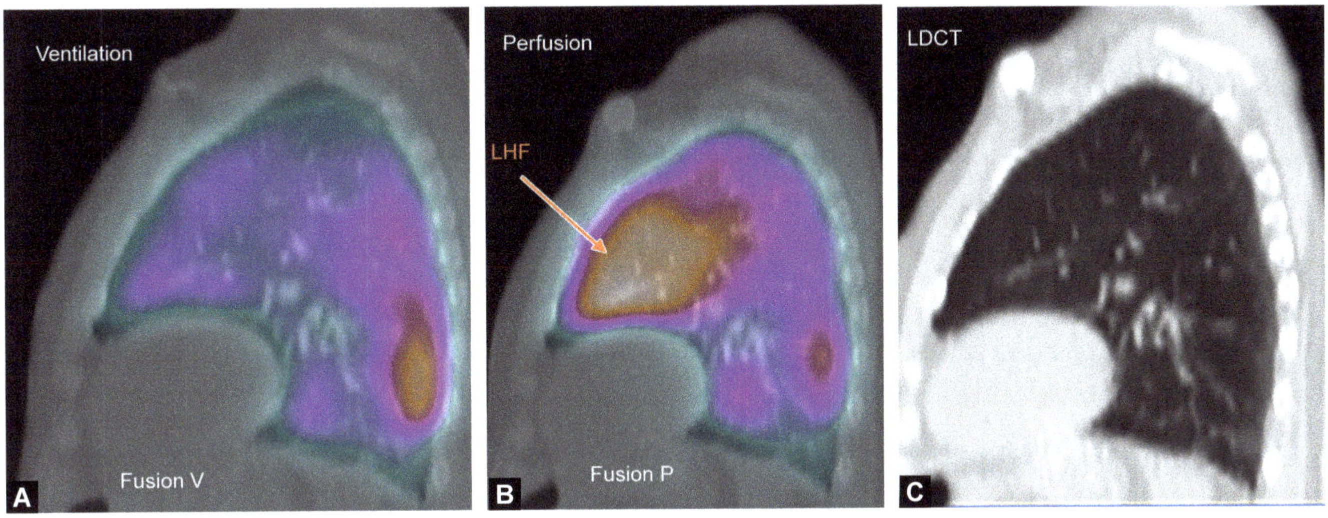

Fig. 24.11: Patient with chronic obstructive pulmonary disease and left heart failure. Sagittal slices; (A) Fusion ventilation and low-dose CT (LDCT) image; (B) Corresponding fusion perfusion and LDCT image, and (C) Corresponding LDCT image.

3. Bajc M, Markstad H, Jarenback L. et al. Grading obstructive lung disease using tomographic pulmonary scintigraphy in patients with chronic obstructive pulmonary disease (COPD) and longterm smokers. Ann Nucl Med. 2015;29:91-9
4. Bajc M, Neilly JB, Miniati M, Schuemichen C, Meignan M, Jonson B, et al. EANM guidelines for ventilation/perfusion scintigraphy: Part 1. Pulmonary imaging with ventilation/perfusion single photon emission tomography. Eur J Nucl Med Mol Imaging. 2009;36(8):1356-70.
5. Bajc M, Neilly JB, Miniati M, Schuemichen C, Meignan M, Jonson B. EANM guidelines for ventilation/perfusion scintigraphy: Part 2. Algorithms and clinical considerations for diagnosis of pulmonary emboli with V/P(SPECT) and MDCT. Eur J Nucl Med Mol Imaging. 2009;36(9):1528-38.
6. Bajc M, Olsson B, Palmer J, Jonson B. Ventilation/perfusion SPECT for diagnostics of pulmonary embolism in clinical practice. J Intern Med. 2008;264(4):379-87.
7. Bajc M, Olsson CG, Palmer J, Jonson B. Quantitative ventilation/perfusion SPECT (QV/P SPECT): a primary method for diagnosis of pulmonary embolism. In: Freeman ML (Ed). Nuclear Medicine Annual. Philadelphia: Lippincott Williams &Wilkins; 2004. pp. 173-86.
8. Bajc M. Potential of hybrid V/P SPECT-low-dose CT in lung diagnostics. Breathe. 2012;9:49-60.
9. Begic E, Opankovic V, Cukic A, Lindqvist M, Miniati M, Bajc Ancillary findings assessed by ventilation/perfusion tomography impact and clinical outcome in patients with suspected pulmonary embolism. Nukleamedizin. 2015;54:223-30. Doi:10.3413/Nukmed-0748-1506
10. British Thoracic Society Standards of Care Committee Pulmonary Embolism Guideline Development Group. British Thoracic Society guidelines for the management of suspected acute pulmonary embolism. Thorax. 2003;58(6):470-83.
11. Carvalho P. Sonographic demonstration of renal tumor extension into the contralateral renal vein. Br J Radiol. 1989;62(744):1093-5.
12. Coco AS, O'Gurek DT. Increased emergency department computed tomography use for common chest symptoms without clear patient benefits. J Am Board Fam Med. 2112;25:33-41.
13. Einstein AJ, Moser KW, Thompson RC, Cerqueira MD, Henzlova MJ. Radiation dose to patients from cardiac diagnostic imaging. Circulation. 2007;116(11):1290-305.
14. Elf JE, Jogi J, Bajc M. Home treatment of patients with small to medium sized acute pulmonary embolism. J Thromb Thrombolysis. 2015;39:166-72. DOI 10.1007/s11239-014-1097-y
15. Freeman LM, Stein EG, Sprayregen S, Chamarthy M, Haramati LB. The current and continuing important role of ventilation-perfusion scintigraphy in evaluating patients with suspected pulmonary embolism. Semin Nucl Med. 2008;38(6):432-40.
16. Friedman WF, Roberts WC. Vitamin D and the supravalvar aortic stenosis syndrome. The transplacental effects of vitamin D on the aorta of the rabbit. Circulation. 1966;34(1):77-86.
17. Garg A, Gopinath PG, Pande JN, Guleria JS. Role of radio-aerosol and perfusion lung imaging in early detection of chronic obstructive lung disease. Eur J Nucl Med. 1983;8(4):167-71.
18. Gruning T, Drake BE, Farrell SL, Nokes T. Three-year clinical experience with VQ SPECT for diagnosing pulmonary embolism: diagnostic performance. Clin Imaging. 2014;38:831-8.
19. Gutte H, Mortensen J, Jensen CV, Johnbeck CB, von der Recke P, Petersen CL, et al. Detection of pulmonary

embolism with combined ventilation-perfusion SPECT and low-dose CT: head-to-head comparison with multidetector CT angiography. J Nucl Med. 2009;50(12):1987-92.

20. Henry JW, Relyea B, Stein PD. Continuing risk of thromboemboli among patients with normal pulmonary angiograms. Chest. 1995;107(5):1375-8.
21. Hurwitz LM, Yoshizumi T, Reiman RE, Goodman PC, Paulson EK, Frush DP, et al. Radiation dose to the fetus from body MDCT during early gestation. AJR Am J Roentgenol. 2006;186(3):871-6.
22. Hurwitz LM, Yoshizumi TT, Goodman PC, Nelson RC, Toncheva G, Nguyen GB, et al. Radiation dose savings for adult pulmonary embolus 64-MDCT using bismuth breast shields, lower peak kilovoltage, and automatic tube current modulation. AJR Am J Roentgenol. 2009;192(1):244-53.
23. Hurwitz LM, Yoshizumi TT, Reiman RE, Paulson EK, Frush DP, Nguyen GT, et al. Radiation dose to the female breast from 16-MDCT body protocols. AJR Am J Roentgenol. 2006;186(6):1718-22.
24. ICRP. Managing Patient Dose in Multi-Detector Computed Tomography (MDCT), ICRP publication 102. Oxford: Elsevier; 2007.
25. ICRP. Radiation Dose to Patients from Radiopharmaceuticals, ICRP publication 53. Oxford: Elsevier; 1988.
26. Jobse BN, Rhem RG, McCurry CA, Wang IQ, Labiris NR. Imaging lung function in mice using SPECT/CT and per-voxel analysis. PloS One. 2012;7(8):e42187.
27. Jögi J, Ekberg M, Jonson B, Bozovic G, Bajc M. Ventilation/perfusion SPECT in chronic obstructive pulmonary disease: an evaluation by reference to symptoms, spirometric lung function and emphysema, as assessed with HRCT. Eur J Nucl Med Mol Imaging. 2011;38(7):1344-52.
28. Jögi J, Jonson B, Ekberg M, Bajc M. Ventilation-perfusion SPECT with 99mTc-DTPA versus Technegas: a head-to-head study in obstructive and nonobstructive disease. J Nucl Med. 2010;51(5):735-41.
29. Jögi J, Markstad H, Tufvesson E, Bjermer L, Bajc M. The added value of hybrid ventilation/perfusion sPeCT/CT in patients with stable COPD or apparently healthy smokers. Cancer-suspected CT findings in the lungs are common when hybrid imaging is used. International Journal of COPD. 2015;10: 25-30.
30. Jögi J, Palmer J, Jonson B, Bajc M. Heart failure diagnostics based on ventilation/perfusion single photon emission computed tomography pattern and quantitative perfusion gradients. Nucl Med Commun. 2008;29(8):666-73.
31. Kan Y, et al. The accuracy of V/Q SPECT in the diagnosis of pulmonary embolism: a metaanalysis. Acta Radiol. 2015; 56(5):565-72. Doi: 10.1177/0284185114533682. Epub 2014 Jan 10.
32. Leblanc M, Leveillee F, Turcotte E. Prospective evaluation of the negative predictive value of V/Q SPECT using 99mTc-Technegas. Nucl Med Commun. 2007;28(8):667-72.
33. Le Duc-Pennec A, Le Roux PY, Cornily JC, Jaffrelot M, Delluc A, de Saint-Martin L, et al. Diagnostic accuracy of single-photon emission tomography ventilation/perfusion lung scan in the diagnosis of pulmonary embolism. Chest. 2012;141(2):381-7.
34. Lemb M, Pohlabeln H. Pulmonary thromboembolism: a retrospective study on the examination of 991 patients by ventilation/perfusion SPECT using Technegas. Nuklearmedizin. 2001;40(6):179-86.
35. Lewczuk J, Piszko P, Jagas J, Porada A, Wojciak S, Sobkowicz B, et al. Prognostic factors in medically treated patients with chronic pulmonary embolism. Chest. 2001;119(3):818-23.
36. Li DJ, Stewart I, Miles KA, Wraight EP. Scintigraphic appearances in patients with pulmonary infection and lung scintigrams of intermediate or low probability for pulmonary embolism. Clin Nucl Med. 1994;19(12):1091-3.
37. Lisbona R, Kreisman H, Novales-Diaz J, Derbekyan V. Perfusion lung scanning: differentiation of primary from thromboembolic pulmonary hypertension. AJR Am J Roentgenol. 1985;144(1):27-30.
38. Mamlouk MD, vanSonnenberg E, Gosalia R, Drachman D, Gridley D, Zamora JG, et al. Pulmonary embolism at CT angiography: implications for appropriateness, cost, and radiation exposure in 2003 patients. Radiology. 2010;256(2):625-32.
39. Miniati M, Bottai M, Monti S, Salvadori M, Serasini L, Passera M. Simple and accurate prediction of the clinical probability of pulmonary embolism. Am J Respir Crit Care Med. 2008;178(3):290-4.
40. Miniati M, Monti S, Bottai M, Scoscia E, Bauleo C, Tonelli L, et al. Survival and restoration of pulmonary perfusion in a long-term follow-up of patients after acute pulmonary embolism. Medicine (Baltimore). 2006;85(5):253-62.
41. Miniati M, Pistolesi M, Marini C, Di Ricco G, Formichi B, Prediletto R, et al. Value of perfusion lung scan in the diagnosis of pulmonary embolism: results of the Prospective Investigative Study of Acute Pulmonary Embolism Diagnosis (PISA-PED). Am J Respir Crit Care Med. 1996;154(5):1387-93.
42. Moores L, Aujesky D, Jimenez D, Diaz G, Gomez V, Marti D, et al. Pulmonary embolism severity index and troponin testing for the selection of low-risk patients with acute symptomatic pulmonary embolism. J Thromb Haemost. 2010;8:517-22.
43. Olsson CG, Bitzen U, Olsson B, Magnusson P, Carlsson MS, Jonson B, et al. Outpatient tinzaparin therapy in pulmonary embolism quantified with ventilation/perfusion scintigraphy. Med Sci Monit. 2006;12(2):PI9-13.
44. Palmer J, Bitzen U, Jonson B, Bajc M. Comprehensive ventilation/perfusion SPECT. J Nucl Med. 2001;42(8):1288-94.
45. PIOPED Investigators. Value of the ventilation/perfusion scan in acute pulmonary embolism. Results of the Prospective Investigation of Pulmonary Embolism Diagnosis (PIOPED). JAMA. 1990;263(20):2753-9.
46. Pistolesi M, Miniati M, Bonsignore M, Andreotti F, Di Ricco G, Marini C, et al. Factors affecting regional pulmonary blood flow in chronic ischemic heart disease. J Thorac Imaging. 1988;3(3):65-72.
47. Reinartz P, Wildberger JE, Schaefer W, Nowak B, Mahnken AH, Buell U. Tomographic imaging in the diagnosis of

pulmonary embolism: a comparison between V/Q lung scintigraphy in SPECT technique and multislice spiral CT. J Nucl Med. 2004;45(9):1501-8.

48. Rizkallah J, Man SF, Sin DD. Prevalence of pulmonary embolism in acute exacerbations of COPD: a systematic review and meta-analysis. Chest. 2009;135(3):786-93.
49. Roach P. V/Q SPECT: the primary imaging test for suspected pulmonary embolism. BMJ. 2013;347:f5119.
50. Roche LM, Niu X, Pawlish KS, Henry KA. Thyroid cancer incidence in New Jersey: time trend, birth cohort and socioeconomic status analysis (1979-2006). J Environ Public Health. 2011;2011:850105.
51. Schonhofer B, Kohler D. Prevalence of deep-vein thrombosis of the leg in patients with acute exacerbation of chronic obstructive pulmonary disease. Respiration. 1998;65(3):173-7.
52. Silverstein MD, Heit JA, Mohr DN, Petterson TM, O'Fallon WM, Melton LJ 3rd. Trends in the incidence of deep vein thrombosis and pulmonary embolism: a 25-year population-based study. Arch Intern Med. 1998;158(6):585-93.
53. Stein PD, Fowler SE, Goodman LR, Gottschalk A, Hales CA, Hull RD, et al. Multidetector computed tomography for acute pulmonary embolism. N Engl J Med. 2006;354(22):2317-27.
54. Stein PD, Hull RD, Ghali WA, Patel KC, Olson RE, Meyers FA, et al. Tracking the uptake of evidence: two decades of hospital practice trends for diagnosing deep vein thrombosis and pulmonary embolism. Arch Intern Med. 2003;163(10):1213-9.
55. Stein PD, Hull RD, Patel KC, Olson RE, Ghali WA, Brant R, et al. D-dimer for the exclusion of acute venous thrombosis and pulmonary embolism: a systematic review. Ann Intern Med. 2004;140(8):589-602.
56. Tunariu N, Gibbs SJ, Win Z, Gin-Sing W, Graham A, Gishen P, et al. Ventilation-perfusion scintigraphy is more sensitive than multidetector CTPA in detecting chronic thromboembolic pulmonary disease as a treatable cause of pulmonary hypertension. J Nucl Med. 2007;48(5):680-4.
57. Van Beek EJ, Kuyer PM, Schenk BE, Brandjes DP, ten Cate JW, Buller HR. A normal perfusion lung scan in patients with clinically suspected pulmonary embolism. Frequency and clinical validity. Chest. 1995;108(1):170-3.
58. Wells PS, Anderson DR, Rodger M, Stiell I, Dreyer JF, Barnes D, et al. Excluding pulmonary embolism at the bedside without diagnostic imaging: management of patients with suspected pulmonary embolism presenting to the emergency department by using a simple clinical model and D-dimer. Ann Intern Med. 2001;135(2):98-107.
59. Worsley DF, Palevsky HI, Alavi A. Ventilation-perfusion lung scanning in the evaluation of pulmonary hypertension. J Nucl Med. 1994;35(5):793-6.

Chapter 25

Positron Emission Tomography: Role in Lung Cancer Evaluation and Management

Laura Serafino-Agrusa, Roberta Catania, Claudio Sorino, Mario Spatafora

OVERVIEW

In recent years, the diagnostic workup of patients with cancer has been improved by the introduction of positron emission tomography (PET). PET is a noninvasive imaging tool to visualize and measure physiological function and biochemical processes (e.g. metabolism) in the living human body. The method is based on the radiolabeling of molecules involved in metabolic processes by short-lived positron-emitting radionuclides. The detection of the radiation caused by the accumulation of these particles in the form of cross sections reflects a qualitative and quantitative image of the corresponding metabolic processes. The small amount of radioactivity needed for the examination induces a low radiation exposure comparable with that of computed tomography (CT) examinations.

The most commonly used tracer for lung cancer (LC) assessment is 18F-fluorodeoxyglucose (18F-FDG), an analog of glucose labeled with fluorine-18, which enters tumor cells due to their increased glucose metabolism. Because of increased expression of glucose transport proteins, cancer cells have an increased cellular uptake of glucose and a higher rate of glycolysis compared to benign cells. As FDG is metabolically trapped and accumulated in tumor cells after phosphorylation by hexokinase, its preferential accumulation may help differentiate benign and malignant tissue. In this regard, a moderate to considerably increased glucose metabolism, as assessed by the standardized uptake value (SUV), may also be noticed in acute inflammatory processes (e.g. active tuberculosis of lymph nodes or sarcoidosis) (Fig. 25.1). Thus, FDG-PET complements anatomic information on standard imaging obtained by CT with "metabolic" information. The development of integrated

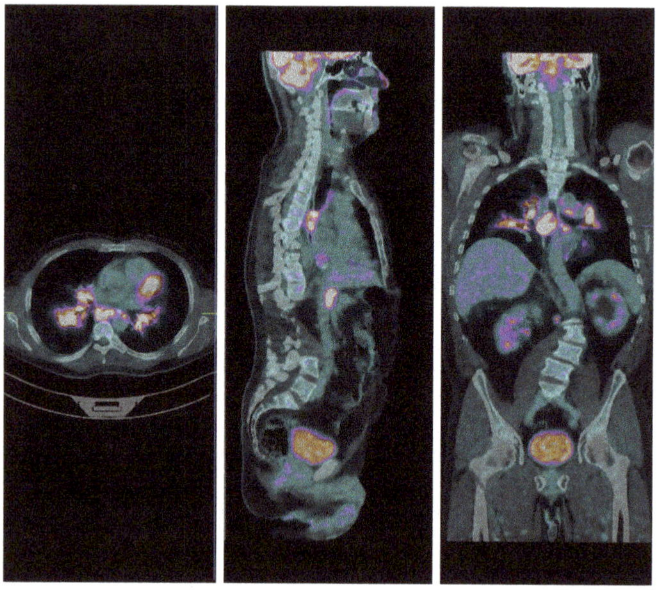

Fig. 25.1: An 18F-FDG-PET/CT scan showing nearly symmetrical increases in FDG uptake in the hilar and mediastinal lymph nodes.

PET/CT has greatly contributed to a more accurate delineation of areas of increased uptake, overcoming the limits of patients repositioning when the two images were acquired independently and fused afterward. The relevance of such combination in everyday practice of clinical oncology cannot be overestimated.

Lung cancer represents the main cause of cancer mortality worldwide, in both men and women, is the second most common cancer in Europe and in the United States and represents a major economic issue for health care systems, accounting for about 12.7% of all new cancer cases per year and 18.2% of cancer deaths. In particular, each year approximately 1.6 million new LC cases are diagnosed and 1.4 million LC-related deaths occur in the world. Despite improvements in survival for many other tumors in recent years, the overall 5-year survival for LC remains relatively poor (around 10%) mainly because LC is diagnosed in advanced stages when treatment options are limited. We will herein review the main applications of FDG-PET in diagnosis, staging and treatment of LC.

ROLE OF PET IN DIAGNOSIS AND STAGING OF LUNG CANCER

Positron emission tomography has been extensively studied in the diagnosis of indeterminate lung lesions. The technique has been proven to be significantly more accurate than CT in differentiating benign from malignant lesions as small as 1 cm. An overall sensitivity of 96% (range, 83–100%), specificity of 79% (range, 52–100%), and accuracy of 91% (range, 86–100%) can be expected. Because a critical mass of metabolically active malignant cells is required for PET diagnosis, false-negative results can occur in subcentimetric lesions. Regardless of size, false-negative results are common in carcinoid (up to 85%) and in patients with lepidic predominant adenocarcinomas (formerly known as bronchoalveolar cell carcinomas), commonly seen on CT with a "ground-glass" opacity pattern. False-positive FDG uptake is seen in inflammatory conditions and granulomatous diseases. Because of its high negative predictive value (NPV), PET excludes malignancy correctly in the vast majority of cases; on the other hand, having a specificity of only 79%, the positive predictive value (PPV) is lower and further investigations are usually required to confirm a diagnosis of malignancy.

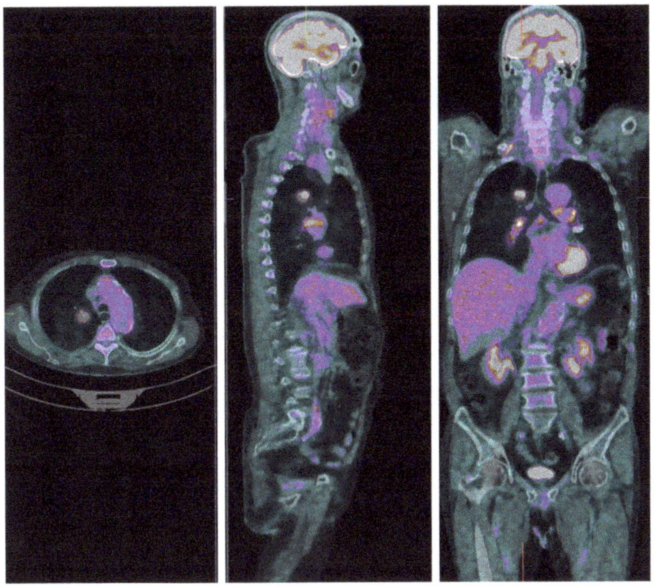

Fig. 25.2: An 18F-FDG-PET/CT scan showing intense radiotracer accumulation (SUV max 22) of a solitary pulmonary nodule in the right upper lobe. The histological examination of biopsy specimen obtained by CT-guided transthoracic fine-needle aspiration revealed a small cell lung cancer.

PET and Solitary Pulmonary Nodule

Solitary pulmonary nodule (SPN), or coin lesion, usually identified in routine chest X-rays of CT scans, is defined as "a non-spiculated round or oval lesion with a diameter smaller than 3 cm surrounded by lung tissue not associated with adenopathy, atelectasis, or pneumonia". Although several risk factors for malignancy, including nodule size, age, history of smoking or asbestos exposure, and concomitant chronic obstructive pulmonary disease (COPD), have been identified, management of patients with SPNs may be challenging. Indeed, accurate diagnosis is important to address patients to prompt resection or, alternatively, to avoid unnecessary surgical procedures in those with benign lesions. FDG-PET is the most accurate, noninvasive imaging modality for the evaluation of SPN. Besides visual image interpretation, semiquantitative analysis with SUVs can be performed to improve accuracy. Dual imaging with PET and CT combines the better image resolution of CT and "biological" information of PET (Fig. 25.2). As a result, PET/CT has been recently reported to have specificity ranging from 70% to 90%, sensitivity ranging from 88% to 96% and an overall accuracy of 83–93% in the assessment of SPN. It should be kept in mind that SPN characterization can be affected by respiratory motion artifacts, especially in lung bases resulting in artifactually decreased SUV levels. In addition, SUV may be influenced by a variety of factors, including patient's body size, blood glucose concentration, and timing of imaging after injection. Because FDG accumulation in tumor is decreased in patients with hyperglycemia, the assessment of SPNs in diabetic patients with the use of PET/CT requires optimal control of blood glucose levels. Abnormal FDG uptake generating false-positive results on PET/CT can also occur in localized inflammatory processes, including granulomas, rheumatoid nodules, acute pyogenic abscess, and so forth. Moreover, the sensitivity of PET to detect malignant lesions is low in small SPNs and those less than 7 mm in diameter will only be seen if they have very high metabolic activity. Therefore, it is not recommended to perform PET scans for lesions less than 1 cm.

In the attempt to improve diagnostic accuracy of PET/CT, new techniques are under active investigation. In this context, dual-phase imaging is a method that acquires two PET/CT data sets for the evaluation of SPN. The first is acquired typically 1 hour after radiotracer injection (initial scan), while an additional PET/CT acquisition is done 1–3 hours later (delayed scan). The rationale of this technique relies on the ability of tumor cells to accumulate FDG for a longer time than nonmalignant lesions. Thus, compared to initial scan, increase in SUV in delayed scan will be suggestive of malignancy. This method, along with the use of alternative radiotracers (such as 18F-fluorothymidine or FFLT and F-fluorocholine) holds promise to improve the accuracy of PET/CT in the diagnostic approach to SPNs.

PET and Staging

Besides providing fundamental prognostic information, the primary goal of staging is to select stage I–IIIA (N0–N2) patients who may be candidate for radical surgery, while those with more advanced stage IIIB (N3) and IV diseases are not. FDG-PET provides useful information in non-small cell lung cancer (NSCLC) staging, particularly in the assessment of regional nodal status (N factor), a crucial and often challenging part of the staging process.

Computed tomography scan has long been used as the routine method to assess N status. However, since lymph node size (cut-off value = 10 mm in short axis) is the only criterion to suspect involvement, both false-positive and false-negative results can be expected. Lymph node size can be increased as a result of inflammatory processes particularly common in disventilated lung districts; on the other hand, microscopic tumor involvement may leave the size of lymph nodes under the selected threshold. Moreover, normal lymph nodes in various parts of the chest may be quite heterogeneous in size. Not surprisingly, CT scan is rather inaccurate in N status assessment, with PPV of 56% and NPV of 83%. In the attempt to improve diagnostic accuracy of CT, visual integration with FDG-PET scan and CT-PET fusion images have been proposed. Several studies confirm that the addition of PET scan to CT scan for mediastinal lymph node staging in potentially operable NSCLC raises sensitivity to 84%, specificity to 89%, PPV to 79% and NPV to 93%. Some studies have suggested that integrated CT-PET fusion images provide slightly more accurate information compared to visual integration of single imaging techniques. Consistent with the concept that inflammatory processes may lead to both enlargement of lymph node size and increased FDG uptake, PET scan is more sensitive but less specific when CT shows enlarged lymph nodes. Due to the high NPV of CT-PET, invasive staging procedures, like endoscopic fine bronchial needle aspiration (FBNA) biopsy or mediastinoscopy, can generally be omitted in patients with negative mediastinal PET images. However, some guidelines specifically recommend invasive staging in some clinical situations, including central tumors, hilar N1 disease, lepidic predominant adenocarcinomas and whenever FDG uptake in primary tumor is low. In addition, it should be kept in mind that the NPV of PET scan in CT-positive mediastinal nodes depends on their size. In this regard, a recent meta-analysis indicates that the post-test probability of unexpected pathologic N2 disease raises from 5% in PET-negative nodes measuring 10–15 mm to 21% in those measuring 16 mm or more, suggesting that invasive mediastinal staging may also be useful in this subset of patients.

M-stage

A significant proportion of LC patients has metastatic disease at the time of diagnosis. In addition, among the patients undergoing curative surgical treatment, around 20% will relapse due to the presence of undetected micrometastasis at the time of initial staging. Since first development, PET has raised much interest as a "one-shot" procedure able to detect unsuspected metastasis in LC and refine diagnostic assessment of suspect lesions detected with other techniques. In this regard, the combination of metabolic imaging with precise anatomic resolution allowed by more recently introduced integrated PET/CT offers the possibility to further refine the search for metastatic disease. Moreover, PET/CT scans are generally extended to body districts, such as skin, pelvis, skeletal muscle, soft tissue, kidney, and pancreas not usually investigated with other conventional procedures routinely used in LC staging.

The ability of PET to allow the detection of unsuspected distant metastasis was originally studied in single-institution or multicenter investigations. While these studies were consistently positive, the percentage of unsuspected metastases revealed by PET was variable, ranging from 10% to 28%. Technical factors and the heterogeneity of samples may explain these discrepancies. In this context, the diagnostic yield of PET in revealing unsuspected metastases may depend both on the presence of clinical predictive factors of metastatic disease and on the percentage of clinical N2-positive stage III disease. These results prompted the conduction of randomized clinical trials aimed at evaluating the cost-effectiveness of a staging strategy based on the addition or anticipation of PET to traditional staging workup. In the PLUS randomized study, it was demonstrated that the addition of PET to conventional staging workup in NSCLC patients almost halves (from 41% to 21%) futile thoracotomies, including explorative thoracotomies and those made on patients with pathological stage IIIA-N2/IIIB or with postoperative relapse or death within 12 months after randomization. In a more recent multicenter randomized trial, the hypothesis that the anticipation of PET (up-front PET strategy) may reduce the number of tests needed and costs of staging in LC patients was tested. While in the overall sample both these endpoints were missed, in patients with stage IV disease a single whole-body PET followed by verification of single decisive lesion was shown to reduce significantly the number of tests needed for staging.

Because the most typical sites of metastatic spread of LC are the adrenal glands, bones, brain or liver, conventional staging includes a CT scan of the chest extended to adrenal glands and liver, whole-body bone scintigraphy and brain imaging. Due to high prevalence of adrenal adenomas in general population, the differential diagnosis with adrenal metastases, occurring in up to 20% of patients with NSCLC, may be troublesome although the chance of malignancy is higher in patients with known IV stage disease or with bigger adrenal lesions. Percutaneous biopsy is a relatively safe and effective procedure to achieve a diagnosis in doubtful cases, and may be mandatory when the histology of the adrenal mass will dictate subsequent management.

Radionuclide bone scintigraphy is the routine method to detect skeletal metastases; however, false-positive scan abnormalities are common due to the uptake of the radionuclide by degenerative and traumatic lesions. In addition, the poor quality of the images limits the possibility of a strategy based on follow-up. PET/CT has been suggested as an alternative method for detection of bone metastases. A recent meta-analysis of on 17 studies (2,940 patients) has shown that both PET and PET-CT are more accurate than bone scintigraphy, with an overall sensitivity and specificity of 92% and 98%, as compared to 86% and 88% of bone scintigraphy, respectively. Biopsy of the suspect lesion is rarely necessary. Similar data have been reported on the accuracy of PET in the search of liver metastases. Besides that most liver lesions seen on CT scan are benign cysts or hemangiomas, one meta-analysis that specifically reviewed hepatic studies derived a pooled yield of 3% for liver metastases in asymptomatic patients with NSCLC. Although data in patients with NSCLC are very limited at present, PET scanning has been shown to detect liver metastases with an accuracy of 92–100% and only rare false-positive findings. In general, PET scanning is not considered to be reliable for detecting brain metastases due the small size of most of them, background brain FDG uptake, and the variable biologic characteristics of brain metastases, which can be either hypermetabolic or hypometabolic. Although sensitivity of conventional 18F-FDG-PET has been reported to be as low as 60%, with occasional false-negative imaging findings of even sizable brain metastases, one study has suggested that the use of alternative tracers, such as 11C-labeled choline, may increase the diagnostic yield of PET scanning for imaging brain metastases. Studies are underway to confirm these preliminary data.

ROLE OF PET IN PROGNOSIS OF LUNG CANCER

The assessment of prognosis is crucial to anticipate the clinical outcome for each individual case and to select the appropriate treatment. While many variables including gender, comorbidity, age, weight loss, laboratory indices [such as, tumor markers, lactate dehydrogenase (LDH) or neutrophil counts] have been investigated, the only universally accepted prognostic indicators in LC are TNM (Tumor, Node, Metastases) stage and performance status. However, TNM staging system is far from being perfect as many of the patients in the early stages eventually die of the disease. Recently, a composite prognostic index generated by the combination of simple tumor, personal and functional variables was developed and validated.

In the continuing search for additional independent prognostic factors in LC, the maximum SUV of the primary tumor on FDG-PET done at time of diagnosis might represent a sound candidate. In addition, it holds the great advantage of being easily repeatable. The prognostic value of FDG-PET at time of diagnosis was evaluated in several studies and was the subject of a systematic review. Despite studies were quite heterogeneous in terms of absolute SUV levels and selected cut-off, typically reflecting median values of single series (range: 2.5–20), in all the 11 studies analyzed patient with "low FDG uptake" in their primary tumors had longer disease-free and overall survival than patients with "high uptake". The problem of the heterogeneous thresholds of the SUV is related to lack of standardization of the acquisition and processing protocols and greatly undermines the applicability of SUV for prognostic estimation purposes. A meta-analysis considering the individual patient data is needed to try to compensate for the large heterogeneity of the reported SUV in different studies. In order to assess whether SUV was an independent prognostic variable, multivariate Cox proportional hazard model was applied. In 2005, Cerfolio et al. published a single-institution retrospective multivariate analysis on 315 prospective patients. Patients with maximum SUV greater than or equal to 10 were more likely to have poorly differentiated tumors and advanced stage disease and were less likely to have their disease completely resected. In addition, maximum SUV was the best predictor of disease-free and overall survival. These promising results were not confirmed in other studies using the same multivariate model. Although statistically significant, SUV max was shown to be inferior to TNM stage and performance status in one study and even not prognostic in another. The degree of FDG uptake by cancer cells clearly reflects their metabolic activity; hence, its prognostic role at initial presentation is indeed conceivable. However, agreement on methods of scanning, SUV measurement and selection of the best cut-off values are needed before this technique can be fully applied in clinical practice for prognostic purposes.

ROLE OF PET IN CHEMOTHERAPY

As most patients with NSCLC are diagnosed in the advanced stage of the disease, the standard primary treatment is cytotoxic chemotherapy with a response rate approaching 40% and limited, though statistically significant, clinical advantage. The assessment of response is currently based upon the application of the Response Evaluation Criteria in Solid Tumors (RECIST) criteria which in turn rely on morphologic imaging techniques. However, since final treatment outcome will be determined more by the biologic aggressiveness of residual tumor than by volume itself, this kind of approach may be inaccurate because residual areas of viable tumor tissue cannot be distinguished from necrotic or fibrotic areas. Due to its ability to assess metabolic activity of tumor, rather than its size, FDG-PET has the potential to overcome this problem and provides information potentially useful to predict clinical advantage early in the course of chemotherapy.

Early studies on patients with breast and colorectal cancer showed that metabolic activity markedly changed within the first week of therapy and that significant tumor response could be reliably anticipated by the observation of a negative PET scan after completion of therapy. The accuracy of this strategy in NSCLC is limited, due to the significant FDG uptake related to tumor metabolic flare secondary to the activation of energy-dependent cellular repair mechanisms and by tumor-infiltrating macrophages. The above false-positive uptake is the main reason behind the proposal, applicable also to radiotherapy (RT), to perform re-evaluation FDG-PET at least 2 weeks after completion of therapy. In any case, consensus is missing on the parameters to be used at time of the response assessment and on the definition of "response" itself. On a practical point of view, when intraindividual comparison of tumor FDG uptake is made using the same protocol in the same institution, a relative decrease in the SUV of the tumor by more than 20% has been suggested as a reasonable definition of metabolic response.

The setting of neoadjuvant chemotherapy appears as the most promising for clinical application of FDG-PET in the evaluation of response. Early prospective studies on neoadjuvant chemotherapy clearly showed that objective response, as assessed by conventional CT scan, is amongst the best predictors of final outcome. However, even when significant response to chemotherapy and/or pathological downstaging of nodal status is achieved, the majority of patients do not survive to the disease. Several studies have addressed the question of whether FDG-PET is more reliable than conventional CT scan to predict final outcome. In a prospective study of 47 patients with stage IIIA-N2 NSCLC, it was shown that a decrease in FDG uptake greater than or equal to 35% after one cycle of neoadjuvant chemotherapy correlates with an increased survival. Less clear-cut observations were made on a similar prospective study by Poettgen et al. on 46 patients with stage III NSCLC. Surprisingly, a wide range of SUV levels after neoadjuvant chemotherapy were observed even in patients with pathologic complete response; since mean SUV was found to strongly correlate with the macrophage counts, the detection of high FDG uptake (and SUV levels) after neoadjuvant chemotherapy may be due to extensive macrophage infiltration, rather than reflecting the presence of residual viable tumor tissue. The concept that postinduction FDG uptake should be interpreted with caution (particularly in larger residual tumor volumes), is further supported by the results of a recent systematic review about the role of FDG-PET for evaluating response after neoadjuvant therapy in locally advanced NSCLC. After selecting for final analysis nine prospective trials, the authors pointed out that, due to the lack of standardized protocols for patient preparation, image acquisition and interpretation, FDG-PET should not be used in clinical practice for selecting patients for surgical resection after neoadjuvant chemotherapy in locally advanced NSCLC.

The same problems due to lack of reproducibility and standardization of the measurement and poor harmonization of response criteria also apply to the clinical setting of the advanced NSCLC. As almost one-third of patients experience early progression during first-line chemotherapy, a reliable predictive method of response could reduce the proportion of patients undergoing toxic therapy without benefit. However, also in this field, the experience with FDG-PET is limited and inconclusive. The most clear-cut observations were made by Weber et al. who repeated PET scan before and after the first cycle of platinum-based chemotherapy in 57 patients with advanced disease to assess whether metabolic response (as defined as a decrease in SUV of 20% or more) is predictive of benefit. Interestingly, metabolic "responders" had longer time to progression (163 days vs 54 days) and median survival (252 days vs 151 days) and higher 1-year survival rate (44% vs 10%) compared to "nonresponders". The ability of pretreatment FDG-PET to predict the response to chemotherapy was confirmed in another study by Lee et al. However, higher response rates did not translate into a survival advantage, due to significantly shorter response duration and time to progression observed in patients with high SUV levels. The authors postulate that high FDG uptake, response to chemotherapy and shorter response duration simply mirror rapid proliferation of hypermetabolic tumor cells and raise concerns on the reliability of response rates as surrogate endpoints for survival. In conclusion, there are some data suggesting that FDG-PET may have a predictive value in neoadjuvant chemotherapy in locally advanced and also in early steps of first-line chemotherapy in advanced NSCLC. However, monitoring tumor response with FDG-PET is still in its infancy. Studies are underway in the setting of targeted therapy and several questions regarding timing with respect to anticancer therapy and technical aspects, including measurement of FDG uptake and thresholds to define metabolic response are unresolved. Therefore, in the absence of prospective multi-institutional studies aimed at the standardization of PET imaging protocols and with prospectively defined response criteria, despite promising, at this time FDG-PET cannot be suggested as a reliable tool for anticipating or monitoring response to chemotherapy.

ROLE OF PET IN RADIOTHERAPY

The FDG-PET is increasingly being used in RT planning in NSCLC and small cell lung cancer (SCLC). RT is a key modality in LC treatment. The main clinical indications in the curative setting are: (1) alternative to surgery in patients with resectable LC refusing surgery or inoperable for medical reasons; (2) local control of relapsed or incompletely-resected NSCLC; (3) combined with chemotherapy in locally advanced unresectable NSCLC and SCLC. In all these clinical circumstances, careful patient selection with appropriate staging and accurate identification of target volume are essential to maximize clinical benefit. An incorrect definition of the gross tumor volume (GTV) (i.e. detectable tumor) or clinical target volume (CTV) (tumor plus a margin of 0.5–0.8 cm for microscopic extension) or an incorrect definition of nodal involvement is a common source of error, which can lead to undertreatment and a reduced probability of tumor control. Alternatively and most importantly, in the case of obstructive bronchial lesions, CT-based distinction between tumor and disventilated normal lung tissue (obstructive atelectasis) may be difficult. In the latter clinical circumstance, one has to decide whether to treat the entire region of combined tumor and atelectatic lung (thereby damaging large volumes of pulmonary tissue) or simply guessing the tumor boundaries with the consequent risk of geographic miss of target.

It has been previously shown that PET-derived GTVs are usually smaller than those suggested by CT scan, leading to reduced total radiation dose and reduced esophageal toxicity. In addition, the ability of PET/CT to allow reliable identification of tumor volume has been confirmed by the striking correlation found with observation made on resected specimens. Moreover, interobserver variability in definition of GTV contours is significantly reduced by adding PET to CT in the preliminary steps of RT planning. Despite all these potential benefits of incorporating PET in RT planning in LC, no randomized phase III trial is available at the moment clearly showing a clinical advantage of PET-assisted planning of RT. In this context, two prospective studies recruited also patients with advanced disease and the only appropriate study to address the question was a nonrandomized trial on patients with locally advanced NSCLC in which a survival benefit was shown in patients treated with PET-assisted planning of RT, compared to conventional CT-assisted planning. Another potential field of application of PET/CT in RT planning is related to its ability to allow identification of areas of resistance to RT to be treated with higher doses. It has long been known that hypoxic tumor cells are much more resistant to RT than well-oxygenated cells and there is strong evidence that LC cells are often hypoxic. Studies are underway to test this hypothesis with the application of alternative tracers, such as 18F-misonidazole or 18F-fluoroazomycin arabinoside, which have the potential to monitor changes in tumor hypoxia during therapy and to allow selective targeting of hypoxic subvolumes with a higher dose of RT.

BIBLIOGRAPHY AND FURTHER READING

1. Allen TL, Kendi AT, Mitiek MO, Maddaus MA. Combined contrast-enhanced computed tomography and 18-fluoro-2-deoxy-D-glucose-positron emission tomography in the diagnosis and staging of non-small cell lung cancer. Semin Thorac Cardiovasc Surg. 2011;23(1):43-50.
2. Blanchon F, Grivaux M, Asselain B, Lebas FX, Orlando JP, Piquet J, et al. 4-year mortality in patients with non-small-cell lung cancer: development and validation of a prognostic index. Lancet Oncol. 2006;7(10):829-36.
3. Borst GR, Belderbos JS, Boellaard R, Comans EF, De Jaeger K, Lammertsma AA, et al. Standardised FDG uptake: a prognostic factor for inoperable non-small cell lung cancer. Eur J Cancer. 2005;41(11):1533-41.
4. Cerfolio RJ, Bryant AS, Ohja B, Bartolucci AA. The maximum standardized uptake values on positron emission tomography of a non-small cell lung cancer predict stage, recurrence, and survival. J Thorac Cardiovasc Surg. 2005; 130(1):151-9.
5. de Geus-Oei LF, van der Heijden HF, Corstens FH, Oyen WJ. Predictive and prognostic value of FDG-PET in non-small-cell lung cancer: a systematic review. Cancer. 2007; 110(8):1654-64.
6. de Langen AJ, Raijmakers P, Riphagen I, Paul MA, Hoekstra OS. The size of mediastinal lymph nodes and its relation with metastatic involvement: a meta-analysis. Eur J Cardio-thorac Surg. 2006;29(1):26-9.
7. De Wever W, Ceyssens S, Mortelmans L, Stroobants S, Marchal G, Bogaert J, et al. Additional value of PET-CT in the staging of lung cancer: comparison with CT alone, PET alone and visual correlation of PET and CT. Eur Radiol. 2007;17(1):23-32.
8. Fischer BM, Mortensen J, Højgaard L. Positron emission tomography in the diagnosis and staging of lung cancer: a systematic, quantitative review. Lancet Oncol. 2001;2(11): 659-66.
9. Goerg C, Schwerk WB, Wolf M, Havemann K. Adrenal masses in lung cancer: sonographic diagnosis and follow-up. Eur J Cancer. 1992;28A(8-9):1400-3.
10. Gould MK, Kuschner WG, Rydzak CE, Maclean CC, Demas AN, Shigemitsu H, et al. Test performance of positron emission tomography and computed tomography for mediastinal staging in patients with non-small-cell lung cancer: a meta-analysis. Ann Intern Med. 2003;139(11):-879-92.
11. Haberkorn U, Morr I, Oberdorfer F, Bellemann ME, Blatter J, Altmann A, et al. Fluorodeoxyglucose uptake in vitro: aspects of method and effects of treatment with gemcitabine. J Nucl Med. 1994;35(11):1842-50.
12. Herder GJ, Kramer H, Hoekstra OS, Smit EF, Pruim J, van Tinteren H, et al. Traditional versus up-front [18F] fluorodeoxyglucose-positron emission tomography staging of non-small-cell lung cancer: a Dutch cooperative randomized study. J Clin Oncol. 2006;24(12):1800-6.
13. Hillers TK, Sauve MD, Guyatt GH. Analysis of published studies on the detection of extrathoracic metastases in patients presumed to have operable non-small cell lung cancer. Thorax. 1994;49(1):14-9.
14. Hoang JK, Hoagland LF, Coleman RE, Coan AD, Herndon JE, Patz EF. Prognostic value of fluorine-18 fluorodeoxyglucose positron emission tomography imaging in patients with advanced-stage non-small-cell lung carcinoma. J Clin Oncol. 2008;26(9):1459-64.
15. Hoekstra CJ, Stroobants SG, Smit EF, Vansteenkiste J, van Tinteren H, Postmus PE, et al. Prognostic relevance of response evaluation using [18F]-2-fluoro-2-deoxy-D-glucose positron emission tomography in patients with locally advanced non-small-cell lung cancer. J Clin Oncol. 2005;23(33): 8362-70.
16. Hustinx R, Paulus P, Jacquet N, Jerusalem G, Bury T, Rigo P. Clinical evaluation of whole-body 18F-fluorodeoxyglucose positron emission tomography in the detection of liver metastases. Ann Oncol. 1998;9(4):397-401.
17. Jadvar H, Alavi A, Gambhir SS. 18F-FDG uptake in lung, breast, and colon cancers: molecular biology correlates and disease characterization. J Nucl Med. 2009;50(11):1820-7.
18. Jemal A, Siegel R, Ward E, Hao Y, Xu J, Thun MJ. Cancer statistics, 2009. CA Cancer J Clin. 2009;59(4):225-49.
19. Jeong YJ, Yi CA, Lee KS. Solitary pulmonary nodules: detection, characterization, and guidance for further diagnostic workup and treatment. AJR Am J Roentgenol. 2007;188(1):57-68.
20. Kanters SD, Lammers JW, Voest EE. Molecular and biological factors in the prognosis of non-small cell lung cancer. Eur Respir J. 1995;8(8):1389-97.
21. Kelloff GJ, Hoffman JM, Johnson B, Scher HI, Siegel BA, Cheng EY, et al. Progress and promise of FDG-PET imaging for cancer patient management and oncologic drug development. Clin Cancer Res. 2005;11(8):2785-808.
22. Kim SK, Allen-Auerbach M, Goldin J, Fueger BJ, Dahlbom M, Brown M, et al. Accuracy of PET/CT in characterization of solitary pulmonary lesions. J Nucl Med. 2007;48(2):214-20.
23. Kolodziejczyk M, Kepka L, Dziuk M, Zawadzka A, Szalus N, Gizewska A, et al. Impact of [18F]fluorodeoxyglucose PET-CT staging on treatment planning in radiotherapy incorporating elective nodal irradiation for non-small-cell lung cancer: a prospective study. Int J Radiat Oncol Biol Phys. 2011;80(4):1008-14.

24. Lee HY, Chung JK, Jeong JM, Lee DS, Kim DG, Jung HW, et al. Comparison of FDG-PET findings of brain metastasis from non-small-cell lung cancer and small-cell lung cancer. Ann Nucl Med. 2008;22(4):281-6.
25. Lee KH, Lee SH, Kim DW, Kang WJ, Chung JK, Im SA, et al. High fluorodeoxyglucose uptake on positron emission tomography in patients with advanced non-small cell lung cancer on platinum-based combination chemotherapy. Clin Cancer Res. 2006;12(14 Pt 1):4232-6.
26. Lorent N, De Leyn P, Lievens Y, Verbeken E, Nackaerts K, Dooms C, et al. Long-term survival of surgically staged IIIA-N2 non-small-cell lung cancer treated with surgical combined modality approach: analysis of a 7-year prospective experience. Ann Oncol. 2004;15(11):1645-53.
27. MacMahon H, Austin JH, Gamsu G, Herold CJ, Jett JR, Naidich DP, et al. Guidelines for management of small pulmonary nodules detected on CT scans: a statement from the Fleischner Society. Radiology. 2005;237(2):395-400.
28. Mac Manus MP, Hicks RJ, Ball DL, Kalff V, Matthews JP, Salminen E, et al. F-18 fluorodeoxyglucose positron emission tomography staging in radical radiotherapy candidates with nonsmall cell lung carcinoma: powerful correlation with survival and high impact on treatment. Cancer. 2001;92(4):886-95.
29. MacManus MP, Hicks RJ, Matthews JP, Hogg A, McKenzie AF, Wirth A, et al. High rate of detection of unsuspected distant metastases by pet in apparent stage III non-small-cell lung cancer: implications for radical radiation therapy. Int J Radiat Oncol Biol Phys. 2001;50(2):287-93.
30. Mac Manus MP, Wong K, Hicks RJ, Matthews JP, Wirth A, Ball DL. Early mortality after radical radiotherapy for non-small-cell lung cancer: comparison of PET-staged and conventionally staged cohorts treated at a large tertiary referral center. Int J Radiat Oncol Biol Phys. 2002;52(2):351-61.
31. Marom EM, McAdams HP, Erasmus JJ, Goodman PC, Culhane DK, Coleman RE, et al. Staging non-small cell lung cancer with whole-body PET. Radiology. 1999;212(3):803-9.
32. Novello S, Giaj Levra M, Vavalà T. Functional imaging in predicting response to antineoplastic agents and molecular targeted therapies in lung cancer: a review of existing evidence. Crit Rev Oncol Hematol. 2012;83(2):208-15.
33. Ost DE, Gould MK. Decision making in patients with pulmonary nodules. Am J Respir Crit Care Med. 2012; 185(4):363-72.
34. Pieterman RM, van Putten JW, Meuzelaar JJ, Mooyaart EL, Vaalburg W, Koëter GH, et al. Preoperative staging of non-small-cell lung cancer with positron-emission tomography. N Engl J Med. 2000;343(4):254-61.
35. Poettgen C, Theegarten D, Eberhardt W, Levegruen S, Gauler T, Krbek T, et al. Correlation of PET/CT findings and histopathology after neoadjuvant therapy in non-small cell lung cancer. Oncology. 2007;73(5-6):316-23.
36. Pretreatment evaluation of non-small-cell lung cancer. The American Thoracic Society and the European Respiratory Society. Am J Respir Crit Care Med. 1997;156(1):320-32.
37. Qu X, Huang X, Yan W, Wu L, Dai K. A meta-analysis of 18FDG-PET-CT, 18FDG-PET, MRI and bone scintigraphy for diagnosis of bone metastases in patients with lung cancer. Eur J Radiol. 2012;81(5):1007-15.
38. Rebollo-Aguirre AC, Ramos-Font C, Villegas Portero R, Cook GJ, Llamas Elvira JM, Romero Tabares A. Is FDG-PET suitable for evaluating neoadjuvant therapy in non-small cell lung cancer? Evidence with systematic review of the literature. J Surg Oncol. 2010;101(6):486-94.
39. Sant M, Allemani C, Santaquilani M, Knijn A, Marchesi F, Capocaccia R, et al. EUROCARE-4. Survival of cancer patients diagnosed in 1995-1999. Results and commentary. Eur J Cancer. 2009;45(6):931-91.
40. Silvestri GA, Gould MK, Margolis ML, Tanoue LT, McCrory D, Toloza E, et al. Noninvasive staging of non-small cell lung cancer: ACCP evidenced-based clinical practice guidelines (2nd edition). Chest. 2007;132(3 Suppl):178S-201S.
41. Toloza EM, Harpole L, McCrory DC. Noninvasive staging of non-small cell lung cancer: a review of the current evidence. Chest. 2003;123(1 Suppl):137S-46S.
42. van Baardwijk A, Bosmans G, Boersma L, Buijsen J, Wanders S, Hochstenbag M, et al. PET-CT-based auto-contouring in non-small-cell lung cancer correlates with pathology and reduces interobserver variability in the delineation of the primary tumor and involved nodal volumes. Int J Radiat Oncol Biol Phys. 2007;68(3):771-8.
43. van Der Wel A, Nijsten S, Hochstenbag M, Lamers R, Boersma L, Wanders R, et al. Increased therapeutic ratio by 18FDG-PET CT planning in patients with clinical CT stage N2-N3M0 non-small-cell lung cancer: a modeling study. Int J Radiat Oncol Biol Phys. 2005;61(3):649-55.
44. Vansteenkiste JF, Stroobants SG. The role of positron emission tomography with 18F-fluoro-2-deoxy-D-glucose in respiratory oncology. Eur Respir J. 2001;17(4):802-20.
45. van Tinteren H, Hoekstra OS, Smit EF, van den Bergh JH, Schreurs AJ, Stallaert RA, et al. Effectiveness of positron emission tomography in the preoperative assessment of patients with suspected non-small-cell lung cancer: the PLUS multicentre randomised trial. Lancet. 2002;-359(9315):1388-93.
46. Weber WA, Petersen V, Schmidt B, Tyndale-Hines L, Link T, Peschel C, et al. Positron emission tomography in non-small-cell lung cancer: prediction of response to chemotherapy by quantitative assessment of glucose use. J Clin Oncol. 2003;21(14):2651-7.

Section 4

Invasive Diagnostic Procedures

Chapter

26 Diagnostic Applications of Flexible Bronchoscopy

Dhruv Joshi, Sergio Agati, Claudio Sorino, Thomas R Gildea

BACKGROUND

Flexible bronchoscopy is a minimally invasive procedure that allows a clinician to explore the airways for diagnostic and therapeutic purposes. The instrument (flexible bronchoscope) uses a long, thin, lighted tube that is inserted through the nose, mouth or, less frequently, tracheostomy.

The tip of the instrument can be oriented, allowing the practitioner to navigate into the bronchi. It causes less discomfort for the patient than rigid bronchoscopy, and offers a better view of smaller airways. The procedure can be performed easily and safely under moderate sedation, without general anesthesia.

The bronchology derives from the experience of Professor Gustav Killian, who in 1897 carried off a piece of pig bone located in the right main bronchus of a pastor with the aid of rigid esophagoscope, under local anesthesia with cocaine, avoiding the usual tracheotomy. Subsequently, in 1905, Chevalier Jackson offered the first standardization of this technique, writing the first systematic treatise and providing technical improvements to the bronchoscope. For about 60 years, bronchoscopists worked with rigid instruments.

The first prototype of the flexible bronchoscope was presented at the 9th International Congress on Diseases of the Chest in Copenhagen in 1966. Since then, the flexible bronchoscope has gone through several iterations. With the addition of several accessories and new technologies, it has now become one the most helpful tools in the hands of pulmonologists for the diagnosis of airway and lung parenchymal diseases.

The first flexible bronchoscope was made by a fiberoptic bundle with a lens on one end and an eyepiece on the other through which the airways were directly viewed.

In the 1980s, the fiberoptic instrument was replaced by a videobronchoscope and this enabled the image to be displayed on a screen. This was accompanied by improvements in the image quality, development of the working channel and improvement in the angulation of the bronchoscope. It is this form of the bronchoscope that is now widely used by bronchoscopists. The ability of the videobronchoscope to project images has also led to its importance as a teaching tool.

EQUIPMENT AND ADVANCES IN BRONCHOSCOPY

The bronchoscope is a lightweight instrument, fully immersible for disinfecting and with bending angles that permit to reach most bronchial branches (Figs. 26.1 and 26.2). It consists of: a central body with the handle; a working channel with a bioptic valve to introduce liquids or operational tools (brushes, forceps, needles); a valve to set the suction, connected to a metal fitting which engages the vacuum tube, and a suction system which, again through the operating channel, allows the suction of secretions, blood and foreign bodies.

The light source may be halogen, incandescent or light-emitting diode (LED). It can be powered by a portable battery or via a cable.

There are bronchoscopes for adults and for children which differ in the distal diameter. In the adult, it is possible to use the standard or a larger model, with distal diameter that can vary from 3.7 mm to 6.4 mm and a working channel which can range from 1.2 mm to 3.2 mm. By virtue of its smaller size, the standard adult model (outer diameter 5.7 mm; working channel 2 mm) is well tolerated and at the same time it allows to practice most

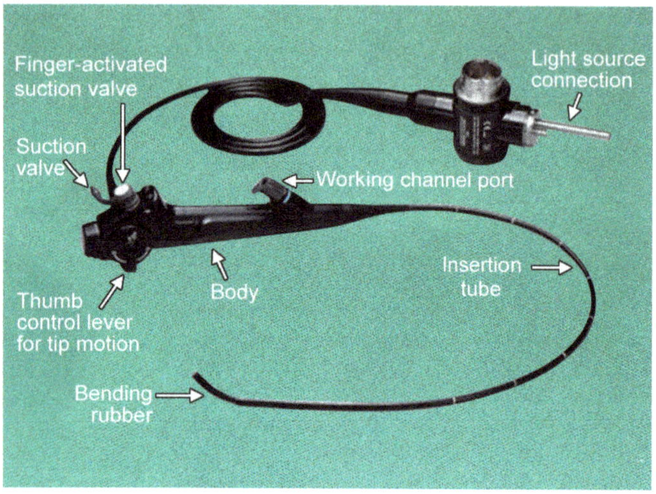

Fig. 26.1: Example of a flexible videobronchoscope with its components. *Courtesy*: Olympus Europa SE & CO. KG.

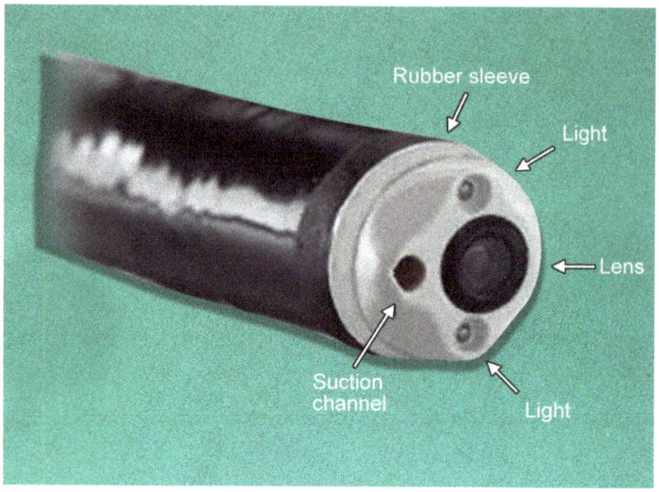

Fig. 26.2: Details of the tip of a flexible bronchoscope.

common techniques, and for this reason it is very versatile. The largest bronchoscopes (outer diameter 6.2-6.4 mm; working channel 3.2 mm) allow the passage of larger instruments, guarantees a more effective suction and it has a wider field of view. The ultraslim model can be used to visualize airways in children. In adults, it enables to visualize thinner bronchi of the lung periphery but it does not allow adequate suction and only very small.

The regular flexible bronchoscope consists in a fiberoptic channel, formed by bundles of optical fibers that transmit light and images, held together by a special adhesive that allows scrolling without any break during flexion. Through a terminal made of an electrical connector, the instrument can be connected to a light source. The vision is directly gotten from an eyepiece on the top of the central body. A camera can be mounted on the lens to visualize the image on a monitor.

To achieve the highest quality of image, the diameter of the optical fibers has been decreased, approaching 5 μm, minimizing the thickness of the adhesive as possible. However, the grid of optical fibers is not completely eliminated, and this is the limit of the fiberoptic bronchoscopy.

Digital technology is responsible for the evolution of these instruments with the extensive spread of videobronchoscope. The fiberoptic channel has been replaced by a video charge-coupled device (CCD) which allows transmission of the image to a video processor and the visualization on a screen.

This technology guarantees to obtain images of much higher quality, easy to edit and to archive. In addition to the improved imaging quality, latest devices such as narrow band imaging (NBI), autofluorescence, and magnification bronchoscopes have propelled bronchoscopic immaging into the 21st century. A wide array of brushes, needles, catheters, and forceps are available to aid with newer diagnostic techniques. In the past decade, endoscopic ultrasound technology bronchoscopies have come to the forefront in the evaluation of endobronchial, mediastinal, and parenchymal lesions.

INDICATIONS FOR DIAGNOSTIC BRONCHOSCOPY (BOX 26.1)

Bronchoscopy is indicated for the diagnosis of various lung diseases in relation to the possibility of a simple inspection or to take samples in the lower airways. Adequate radiological documentation must precede the maneuver, with the purpose of identifying correctly the seat of the pathological process and to choose the most appropriate procedure.

Particularly bronchoscopy is commonly used in the definition of pulmonary infiltrates of unknown nature. In patients with signs and symptoms of infection of lower airways, it allows to recover microbiological samples, especially when sputum is not present. In this way, it is possible to define the etiology and choose a more targeted antibiotic therapy. The examination should be performed routinely in immunocompromised patients for diagnosing opportunistic infections. Sampling of the lower airways is also indicated in pneumonia with slow or incomplete healing.

Box 26.1: Indications for diagnostic bronchoscopy.

- Malignancy
  - Diagnosis of bronchogenic carcinoma
  - Staging of bronchogenic carcinoma
  - Restaging after therapy and/or initial mediastinoscopy
  - Abnormal sputum cytology
  - Follow-up after treatment of carcinoma
  - Evaluation of patients with head and neck malignancy
  - Evaluation of patients with esophageal malignancy
  - Metastatic carcinoma
  - Mediastinal mass
- Infection
  - Recurrent or unresolved pneumonia
  - Infiltrate in an immunocompromised patient
  - Cavitary lesion
- Unexplained lung collapse
- Interstitial lung disease
- Hemoptysis
- Unexplained chronic cough
- Localized wheezing
- Stridor
- Foreign body aspiration
- Chest trauma
  - Blunt or penetrating
  - Chemical
  - Thermal
- Unexplained pleural effusion
- Evaluation of the patient after lung transplantation
- Endotracheal intubation
  - Confirm tube position
  - Evaluate for tube-related injury
  - Confirm position of transtracheal oxygen catheter
- Tracheobronchial stricture and stenosis
- Hoarseness or vocal cord paralysis
- Superior vena cava syndrome
- Fistula
  - Bronchopleural
  - Tracheo- or bronchoesophageal
  - Tracheo- or bronchoaortic
- Persistent pneumothorax
- Postoperative assessment of tracheal, tracheobronchial, bronchial, or stump anastomosis
- Bronchography

In the case of centrally localized masses or nodules, bronchoscopy is an essential diagnsotic tool for cyto-and histopathological analysis.

In the case of peripheral lesions, particularly of small dimensions, fluoroscopic guidance, electromagnetic navigation guidance, or radial probe ultrasound guidance permit to sample blindly even in the absence of a direct endoscopic view. Flexible bronchoscopes with a thin diameter (between 2.8 mm and 3.5 mm) permit to reach smaller peripheral airways, but the image quality and the small size of the operating channel often do not ensure adequate collecting.

Transbronchial needle aspiration (TBNA) is a tool to sample enlarged mediastinal or hilar lymph nodes or masses. TBNA with ultrasound guidance [endobronchial ultrasound-guided transbronchial needle aspiration (EBUS-TBNA)] is safer and is very effective not only in diagnosis but also in the nodal staging of lung cancer. The EBUS-TBNA is less invasive than mediastinoscopy and may displace it in a growing number of cases.

In the case of hemoptysis, bronchoscopy is used to confirm a source of bleeding from the lower airways through a direct visualization of the area from which the blood comes. At the same time it is possible to provide for a local management of the leak via laser, argon plasma coagulation (APC), balloon tamponade, or selective occlusion of the suspected bronchus with a blockade catheter. In case of massive bleeding, the use of rigid bronchoscopy is the most indicated.

In patients presenting with persistent, not yet identified atelectasis, or possible bronchial obstruction, bronchoscopy allows to identify the site of the obstruction and eventually its removal (e.g. mucus plug, foreign body).

An inspection of the airways is useful in patients scheduled for lobectomy or pneumonectomy and to control the anastomosis after surgery. Again with the aim of checking airways, the bronchoscopy is used when tracheostomy tubes are placed (to point out any complications as displacement or percutaneous insertion), when tracheobronchial or bronchopleural fistulas are suspected and after blunt or open chest and neck trauma.

Even in the diagnosis of not yet justified symptoms such as coughing or wheezing or in the case of persistent pneumothorax, lower airways endoscopic exploration is recommended.

In a patient undergoing lung transplant, bronchoscopy is performed to assess possible rejection, its severity, and to diagnose opportunistic infections. Even the lung donor undergoes endoscopic control before explantation, to assess the condition of the airways and to reveal any infectious states.

Bronchoscopy is the gold standard in the dynamic assessment of the airways, in the diagnosis of tracheomalacia and tracheobronchomalacia.

The use of flexible bronchoscopy with autofluorescence or NBI in the early detection of precancerous lesions of trachea and more proximal airways is still controversial.

CONTRAINDICATIONS TO FLEXIBLE BRONCHOSCOPY (BOX 26.2)

A careful planning is required before performing any endoscopic maneuver, considering the goal to be achieved, in order to choose the most suitable procedure with the highest chance of diagnstic success and the lowest risk. Pre-existing comorbidities should be previously assessed since they may increase the risk.

Bronchoscopy is not indicated when there is a high probability of complications related to the procedure itself or to the sedation. The partial airway obstruction and the sedation are able to affect gas exchange also in normal subjects.

The contraindications to endoscopic maneuvers might be absolute or relative. Considering that in bronchoscopy the major complications are rare, absolute contraindications are few. The lack of informed consent is the most relevant, especially in the case of elective examinations. The patient must provide consent after adequate information about indication, risks, and diagnostic alternatives. If he cannot provide it, because unconscious or sedated, it is used to proceed only in the case of clear danger for his survival. The examination should be also avoided if there are not proper conditions for adequate oxygenation or if equipment malfunctions are known.

Bronchoscopy may have systemic effects on the cardiovascular system such as an increase in mean systemic pressure, changes in cardiac index and abnormal rhythms. Not-urgent procedures should not be performed in the course of an acute myocardial infarction (MI) or unstable angina and should be reprogrammed after 6 weeks. Even in patients with severe hypertension/hypotension or uncontrolled rhythm disturbances (tachycardia/bradycardia), the risks and the benefits of the procedures should be weighed.

Box 26.2: Contraindications to flexible bronchoscopy.

- Absolute contraindications
  - Inadequate oxygenation during the procedure
- Relative contraindications
  - Malignant arrhythmia
  - Unstable cardiac status
  - Refractory hypoxemia
  - Bleeding diathesis or severe thrombocytopenia (if biopsy is anticipated)
- Factors associated with increased risk of complications
  - Uncooperative patient
  - Recent or unstable angina
  - Unstable asthma
  - Moderate to severe hypoxemia
  - Hypercarbia
  - Uremia
  - Thrombocytopenia
  - Pulmonary hypertension
  - Lung abscess
  - Immunosuppression
  - Superior vena cava obstruction
  - Debility, advanced age, or malnutrition
  - Recent use of clopidogrel

A severe hypoxemia [partial pressure of oxygen (PaO_2) < 60 mm Hg or saturation < 90%, with a fraction of inspired oxygen (FiO_2) > 60%] is a high-risk condition and when bronchoscopy is absolutely indispensable (for example, in the presence of endobronchial foreign body), it is possible to proceed with the support of noninvasive ventilation (NIV) or after placement of laryngeal mask airway (LMA) or orotracheal tube. In these cases, the patients must be well-informed about the risks, especially for elective intubation.

In patients with respiratory failure and hypercapnia, it must be paid attention to the amount of oxygen delivered, as it can further worsen the blood gas analysis profile. The NIV provides better control of gas exchanges than the Venturi mask, but it seems to increase the risk for orotracheal intubation after the examination.

Patients with severe chronic obstructive pulmonary disease (COPD) [forced expiratory volume in the first 1 second of expiration (FEV1) < 1.2 L; FEV1/forced vital capacity (FVC) < 50%], unstable asthma or with previous intensive care unit (ICU) admission are at high risk for events of moderate to severe bronchospasm. The premedication with bronchodilators and a good control of asthma symptoms minimize this risk.

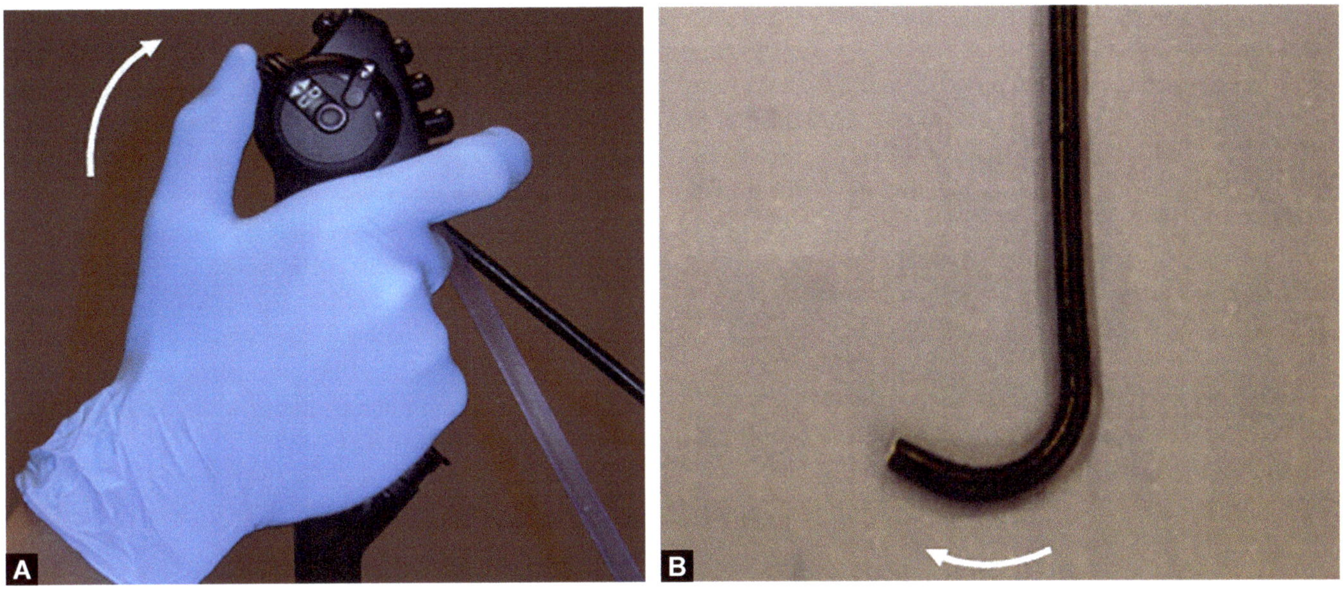

Figs. 26.3A and B: Movements of the distal tip of the bronchoscope. When the thumb pushes up the control level, the tip of the bronchoscope is extended backward up to 110° (extension). On the opposite, if the lever is pushed down, the tip of the bronchoscope is flexed forward up to 130° (flexion).

In patients with anticoagulation, antiplatelet or thrombocytopenia, coagulopathies, severe uremia and pulmonary hypertension, the risk of bleeding is higher in procedures involving brushings, biopsies, or needle aspirations. Risk can be minimized by the timely suspension of current therapies and replacement with low molecular weight heparins. High-risk conditions are: platelet count of 50,000 platelets/mm^3 or lower, an international normalized ratio (INR) of 1.3 or greater or an elevated partial thromboplastin time (PTT) 1.5 times baseline and blood urea nitrogen (BUN) greater than 30 mg/dL. The infusion of platelets or fresh frozen plasma (FFP) should be indicated before the endoscopies, to correct the abnormalities.

Bronchoscopy is safe in older subjects, in which it is very important to take care to sedation. Non-urgent procedures should be avoided in pregnant women and postponed after birth or at least after 28 weeks of gestation. If indispensable, proceeding under general anesthesia should be indicated.

TECHNIQUE

Before starting the examination, it is necessary to choose the most suitable bronchoscope, which depends on the patient's condition and the purpose of the procedure.

The bronchoscope was designed to be used with the left hand guiding the bronchoscope, while the other is used to operate the suction channel and the lever. A right-handed operator often prefers to guide the bronchoscope with right hand. The control lever, which controls the tip, is moved with the thumb and it only permits movement in a vertical plane (Figs. 26.3A and B). Two wires extend from the handle to the tip, in the insertion cord. Moving the lever down, moves the tip up and moving the lever up, points the tip down. Side to side movement is accomplished by rotation of the body of the bronchoscope with the operator's wrist and shoulder.

The flexible bronchoscope can be usually inserted via the nose or via the oral route. The nasal route offers a better view of the nasal cavity, pharynx, and larynx. It allows more stability of the instrument when passing through the vocal cords, avoids bite damage and ensures less stimulation of the gag reflex, maneuvering with precision.

The oral route is preferable in the risk of bleeding, in the case of removal of foreign bodies, septal deviation, polyps, trauma. In patients who have tracheotomies, the airway can be directly assessed by inserting the flexible bronchoscope via the stoma site.

POSITIONING AND ROUTES OF ACCESS

For the bronchoscopist to safely and adequately perform the procedure, it is essential to have a good understanding of the anatomy and to properly position the patient. The supine position is more comfortable for the patient and for the operator and easier and safer in emergency procedures or in the event of complications. However, a semisupine or sitting position may also be used if supine positioning cannot be performed. The operator can stand in front of or behind the head of the patient, depending on his experience. Standing in front of the patient, the vision will appear inverted. Ahead there is the back wall and the right of the patient will correspond to the left of the operator and vice versa. Behind the head there will be a more easy understanding through the precise correspondence between the various anatomical structures with opertaor point of view.

If necessary, flexible bronchoscopy may be performed after endotracheal intubating the patient. In this method, the endotracheal tube is initially inserted into the trachea and then the bronchoscope is advanced through the lumen of the tube, directly into the trachea and the major airways. This is suggested for unstable patients, including those with altered cognitive status unable to protect their airway, and those with significant hypoxia, in order to ensure a stability of the airways. Endotracheal intubation is also used in subjects with hemoptysis when the placement of endobronchial blockers or unilateral main-stem intubation may be required, and very rarely when patients are unable to cooperate due to severe anxiety. If a standard 5.7-mm bronchoscope is used, the endotracheal tube should have an internal diameter of at least 8 mm.

PREPARATION

Preparation is a crucial moment on which depends, in a large part, the success of bronchoscopy. It aims to reduce risks and discomfort for the patient.

The discomfort may be due to several causes: the anxiety connected with the condition of the disease, the lack of information on health status, the modalities of the examination.

Usually, there is a discrepancy between medical staff and patients in the evaluation of suffering. Physicians tend to underestimate the discomfort and then to treat it improperly.

The best possible psychological support should be given. There should be a welcoming environment and a professional personnel. The room must be equipped for emergencies. Information should be accurate, explaining the procedure in all steps. It should be explained that the transition from the nose can give pain; passing through the vocal cords and the trachea gives a feeling of suffocation and contact with the bronchial mucosa can give a cough.

A good practice would provide the use of a checklist, to focus attention on all the issues to be considered before starting the procedure. It could be written down important information such as the medical history: possible smoking status, allergies, significant diseases (such as heart or lung disease), previous surgeries.

The examination should be performed fasting to reduce the volume and the acidic contents of the stomach. This is to reduce the possible risk of regurgitation and aspiration of gastric material. The British guidelines suggest four hours of fasting. The prescribed therapy should be taken with a minimal amount of water always 4 hours before the examination, if possible.

It should be useful to know the value of some blood tests, such as hemoglobin and platelet counts, particularly in the case of biopsies, and liver and kidney function for sedation. In patients with oral anticoagulation therapy (OAT), it is recommended to ensure that the INR is below 1.3.

In view of the execution of biopsy, it is necessary to verify the correct interruption of any antiplatelet or anticoagulation therapy. The management of these treatments is very delicate because it is essential to correlate the bleeding risk with the risk of thrombotic events.

Due to the long duration of their action, vitamin K antagonists (VKA) require their replacement with low molecular weight heparins (the so-called "bridging"), exploiting their short duration. The treatment should be stopped at least 3 days before the procedure. Even if not supported by randomized trials, this behavior is common practice for years and has proved safety and efficacy. Therapy with subcutaneous low molecular weight heparin should be suspended in the past 12 hours.

In theory, the *novel oral anticoagulants (NOACs)* have advantages compared to VKA, due to their short blood half-life and their rapid anticoagulant effect. It is feasible that a brief interruption during surgery is sufficient, without the need to perform bridging with heparins. The data to support this behavior are still very limited as regards evidence to support and clinical experience. The only recommendations currently applicable are derived from expert opinion, so it is essential that all local reality may work in close collaboration with prescriber centers to implement a more accurate monitoring of clinical effects.

In patients with normal renal function, the European Heart Rhythm Association (EHRA) experts suggest to schedule the procedure at least 24 hours after the last dose of NOAC. In case of impaired renal function, the procedure should be planned. In patients treated with dabigatran: if high glomerular filtration rate (GFR) is lower than 80 mL/minute, at least 36 hours after the last dose; if GFR is lower then 50 mL/minute, at least 48 hours after the last dose. In patients treated with apixaban and rivaroxaban: if GFR is between 15 mL/minute and 30 mL/minute, at least 36 hours after the last dose.

For endoscopic procedures without biopsy and low-risk interventions, in which you can provide a good local hemostasis, EHRA experts suggest not to interrupt the NOAC, performing the bronchoscopy preferably as late as possible after the last administration (12 hours after the last dose of dabigatran or apixaban, 24 hours after the last dose of rivaroxaban). Such behavior is common practice in patients treated with low molecular weight heparin or fondaparinux.

As for antiplatelet therapy, an adequate suspension of the drug must be provided. Ticlopidine has rapid action and it is active 1-2 hours after ingestion and removed after 24-96 hours. The clopidogrel antiplatelet action reaches its maximum effect after 4-7 days.

It is better to suspend ticlopidine and clopidogrel respectively 3-4 days and 6-7 days before the bronchoscopy. For Cardio Aspirin, the suspension it is recommended 48 hours before the examination.

In the case of biopsies in patients with heart valves or with a history of rheumatic valvular endocarditis, it might be useful an antibiotic prophylaxis.

Each patient undergoing bronchoscopy should have heart rate, respiratory rate, blood pressure and oxygen saturation recorded before, during and after the procedure.

The onset of hypoxemia during bronchoscopy is relatively common and it may persist for a few hours. There are different causes such as excessive sedation, bronchospasm, suction maneuvers with removal of oxygen and lung volume reduction below the functional residual capacity, and alveolar collapse by bleeding or instillation of liquid.

To reduce the risk of hypoxemia-related complications, oxygen supplementation should be used when pulse oximeter oxygen saturation is less than 90% or it reduces more than 4% for a prolonged time (> 1 minute). It is also recommended in old patients (> 65 years), heart diseases, pulmonary fibrosis, obstructive airway diseases with FEV1 less than 1 L. On the contrary, oxygen may be not administered in stable patients with pulse oximeter oxygen saturation greater than 90% (or PaO_2 > 60 mm Hg) and normal FEV1, because significant events of desaturation are rare in such patients.

Oxygen should be kept for 1-2 hours after the end of the examination in patients with chronic lung or heart disease or when a deep sedation has been performed. Moreover, in the case of heart diseases, the patient should undergo continuous ECG monitoring. A peripheral venous access must always be recovered to ensure the possibility to administer endovenous drugs during the examination or at the end, if necessary.

SEDATION

Bronchoscopic procedures performed under sedation are equally safe than those performed in the awake patient. However, the patient's satisfaction and procedure tolerance are improved with the use of sedation. Minimal, moderate, deep sedation or general anesthesia may be used, depending on several factors such as the setting, the complexity of procedure being performed, the anticipated length of the procedure and the patient's preference. Benzodiazepines and opioids are suggested for mild to moderate sedation. Short-acting agents, such as Midazolam and Fentanyl, are usually chosen to minimize the recovery time. Propofol is an altemative drug that may be used. It has an adverse events profile, an anesthetic effect, and a patient tolerance similar to combined benzodiazepines and opioids, whereas it has the advantage of a shorter recovery time.

Topical anesthesia is used as an adjunctive tool prior to and during the procedure as it helps decrease the cough and amount of systemic sedation needed to perform flexible bronchoscopy. Lidocaine is the preferred agent for topical anesthesia. It may be administered as a gel, solution or spray. Lidocaine has a good safety profile, but the minimum effective dose should be used. At high doses, it may have cardiac and neurologic toxicity, mainly in patients with advanced age, liver disease and heart failure. The maximum recommended dose based on the patient's weight is 4.5 mg/kg.

Anticholinergic agents such as atropine and glycopyrrolate have been routinely used by bronchoscopists to reduce coughing, airway secretions and prevent vasovagal episodes. However, the use of these agents has shown no significant benefit in the reduction of coughing, secretions, complication rates or improvement of patient tolerance. Differently, the use of atropine resulted in greater fluctuations of hemodynamic parameters, including increased blood pressure and pulse. Following that, these agents are no longer used for premedication prior to bronchoscopy.

ANATOMY OF AIRWAYS

Upper Airways

To perform bronchoscopy, it is useful to know the anatomical structures that will be encountered. When introducing the instrument through the nose, the upper respiratory tract appears. The nasal vestibule is the entrance of the nasal cavity. It is a channel with an inner skin, where hairs, called vibrissae, are implanted. It consists of a superficial orifice, through which the nasal cavity communicates with the outside, and a deep orifice, which constitutes effectively the beginning of the nasal cavity and therefore of the upper airways (Fig. 26.4). The *nasal cavity* comprises several structures:

- *Floor*: It has the form of a canal which extends laterally through the lower meatus and it is bordered medially by the septum and posteriorly by the choanae. It consists of the upper surface of the hard palate and separates the oral cavity from the nasal cavity.
- *Top wall*: It consists of different bones: the nasal spine of the frontal bone and the nasal bones (in the front); the cribriform plate of the ethmoid (medially); the horizontal process of the frontal bone (laterally); the body of the sphenoid (posteriorly).
- *Medial wall*: It corresponds with the nasal septum and it is constituted by a cartilaginous part (quadrangular cartilage) and a rear bony part.
- *Side wall*: It is extremely complex and has three bony protrusions called nasal turbinates respectively upper, middle and lower (sometimes could be a supreme one).

The side wall with the three turbinates delimitate three anatomical spaces called nasal meatuses (lower, middle, upper).

The *nasal pharynx* is a purely aerial portion of the pharynx, in direct relation with the nasal passages, at the top, and with the oropharyn, inferiorly.

Located in front of the cervical spine and below the base of the skull, it has a roughly hexagonal shape in adults. The upper wall, inclined downward and backward, has a bony skeleton made from the articulation of different bones. The back wall is in contiguity with bands of loose connective (retropharyngeal space) and with the superior pharyngeal constrictor muscle. The side wall is formed by the long muscles of the head, forming two wall reliefs. In the middle, it is possible to find the orifice of the eustachian tube, which has a triangular shape and is reduced to a simple slit at rest. This tube presents a front lip and a most protruding near lip. The pharyngeal recess is a deep depression located between the rear lip ostium

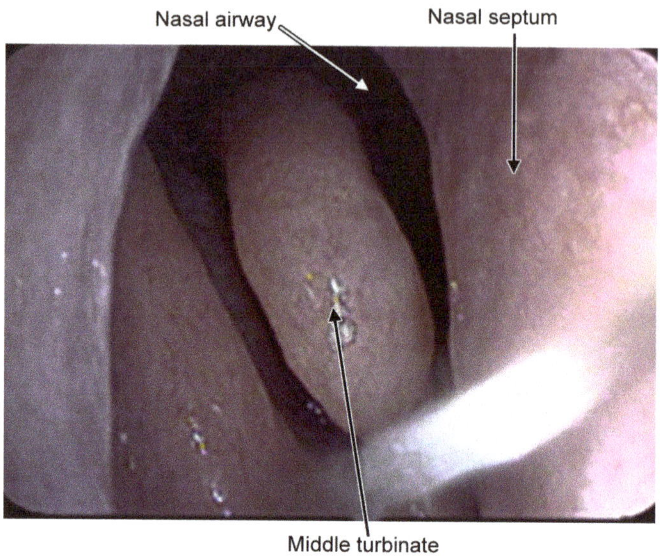

Fig. 26.4: Endoscopic view of nasal airway.

of the tube and the back wall. The front wall is formed by the choanae, empty areas that connect nasal cavity with nasal pharynx. The lower wall is formed by the dorsal surface of the soft palate and, behind the veil of the palate, the intrapharyngeal ostium connects nasopharynx and oropharynx.

The *oropharynx* opens to the outside through the isthmus of the mouth and communicates at the top with the nasopharynx, down with the larynx.

The upper wall of the oropharynx consists of the bottom surface of the soft palate, a large mucosa fold, placed posterior to the hard palate. Inferiorly, from the soft palate, a drop-shaped process descends, called uvula, formed internally by small muscle uvula. The side walls consist of two arches, the palate-pharyngeal and the palate-glottic, which originate from the soft palate, respectively posteriorly and in the front. They contain homonyms muscles. Ipsilateral between the two arches an alcove is formed, the tonsillar fossa, where the palatine tonsil can be found. The rear wall is continuing with that of the rhinopharynx.

The *larynx* is comprised between the upper margin of the epiglottis and the lower border of the cricoid cartilage. The front wall of the upper portion of the laryngopharynx is ideally the laryngeal entry, the cavity access to the larynx. The entry laryngeal is superiorly and anteriorly bordered by the bottom surface of the epiglottis. Laterally there are two recesses, the pyriform fossas, whcih are limited medially by the aryepiglottic folds and laterally by the margins of the thyroid cartilage.

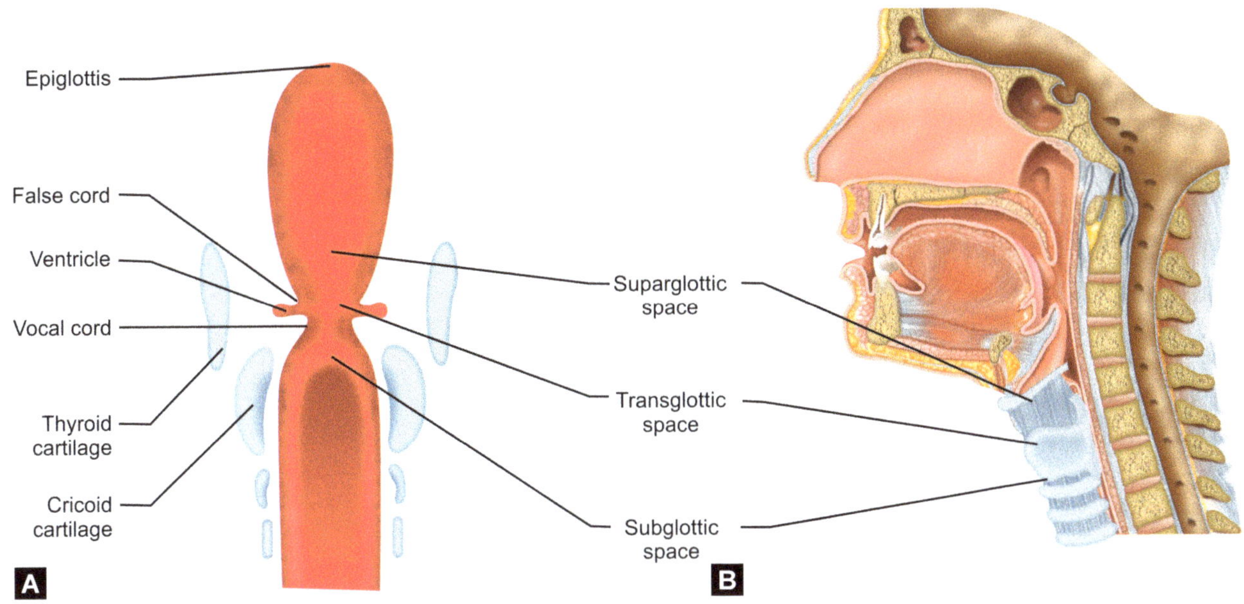

Figs. 26.5A and B: Anatomy of the larynx.

Larynx is divided into three major areas (Figs. 26.5A and B):

1. Supraglottic space, containing epiglottis, aryepiglottic folds, arytenoids, laryngeal ventricle, and ventricular bands.
2. Transglottic space, containing the vocal cords and the anterior and posterior commissures.
3. Subglottic space, which extends from the vocal folds to the cricoid cartilage.

Lower Airways

The airways are empty tubes through which air reaches the lungs, where the exchange of respiratory gases occurs. Trachea is the first structure of the lower airways. It is divided at the carina level (Fig. 26.6) into the two main bronchi, right and left. In any side, main bronchus divides gradually into lobar, segmental, subsegmental branch, continuing to branch out until the 19th division, when they end into terminal bronchioles.

Bronchi are covered by a mucous membrane which raises in longitudinal folds and it is constituted by columnar, ciliated, pseudostratified epithelium supported by a basement membrane. The epithelium is higher in the large airways and it becomes thin toward periphery. Immediately below this membrane, elastic fibers are gathered into thin bundles.

The rest of the wall includes the submucous tunica, which consists of loose connective tissue containing various accessory structures, such as the submucosal glands, blood vessels, lymph vessels and nerves, together with a muscular layer.

More externally there is the fibrous tunica, made of connective tissue, rich in elastic fibers. In the trachea, main and intermediate bronchi, the fibrous tunica wraps semilunar, horseshoe-shaped cartilages. The back wall of these structures is defined "pars membranous". It is rich in smooth muscle and has no cartilage. The gradual bronchial branching is associated with a progressive decrease of semilunar cartilages, until they are replaced with intermittent, cartilaginous plates, gradually less numerous. Downstream the last plate of cartilage the bronchioles originate. The layer of elastic fibers between mucosal epithelium and submucosa is gradually replaced by smooth muscle, which arranges in rings, surrounding the entire circumference of the bronchi. Some of the elastic fibers are consolidated in beams between mucosal epithelium and smooth muscle and appear as crests with a longitudinal course.

The endoscopic appearance of the bronchial mucosa varies according to age and could be influenced by environmental factors. In a young person, it has a reddish color and it is raised in clearly visible and well-defined folds, up to the subsegmental branches. The cartilaginous rings are overall slightly prominent.

With increasing age, profiles become less clear, for the reduction of elastic fibers, while the increase of collagen fibers makes cartilages more prominent.

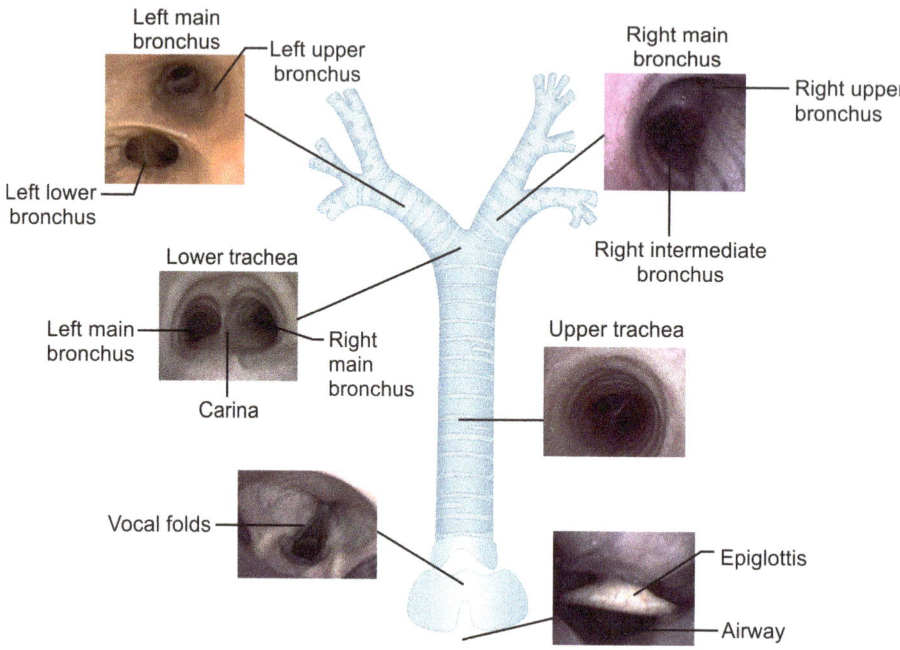

Fig. 26.6: Endoscopic anatomy of trachea and main bronchi.

In subjects with smoking or occupational exposure, bronchial mucosa presents deposits of inhaled substances and it could appear blackish.

Bronchial Nomenclature

Knowing the bronchial nomenclature is very important to be able to pinpoint the location of pathological processes in the radiology images and to be able to orientate correctly within the airways. The nomenclature has been reviewed and published in 1950 by an international committee and since then it is commonly used by all bronchoscopists (Table 26.1).

PROCEDURES

Regular flexible bronchoscopy has traditionally been used to perform procedures such as bronchial washing, bronchoalveolar lavage (BAL), bronchial brushing, bronchial biopsy, transbronchial biopsy, and TBNA. Such procedures, below briefly described, have been extensively addressed in dedicated chapters of this book.

Bronchial washing allows the clearance of the airway from mucus or blood. This technique involves the instillation of 5–30 mL of saline in the area of concern and the subsequent suction of fluid into a suction trap. This is usually sent for microbiological and cytological evaluation.

It should be noted that such microbiological examination may be hampered by contamination of the respiratory flora, whereas the cytological study for the detection of tumor cells on samples obtained by bronchial washing alone has a poor diagnostic yield, thus a combination of washings, brushings and biopsies is recommended.

Bronchoalveolar lavage is performed by a gentle instillation of normal saline through the scope and into the airway. The fluid is then suctioned back through the scope into a container where it can be sent to the lab for diagnostic testing.

Bronchial brushing is performed through a small brush which is introduced into the bronchoscopic working channel and the airways. It is then advanced back and forth in order to obtain an adequate sample to be sent to the lab for diagnostic testing (cytological and microbiological).

Endobronchial biopsy is performed through forceps that are then advanced through the bronchoscope to obtain tissue from visible bronchial lesions.

Transbronchial lung biopsy is a useful procedure for the diagnosis of peripheral lung lesions that cannot be directly visualized. In this technique, the bronchoscope is wedged as distally as possible and then small forceps are advanced via the working channel toward the target lesion. Small samples of lung tissue are removed to be sent to the lab for diagnostic testing. It is performed

Table 26.1: Summary of bronchial nomenclature.

Right lung			
Superior lobe	B1: apicalis		a. apicalis proprius
			b. (subapicalis) ventralis
	B2: (lobi superioris) dorsalis		a. (subapicalis) dorsalis
			b. (lobi sup.) horizontalis
	B3: (lobi superioris) ventralis		a. (lobi sup. ventr.) lateralis
			b. (lobi sup. ventr.) medialis
Intermediate lobe	B4: medius lateralis		a. lateralis
			b. medialis
	B5: medius medialis		a. latralis
			b. medialis
Inferior lobe	B6: (lobi inferioris) superior		a. superior
			b. lateralis
			c. medialis
	B*: (lobi inferioris) subsuperior		
	B7: mediobasalis		a. dorsalis
			b. ventralis
	B8: ventrobasalis		a. lateralis
			b. basalis
	B9: laterobasalis		a. lateralis
			b. basalis
	B10: dorsobasalis		a. dorsalis
			b. lateralis
			c. medialis
Left lung			
Superior lobe	Sup. division bronchus	B1+2: apicodorsalis	a. apicalis
			b. (subapicalis) dorsalis
			c horizontalis
		B3: (lobi superioris) ventralis	a. (lobi sup. ventr.) lateralis
			b. (lobi sup. ventr.) medialis
			c. (lobi sup. ventr.) superior
	Inf. division bronchus	B4: lingualis superior	a. lateralis ventralis
			b. (lobi sup.) ventralis
		B5: lingualis inferior	a. superior
			b. inferior
Inferior lobe		B6: (lobi inferioris) superior	a. superior
			b. lateralis
			c. medialis
		B*: (lobi inferioris) subsuperior superior	
		B8: ventrobasalis	a. lateralis
			b. basalis
		B9: laterobasalis	a. lateralis
			b. basalis
		B10: dorsalis	a. dorsalis
			b. lateralis
			d. medialis

under fluoroscopic guidance to help guide the operator toward the target lesion and minimize complications such as pneumothorax. Newer technologies such as radial transducer probes EBUS-guided, and electromagnetic navigation can be used to help access smaller and more peripheral target lesions and have improved diagnostic yield.

Transbronchial needle aspiration is a technique used to diagnose mediastinal and hilar pathology. A small needle is passed through the bronchoscope and through the bronchial wall to sample lymph node or lung tissue. EBUS may improve the diagnostic yield of TBNA by allowing real-time visualization of mediastinal and hilar structures.

RISKS AND COMPLICATIONS

Generally flexible bronchoscopy is a safe procedure, with a described mortality less than 0.04% and a major complication rate less than 0.5%. Complications may occur at different times of the procedure. Anesthesia and premedication may be associated with: allergies, arrhythmias, dyspnea, bronchospasm. Complications that may arise during the endoscopic maneuver are: aspiration, hypoxemia, arrhythmias, vasovagal syndrome, pulmonary edema, bleeding, pneumothorax, seizures, tremors, fainting. *Discomfort and coughing* are the most frequent unwanted events, which may occur while the bronchoscope is passed through the nose, throat and airways. It may be reduced with local anesthetics or sedatives.

Transbronchial biopsy is the procedure most frequently burdened by complications, with a risk rated up to three times higher than a normal bronchial biopsy, especially in patients with severe underlying diseases (e.g. emphysema, coagulopathies).

Pneumothorax is not common, but it may occur if the lung is punctured during biopsy or if very inflamed or diseased airways are damaged by the bronchoscope. *Bleeding* after a biopsy is common, but it is usually minor and stops on its own. Sometimes cold saline or a medication (e.g. epinephrine) can be given through the bronchoscope to stop bleeding.

Hypoxemia during bronchoscopy may occur for several reasons, including the obstruction of airways due to the instrument, and the liquids injected into the lungs during the procedure. Suction during bronchoscopy causes a reduction in the fraction of inspired oxygen (FiO_2). This may lead to decreased partial pressure of oxygen (PaO_2) in arterial blood. Consequently, suction should be applied for a short time.

Other complications which may arise later, after performing the endoscopic procedure, include atelectasis, respiratory failure, infectious disease, heart failure.

Post bronchoscopy fever has been described with an incidence of 3–30% and is usually a self-limiting condition that resolves within 24 hours and does not require any treatment.

Prophylactic antibiotics are generally not required for the performance of flexible bronchoscopy.

Bronchoscopy is basically secure and with low risk of complications provided it is done in the best possible conditions.

CLEANING AND REPROCESSING FLEXIBLE BRONCHOSCOPES

According to the Spaulding classification of instruments, the flexible bronchoscope comes under the category of semicritical instruments. As such they must be free of all microorganisms with the exception of low numbers of bacterial spores. The minimum recommended practice for these instruments is high-level disinfection with a liquid sterilant/disinfectant. This is not the same as sterilization which includes the destruction of all living organisms including spores. Most surgical and sharp instruments require sterilization. Despite often using needles and forceps to biopsy lesions, suction blood and pierce the lining of the airways all of which often contaminate the working channel, the flexible bronchoscope is still considered a semicritical instrument. The high-level disinfectant required for cleaning bronchoscopes must possess certain characteristics including broad antimicrobial spectrum, rapid activity, material compatibility, lack of human or environmental toxicity, unscented, nonstaining, prolonged reuse and shelf life, ease of use and cost-effectiveness.

BIBLIOGRAPHY AND FURTHER READING

1. Du Rand IA, Blaikley J, Booton R, Chaudhuri N, Gupta V, Khalid S, et al. British Thoracic Society guideline for diagnostic flexible bronchoscopy in adults: accredited by NICE. Thorax. 2013;68:i1-i44.
2. Ernst A, Eberhardt R, Wahidi M, Becker HD, Herth FJ. Effect of routine clopidrogrel use on bleeding complications after transbronchial biopsy in humans. Chest. 2006;129(3):734-7.
3. Heidbuchel H, Verhamme P, Alings M, Antz M, Hacke W, Oldgren J, et al. European Heart Rhythm Association Practical Guide on the use of new oral anticoagulants in patients with non-valvular atrial fibrillation. Europace. 2013;15:625-51.

4. Hertz FJ, Becker HD, Ernst A. Aspirin does not increase bleeding complications after transbronchial biopsy. Chest. 2002;122(4):1461-4.
5. Jackson CL, Huber JF. Correlated applied anatomy of the bronchial tree and lungs with a system of nomenclature. Dis Chest. 1943;9:319-26.
6. Jin F, Mu D, Chu D, Fu E, Xie Y, Liu T. Severe complications of bronchoscopy. Respiration. 2008;76(4):429-33.
7. Nomenclature of broncho-pulmonary anatomy: an international nomenclature accepted by the thoracic society. Thorax. 1950;5:222-8.
8. Panchabhai TS, Mehta AC. Historical perspectives of bronchoscopy. Connecting the dots. Ann Am Thorac Soc. 2015;12(5):631-41.
9. Patrono C, Coller B, FitzGerald GA, Hirsh J, Roth G. Platelet-active drugs: the relationships among dose, effectiveness and side effects: the seventh ACCP Conference on atithrombotic and thrombolytic therapy. Chest. 2004;126(3 Suppl):234S-64S.
10. Pue CA, Pacht ER. Complications of fiberoptic bronchoscopy at a university hospital. Chest. 1995;107(2):430-2.
11. Schulman S, Bijsterveld NR. Anticoagulants and their reversal. Transfus Med Rev. 2007;21:37-48.
12. Wahidi MM, Rocha AT, Hollingsworth JW, Govert JA, Feller-Kopman D, Ernst A. Contraindications and safety of transbronchial lung biopsy via flexible bronchoscopy. A survey of pulmonologists and review of the literature. Respiration. 2005;72(3):285-95.
13. Woodhouse C, Evans G, Muller AF. The new oral anticoagulants: practical management for patients attending for endoscopic procedures. Frontline Gastroenterol. 2013;4:213-8.

Chapter

27

Bronchial Brushing and Biopsy

Debabrata Bandyopadhyay, Thomas R Gildea, Sergio Agati, Claudio Sorino

Several procedures have been developed with the aim of obtaining tissue samples during bronchoscopy. The main utility of sampling of tissue is the diagnosis of cancer, but it can give information about other cause of bronchopulmonary lesions and processes.

BRONCHIAL BRUSHING

Bronchial brushing is an endoscopic technique aimed at sampling superficial cells from a pathological lesion or, in diffuse disease, from the affected mucosa. The samples obtained are usually sent for cytological and microbiological examination.

The main application of bronchial brushing in adults is the diagnosis of malignant lesions, whereas in children it is more often employed to sample material for cytological analysis of inflammation or for the assessment of infection (e.g. tuberculosis) or to obtain viable cells for ciliary studies.

Procedure

The procedure is performed by advancing a small brush (Figs. 27.1A and B) through the bronchoscopic working channel within the protective sheath. Once the sheath protrudes from the distal end of the bronchoscope, the brush is released in the direction of the target lesion or suspect area by an assistant, with the brush extending approximately 3 cm from the bronchoscope (Fig. 27.2).

It is then advanced back and forth and in rotating motions till an adequate sample is obtained. Subsequently

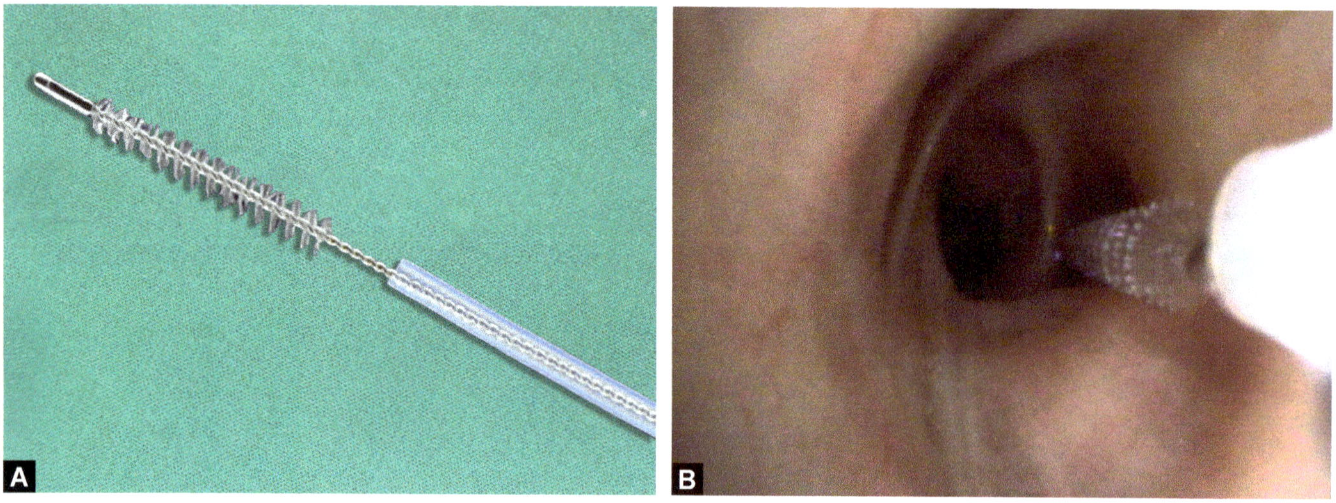

Figs. 27.1A and B: (A) Example of cytology brush and (B) its endoscopic view when advanced out of the catheter at the distal end of the bronchoscope.

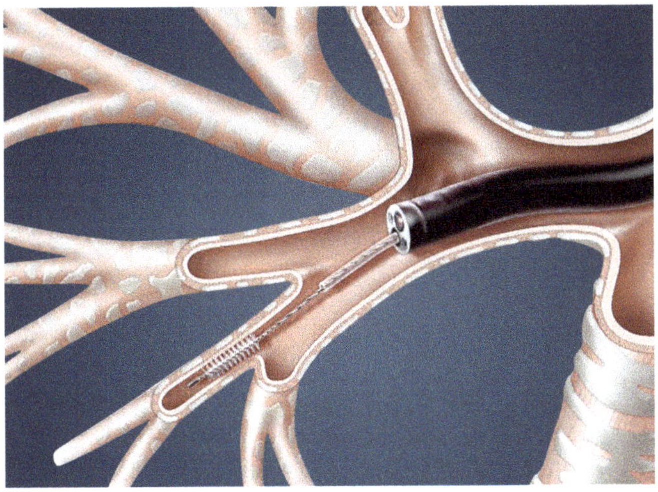

Fig. 27.2: Bronchial brushing. Exemplification of the procedure. *Courtesy*: Olympus Europe SE & CO. KG.

it is drawn back into the sheath and finally retracted out of the bronchoscope. This can either be performed under direct visualization for endobronchial lesions or under fluoroscopic guidance for peripheral lesions. In such a case, a metal tip of the brushes allows good visibility under fluoroscopy and leads to atraumatic brushing. After brushing the lesion or suspected area, the brush is withdrawn and the material cells are transferred directly onto microscope glass slides previously labeled with the patient identification.

The brushing technique may differ according to the size of employed bronchoscope and its working channel. A standard protected brush technique can be used with the bronchoscopes with 2.2 mm channel. Thinner pediatric bronchoscopes (e.g. 3.6 mm and 2.9 mm scopes) have a 1.2 mm channel, thus only unprotected thin brushes can be used. To prevent losing of the sampled material during the withdrawal of the brush through the channel, the unprotected brushing is usually left as a last procedure during bronchoscopy and after sampling the brush is only just withdrawn into the channel and removed together with the bronchoscope. Then the brush can be pushed out again to remove the sampled material for further processing.

Smear Preparation

To prepare the smears, the bristles of the brush are pressed and rolled against one or more glass slides, with the aid of pressure from a syringe. Cellular morphology should be preserved and air drying avoided. This is more likely to occur at the edges of the smear, so circular motion is preferred to a back and forth stroking of the brush against a glass slide. The samples should then be fixed as quickly as possible. There are different fixation techniques available for cytology specimens that are submitted on a slide. They include the immersion of the slide in a jar filled with 95% ethyl alcohol or the use of a cytology fixative spray. The spray bottle should be held 6–8 inches away from the slide and the entire cell smear should be evenly sprayed by depressing the plunger one to three times. You should allow the smear to dry thoroughly before staining, performing cytochemical or other molecular biological detection analyses or sending the slide to the lab.

ENDOBRONCHIAL BIOPSY

Endobronchial targeted biopsy is extremely useful in the evaluation of abnormal intrabronchial structures or masses. It is performed though suitable forceps under direct bronchial visualization (Figs. 27.3A to C). Endobronchial biopsy is a relatively easy technique for lesions which are visible through bronchoscope and located straight ahead. For lesions in difficult locations (e.g. lateral wall), the tip of the bronchoscope is flexed as far as possible so that opened forceps could be jammed against the surface of the abnormal structure. Some particular forceps help to biopsy this kind of lesions and avoids the extensive flexion of the instrument (Fig. 27.4). Differently from brushing, the aim of endobronchial biopsy is to get a small piece of tissue with all the relevant structures and cells for proper histological analysis.

The site for bronchial biopsy is derived from the expected pathology and visual assessment.

In the absence of visible localized pathologies, the site of biopsy is usually chosen in relation to the accessibility and possibility of a good grasp by the forceps. The majority of the interbronchial carinas are good sites for biopsy.

Procedure

Figures 27.3A to C show the main steps of endobronchial biopsy. The bronchoscope is advanced just proximal to the target lesion. The forceps are then advanced via the working channel till their distal end is visible outside the bronchoscope. The forceps are then opened and directed toward the lesion. To optimize the positioning of the forceps, the bronchoscope may be rotated. Once the forceps are well anchored to the target lesion, they are closed firmly. To preserve proper cell structure, it is important to cut out the sample rather than tearing it from the tissue. Then the forceps are withdrawn thoroughly through the working

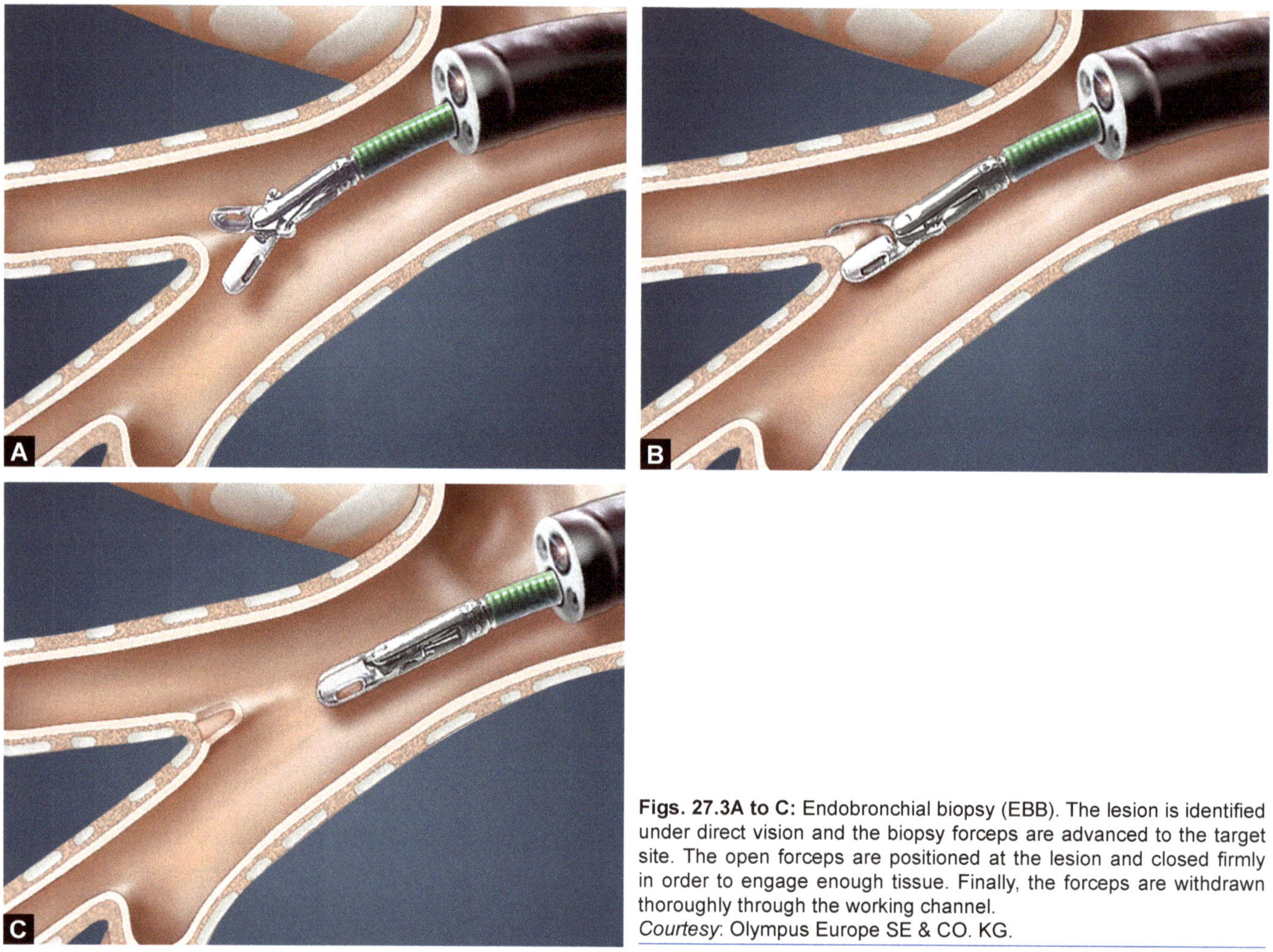

Figs. 27.3A to C: Endobronchial biopsy (EBB). The lesion is identified under direct vision and the biopsy forceps are advanced to the target site. The open forceps are positioned at the lesion and closed firmly in order to engage enough tissue. Finally, the forceps are withdrawn thoroughly through the working channel.
Courtesy: Olympus Europe SE & CO. KG.

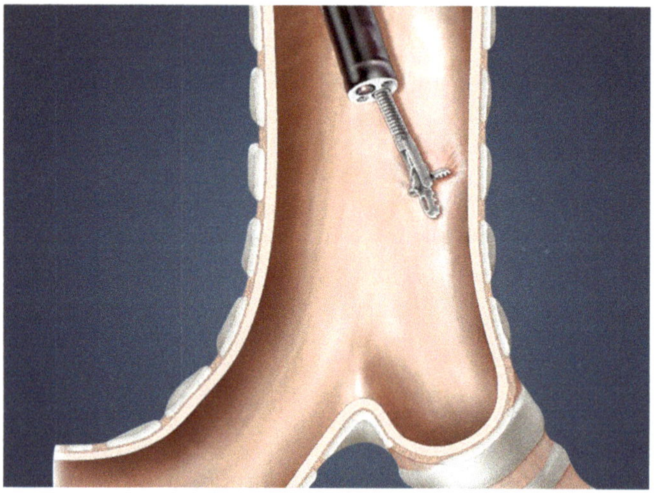

Fig. 27.4: Bronchial biopsy with tangential biopsy forceps.
Courtesy: Olympus Europe SE & CO. KG.

channel and the collected specimen is prepared for further processing (it is usually transferred to a test tube/jar containing 10% formalin) and sent for histopathological examination. One variant of this technique is the *push biopsy* in which following the closure of the forceps, these and the bronchoscope together are pushed distally stripping a larger sample. The entire procedure can be repeated several times till adequate samples are obtained. Three or four biopsies are usually taken in each visible lesion to ensure that at least one is suitable for analysis. If circumstances permit, it would be optimal to run up to seven withdrawals to ensure sufficient material for immuno-histochemical analysis. Biopsy specimens of good quality should be composed of a subepithelial area (without crushed artifacts, cartilage and blood clots) of 0.3–0.5 mm^2. Very gentle manipulation of the samples from the forceps to vials is required.

The most widely used type of forceps for endobronchial biopsy is the fenestrated long oval cup forceps, which are usually able to provide enough large sample for the histological evaluation (Fig. 27.5). When a bronchoscope with a large operative channel is used (2.2 mm or greater), different types of reusable or single-use forceps are available. When pediatric bronchoscopes with a channel of 1.2 mm in diameter are used, only few models of thin forceps can be used and due to their very small sizes, the bioptic samples are often inadequate.

TRANSBRONCHIAL BIOPSY

Transbronchial lung biopsy (TBB or TBLB) is one of the most important sampling procedures performed during flexible bronchoscopy, and is also known as *bronchoscopic lung biopsy* (BLB) (Figs. 27.6A and B). The principal aim of the diagnostic bronchoscopy is to obtain tissue specimens for cytological, histopathological, and microbiological analysis. Many sampling instruments have been used to achieve this goal. Dr Anderson was the first physician to perform lung biopsy via rigid bronchoscopy in 1965 and Levin et al. published their experience with TBB using flexible bronchoscopy in 1974. Since then pulmonologists have been routinely performing TBB to diagnose many diffuse and localized lung diseases.

Even the distal peripheral lesions can be accessed from the bronchial lumen by this technique often with the help of fluoroscopy. Complications resulting from the TBB are exceedingly rare but can be lethal. Risk factors predisposing to these complications should be identified and rectified prior to the procedure. This technique provides a high diagnostic yield in focal lesions as well as many diffuse parenchymal lung diseases. It precludes the need for more invasive diagnostic procedures. Although it is a widely employed technique, it is paramount to be aware of its applications and limitations, and to properly select patient by evaluating risks and benefits. This will minimize the chances of complications and enhance outcomes of the procedure.

It is important to recognize that in some literature the term of TBB is also referred to other tools such as brush,

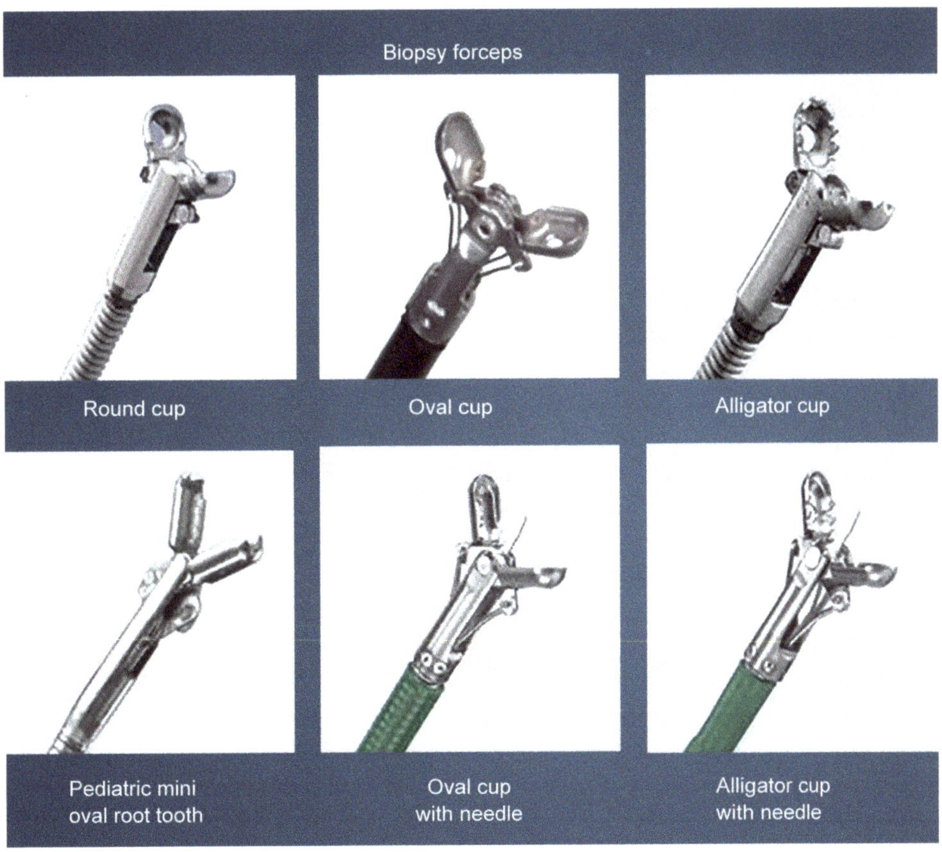

Fig. 27.5: Different varieties of biopsy forceps used for transbronchial biopsy.

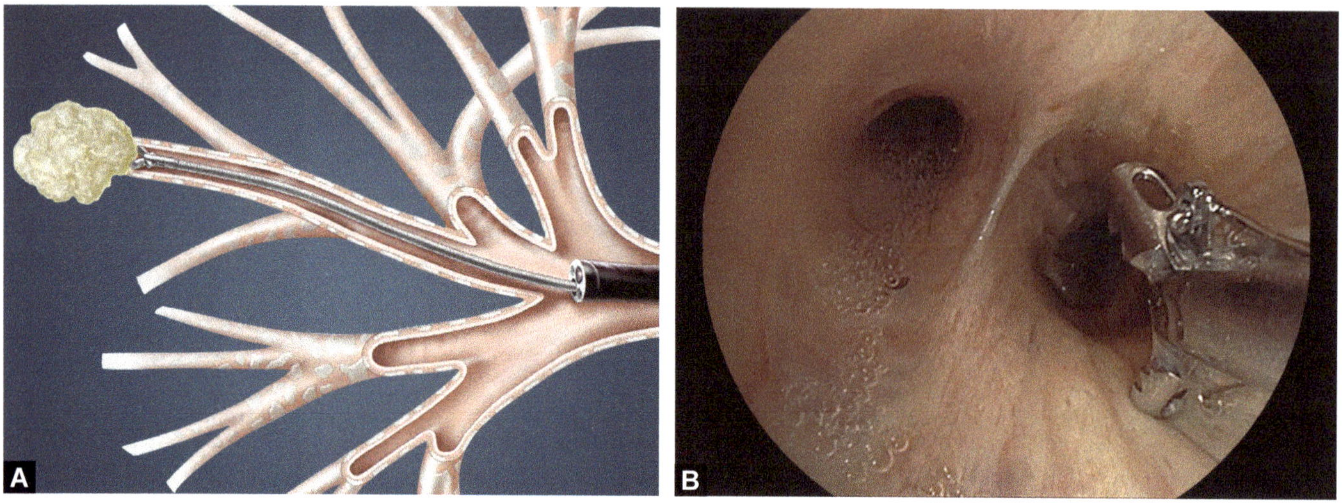

Figs. 27.6A and B: Transbronchial lung biopsy (TBLB). (A) The endoscope is advanced as far as possible into the target area. (B) Endoscopic view of TBLB forceps.
Courtesy: Olympus Europe SE & CO. KG.

needle, needle-brush, etc. The term *peripheral transbronchial needle aspiration* (P-TBNA) is preferred to indicate the sampling of peripheral lesions through needles commonly used for TBNA (usually a 21 G needle, preferably under fluoroscopic, endoscopic or electromagnetic guidance). The diagnostic yield of P-TBNA was found to be superior to any other procedure in particular in lesions greater than 2 cm and localized in the middle lobe, even in the absence of the "bronchus sign". In this chapter, we will refer to the classic TBB with biopsy forceps for illustrative purposes.

Indications and Contraindications

The TBB is indicated in the diagnosis of peripheral lesions and in the case of diffuse parenchymal lung diseases.

In the case of a peripheral lesion of possible neoplastic nature, the diagnostic sensitivity is strongly influenced by the size. The yield is less than 25% below 2 cm, while for lesions greater than 2 cm it will range between 30% and 75%, to more than 80% above the 4 cm. Moreover, this procedure may be significantly conditioned by the presence of a direct relationship between the lesion and the tracheobronchial tree. Radiologically such a relationship is suggested by the presence of the so-called "bronchus sign", i.e. the recognition of a bronchus that leads to the lesion to be sampled or that is contained within the lesion itself. The diagnostic yield is furthermore improved by the assessment of rapid on-site cytopathological evaluation and by the use of a radiological guidance. In this regard, biopsy performed under the guidance of multislice computed tomography (CT) chest, with specific low-dose protocol, it is more sensitive than under the classical fluoroscopic guide.

In the case of diffuse lung diseases, TBB should be considered the first choice during a bronchoscopic investigation. Through bronchial lumen it is possible to reach peripheral centrilobular regions and, for this reason, this method of sampling is extremely effective in a wide range of diseases. Tissue may be collected tissue samples in localized disorders all around terminal and respiratory bronchioles, involving these districts or spread through lymphatics. The TTB may be diagnostic in cases of carcinomatous lymphangitis, sarcoidosis, Langerhans cell histiocytosis, pulmonary lymphangioleiomyomatosis (LAM), alveolar proteinosis, lymphoproliferative processes, infections (if more than the typical morphology it is also possible to isolate pathogen from tissue) and pneumoconiosis, especially silicosis.

Because histological findings are not very specific in small fragments of lung parenchyma, the small samples recovered with TBB are not sufficient in diseases which require a morphological characterization of large volumes such as *nonspecific interstitial pneumonia* (NSIP), usual *interstitial pneumonia* (UIP), *desquamative interstitial pneumonia* (DIP). It is very often necessary to integrate pathological, clinical, radiological, and laboratory findings.

The cellular variant of NSIP has a characteristic morphological pattern and generous TBB can provide adequate samples in some cases, such as drugs toxicity, or in idiopathic forms, when integrated with clinical and radiological findings. It has been reported that the typical UIP pattern of *idiopathic pulmonary fibrosis* (IPF) (irregular fibrosis, fibroblastic foci, honeycombing) was detected in samples taken with TBB, in 32% cases. Anyway, surgical biopsy would remain the most appropriate procedure to identify IPF.

In vasculitis, the role of TBB is still debated. Episodic cases of samples with lesions morphologically consistent with granulomatosis with polyangiitis (Wegener's granulomatosis) and eosinophilic granulomatosis with polyangiitis (EGPA) or Churg-Strauss syndrome are reported. However, histological aspects could be different and patterns, at most suggestive, frequently need to be integrated, particularly, with laboratory data.

In *hypersensitivity pneumonitis* (extrinsic allergic alveolitis), the diagnostic yield ranges from 20% to 90%, according to histological criteria adopted, number of samples and type of disease. For example, even if more than 300 etiological agents are known, the typical granulomas are more easily found in the "Farmer's lung".

Transbronchial biopsy has a role in immunocompromised patients, where pulmonary complications are common. These include opportunistic infections, toxic effects of chemotherapy, radiation therapy, graft-versus host disease, acute or chronic rejection, idiopathic pulmonary disorders, collagen vascular diseases. Early detection of these conditions affects survival. In the presence of pulmonary infiltrates, the first diagnostic step involves the use of noninvasive methods, which are inconclusive in 40% of cases. Bronchoalveolar lavage (BAL), when possible, should always be performed for the large amount of information that can be provided in case of infectious and noninfectious etiology. If there are no contraindications, selected patients should be subjected to TBB before proceeding to surgical procedures. The samples obtained with TBB often detect nonspecific lesions, but may contribute to the diagnosis or affect treatment decisions in the context of a specific clinical presentation and of a particular radiological pattern. After lung transplantation, TBB is used as a method of sampling in bronchoscopy for the detection of acute lung rejection. Regarding the infectious disease, samples of TBB result little specific and always require the use of special stains. The addition of TBB and BAL lets achieve a diagnostic sensitivity of up to 83% in many cases such as Pneumocystis jiroveci or mycobacterial infections.

Transbronchial biopsy is a procedure that can be practiced in patients undergoing mechanical ventilation. Although there is a higher incidence of pneumothorax (PNX) in ventilated patients (13%) compared to nonventilated (5%), it is considered sufficiently safe and able to provide information that will change the management in a significant proportion of patients (65% of medical patients and 25% of patients with lung transplantation).

Contraindications to the performance of TBB are similar to the classic contraindications to flexible bronchoscopy, taking into consideration that the majority of complications are associated with this procedure. In general, contraindications are related to the risk of causing tachycardia, hypoxemia and bronchospasm.

In particular, when a TBB is planned, it is important to pay attention to the risk of bleeding related to the use of antiplatelet agents and anticoagulants. So patient must have suspended antiplatelet drugs by at least 5 days and low molecular weight heparin by 12 hours. It is not possible to exclude that the risk of bleeding is related to the drug used, since there is evidence that taking Cardio Aspirin is not associated with an increased bleeding. Moreover, platelets must be higher than 50,000/mm^3, the international normalized ratio (INR) lower than 1.3 and partial thromboplastin time (PTT) not elevated. In patients receiving platelets or fresh frozen plasma, it is indicated to check that the abnormalities are corrected before proceeding.

The TBB should not be practiced in patients with acute respiratory failure (PO_2 < 60 mm Hg or digital oxyhemoglobin saturation < 90%), with the support of high-flow oxygen (FiO_2 > 50%) and in patients with acute myocardial infarction and life-threatening arrhythmias in the last 6 weeks. Finally, it is appropriate to postpone the examination in patients with an exacerbation of asthma or chronic bronchitis and decompensated heart failure.

Relative contraindications of TBB are shown in Table 27.1.

Required Tools

The term TBB refers not only to sampling of lung tissue through biopsy forceps, but it also includes the use of various other instruments.

As regards the biopsy forceps, there are different types (*see* Fig. 27.5). The classical cup forceps possesses smooth and sharp margins and can be fenestrated or not-fenestrated, with the presence of a hole on both valves in order to reduce artifacts from crushing. Toothed forceps ("crocodile teeth" or "alligator") have a greater capacity to berth and a stronger grip. The pliers can also have a needle between the shells that favors the anchoring on the

Table 27.1: Relative contraindications of transbronchial biopsy.

Contraindications	*Comments*
Thrombocytopenia	Procedure is regarded safe with platelet count more than 50,000. However, bleeding complication has been reported even with higher platelet count up to 100,000
Uremia	Uremia increases bleeding risk during the procedure. Some centers use nasal or intravenous desmopressin (DDAVP) 30 minutes prior to the procedure in this situation*
Mild to moderate pulmonary hypertension	Higher risk of hemorrhage than control although limited data suggest it is a probably a safe procedure†
Mechanical ventilation	Should be done cautiously because of poor diagnostic yield (< 50%) and higher complication rates (30%)††
Myocardial infarction	Bronchoscopy within 30 days is associated with 5% mortality due to active ischemia
Medications	Heparin infusion should be withheld for 6 hours and low molecular weight (LMW) heparin 12 hours prior to the procedure. Warfarin should be discontinued for 5 days with a goal to reduce the international normalized ratio (INR) below 1.5. Aspirin can be continued but clopidogrel needs to be stopped 5–7 days prior to the procedure. Similarly prasugrel, dabigatran, rivaroxaban should be withheld 5–7 days prior to the procedure. Antibiotics prophylaxis against endocarditis is not required

*Shapiro MD, Kelleher SP. Intranasal deamino-8-D-arginine vasopressin shortens the bleeding time in uremia. Am J Nephrol. 1984;4(4):260-1.
†Diaz-Guzman E, Vadi S, Minai OA, Gildea TR, Mehta AC. Safety of diagnostic bronchoscopy in patients with pulmonary hypertension. Respiration. 2009;77(3):292-7.
††British Thoracic Society Bronchoscopy Guidelines Committee. British Thoracic Society guidelines on diagnostic flexible bronchoscopy. Thorax. 2001;56:i1-21.

selected target, preventing slipping on the bronchial wall. Forceps may be of various sizes and typically must have a diameter of at least 0.2 mm, lower than the operating channel of the endoscope used.

It is shown that the diagnostic yield of larger samples is greater as these contain higher amounts of tissue, especially more alveolar tissue. The cup forceps are those that recover the smaller fragments, and for this reason, "alligator" pliers are commonly most used because they allow the recovery of more abundant samples. If the clamps are not closed within the biopsy channel, it will be fewer artifacts from crushing. It can be used larger pliers, without pulling them out of the working channel after the seizure, but removing them together with the bronchoscope. This procedure should be practiced in deep sedation, after intubation with a rigid bronchoscope, using gastroenterological origin pliers, adapted for bronchoscopy ("jumbo" pliers).

Association of the classical biopsy procedure with suction through a suction catheter provides a diagnostic sensitivity higher than the methods isolated. The suction catheter is introduced through the working channel and, once placed, it is mobilized with gentle movements up and down to allow the recovery of the pathological tissue by applying continuous suction with a syringe of 10 mL. An emerging method of sampling involves the use of flexible cryoprobes. The patient should be intubated with an endotracheal tube, laryngeal mask or, even better, with a rigid bronchoscope. The cryoprobe is introduced into the working channel of the bronchoscope and conducted in contact with the tissue to be sampled. The freezing effect promotes the adhesion of the frozen tissue to the probe itself and, applying a gentle traction, it can be torn away. The probe should not be removed from the biopsy channel and the bronchoscope be removed simultaneously with the probe itself.

The use of fluoroscopy or endoscopic guidance is essential to reduce complications, in particular the occurrence of PNX. The efficacy and safety of this procedure are under discussion. Recent studies are encouraging as they confirm the safety and high diagnostic yield, linked to the ability to recover most bulky samples, both in diffuse lung diseases and in tumors.

Procedure

Before starting bronchoscopy, a recent high-resolution chest CT must be available for consultation. In certain clinical settings, CT provides indications suggestive for the diagnosis, as in the case of sarcoidosis, UIP or LAM. In other cases, it allows visualization of central or peribronchovascular lesions that may be more accessible to a bronchial biopsy. Finally, even if the CT does not prove specific diseases, it enables us to identify the areas whereas the execution of TBB would be more effective (bronchus sign, centrilobular nodules, ground-glass opacity).

The preparation of the patient involves local anesthesia of the nose and the oropharynx, and conscious sedation (*see* Chapter 26 on flexible bronchoscopy).

After an extensive inspection of the airways by flexible bronchoscopy, the TBB is performed using a biopsy forceps. Three different types of biopsy forceps are more often used: (1) cup forceps, (2) toothed (alligator forceps), and (3) needle forceps. Alligator forceps is most commonly employed because of its propensity to get a larger tissue specimen.

In order to perform TBB, the tip of the bronchoscope is advanced to wedge in the subsegmental airway leading to the lesion. The biopsy forceps is introduced via working channel of the bronchoscope and a mild resistance is felt when forceps reaches the distal end of the scope. Occasionally a greater resistance may be sensed at this point, particularly if bronchoscope is placed inside upper lobes or superior basal segments. In that situation, the distal end of the scope should be gently straightened in order to prevent damage of the scope before forcing the forceps through. If this is not successful, the bronchoscope may be withdrawn to the lobar bronchus and the forceps positioned at few centimeter beyond the tip of the scope inside the desired airway. Subsequently the scope is wedged using forceps as a guidewire. At this point, rotating fluoroscopy may be used to confirm the position of the scope and forceps. Rest of the procedure can be performed under fluoroscopic guidance. Figures 27.7A to D illustrate the positions of forceps in fluoroscopy for biopsy at different sites.

The biopsy forceps is gently advanced into lung parenchyma until a resistance is met, which signifies reaching to the pleural surface. The forceps is then withdrawn approximately 1.5–2 cm proximally. The patient is asked to take a deep inspiration, which opens up the airways, while the forceps cusps are opened. Subsequently the patient is advised to exhale as the forceps with open cusps is gently advanced and cusps are closed at the end of expiration. Finally, the forceps is pulled out with a single sharp but gentle movement. A tug is usually felt as the lung tissue is snipped off. It is important to note, this whole process is painless. If patient complains of chest pain at any time, the biopsy should be abandoned from that site due to possibility of pleura being pinched. Similarly the forceps should be withdrawn temporarily during bouts of cough to avoid occurrence of PNX.

For focal mass lesion, the forceps is advanced to the margin of the lesion until a resistance is felt and the

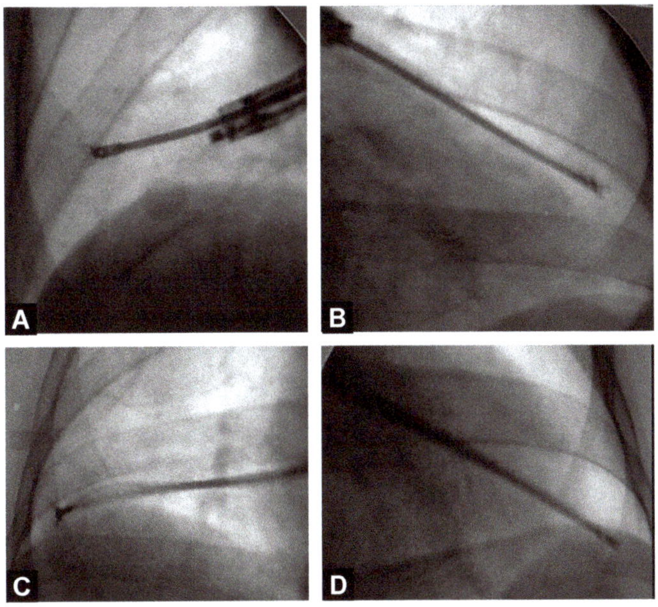

Figs. 27.7A to D: Position of bronchoscope and biopsy forceps. (A) Right middle lobe bronchus. (B) Lingular bronchus. (C) Right lower lobe bronchus. (D) Left lower lobe bronchus.

forceps cannot be advanced further. The position should be checked by fluoroscopy and procedure is continued with its guidance. After confirming the position, forceps is retracted back by 1–2 cm and the cusps are opened. Thereafter, the biopsy forceps is advanced firmly against the mass as the cusps are closed. The forceps is then pulled back in a similar way.

This process is repeated multiple times to obtain enough tissue without breaking the wedge.

Sampling of solitary pulmonary nodules (SPNs) can be time consuming and radiation intensive for the patient. A minimal invasive alternative is the guide sheath technique (Fig. 27.8). At the beginning, the guide sheath can be advanced and placed at the center of a SPN either under X-ray or with ultrasonic guidance. Once positioned, the guide sheath acts like an extended working channel, allowing safe and repeated access to the lesion for taking multiple samples with the help of biopsy forceps, a cytology brush or TBNA needles.

After performing biopsies, the forceps are withdrawn but the bronchoscope is kept wedged for about 4 minutes (normal bleeding time) to stop bleeding. It is important to avoid suction and simply keep the scope wedged and it will contain bleeding even if the lens is totally obscured. If excessive bleeding is suspected, 10–15 mL aliquot of iced-cold saline instillation is recommended. Alternatively lower

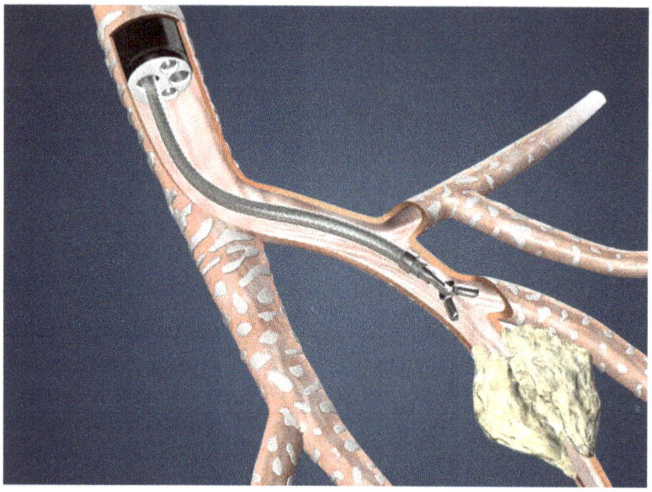

Fig. 27.8: Sampling of periphery pulmonary coin lesion by a guide sheath technique. The guide sheath is placed at the center of a SPN either under X-ray or with ultrasonic guidance, allowing safe and repeated access to the lesion.
Courtesy: Olympus Europe SE & CO. KG.

concentration of epinephrine at 1:100,000, 2 mL aliquot can be used with close monitoring for cardiac arrhythmia. Subsequently bronchoscope is pulled back without suctioning the blood clot and after closely observing for any fresh bleeding. This is just one technique and we are aware that there are others that use continuous suction to deal with post biopsy hemorrhage.

Other techniques for managing hemorrhage can be to position the patient with dependent lung down to contain the bleeding, and the use a balloon for tamponade. There are other procoagulant drugs described in rare circumstances. The key is to be prepared as the patient with massive bleeding is at risk for asphyxiation from central airway occlusion with clot rather than exsanguination.

Guidelines recommend obtaining four to six samples for diffuse lung disease and seven to eight specimens for focal lung condition. The tissue sample is collected in either 10% formalin or normal saline. A fluoroscopic examination is performed after the procedure to detect any PNX. Chest X-ray is not routinely indicated unless patient develops symptoms such as chest discomfort, shortness of breath, hypoxemia and massive hemoptysis. Patients should be observed in recovery room for at least 2 hours post procedure.

Possible Complications

Major complications are rare after TBB (2%) (Table 27.2) and the mortality rate is low (0.12%). In addition, adverse events may occur in relation to the use of sedation and local anesthetic.

Table 27.2: Major complications after transbronchial biopsy.

Major complications	*Comments*
Bleeding	Clinically significant in 1.8% procedures
Pneumothorax	Incidence 1–6%; more common in diffuse disease, age, number of biopsies. It can occur irrespective of the use of fluoroscopy. In 40% cases, the process may be delayed by 2 hours
Cardiac arrhythmia	Atrial arrhythmia is more common, related to hypoxia
Hypoxemia	Common with use of sedatives, noticed in 10% of cases, usually transient. Can precipitate cardiac complications

PNX and bleeding are the most frequent complications. The PNX occurs in 1–6% of patients undergoing the procedure with an increased risk in diffuse lung diseases and in relation with age and number of withdrawals. It occurs even if the guide with fluoroscopy is used and in the 40% of cases it can occur at a distance of 2 hours from the conclusion of the examination.

The X-ray control is not indicated and the extent of the PNX is related to the symptoms.

A significant bleeding is observed in 2–9% of patients and is a major obstacle to the collection of a sufficient number of samples.

The use of sedatives may lead to a condition of hypoxemia, generally transient, but which can precipitate cardiac complications as atrial arrhythmia.

BRONCHIAL WASHING

The bronchial lavage is a procedure used to obtain cytology samples from the airways, usually as complementary tool to other diagnostic techniques. It consists in instilling isotonic saline in the bronchi and bronchioles (usually 5–30 mL each time) and its subsequent aspiration through the bronchoscope channel. This can cleanse the tubes from secretions before biopsies, and remove blood, cells and small tissue fragments resulting from previous biopsies.

The instillation may be repeated several times, provided that vital signs and oxygen saturation of the patient is stable; however, it is advisable not to exceed 120 mL of saline injected. The fluid recovered is collected and undergo to cytological and microbiological analysis. Few milliliters are usually enough for each study. It is preferable to use the excess amount for the cell search.

The additional diagnostic yield of bronchial lavage for diagnosis of pulmonary malignancy during bronchoscopy is relatively low. However, it remains a cost-effective technique in the diagnostic workup of patients with such a clinical suspicion.

BIBLIOGRAPHY AND FURTHER READING

1. Andersen HA, Fontana RS, Harrison EG Jr. Transbronchoscopic lung biopsy in diffuse pulmonary disease. Dis Chest. 1965;48:187-92.
2. Anders GT, Johnson JE, Bush BA, Matthews JI. Transbronchial biopsy without fluoroscopy. A seven-year perspective. Chest. 1988;94(3):557-60.
3. British Thoracic Society Bronchoscopy Guidelines Committee. British Thoracic Society guidelines on diagnostic flexible bronchoscopy. Thorax. 2001;56:i1-21.
4. Gasparini S. Conventional biopsy techniques. In: Ernst A, Herth FJ (Eds). Principles and Practice of Interventional Pulmonology. New York: Springer; 2013. p. 156.
5. Gilman MJ, Wang KP. Transbronchial lung biopsy in sarcoidosis. An approach to determine the optimal number of biopsies. Am Rev Respir Dis. 1980;122(5):721-4.
6. Hautmann H, Henke MO, Bitterling H. High diagnostic yield from transbronchial biopsy of solitary pulmonary nodules using low-dose CT-guidance. Respirology. 2010;15(4):677-82.
7. Jain P, Hadique S, Mehta AC. Transbronchial lung biopsy. In: Mehta AC, Jain P (Eds). Interventional Bronchoscopy: A clinical Guide. New York: Springer; 2013. p. 15.
8. Khoo KL, Lee P, Mehta AC. Endobronchial epinephrine: confusion is in the air. Am J Respir Crit Care Med. 2013;187(10):1137-8.
9. Levin DC, Wicks AB, Ellis JH Jr. Transbronchial lung biopsy via the fiberoptic bronchoscope. Am Rev Respir Dis. 1974;110:4-12.
10. Patel RR, Utz JP. Bronchoscopic lung biopsy. In: Wang KP, Mehta AC, Turner JF (Eds). Flexible Bronchoscopy, 3rd edition. Oxford, UK: Wiley-Blackwell; 2012. p. 118.
11. Rittirak W, Sompradeekul S. Diagnostic yield of fluoroscopy-guided transbronchial lung biopsy in non-endobronchial lung lesion. J Med Assoc Thai. 2007;90 (Suppl 2):68-73.
12. Stover DE, Zaman MB, Hajdu SI, Lange M, Gold J, Armstrong D. Bronchoalveolar lavage in the diagnosis of diffuse pulmonary infiltrates in the immunosuppressed host. Ann Intern Med. 1984;101:1-7.
13. Thirumala RD, Lessnau KD, Mosenifar Z. (2014). Transbronchial biopsy. [online] Available from http://emedicine.medscape.com/article/1894323-overview#a1. [Accessed December, 2015].
14. Tsushima K, Sone S, Hanaoka T, Takayama F, Honda T, Kubo K. Comparison of bronchoscopic diagnosis for peripheral pulmonary nodule under fluoroscopic guidance with CT guidance. Respir Med. 2006;100(4):737-45.

Chapter

28

Transthoracic Needle Biopsy

Zafar Neyaz, Dilip Kumar MP, Claudio Sorino

OVERVIEW

Transthoracic needle biopsy (TNB) is a minimally invasive technique for establishing diagnosis in many intrathoracic diseases, and constitutes a valid alternative to more invasive surgical procedures. In the past TNB was performed under fluoroscopic guidance; however, nowadays computed tomography (CT) scan and ultrasound are mostly used. The overall diagnostic yield of TNB ranges from 88 to 97%. Although TNB has low risk of significant complications, detailed knowledge of anatomy and technical aspects of biopsy procedure is necessary. Due to its relative safety, TNB can also be performed on outpatient basis by using local anesthesia with or without conscious sedation.

Various aspects of TNB of pulmonary, mediastinal and pleural lesions have been discussed. As CT scan is the preferred imaging guidance for TNB, this chapter mainly focuses on the technical aspects of percutaneous CT-guided needle biopsy.

INDICATIONS AND CONTRAINDICATIONS

Transthoracic needle biopsy can be used to investigate any lesion of lung, mediastinum or pleura provided it is accessible to needle. However, a bronchoscopic approach is preferred for hilar and central lung lesions, as the transthoracic approach will be long with relatively high risk of vascular injury. Although TNB may be used to obtain sample in interstitial lung disease, usually a thoracoscopic or open lung biopsy is performed to minimize the risk of pneumothorax and to obtain larger samples. Common indications are pulmonary nodule or mass, persistent pulmonary infiltrate, mediastinal mass, and focal or diffuse pleural thickening. In patients at high risk for lung cancer who develop a resectable solitary pulmonary nodule with imaging characteristics typical of primary lung cancer, surgery can be the appropriate first step.

For TNB, patient has to lie still and maintain prone, supine or decubitus position. For small lung lesion, breath holding is needed for successful lesion targeting. An uncooperative patient is one of the major contraindications for TNB. Vascular lesions such as aneurysm or arteriovenous malformation should never be subjected to biopsy. Prothrombin time (PT) or activated partial thromboplastin time (APTT) ratio of more than 1.4 and a platelet count below 100,000/mL are relative contraindications for TNB. For lung biopsy, other relative contraindications are bulla or severe emphysema in biopsy path, a solitary lung caused by contralateral pneumonectomy, positive pressure ventilation, forced expiratory volume in 1 second (FEV1) less than 35% and pulmonary hypertension.

BIOPSY PLANNING

Careful planning and assessment of the risk factors is the key for successful biopsy. Patient should be explained about the procedure, its benefits and possible complications in detail.

Oral anticoagulant medication should be discontinued at least 4 days before the procedure. There are no definite guidelines for stopping antiplatelet medication; however, it is recommended to discontinue aspirin at least 5 days before the procedure. If the patient has intractable cough, cough suppressants should be prescribed.

An adequate blood coagulation capacity should be proved before the procedure. Particularly, recent PT and an international normalized ratio (INR) should be obtained in patients with known or suspected liver disease and in patients taking warfarin. APTT should be measured in patients receiving heparin. A complete blood count is also recommended before the biopsy in order to determine platelet count and the baseline hemoglobin concentration.

Recent contrast-enhanced CT scan and other previous radiological investigation should be reviewed. Appropriate imaging guidance and needle for TNB is chosen based on the lesion location, size, vascularity and important structures located in the anticipated biopsy path. CT guidance is used for most of TNB procedures; however, ultrasound guidance may be used for pleural, large anterior mediastinal and large peripheral lung lesions. CT scan not only allows clear visualization of intrathoracic structures, complications such as pneumothorax and hemothorax could be identified at the earliest. CT fluoroscopy is a recent advancement that in available in many standard CT scanners. Rapid image reconstruction with an in-room control panel and monitor permits the radiologist, to perform biopsy while visualizing the lesion and needle in real-time. Although this technique is associated with a small radiation to the operator, it is very useful for targeting small lung nodules and lower lobe lesions which move significantly with respiration. TNB under CT fluoroscopy could be performed in much less time and rapid diagnosis of complications is possible.

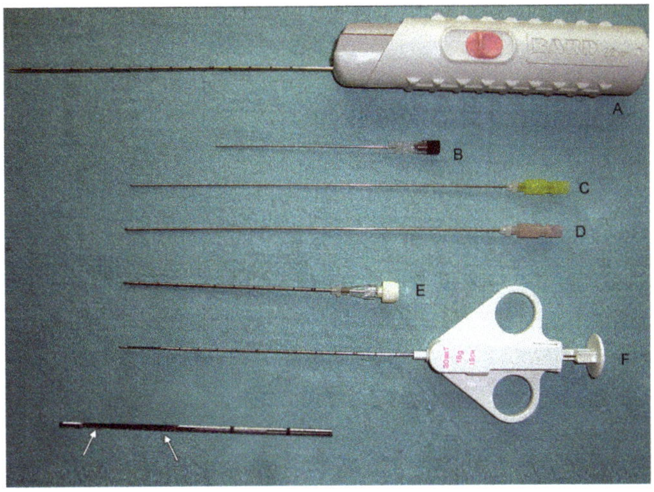

Figs. 28.1A to F: Various aspiration and cutting biopsy needles: (A) Spring load core biopsy system 18-gauge 16 cm long (BARD, AZ, USA) used mostly for ultrasound-guided procedures. (B) 22-gauge 89 mm long spinal needle. (C) 20-gauge 20 cm long Chiba needle. (D) 18-gauge 20 cm long Chiba needle. (E) 16-gauge outer guiding needle with stylet inside. (F) 18-gauge 15 cm long light weighted automated core biopsy needle which may be used coaxially with the 16-gauge guiding needle (Quick-Core biopsy needle, Cook, Bloomington, IN, USA). Inset specimen notch (arrowheads) of the biopsy needle for collecting specimen.

NEEDLE TYPES

Broadly there are two types of needles used for TNB: (1) aspiration and (2) cutting needles. Aspiration needles are usually 18–25 gauge (G) and used for retrieval of specimens for cytological and microbiological evaluation. Commonly available aspiration needles are Chiba and spinal needles. The cutting needles are used for retrieval of specimens for histopathological evaluation. There are some modified aspiration needles available which obtain tissue fragments for histology in addition to aspiration material. Two commonly used such needles are the Franseen and Westcott needles. Automated core biopsy needles are spring-loaded devices which retrieve a linear tissue core. These needles are usually larger in caliber and stiffer than aspiration needles; however, nowadays thinner caliber (18–20 G) automated biopsy needles are available (Figs. 28.1A to F).

Transthoracic needle biopsy can be done with a single needle or coaxial technique. In coaxial technique initially an outer guiding needle is placed to the edge of lesion and specimen is obtained by inserting a thinner gauge needle through it. For sampling the lesion, the inner biopsy needle is usually 2–3 cm longer than the outer guiding needle. The advantage of coaxial technique is that multiple samples can be taken from a single puncture which results in a short procedure time. While coaxial technique offers many advantages, a slight disadvantage is that a larger caliber outer guiding needle is used for initial puncture. If both aspiration and core biopsy specimens are needed, they can be obtained through the same outer guiding needle.

Selection of needle in a particular case depends on many factors, including size, location and suspected nature of lesion, intervening structures in the biopsy path, status of the underlying lung, experience of the radiologist, type and amount of specimen needed for diagnosis. For CT-guided procedures, a light weighted automated biopsy device is preferred as it can be left attached to the patient while taking check scans; however, heavy biopsy devices may used if ultrasound guidance is used. Length of needle or biopsy device should be enough to reach the lesion but not too long otherwise it will not fit in the CT gantry. Some biopsy needles like Quick-Core biopsy needle (Cook, USA) allows advancement of inner specimen notch into the lesion before firing and exact site of sampling could be ascertained.

Fine needle aspiration cytology has up to 95% accuracy for malignant lesions; however, the yield is much lower in benign lesions. Aspiration cytology is also less reliable than histology in differentiating cell type of malignant lesions. In suspected lymphoma cases, adequate size tissue cores are needed for histological classification by immunohistochemistry. Complications of small gauge cutting needles are similar or slightly higher than aspiration needles. For these reasons, an 18–20 G cutting needle with coaxial technique is preferred especially if an onsite cytopathologist is unavailable. Needle gauge does not affect complications rates if needles of 18 G or lesser are used; however, a thinner gauge needle may be preferred if chances of complication are high.

PREBIOPSY PREPARATION AND GENERAL BIOPSY TECHNIQUE

Informed consent should be obtained from the patient. Patient should be taken for biopsy after reviewing the imaging and coagulation profile. All necessary equipment and adequate staff should be available for monitoring the patient and to deal with any emergency. An 18-G or 20-G intravenous cannula should be placed. Blood pressure, pulse rate and oxygen saturation of the patient are monitored during and after the procedure. In hypertensive patients, blood pressure should be adequately controlled as the anxiety and pain associated with biopsy procedure may further increase the blood pressure.

The procedure is performed under local anesthesia (1–2% lidocaine). Sedation is generally not given as the patient has to lie still and follow breath hold instructions. However, in apprehensive patients, 0.25 mg oral alprazolam or 1 mg intravenous midazolam can be given. Pain during TNB occurs mainly during administration of local anesthesia, puncturing of parietal pleura and due to lying in one position on the CT table. Pain medication should be given if required.

Patient positioning mainly depends on the lesion accessibility and the safest path to the lesion. Usually the needle puncture site is kept upward. As the same position must be maintained throughout the procedure, adequate padding and adjustments in positioning should be done to ensure patient's comfort. A prone position is preferred during lung biopsy as it allows least chest wall motion and a comfortable supine "puncture site down" post biopsy positioning. Supine and lateral decubitus positions are associated with moderate and maximum chest wall motion respectively. If a pulmonary abscess is suspected, the lateral decubitus position can help prevent flooding the contralateral lung with infected material during the procedure.

Most mediastinal, pleural and upper lobe lung lesions can be biopsied during gentle free breathing. However, small lung lesions and those close to diaphragm may show significant respiratory motion and breath holding is important for targeting these lesions. Patient must hold breath in the same degree of inspiration or expiration each time to maintain needle and lesion alignment. Additionally patient is advised not to take deep inspirations while needle is in the lung, as significant needle movement will increase chances of pleural tearing and needle dislodgment.

After positioning the patient on CT table, CT sections are taken for marking the needle entry site. Nonenhanced CT sections are usually sufficient for planning if a recent contrast-enhanced CT is available for review. However, if there are vascular structures near the needle path or the previous CT is old, intravenous contrast agent should be given. Biopsy is planned on the axial image which has a safe route for needle insertion (Figs. 28.2A and B). Patient is moved into the CT gantry at the table position of this axial section and a horizontal line is drawn over the patient's skin by following the laser light emitted from the scanner. On axial CT image the distance between the planned needle entry site and a bony landmark like vertebral spinous process is measured. Now this bony landmark is felt on the patient's skin and the needle entry site is marked at the measured distance. If there is no bony landmark nearby, a small radiopaque marker may be stick on patient's skin on the horizontal line already drawn and this reference may be used for skin marking.

Needle entry site should be marked by an inedible marker otherwise it will be washed during cleaning process. If inedible marker is not available, a small impression may be created by pressing the back of a needle hub over the skin. Now the site is cleaned with povidone-iodine or chlorhexidine solution and draped. Local anesthetic is injected at the needle entry point and a small nick is made over the skin with number 11 scalpel. Further biopsy technique is discussed in the respective sections. It is important to have material for transporting the biopsy specimen like formalin vial, saline vial, slides, routine fixatives and microbiological culture media in selected case.

Many commercial devices are also available for planning the needle entry site. Some are needle positioning devices which hold the needle in exact location and angulation, while others have a laser light which points the exact plane of needle insertion. However, with little experience these equipments are not necessary. Sometimes

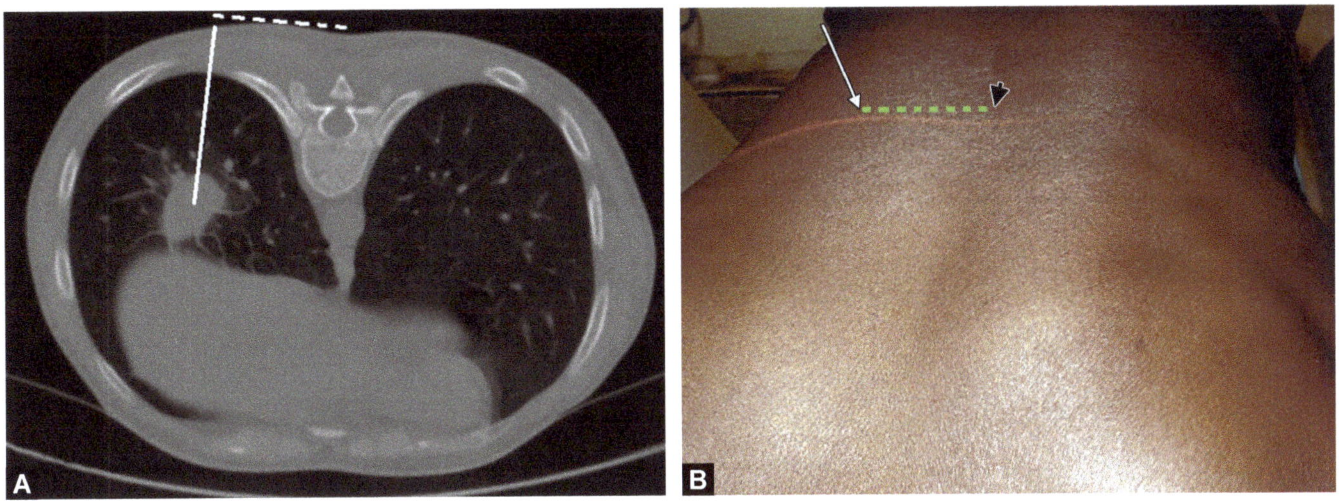

Figs. 28.2A and B: Technique of marking the needle entry site (A) The needle trajectory has been drawn on the CT image and the distance (dotted line) between the needle entry site and vertebral spinous process has been measured. (B) Patient has been moved into the CT gantry at the same table position. Location of this particular CT section is indicated by the laser light. The needle entry site (white arrow) is marked at the measured distance from the spinous process (arrowhead).

needles are to be maintained in desired needle angulation prior to complete insertion. For this a sterile drape may be fashioned to support this needle in desired angulation (Figs. 28.3A to C).

If a bony structure blocks access to a lesion, changing position of patient's arm, rotating the patient or choosing another needle path may be helpful. An angled needle insertion in z-axis may also be used to approach such lesion while avoiding the intervening bone. During the angled needle insertion, the CT gantry may be titled in the plane of needle and the resulting CT image will show the entire needle over a single image. Sagittal CT reconstructions are very useful during angled needle insertion for estimating the needle angulation in z-axis and needle entry site (Figs. 28.4A to C). During the TNB, repeated check CT sections are taken to look for needle position and for detection of any complication. To minimize radiation dose to patient, tube current should be reduced to 30–50 mAs and 2.5–5.0 mm sections are taken in sequential mode. However, adequate number of CT sections must be taken to visualize the needle tip clearly.

BIOPSY TECHNIQUE FOR PULMONARY, MEDIASTINAL, AND PLEURAL LESIONS

Pulmonary Lesions

Overall diagnostic yield of lung biopsies varies from 92% to 95%. Generally the shortest intercostal route should be taken during lung biopsies, avoiding fissures, large pulmonary vessels, bulla and emphysematous areas. Special care should be taken during biopsy of central lesions, lower lobe lesions and small subpleural nodules. If a lung lesion could be accessed without puncturing the aerated lung, possibility of post biopsy pneumothorax could be minimized. It may be done by placing needle through an area of contact of mass with the pleura or mediastinal fat, pleural effusion, collapsed or consolidated portion of lung (Figs. 28.4 to 6). Sampling of associated collapsed or consolidated lung should be avoided and intravenous contrast may be helpful for identification of the true extent of mass lesion (Figs. 28.4A to C).

During lung biopsies, needle should be aligned with lesion while it is still in the chest wall. The aim is to reach the lesion in a single pleural puncture and to minimize needle manipulation inside the lung parenchyma. Once the needle is perfectly aligned then only it should be advanced through the pleura. If a lesion is in peripheral location, it may be reached in one stroke. For deeper lesions initially needle is advanced into the outer 1–2 cm of lung and a check scan is taken. If the needle is in alignment with lesion then it is advanced till the lesion margin. During biopsy of lower lobe lesions, at least 1–2 cm of needle should be left inside the lung parenchyma during free breathing to avoid needle dislodgment and pleural tearing. After piercing lung, the needle should be left to rock freely with respiration and should be manipulated only during the designated breath hold.

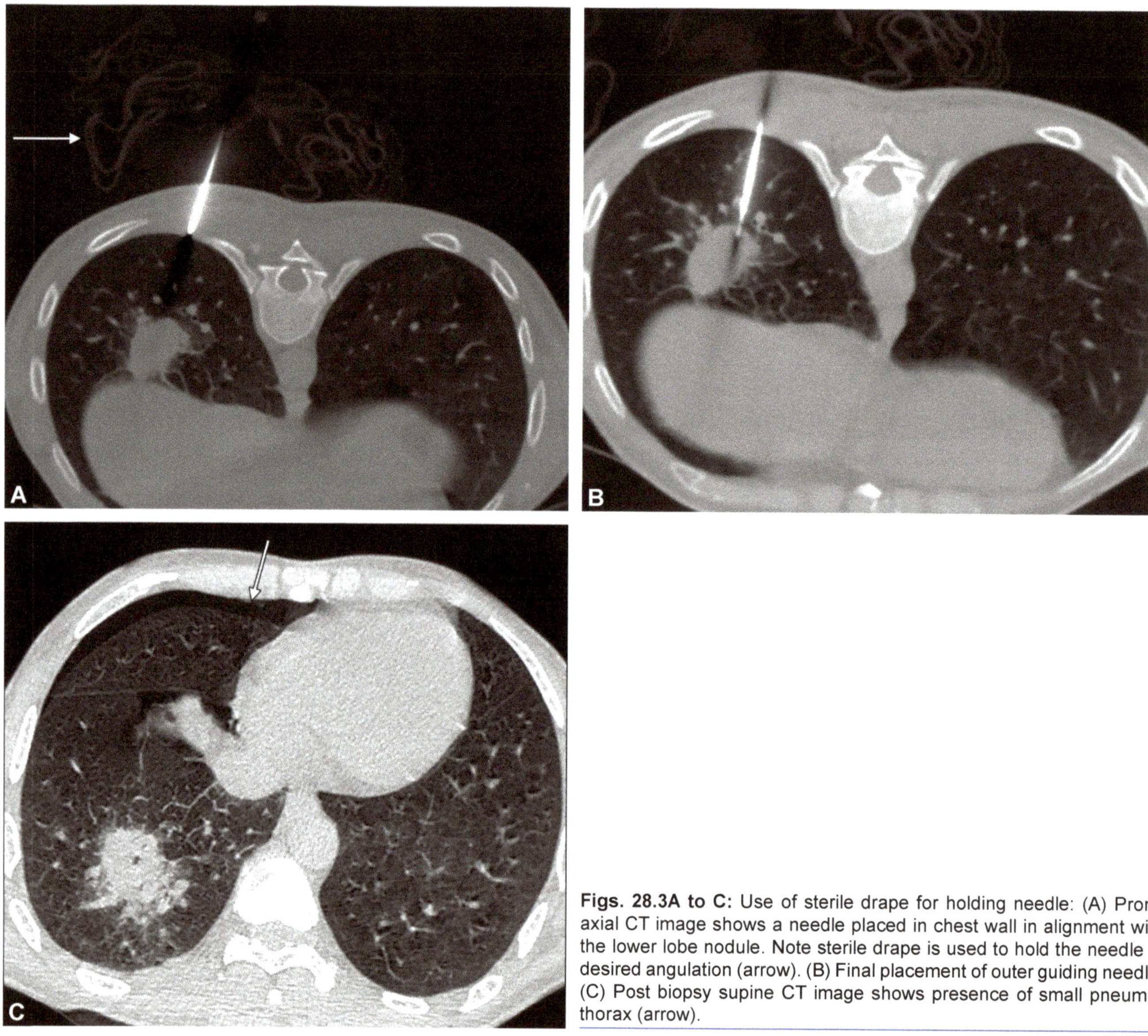

Figs. 28.3A to C: Use of sterile drape for holding needle: (A) Prone axial CT image shows a needle placed in chest wall in alignment with the lower lobe nodule. Note sterile drape is used to hold the needle in desired angulation (arrow). (B) Final placement of outer guiding needle. (C) Post biopsy supine CT image shows presence of small pneumothorax (arrow).

Small subpleural lesions are also very difficult to target because there is very little space for needle manipulation without a repeat pleural puncture and a short needle length inside the lung can easily dislodge due to respiratory motion. Moore EH has suggested that initially the needle should be placed through the whole diameter of the subpleural nodule and then the patient should be allowed to breathe. Then the needle tip is moved into the center of nodule and deeper half of nodule is sampled during a single breath hold. The rationale of this technique is to leave a longer length of needle inside lung during breathing for a better anchoring. A tangential path has been advocated by some authors rather than a right angle path for sampling the subpleural nodules as it provides greater needle stability and more room for needle correction. Some authors suggest that multiple pleural punctures during lung biopsy increase the chances of pneumothorax and procedure failure, while in other studies no correlation between number of needle passes and incidence of pneumothorax have been demonstrated. Biopsy procedure is usually abandoned if significant pneumothorax develops; however, if pneumothorax is small and not progressing, biopsy could be completed (Figs. 28.7A to C). In presence of pneumothorax, the lung becomes more mobile, and less stretched pleura is difficult to puncture.

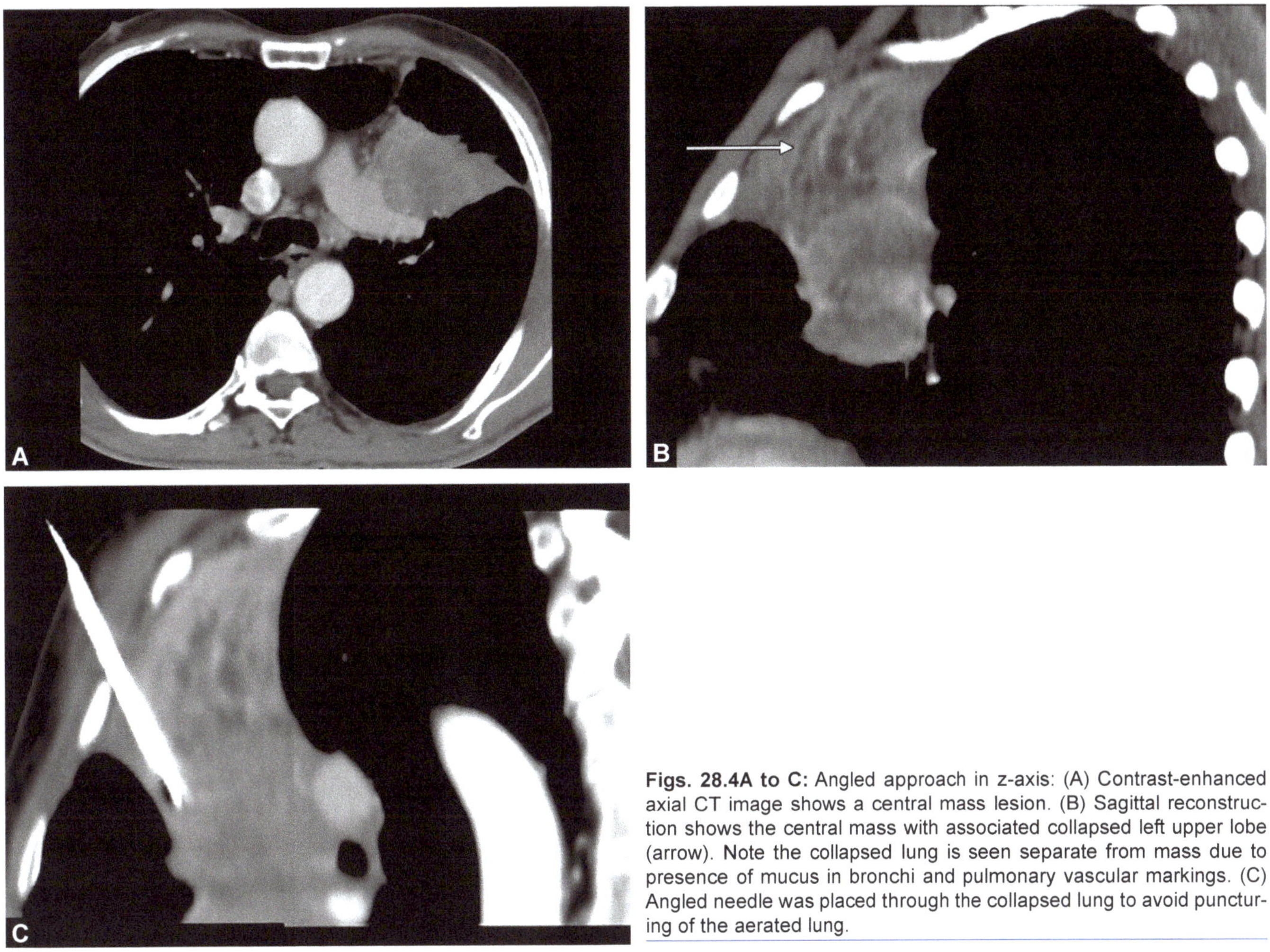

Figs. 28.4A to C: Angled approach in z-axis: (A) Contrast-enhanced axial CT image shows a central mass lesion. (B) Sagittal reconstruction shows the central mass with associated collapsed left upper lobe (arrow). Note the collapsed lung is seen separate from mass due to presence of mucus in bronchi and pulmonary vascular markings. (C) Angled needle was placed through the collapsed lung to avoid puncturing of the aerated lung.

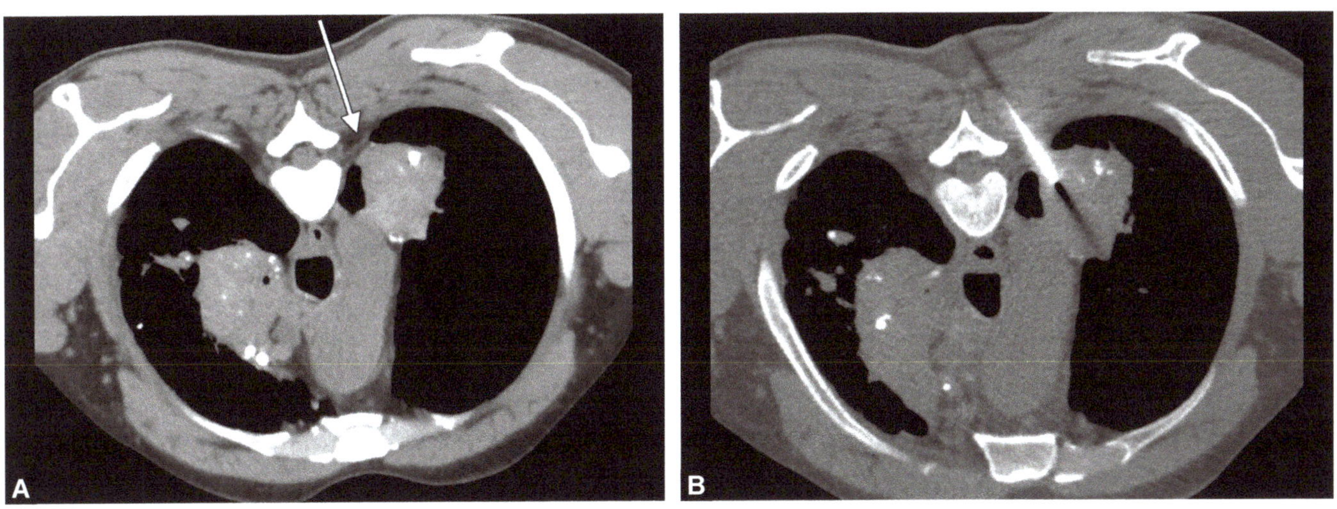

Figs. 28.5A and B: Avoiding aerated lung by placing needle through pleural contact: (A) Axial CT scan shows a mass lesion in left lung with a small contact between the mass and pleura (arrow). (B) Guiding needle is placed through this area of contact without transgressing the aerated lung.

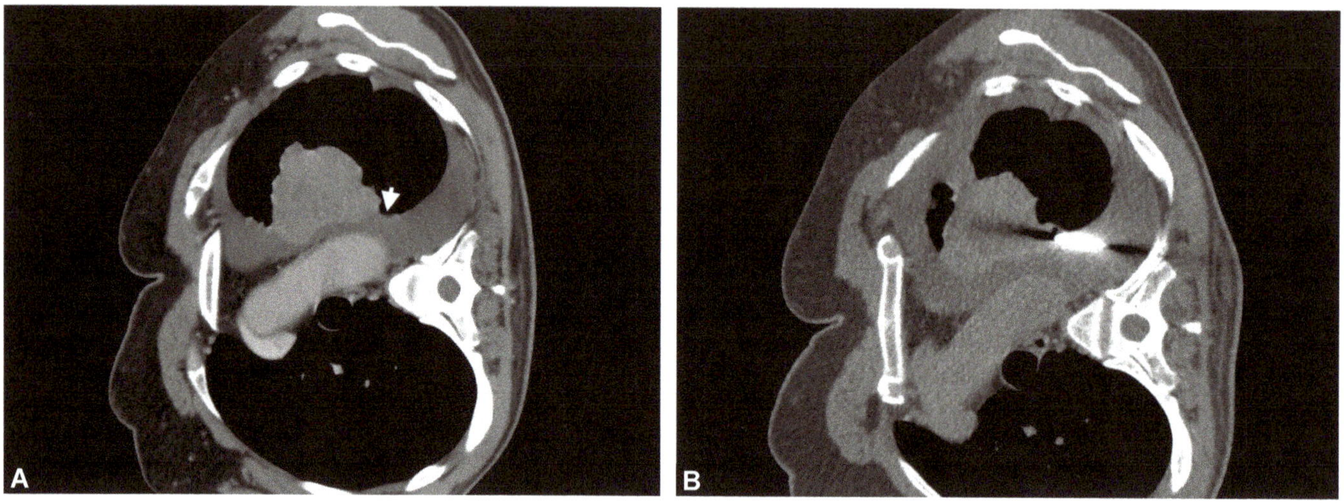

Figs. 28.6A and B: Avoiding aerated lung by placing needle through pleural effusion: (A) CT section taken in lateral decubitus reveals a small window to the mass through the pleural effusion (arrowhead). (B) Biopsy needle placed through the effusion.

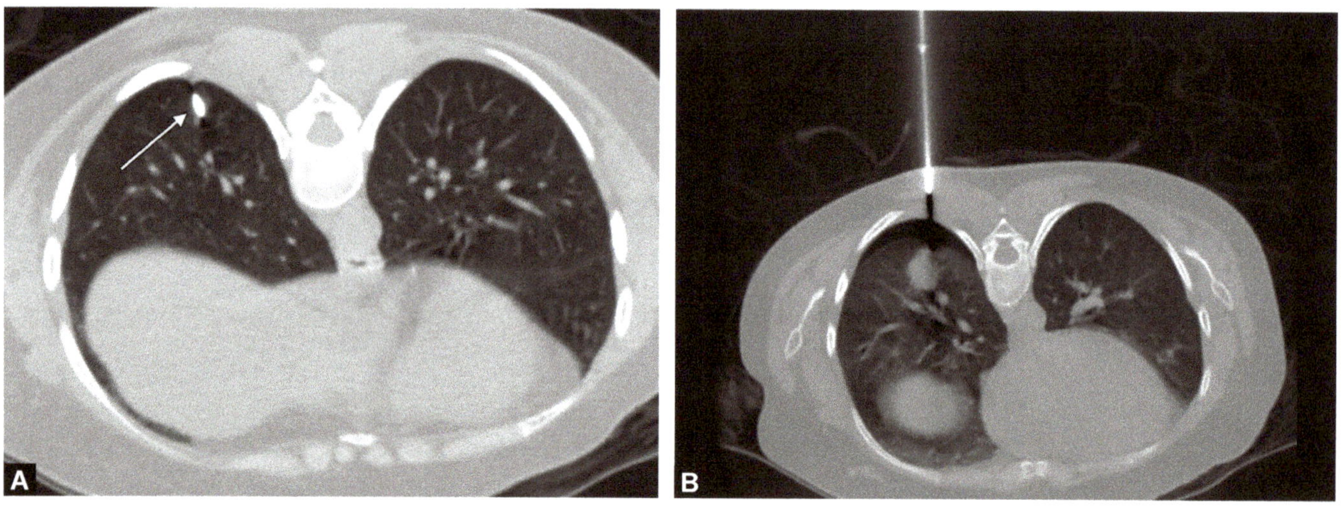

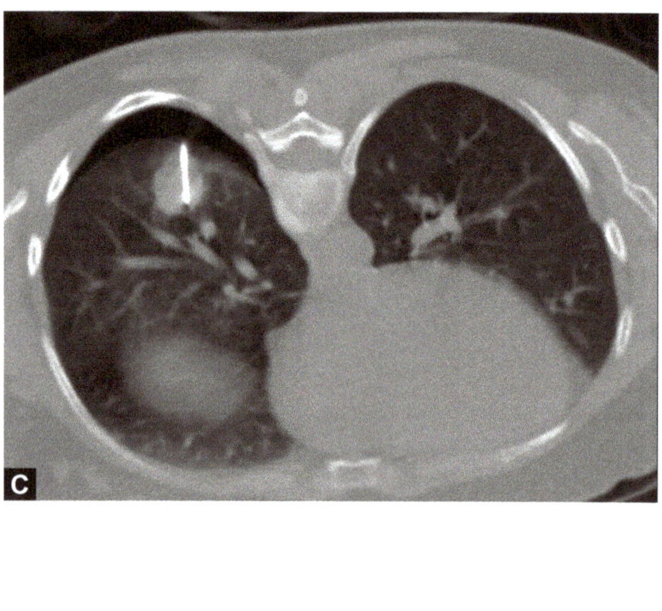

Figs. 28.7A to C: Biopsy under stable pneumothorax. (A) During initial puncture, the needle tip (arrow) reached caudal to the lesion due to inconsistent breath hold. After the needle was removed, a small pneumothorax developed. (B) After observation, a repeat puncture was performed through the stable pneumothorax. (C) Final position of needle into the lesion.

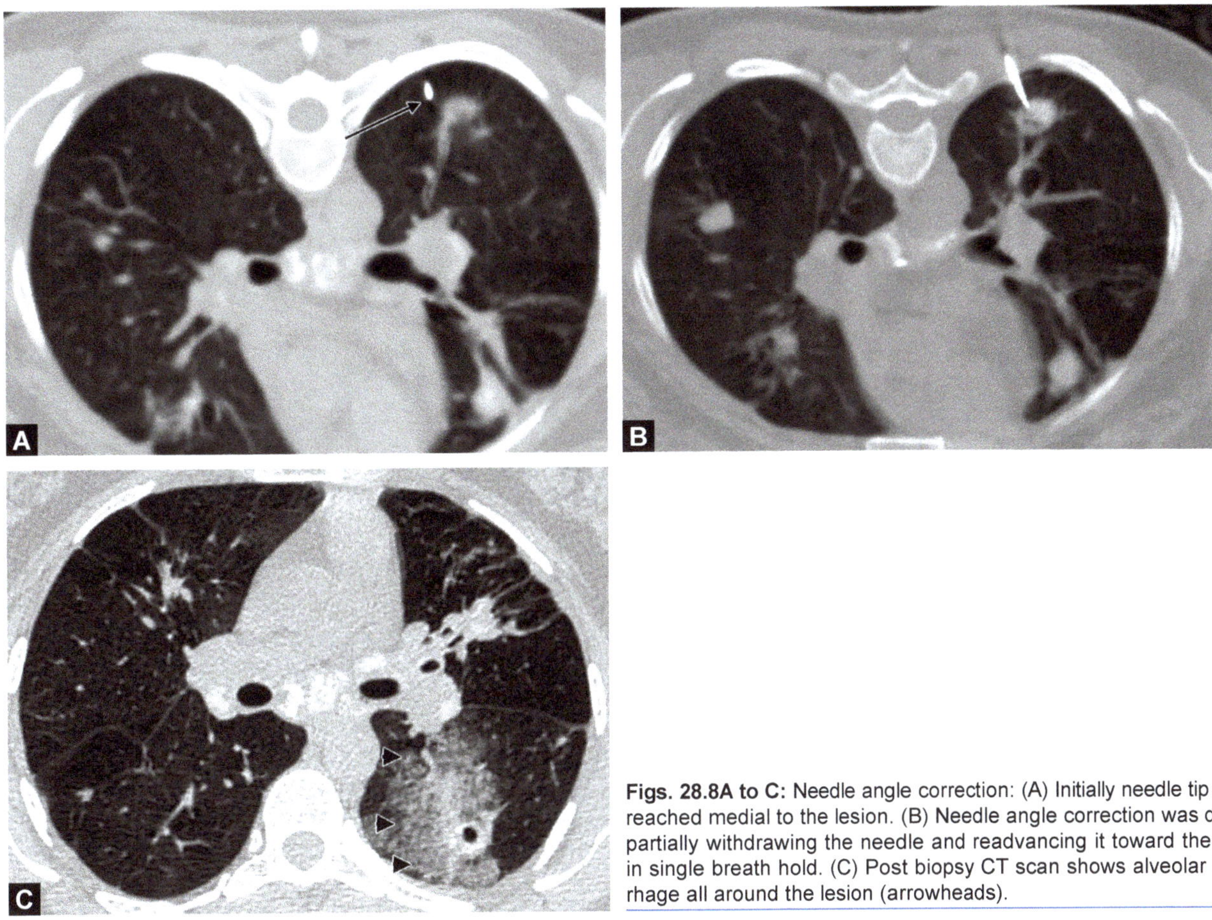

Figs. 28.8A to C: Needle angle correction: (A) Initially needle tip (arrow) reached medial to the lesion. (B) Needle angle correction was done by partially withdrawing the needle and readvancing it toward the lesion, in single breath hold. (C) Post biopsy CT scan shows alveolar hemorrhage all around the lesion (arrowheads).

Sometimes the direction of needle needs correction if there is change in lesion location due to respiratory or patient's movement. If the lesion has moved significantly, a new skin puncture may also be required. To correct the needle angle, the needle is partially withdrawn and needle tip is redirected by pushing the hub in the desired direction. Then it is readvanced toward the lesion while maintaining it in desired angulation (Figs. 28.8A to C). However, while manipulating, the needle tip should be kept inside lung parenchyma and repeated pleural puncture should be avoided.

Sometimes the final position of coaxial needle is on the periphery of lesion rather the central portion. In such cases, a small amount of needle direction correction could be achieved at the time of sampling. The hub of the guiding needle is pushed in the desired direction and then sampling with inner biopsy needle is completed while maintaining the desired angulation (Figs. 28.9A and B). This technique named "final manipulation" is particularly useful during sampling of smaller nodules and to avoid vascular structures. If one is using coaxial technique, similar small tilting movements at the time of sampling may be used to obtain specimen from a slightly different areas of the lesion. During obtaining the specimen, usually the patient is asked to hold breath. Another important thing is to grasp the needle between thumb and index finger while resting the side of the hand on the patient, and the other hand is used for attaching syringe for suction or inserting inner coaxial biopsy needle. This stabilizes the needle and prevents inadvertent advancement or withdrawal of needle tip from the lesion.

Mediastinal Lesions

Transthoracic needle biopsy is an effective tool for assessment of patients with mediastinal masses. Most commonly a parasternal or posterior paravertebral approach is used, but sometimes needle placement through the suprasternal notch or subxiphoid space is required. For biopsy of mediastinal lesions generally an extrapleural approach is

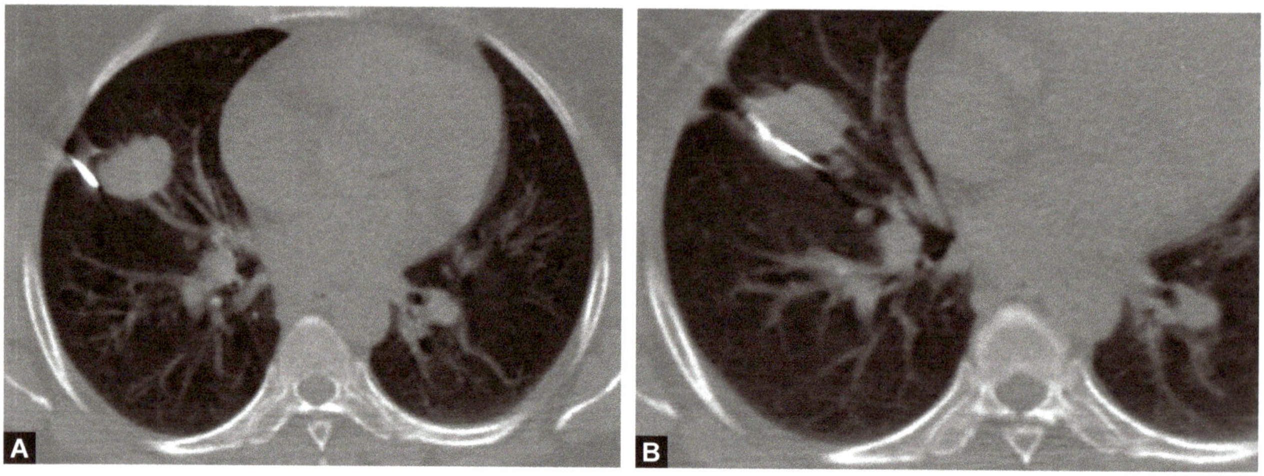

Figs. 28.9A and B: Final manipulation technique: (A) The tip of outer guiding needle is touching the margin of lesion rather than the central portion. While advancing the specimen notch of the inner biopsy needle, the guiding needle was angulated toward the center of lesion. (B) Final position of inner biopsy needle inside the lesion.

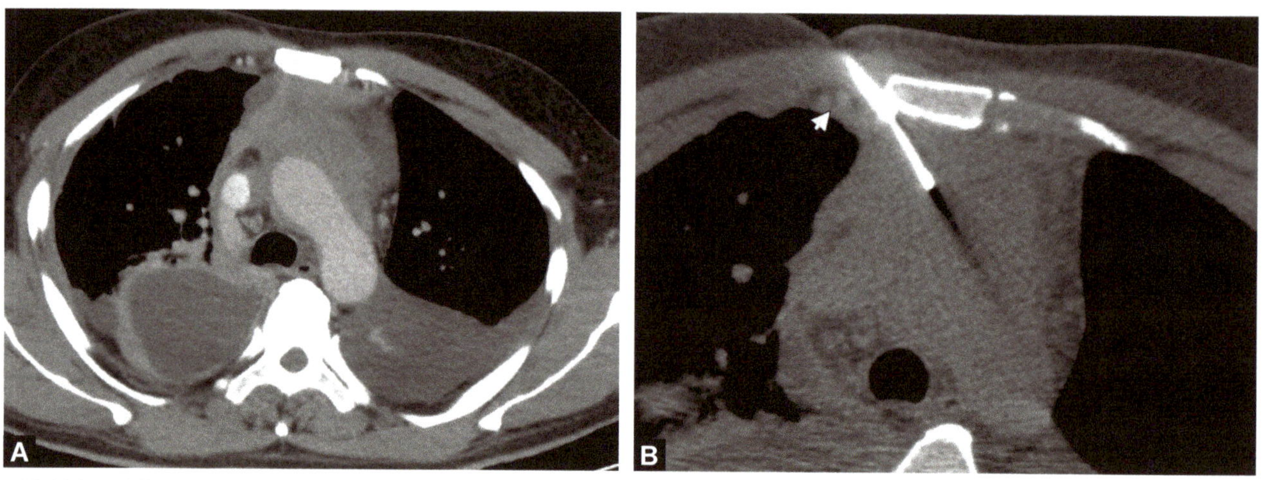

Figs. 28.10A and B: Anterior parasternal approach to mediastinal lesions: (A) Contrast-enhanced CT image shows anterior mediastinal mass and bilateral pleural effusion. (B) Needle is placed from the right parasternal approach just lateral to the sternal margin. Care was taken to avoid injury to the internal thoracic vessels (arrowhead).

preferred avoiding needle insertion through the lung and pleura. In addition, care should be taken to avoid injury to various vascular structures, esophagus, and nerves.

Transthoracic needle biopsy from a parasternal approach is performed by placing the patient in supine or lateral decubitus position. In this approach, the needle is inserted in the space between the lateral sternal margin and internal mammary vessels (Figs. 28.10A and B). This approach is suitable for anterior mediastinal lesions which are directly in contact with anterior chest wall or a safe parasternal window is available through the mediastinal fat. A posterior paravertebral approach is used for middle mediastinal, posterior mediastinal, and subcarinal lesions. Patient is placed in prone, prone oblique or lateral decubitus position. The needle is inserted immediately lateral to the vertebral body between the endothoracic fascia and parietal pleura. Needle is usually placed on right side as presence aorta makes this approach difficult from left side. If the extrapleural space is too thin for safe needle placement then normal saline or diluted contrast may be injected to widen this space (Figs. 28.11A to D). Similarly, when an extrapleural parasternal window is lacking, injection of saline solution or dilute contrast medium may be used to create an artificial extrapleural path for needle placement.

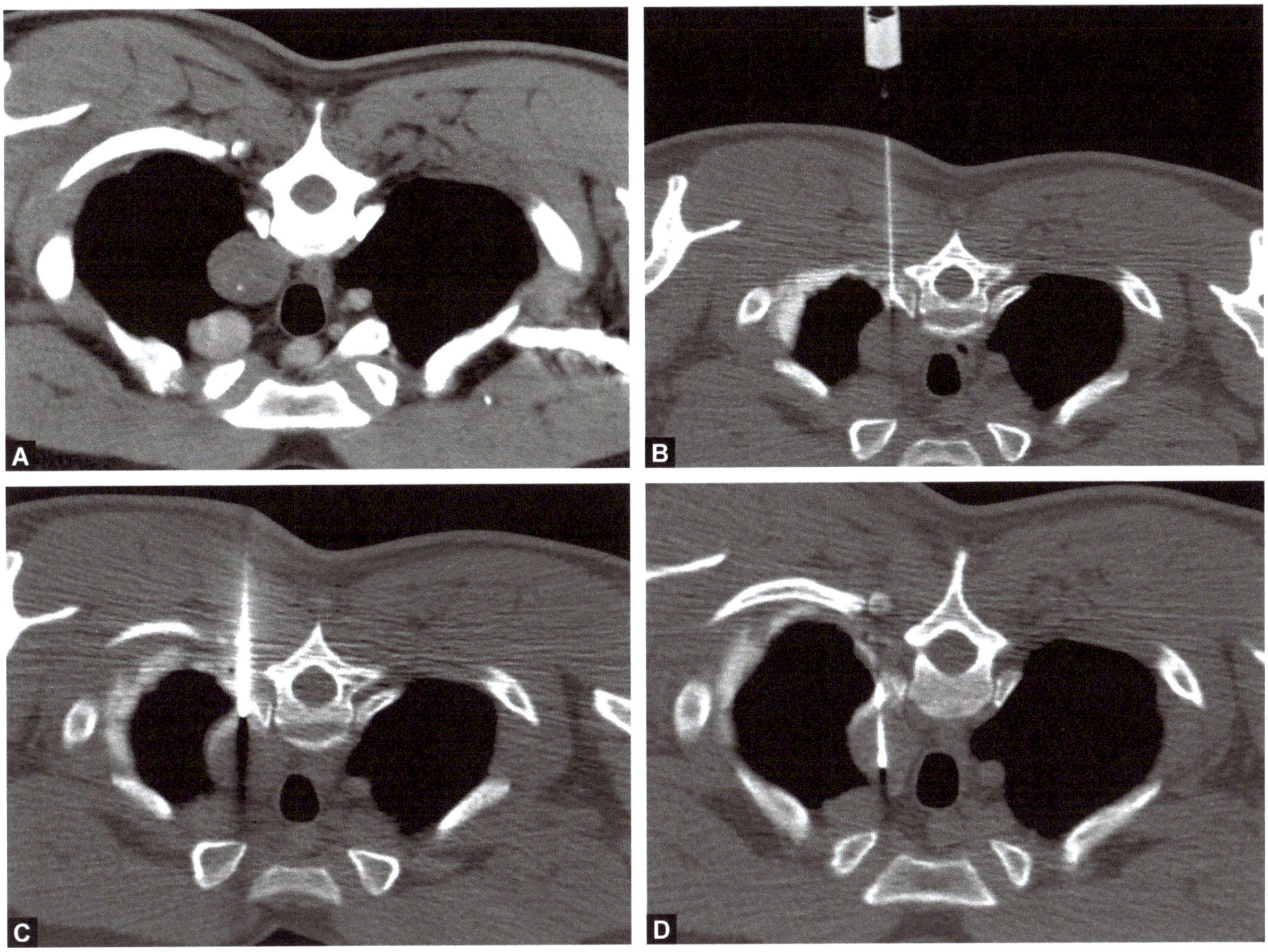

Figs. 28.11A to D: Posterior paravertebral approach with saline instillation: (A) Contrast-enhanced CT scan shows a rounded mass in middle mediastinum and no extrapleural window is available. (B) A 22-gauge Chiba needle is advanced into the paravertebral space and contrast-saline solution is injected. (C) After widening the paravertebral space a safe window is created and the guiding needle is advanced through this space. (D) Final positioning of the biopsy needle into the mass. Biopsy was suggestive of schwannoma.

A transpulmonary approach may be used for biopsy of a mediastinal lesion when it is not accessible with an extrapleural approach. However, the needle passes through the lung parenchyma and two layers of visceral pleura, and complications like pneumothorax and alveolar hemorrhage may occur. In transsternal approach, initially a bone biopsy system or an 18-G guiding needle is used to penetrate the sternal bone and a thinner gauge biopsy needle is placed coaxially to obtain the specimen. For lesions hidden behind the sternum, a suprasternal or subxiphoid approach may be used depending on location. Either ultrasound or CT guidance may be used. Needle angulation in z-axis is required for both these approaches and special care should be taken to avoid vascular structures.

Pleural Lesions

For pleural lesions either a single or coaxial needle technique may be used, as needle placement is relatively easy (Fig. 28.12). If lesion is clearly visible on ultrasound, biopsy can be done under ultrasound guidance.

POSTPROCEDURAL PRECAUTIONS

Most complications occur immediately or within the first hour of TNB; however, delayed pneumothorax has been reported. Whenever the lung is punctured, after needle removel, patient should be gently rolled in a "puncture site down" position and oxygen is supplemented through nasal mask. However, some authors report no benefit of

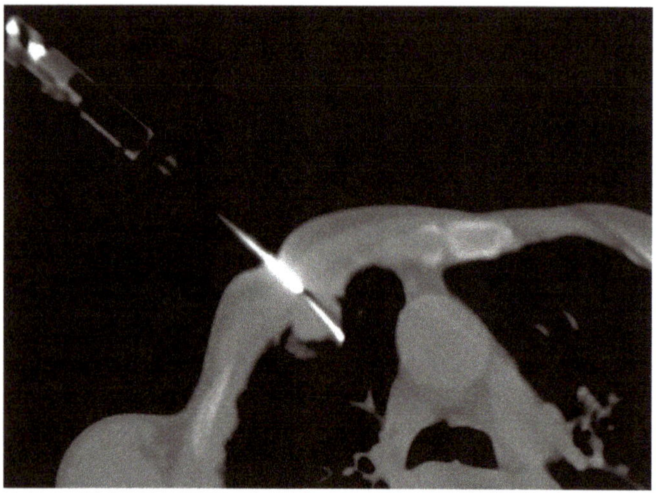

Fig. 28.12: Biopsy of pleural mass under CT guidance. Axial CT image showing biopsy needle placed into a pleural nodule.

putting patients in such a position. If the biopsy has been performed under CT guidance, an immediate post biopsy scan is taken to check for complications. Following a biopsy performed under fluoroscopy or ultrasound, an upright expiratory chest film is immediately obtained to look for pneumothorax, alveolar or pleural hemorrhage. If post biopsy CT scan or chest X-ray shows no significant complication and patient is asymptomatic, patient is shifted to recovery area on a stretcher. The patient is advised to remain in recumbent position and vitals are monitored for 2 hours. Patient should be instructed not to talk, cough or breathe deeply after the procedure. An expiratory chest X-ray is done 2 hours after biopsy and if no complication is detected, the patient could be discharged. Patient is advised to visit to nearest emergency department if dyspnea or chest pain develops and any strenuous physical activity should be avoided for 3 days.

If the patient has developed small pneumothorax immediate after biopsy or during observation period and the patient is asymptomatic, expiratory chest X-rays are taken at 1 hour intervals. If the pneumothorax remains small and patient does not develop any symptoms 3 hours after biopsy, patient may be discharged. However, clinical condition of the patient and home circumstances should be taken into consideration before discharging. Immediate chest X-ray or CT scan should be performed if patient becomes symptomatic. A pneumothorax should be treated if it is increasing or large in size (more than 30%) or if patient has symptom attributed to pneumothorax. All symptomatic patients and those with large pneumothorax should be admitted for observation.

POSSIBLE COMPLICATIONS

Despite careful biopsy planning and proper technique, complications sometimes happen. Complications are usually related to transgression of lung, pleura or a vascular structure. Pnemothorax, alveolar hemorrhage, hemothorax and chest wall hematoma are the most common complications. Other less commonly reported complications are infection, air embolism, hemomediastinum, nerve injury and malignant seeding of needle tract.

Incidence of pneumothorax after transthoracic needle lung biopsy is 15–25% and only 4–6% required chest tube insertion. Incidence is much less common after mediastinal biopsies; however, small pneumothorax is reported in 4.8–5.5% cases. Risk factors for pneumothorax are chronic obstructive pulmonary disease (COPD), long needle path, small lesion size, multiple pleural punctures and wider needle insertion angle (Figs. 28.13A to C). If pneumothorax develops during the procedure, it can be manually aspirated by the guiding needle if it is still inside or by putting another needle into the pleural space. Patient should be placed in "puncture site down" position and oxygen should be given with nasal cannula. If pneumothorax is increasing and becomes symptomatic, a 6- to 9-French catheter can be easily placed under CT guidance.

Alveolar hemorrhage around needle path is seen in about 29% cases on immediate post biopsy CT. However, only 3.4% of these patients experience hemoptysis and less than 1% of biopsy-related hemoptysis are significant enough to require medical treatment (*see* Figs. 28.8A to C). In fact, small amount of hemorrhage along the needle track is associated with lower incidence of pneumothorax. Small lesion size, greater lesion depth, pulmonary arterial hypertension are some of the risk factors for hemorrhage. If risk of hemorrhage is high, a small caliber needle may be preferred. If hemoptysis occurs, patient should be reassured and placed in "puncture site down" position to prevent spillage of blood into opposite lung. Fortunately, most of time hemoptysis resolves with conservative treatment. Massive hemoptysis is an emergency condition and may require intubation with a double-lumen endotracheal tube.

Systemic arterial air embolism is a very rare complication of TNB of lung. As the pulmonary venous pressure decreases during inspiration, if a biopsy needle is left open while it is puncturing a pulmonary vein, ambient air may be pulled in. Secondly when a needle traverses both a pulmonary vein and adjacent airway, it may result in a bronchovenous fistula and increased airway pressure, as during coughing may lead to air embolism. While air embolism to

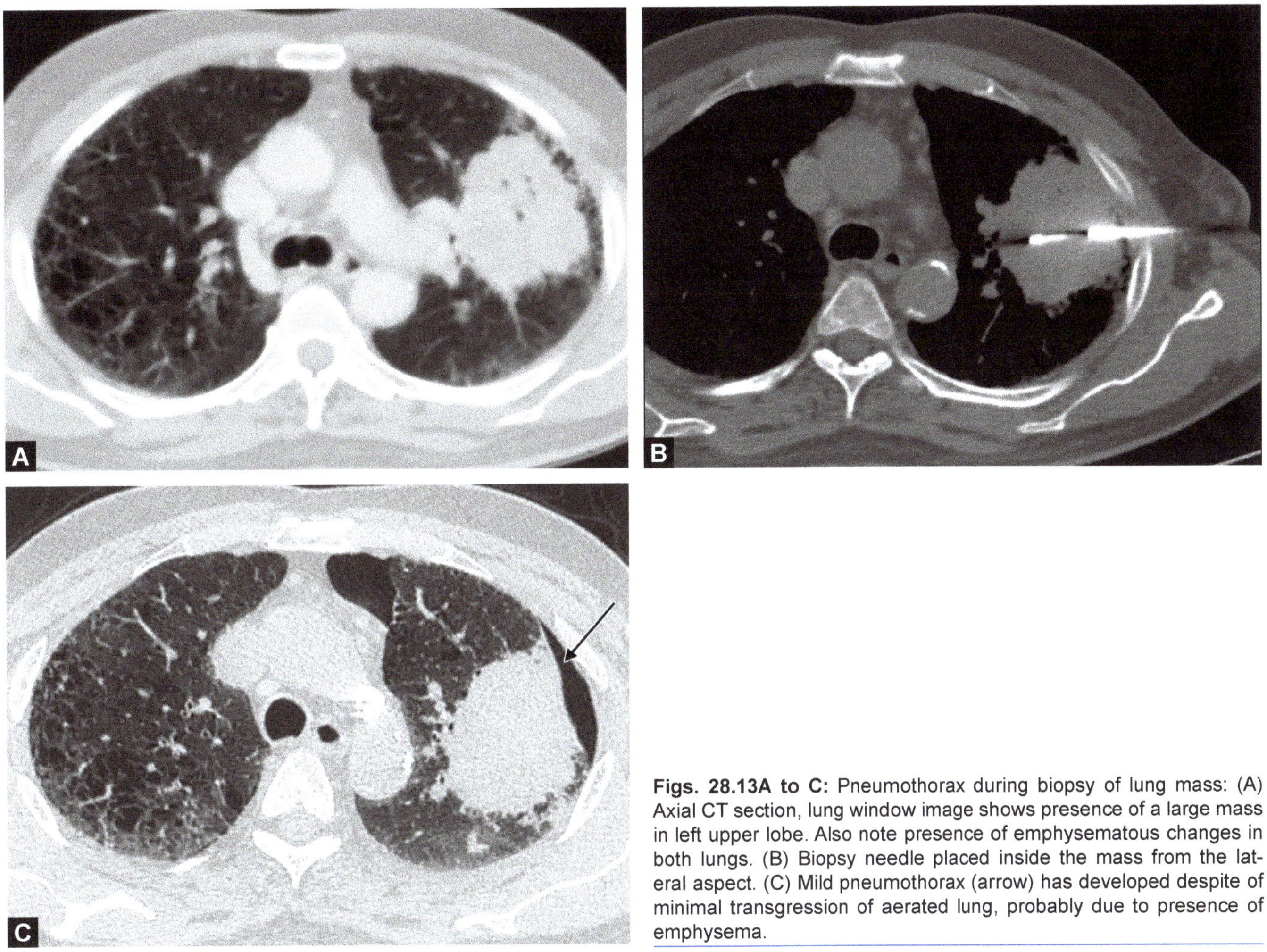

Figs. 28.13A to C: Pneumothorax during biopsy of lung mass: (A) Axial CT section, lung window image shows presence of a large mass in left upper lobe. Also note presence of emphysematous changes in both lungs. (B) Biopsy needle placed inside the mass from the lateral aspect. (C) Mild pneumothorax (arrow) has developed despite of minimal transgression of aerated lung, probably due to presence of emphysema.

skeletal muscles and viscera is well tolerated, involvement of cerebral and coronary circulation may have serious consequences. Factors which predispose for air embolism are coughing during the biopsy, coaxial technique, biopsy of consolidated lung, cavitary or cystic lesions and an associated vasculitis. To minimize chances of air embolism, hub of guiding needle should always be occluded with inner stylet or finger, and patient should be instructed to avoid breathing deeply and coughing during biopsy. In event of suspected air embolism, patient should be placed in right lateral decubitus position and high-flow oxygen must be started.

Hemothorax and chest wall hematoma are infrequent but may develop if an intercostal or internal mammary artery is injured during TNB. A hemothorax is diagnosed if a new 30–40 Hounsfield Unit (HU) fluid collection develops in pleural space during or after biopsy. To avoid injury to intercostal vessels, the biopsy needle should be placed along the superior edge of the rib. Tumor seeding along the needle track is an extremely rare complication with a reported incidence of 0.01–0.06% in literature. Pleural mesothelioma has a higher incidence of needle track seeding.

BIBLIOGRAPHY AND FURTHER READING

1. Birchard KR. Transthoracic needle biopsy. Semin Intervent Radiol. 2011;28(1):87-97.
2. Cham MD, Lane ME, Henschke CI, Yankelevitz DF. Biopsy procedures of the lung, mediastinum, and chest wall. In: Kandarpa K, Machan L (Eds). Handbook of Interventional Radiologic Procedures, 4th edition. Philadelphia, USA: Wolters Kluwer/Lippincott Williams & Wilkins; 2011. pp. 478-85.
3. Cham MD, Lane ME, Henschke CI, Yankelevitz DF. Lung biopsy: special techniques. Semin Respir Crit Care Med. 2008;29(4):335-49.

4. Cheng HM, Chiang KH, Chang PY, Chou YF, Huang HW, Chou AS, et al. Coronary artery air embolism: a potentially fatal complication of CT-guided percutaneous lung biopsy. Br J Radiol. 2010;83(988):e83-5.
5. Collings CL, Westcott JL, Banson NL, Lange RC. Pneumothorax and dependent versus nondependent patient position after needle biopsy of the lung. Radiology. 1991;181(2):385-7.
6. Cox JE, Chiles C, McManus CM, Aquino SL, Choplin RH. Transthoracic needle aspiration biopsy: variables that affect risk of pneumothorax. Radiology. 1999;212(1):165-8.
7. De Filippo M, Saba L, Silva M, Zagaria R, Concari G, Nizzoli R, et al. CT-guided biopsy of pulmonary nodules: is pulmonary hemorrhage a complication or an advantage? Diagn Interv Radiol. 2014;20(5):421-5.
8. Gupta S, Seaberg K, Wallace MJ, Madoff DC, Morello FA Jr, Ahrar K, et al. Imaging-guided percutaneous biopsy of mediastinal lesions: different approaches and anatomic considerations. Radiographics. 2005;25(3):763-86.
9. Hare SS, Gupta A, Goncalves AT, Souza CA, Matzinger F, Seely JM. Systemic arterial air embolism after percutaneous lung biopsy. Clin Radiol. 2011;66(7):589-96.
10. Klein JS, Salomon G, Stewart EA. Transthoracic needle biopsy with a coaxially placed 20-gauge automated cutting needle: results in 122 patients. Radiology. 1996;198(3):715-20.
11. Klein JS, Zarka MA. Transthoracic needle biopsy. Radiol Clin North Am. 2000;38(2):235-66.
12. Kulkarni S, Kulkarni A, Roy D, Thakur MH. Percutaneous computed tomography-guided core biopsy for the diagnosis of mediastinal masses. Ann Thorac Med. 2008;3(1):13-7.
13. Lal H, Neyaz Z, Nath A, Borah S. CT-guided percutaneous biopsy of intrathoracic lesions. Korean J Radiol. 2012; 13(2):210-26.
14. Loh SE, Wu DD, Venkatesh SK, Ong CK, Liu E, Seto KY, et al. CT-guided thoracic biopsy: evaluating diagnostic yield and complications. Ann Acad Med Singapore. 2013;42(6):285-90.
15. Loubeyre P, Copercini M, Dietrich PY. Percutaneous CT-guided multisampling core needle biopsy of thoracic lesions. AJR Am J Roentgenol. 2005;185(5):1294-8.
16. Manhire A, Charig M, Clelland C, Gleeson F, Miller R, Moss H, et al. Guidelines for radiologically guided lung biopsy. Thorax. 2003;58(11):920-36.
17. McSweeney SE, O'Regan KN, Mc Laughlin PD, Crush L, Maher MM. Evaluation of the efficacy and safety of percutaneous biopsy of lung. Open Respir Med J. 2012;6:82-8.
18. Moore EH, LeBlanc J, Montesi SA, Richardson ML, Shepard JA, McLoud TC. Effect of patient positioning after needle aspiration lung biopsy. Radiology. 1991;181:385-7.
19. Moore EH. Technical aspects of needle aspiration lung biopsy: a personal perspective. Radiology. 1998;208(2):303-18.
20. Morrissey B, Adams H, Gibbs AR, Crane MD. Percutaneous needle biopsy of the mediastinum: review of 94 procedures. Thorax. 1993;48(6):632-7.
21. Mullan CP, Kelly BE, Ellis PK, Hughes S, Anderson N, McCluggage WG. CT-guided fine-needle aspiration of lung nodules: effect on outcome of using coaxial technique and immediate cytological evaluation. Ulster Med J. 2004;73(1):32-6.
22. Ofiara LM, Navasakulpong A, Beaudoin S, Gonzalez AV. Optimizing tissue sampling for the diagnosis, subtyping, and molecular analysis of lung cancer. Front Oncol. 2014;4:253.
23. Priola AM, Priola SM, Cataldi A, Ferrero B, Garofalo G, Errico L, et al. CT-guided percutaneous transthoracic biopsy in the diagnosis of mediastinal masses: evaluation of 73 procedures. Radiol Med. 2008;113(1):3-15.
24. Richardson CM, Pointon KS, Manhire AR, Macfarlane JT. Percutaneous lung biopsies: a survey of UK practice based on 5444 biopsies. Br J Radiol. 2002;75(897):731-5.
25. Tsai IC, Tsai WL, Chen MC, Chang GC, Tzeng WS, Chan SW, et al. CT-guided core biopsy of lung lesions: a primer. AJR Am J Roentgenol. 2009;193(5):1228-35.
26. Wallace AB, Suh RD. Percutaneous transthoracic needle biopsy: special considerations and techniques used in lung transplant recipients. Semin Intervent Radiol. 2004;-21(4):247-58.
27. Wallace MJ, Krishnamurthy S, Broemeling LD, Gupta S, Ahrar K, Morello FA Jr, et al. CT-guided percutaneous fine-needle aspiration biopsy of small (< or = 1-cm) pulmonary lesions. Radiology. 2002;225(3):823-8.
28. White CS, Meyer CA, Templeton PA. CT fluoroscopy for thoracic interventional procedures. Radiol Clin North Am. 2000;38(2):303-22.
29. Wiener RS, Wiener DC, Gould MK. Risks of transthoracic needle biopsy: how high? Clin Pulm Med. 2013;20(1):29-35.
30. Wong ET, Dunham C, Patsios D. Qualitative assessment of pain management in patients undergoing computed tomography-guided transthoracic lung biopsy. Pain Res Manag. 2014;19(3):149-52.
31. Wu CC, Maher MM, Shepard JA. Complications of CT-guided percutaneous needle biopsy of the chest: prevention and management. AJR Am J Roentgenol. 2011;196(6):W678-82.
32. Yamagami T, Kato T, Iida S, Hirota T, Nishimura T. Percutaneous needle biopsy for small lung nodules beneath the rib under CT scan fluoroscopic guidance with gantry tilt. Chest. 2004;126(3):744-7.
33. Yang PC. Ultrasound-guided transthoracic biopsy of the chest. Radiol Clin North Am. 2000;38(2):323-43.
34. Yankelevitz DF, Vazquez M, Henschke CI. Special techniques in transthoracic needle biopsy of pulmonary nodules. Radiol Clin North Am. 2000;38(2):267-79.

Chapter

29 Conventional Transbronchial Needle Aspiration

Claudio Sorino, Danai Khemasuwan, Thomas R Gildea, Stefano Gasparini, Atul C Mehta

OVERVIEW OF TRANSBRONCHIAL NEEDLE ASPIRATION AND MAIN INDICATIONS

Transbronchial needle aspiration (TBNA) is a diagnostic technique that allows obtaining tissue from the deeper submucosa and beyond the confines of the endobronchial tree in a minimally invasive manner (Figs. 29.1A and B). It is used mainly for the diagnosis and staging of lung cancer and other mediastinal lesions. Its further indications include the diagnosis of granulomatous, inflammatory and infectious diseases involving the mediastinal lymph nodes.

Conventional TBNA (C-TBNA) is performed after thoroughly reviewing the computed tomography (CT) scan of the chest. TBNA is a convenient, cost-effective and minimally invasive alternative to the mediastinoscopy for the majority of mediastinal pathologies including lung cancer, sarcoidosis, lymphoma. In addition, C-TBNA skills are easy to acquire and has a steep learning curve. Besides it does not require advanced imaging technique except for a CT scan of the chest.

Endobronchial needle aspiration (EBNA) is the technique in which the transbronchial needle is used to obtain cytology specimen from the core of an endoscopically visible lesion such as endobronchial masses, and for drainage of cystic lesions adjoining the tracheobronchial tree.

Peripheral transbronchial needle aspiration (P-TBNA) is a simple technique to obtain, under fluoroscopic guidance, the cytology specimen from peripheral lung nodules larger than 2 cm in size and with a negative bronchus sign. In this chapter, we review the planning, technique, and limitations of C-TBNA, EBNA, and P-TBNA.

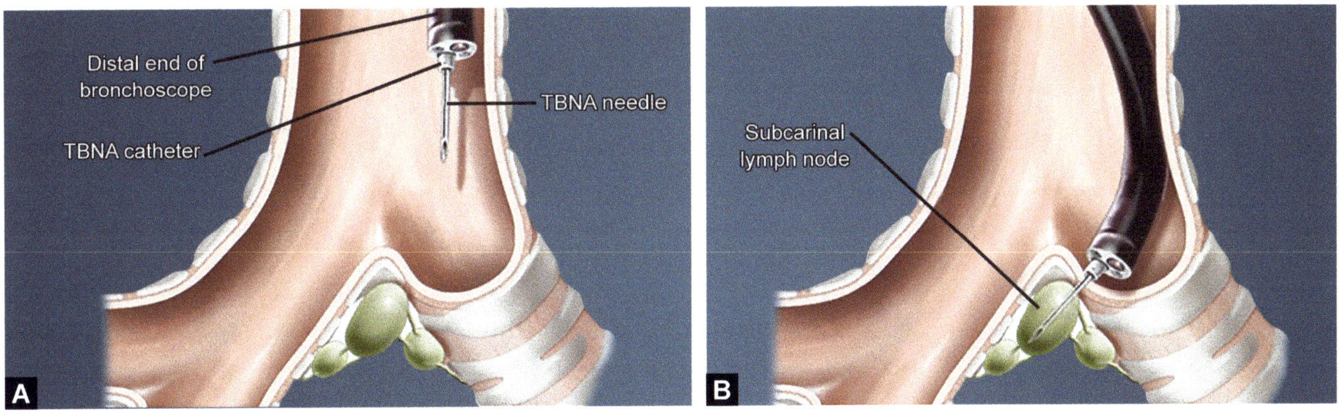

Figs. 29.1A and B: Schematic presentation of TBNA. (A) At the distal end of the bronchoscope is visible the metal hub which emits the TBNA needle. (B) The needle is pushed through the bronchial wall penetrating the lymph node for sampling. (TBNA: Transbonchial needle aspiration). *Courtesy*: Olympus Europe SE & CO. KG.

PLANNING OF C-TBNA AND CHEST IMAGING STUDY

Conventional TBNA procedures should be performed only following a thorough clinical and radiological evaluation including a CT scan of the chest. All elective TBNA must be performed after a thorough review of the CT scan of the chest. This is to properly select the target site and avoid injury to surrounding vascular structures. A contrast-enhanced CT is preferred over the noncontrast one. A positron emission tomography (PET) scan can also be used as guidance to perform the C-TBNA. From a technical perspective, however, PET scan affords no specific advantage over the standard CT in navigating to the target lymph node. The assistants must be instructed about the procedure and the potential adverse events and their management.

Prior to a staging procedure, a number of slides should be labeled with patient's identification. The lymph node station from which specimen is obtained should be marked on the slides for accurate processing and reporting. Lung cancer staging with C-TBNA is performed by sampling the higher stations before the lower ones, i.e. N3, before N2, and finally N1. While performing the C-TBNA, the high right paratracheal region is avoided to reduce the risk of pneumothorax and over staging of the lung cancer, from T1 to N3. The right upper lobe apical segment is in close proximity of the upper right paratracheal wall increasing the possibility of pneumothorax if a C-TBNA is performed in this location. Similarly, the inadvertent aspiration of a mass lesion in the right upper lobe (T1) could be falsely interpreted as N2 or N3 disease is the C-TBNA is performed in this location.

MAPPING SYSTEMS OF THE LYMPH NODES

In order to facilitate the selection of the target for the needle insertion, Wang first proposed a classification of hilar-mediastinal lymph nodes accessible by TBNA. Accordingly, 11 lymph node stations were identified, and guidance on how to identify and sample the lymph node is provided for each station (Fig. 29.2A). More recently, the International Association for Study of Lung Cancer (IASLC) proposed an updated method of grouping the lymph node stations together into "stations", based on their surgical anatomical location. According to the IASLC classification, hilar-mediastinal lymph nodes can be categorized into three groups: (1) carinal region, (2) subcarinal region, and (3) hilar region (Fig. 29.2B). Based on this mapping system, C-TBNA is most suitable for sampling stations 4R, 4L, 7, 10R, 11R, 10L, and 11L (Figs. 29.3A to D).

Even though the two mentioned mapping systems are closely related, Wang's method has some advantages over IASLC's system. In particular, most IASLC lymph node stations are identified through surgical anatomic landmarks including aorta, pulmonary vein, and esophagus. The relationships among these structures may be difficult to be evaluated by the bronchoscopist during TBNA procedures even under ultrasonic guidance. On the contrary, Wang's classification identifies different stations by endoscopic and radiological landmarks, thus making it easy to recognize the target sites. IASLC classification does provide much needed standardization in lung cancer mapping.

REQUIRED TOOLS

A system for obtaining a tissue sample by TBNA includes: (1) a flexible needle with a more flexible proximal region able to bend together with the bronchoscope tube, and a less flexible distal region with a tip able to penetrate the tissues; (2) a catheter with an interior lumen, within which the flexible needle can slide and a distal metal hub; (3) a suction source in fluid communication with the flexible needle (Fig. 29.4).

There are several flexible needles which can be used for the execution of the TBNA, with diameter varying from 19 gauge to 22 gauge. In order to be suitable for sampling from the hilar-mediastinal region, a flexible TBNA needle should have certain characteristics: first, the needle must be retractable in nature to be pulled back within the plastic catheter to prevent the damage to the bronchoscope during the passage of the instrument through the working channel. The sharp end of the beveled needle is housed within the distal metal hub in a fully retracted position during its insertion through the working channel. Second, the needle should be sufficiently long (13–15 mm) in order to allow its position on to the core of the mediastinal lymph node through the tracheobronchial wall. A 22-gauge TBNA needle is used for obtaining a cytological sample, while a 19-gauge needle for histology. The needle catheter can be easily delivered through the most flexible bronchoscopes with a working channel diameter of more than 2.2 mm in diameter (Figs. 29.5A to D). The proximal end of the needle is used to advance and to retract the needle. The suction can be applied through the proximal suction port using a 20 mL or 50 mL syringe.

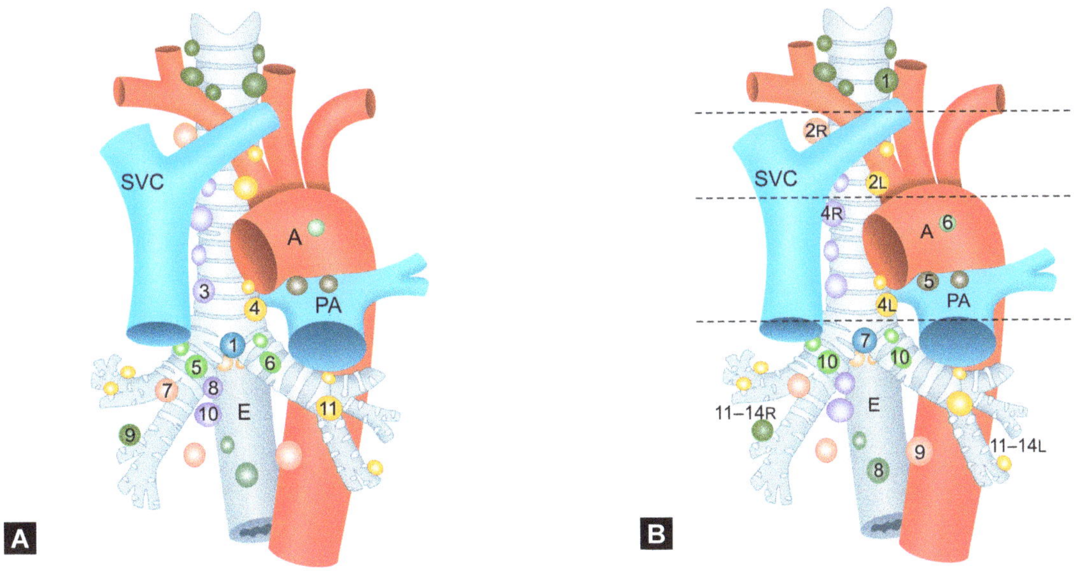

1 Anterior carina
2 Posterior carina
3 Right paratracheal
4 Left paratracheal
5 Right main bronchus
6 Left main bronchus
7 Right upper hilar
8 Subcarina
9 Right lower hilar
10 Sub-subcarinal
11 Left hilar

1 Highest mediastinal
2 Upper paratracheal
3 Prevascular and retrotracheal
4 Lower paratracheal
5 Subaortic
6 Para-aortic
7 Subcarinal
8 Paraesophageal
9 Pulmonary ligament
10 Hilar
11 Interlobar
12 Lobar
13 Segmental
14 Subsegmental

Figs. 29.2A and B: Lymph nodes classification according to (A) Wang and (B) to the International Association for Study of Lung Cancer (IASLC). All the lymph node stations described by Wang are accessed via TBNA. The corresponding stations according to the IASLC classification are 4R, 4L, 7, 10R, 11R, 10L, and 11L.(SVC: Superior vena cava; A: Aorta; PA: Pulmonary artery; E: Esophagus; TBNA: Transbonchial needle aspiration; R: Right; L: Left).

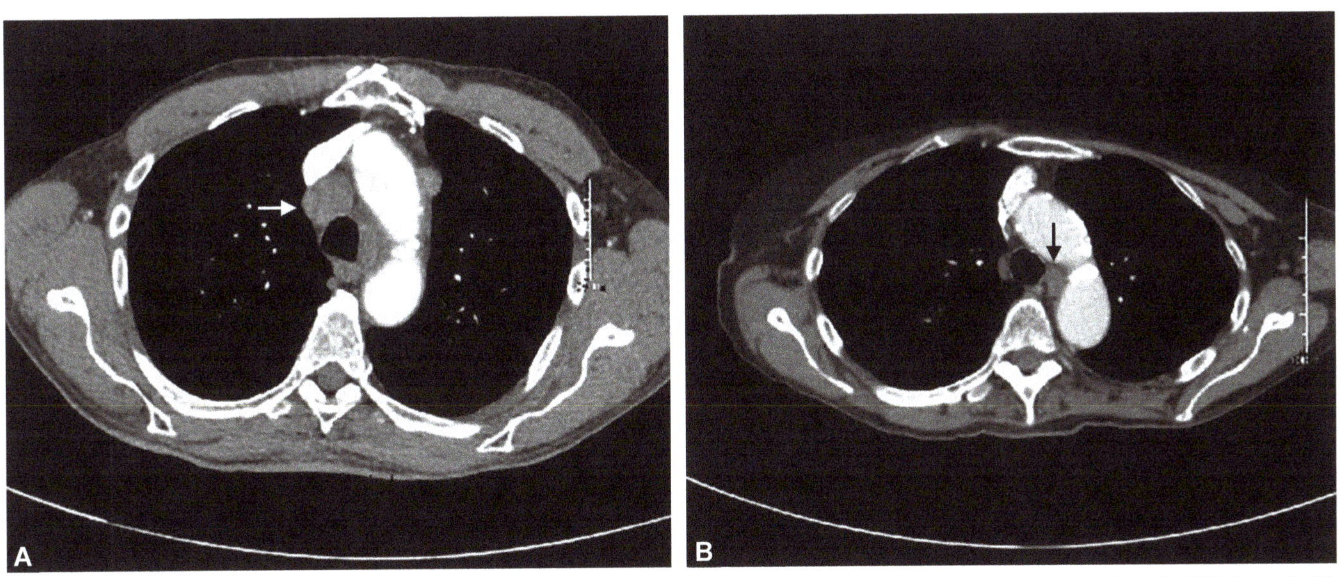

Figs. 29.3A and B: CT images demonstrating enlarged mediastinal and hilar lymph nodes. (A) Right paratracheal lymph node (4R) (arrow). (B) Left paratracheal lymph node (4L) (arrow).

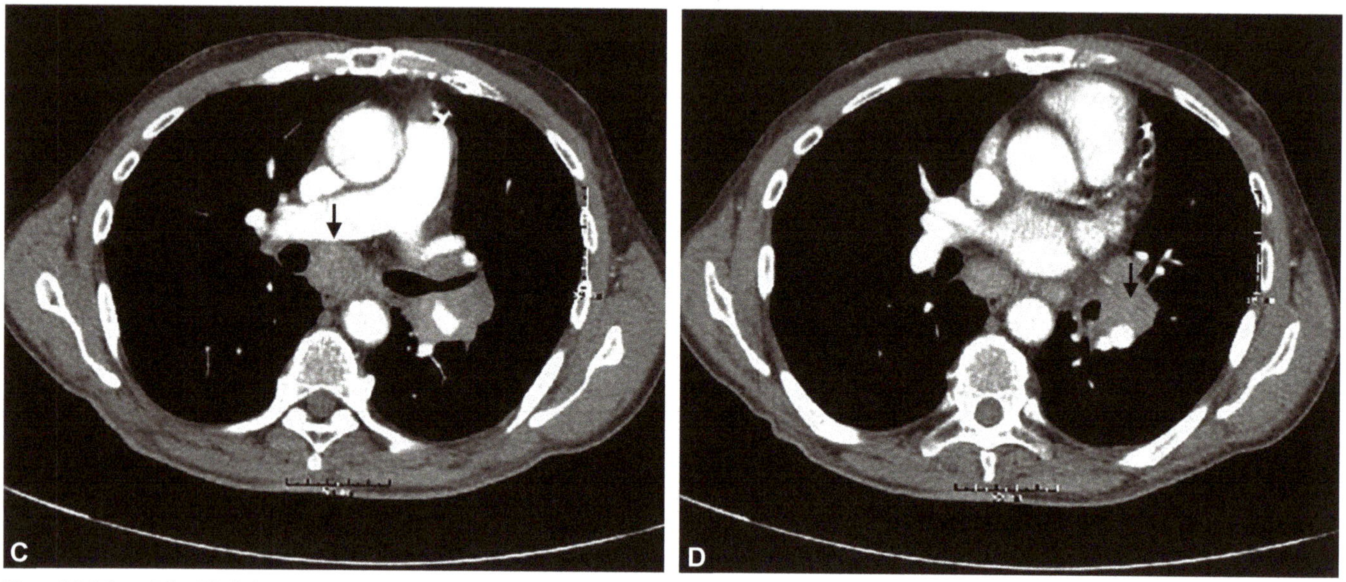

Figs. 29.3C and D: (C) Subcarinal lymph node (7) (arrow). (D) Left interlobar lymph node (11L) (arrow).

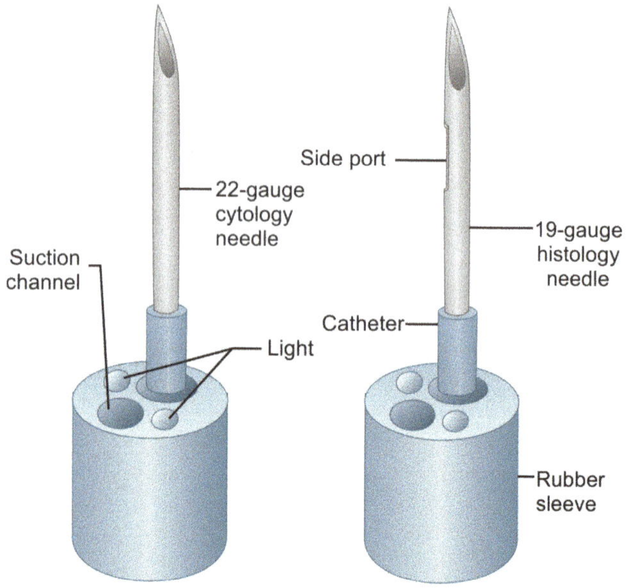

Fig. 29.4: Distal end of bronchoscope with two different TBNA needles within their catheters. (TBNA: Transbronchial needle aspiration).

TECHNIQUE

The procedure of TBNA can be performed either through the nasal or the oral route. The airways, especially the puncture site, should be clear of any secretion to avoid false-positive results from contamination with bronchial secretions. The first step toward performing TBNA is to choose the target site where the needle is to be inserted (Figs. 29.6A to D). Once the target site is identified, the needle-catheter is inserted into the working channel of the bronchoscope while keeping the instrument as straight as possible keeping the needle tip is completely retracted and protected inside the metal hub in order to avoid any damage to the bronchoscope.

In the proximity of the target site, the catheter is advanced beyond the distal end of the bronchoscope keeping the latter's distal end in a neutral, forward viewing position. Once the position of the distal hub is confirmed beyond the tip of the scope, the needle is projected out of its catheter. In order to avoid the catheter from being kinked during the procedure, the metal hub is kept as close to the tip of the bronchoscope as possible.

The ideal position of the needle is keeping it close to the tip of the scope without the beveled end entering the channel. This position provides full control over the movement of the needle and avoids kinking of the catheter.

At this stage the goal is to insert the needle at the target site to its fullest length at an angle no less than 45° to the tracheobronchial wall. This can be carried out using any one of the following methods.

Several deployment techniques used to insert the needle into the airway wall are described:

1. *Jabbing method* (Fig. 29.7A): As the term describes, this method involves inserting the extended needle at the target site by giving a firm jab to the catheter at the proximal end of the working channel while

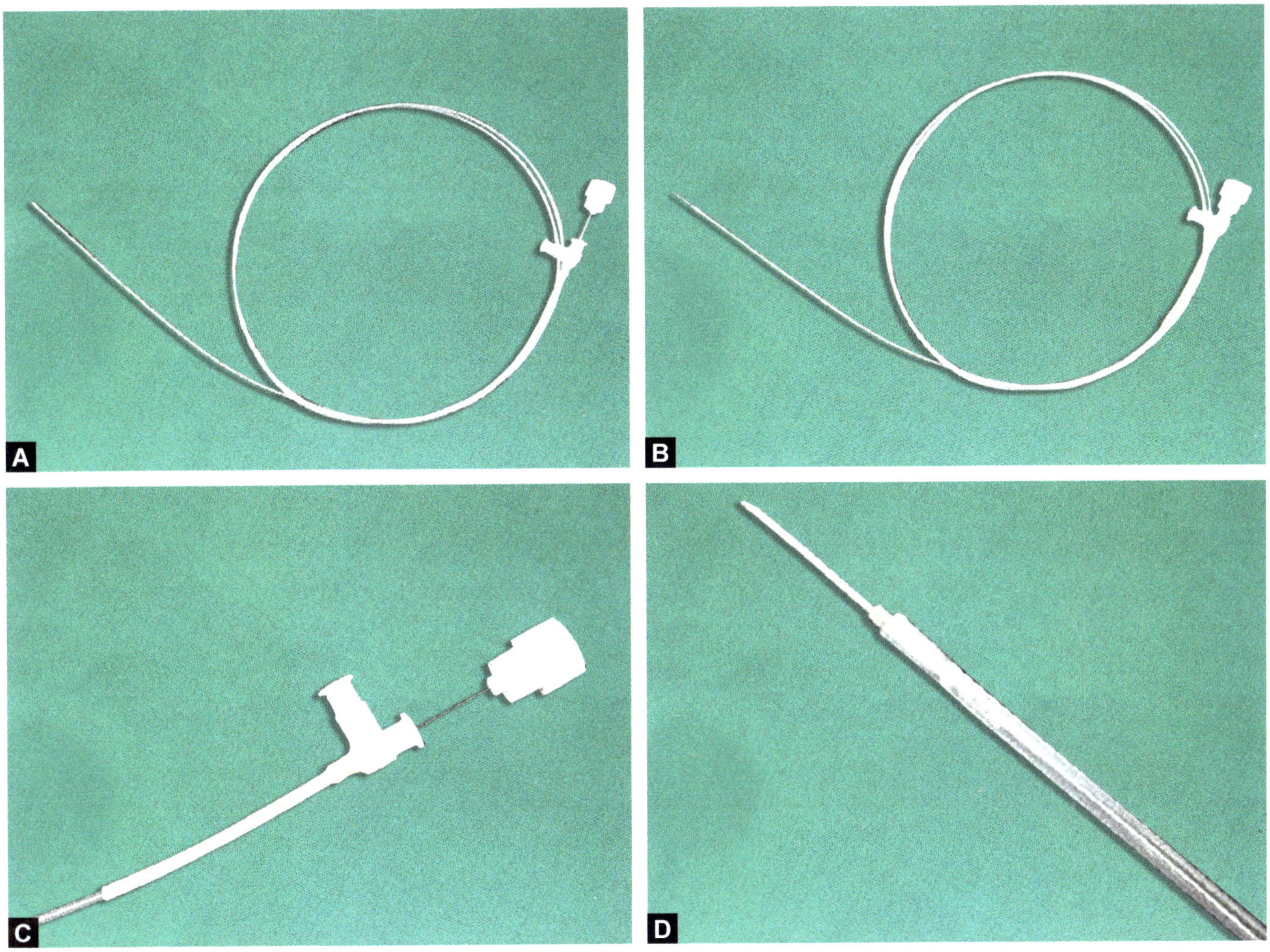

Figs. 29.5A to D: A MW-122 needle with distal 22-gauge TBNA needle. (A) Needle fully within metal hub. (B) The proximal control device is advanced and locked in place to deploy the TBNA needle. (C) Proximal control device. (D) Needle after full deployment. (TBNA: Transbronchial needle aspiration)

firmly holding the bronchoscope (usually the bronchoscope is held in position by the assistant either at the nose or mouth). A caution is required to accurately anchor the bevel of the needle at the target site between the tracheal rings. If the needle is placed against a cartilage, there is a risk of kinking the catheter.

2. *Pushing or Piggyback method* (Fig. 29.7B): The principle behind this method is to stabilize the needle catheter at the proximal end of the working channel and then pushing the scope forward along with the needle in a piggyback fashion to its fullest insertion. Little finger can be used to stabilize the TBNA catheter at the biopsy port of the working channel. The bronchoscope, catheter and needle are advanced *enbloc* into target puncture site at a 90° angle, such that the needle penetrates the airway wall.
3. *Hub against the wall method* (Fig. 29.7C): The catheter is advanced until its distal metal hub is visualized. The hub is placed against the target site at a 45–90° angle with the airway wall. The assistant is asked to keep the bronchoscope in a stable position and the TBNA needle is pushed for penetrating the airway wall. This method requires good coordination between the bronchoscopist and the assistant.
4. *Cough method* (Fig. 29.7D): The bronchoscope is positioned close to the target puncture site. The bevel end of the needle is deployed and anchored there at the target site. The patient is asked to give a loud

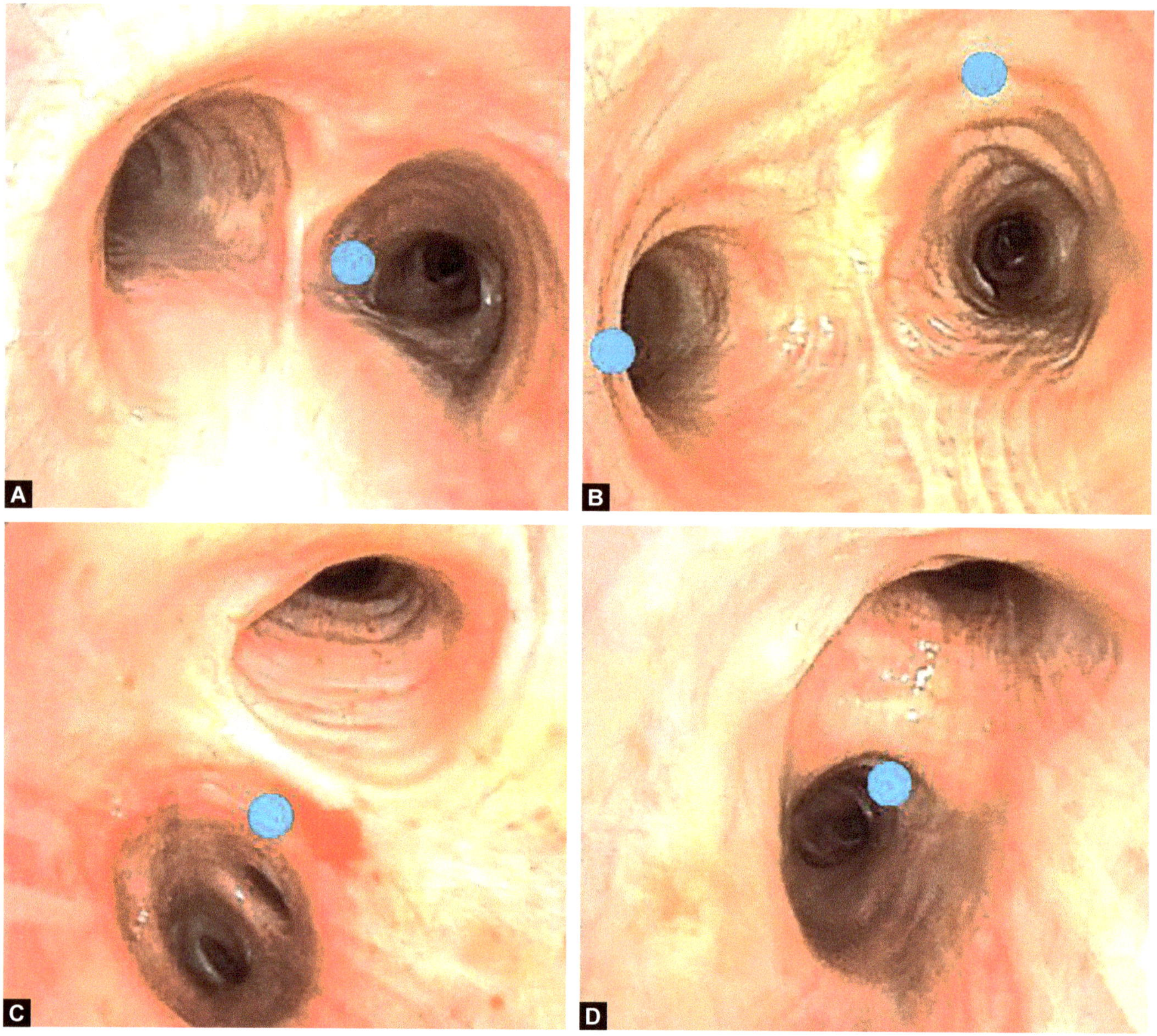

Figs. 29.6A to D: Endoscopic view: (A) TBNA site for station 7 lymph nodes is 3–5 mm below either side of the primary carina with the needle pointing in inferomedial direction. (B) The site for station 4R is about 2 cm about main carina between 1 and 2 o'clock position, site for station 4L is at lateral wall of trachea and left main bronchus at the level of carina at 9 o'clock position. (C) TBNA site for 11L is at the secondary carina between left upper and lower lobe bronchus at 12 to 2 o'clock position. (D) TBNA site for 11R is immediately below the origin of right upper lobe bronchus at 3 o'clock position on lateral wall of bronchus intermedius. (TBNA: Transbronchial needle aspiration).

cough. The inward movement of airway wall toward the needle facilitates its penetration into the airway wall and the lesion.

There are no comparative studies to identify the superiority of any of these methods over the others. The choice of technique is strictly at the discretion of the bronchoscopist. Ideally the bronchoscopist should be expert in several of the techniques. Once the needle is inserted at the target site to its fullest extent, suction is applied at the proximal end using a syringe (preferably with a dual lock system). While maintaining the suction, the catheter, and thus the needle, is agitated to obtain loose cells for cytological examination. Usually the operator grips the proximal part of the catheter (approximately a couple of centimeters

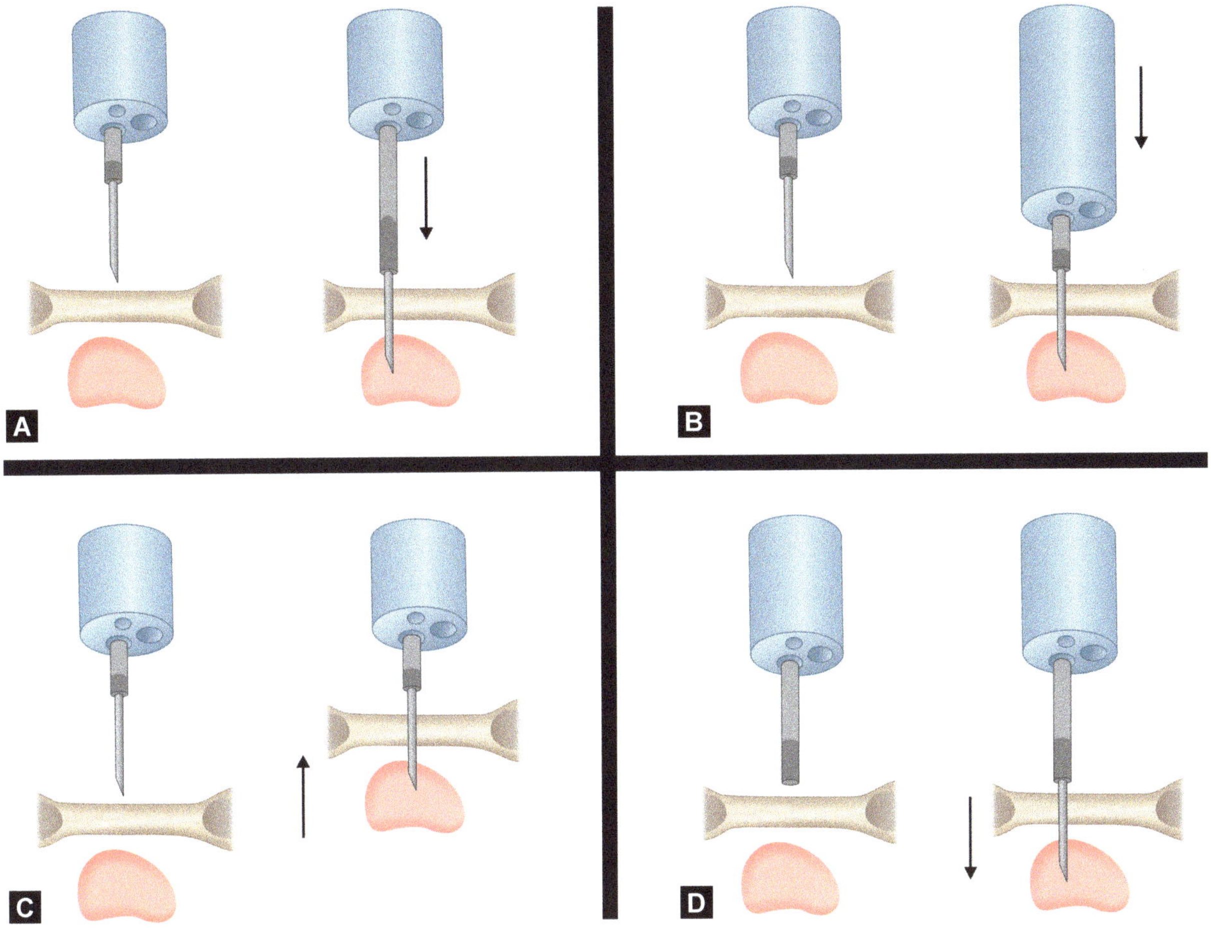

Figs. 29.7A to D: Four different techniques used for insertion of TBNA needle into the airway wall. (A) Jabbing method. (B) Piggyback method. (C) Cough method. (D) Hub against the wall method. (TBNA: Transbronchial needle aspiration).

above the entry port of the bronchoscope) and pushes it quickly and repeatedly (8–10 times are sufficient), being careful not to fully pull out the needle from the place of sampling.

To obtain a specimen for histological examination, a larger (19 gauge) needle is moved back and forth by 2–3 mm several times without removing it completely from the target site. The motion should be slow and deliberate with the intent of "coring" a piece of tissue for histology. The aspiration maneuver should be maintained no longer than 10 seconds to avoid the possible coagulation of the blood in the needle.

After obtaining the specimen and before withdrawing the needle through the tracheobronchial wall, the suction is released. The needle is pulled out of the wall and retracted back into the catheter. It is important to *release the suction before the removal of the needle* from the wall to prevent contamination of the specimen with the bronchial cells and respiratory secretions. Then, the catheter can be withdrawn from the bronchoscope in a single smooth motion avoiding needle trauma to the working channel.

After the needle is removed from the endoscope, the aspirated material is expelled and smeared on glass slides for a cytological evaluation. Three to four satisfactory specimens are obtained from each site to optimize the diagnostic yield. The final specimen is rinsed into Cytolyt® which is a methanol-based preservative solution. Slides typically also get placed in an alcohol-based fixative.

The highest sensitivity of TBNA is obtained with a cytopathologist in the examination room for a *rapid on-site cytological evaluation (ROSE)*. If this is not possible, the operator should verify that smears contain visible tissue or cells and not only blood. Cell clots can be visible as tiny white spots and usually give a feeling of consistency when the operator smears the two glass slides against each other.

The ROSE is a comparable technique to the intra-operative frozen section. This technique can be used during the bronchoscopy to provide an immediate preliminary result to the operator on the quality of C-TBNA specimen. If available, ROSE is preferred to reduce the number of passed required and the duration of the procedure. Histology specimens are directly preserved into the alcohol solution for centrifugation and cell block formation.

The drawback of the ROSE is the additional cost for the time spent by cytopathologist. In addition, a prospective study did not support a routine use of ROSE for the purpose of improving the diagnostic yield. However, a study has demonstrated that the patients who were assigned to the ROSE group had lower rate of complications. Therefore, ROSE may have a role in high-risk patients. Recent studies support the notion that with a short course of proper training, a bronchoscopist could become proficient in interpreting malignant cytology specimen overcoming total reliance on the cytopathologist.

CONTRAINDICATIONS AND POSSIBLE COMPLICATIONS

A severe coagulopathy with platelets less than 50,000/mm^3, international normalized ratio (INR) of more than 1.3 and/or a prothrombin time (PT) exceeding 30 seconds is absolute contraindications to the execution of TBNA. The other high-risk conditions are similar to those for a routine bronchoscopy (severe cardiac arrhythmias, unstable ischemic heart disease, severe respiratory failure with hypercapnia or hypoxemia unresponsive to oxygen support, severe tracheal stenosis, severe pulmonary hypertension, ongoing bronchospasm).

Many studies have confirmed that TBNA is a safe procedure with minimal rate of complications (0.3%). Although infrequent, the potential complications of TBNA include pneumothorax, pneumomediastinum, bacteremia, pericarditis and mediastinal or intratracheal bleeding due to the inadvertent puncture of a major intrathoracic blood vessel during the procedure. In that event, blood is seen filling the catheter. The suction should be immediately released and the needle retracted back out of the wall and into the catheter. Bleeding after TBNA procedure is usually minimal and resolves spontaneously. The hemorrhagic specimen is collected and process in a usual fashion. On occasion, a heparin flush through the catheter may be required to unclog it prior to its reuse. The complications described in the literature have not been associated with significant clinical consequences and there is no report of direct procedure-related mortality.

Box 29.1: Factors influencing the diagnostic yield of transbronchial needle aspiration.

- Enlarged lymph nodes seen on CT scan
- Position of the lymph node to be sampled (station 7 and 4R > 4L)
- Size of the lymph node
- Presence of erythema at the target site
- Widened carina
- Type of needle used (histology > cytology)
- Number of samples obtained
- Availability of extemporaneous cytology (ROSE)
- Nature of lymph node disease (malignant > benign)
- Skills and experience of the operator
- Ultrasound-guided sampling

DIAGNOSTIC YIELD OF TRANSBRONCHIAL NEEDLE ASPIRATION

Transbronchial needle aspiration has an extremely high diagnostic specificity for neoplastic diseases, ranging from 96 to 100%, and with rare reported false positives. In contrast, the sensitivity of TBNA is highly variable and can range from 15 to over 85% based on the prevalence of the lung cancer in the study population. The studies have also shown that the sensitivity of the technique may improve with training and experience. As shown in Box 29.1, several factors may influence the diagnostic yield of the procedure, the main of which are the size and location of the targeted lymph node, the operator's skill and the number of needle passes. Studies on TBNA yield have shown that a positive cytology sample is obtained with the first aspirate in more than 42% of the procedures, whereas there was no further improvement in the diagnostic yield after the seventh aspirate. Overall, the first needle pass consistently contributed greater than or equal to 50% toward the diagnostic yield, three passes provided greater than or equal to 89% and five passes yielded greater than or equal to 98% at all sites. Three transbronchial needle passes per site can be considered appropriate when only a tissue diagnosis is sought and when alternative sites or sampling modalities are available. At least four or five passes should be carried out at lymph node stations critical for the staging of lung cancer. As expected, the yield of TBNA for sarcoidosis is the greatest in stage I (50–80%), where only adenopathy is present.

ENDOBRONCHIAL NEEDLE ASPIRATION

Endobronchial needle aspiration is the technique in which the transbronchial needle is used to obtain cytology specimen from an endoscopically visible lesion. The added diagnostic yield of EBNA mainly concerns patients with submucosal and exophytic mass lesions (Fig. 29.8). The major advantage of EBNA over the forceps biopsies is the elimination of the crush artifact in the histologic specimen. In addition, forceps biopsy and brushing are more likely to sample the superficial mucosa and potentially miss the submucosal disease. EBNA technique is easier to penetrate deeper layers of bronchial wall to obtain the specimens from the submucosal and even peribronchial lesions. In patients with exophytic mass lesion, surface biopsies and brush may not be sufficient to provide a tissue diagnosis if the lesion is necrotic in nature. Endobronchial needle can penetrate to the core of the lesion and provide viable tissue rather than necrotic tissue from the surface of the lesion. In addition, EBNA is considered as a preferred technique for obtaining specimens from endobronchial and particularly hemorrhagic lesions, since the risk of bleeding appears to be lower with EBNA compared to other biopsy techniques. In terms of diagnostic yield, the average diagnostic yield of EBNA from several studies was 80% (range 68–91%). Overall, diagnostic yield of bronchoscopy can be increased by adding EBNA to conventional sampling procedure for submucosal and peribronchial lesions.

Endobronchial needle aspiration technique is usually performed with a transbronchial 22-gauge needle. The cytologic specimen from submucosal lesion can be obtained by introducing the needle into the lesion at an oblique angle of approximately 30–45°. Meanwhile, in case of exophytic mass, the needle should enter the lesion at 90° angle at the base of the mass. The number of passes is not well-studied; however, two to three passes should be adequate in most cases. Overall, routine use of EBNA in combination with conventional technique appears to be useful in patients with submucosal lesions.

PERIPHERAL TRANSBRONCHIAL NEEDLE ASPIRATION

Peripheral transbronchial needle aspiration is a simple and widely used technique to obtain the cytology specimen from peripheral pulmonary nodules (PPNs) typically under fluoroscopic guidance. P-TBNA provides a high diagnostic yield especially if the bronchus is compressed and displaced by the tumor mass with intact bronchial

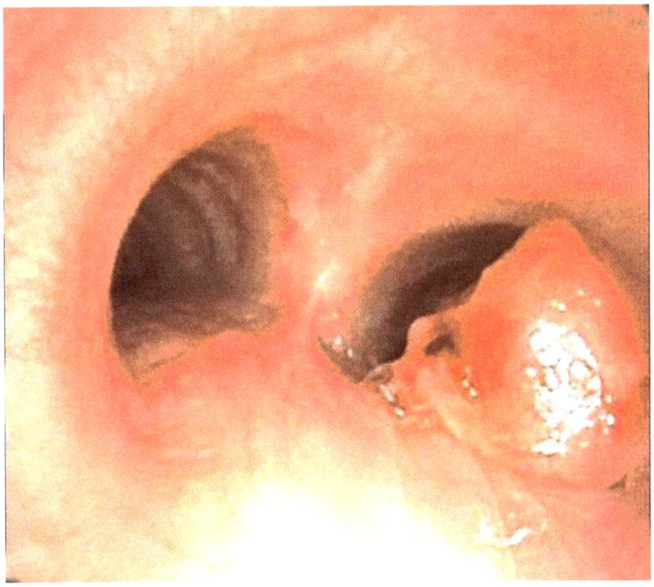

Fig. 29.8: Round, exophytic mass lesion at right main stem bronchus.

mucosa. In this type of lesion, P-TBNA provides relatively high diagnostic tissue (>70%) compared with transbronchial biopsy (19%). Size is one of the most important factors affecting the diagnostic yield of P-TBNA. There is no evidence that P-TBNA increases the diagnostic yield of bronchoscopy over the conventional diagnostic biopsy techniques in peripheral tumors that are smaller than 2 cm in diameter or have a positive bronchus sign (Fig. 29.9A).

The procedure is usually performed using 22-gauge (cytology) needle. The lesion is identified on a chest CT scan. The exact location of the nodule in the peripheral bronchus may also be confirmed by radial probe endobronchial ultrasound (EBUS) or electromagnetic navigation (Fig. 29.9B). Meanwhile, fluoroscopy is used as a real-time guidance to the lesion.

The TBNA needle is passed through the working channel of the bronchoscope making sure that the distal end of the needle is fully retracted within the metal hub. Once, the hub is visualized outside the distal end of the bronchoscope into the endobronchial tree the catheter is advanced toward the lesion. Excessive force is avoided during this stage procedure to avoid acute bending of the catheter. At this stage, the catheter is further guided toward the lesion using fluoroscopic guidance. Once the metal hub is placed in the close proximity of the lesion, the 22-gauge needle is deployed and pushed into the lesion. Suction is applied in a usual fashion by using a syringe and the catheter is agitated to obtain the specimen. Then, the needle is pulled back into the hub and the catheter is removed with a

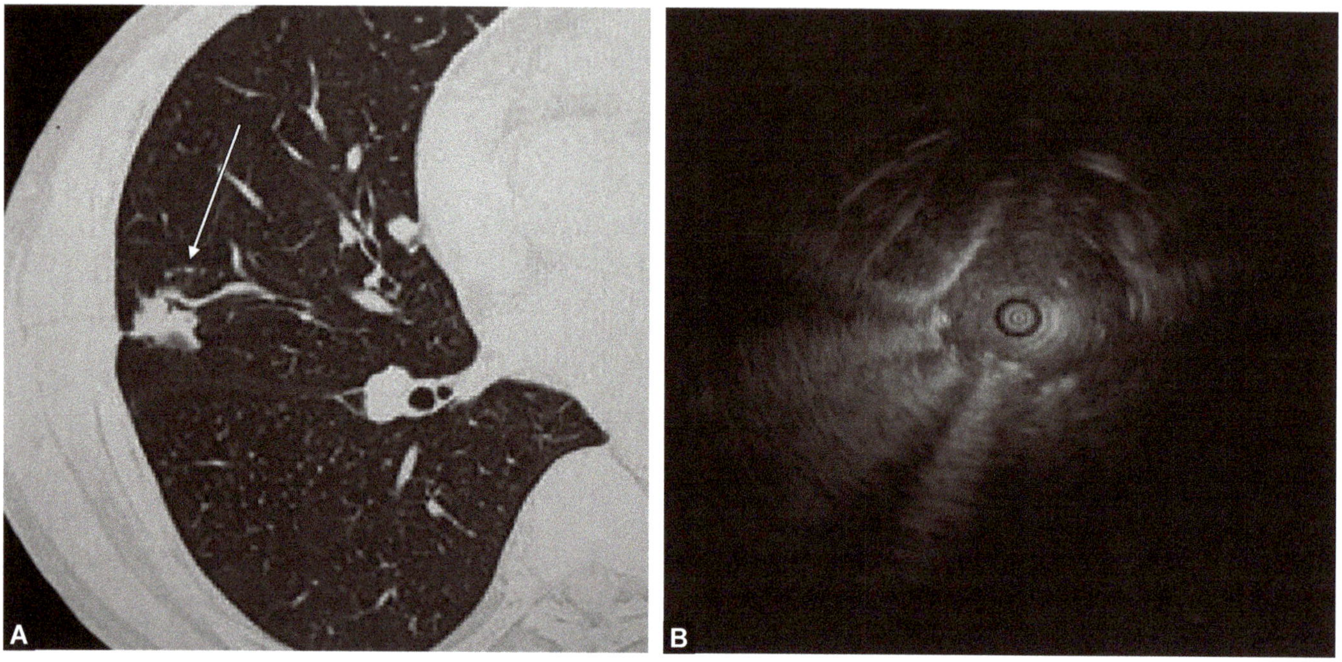

Figs. 9A and B: (A) CT scan showing a pulmonary nodule (diameter of 18 mm) in the right middle lobe (arrow). (B) Radial probe endobronchial ultrasound (EBUS) image showing a hypoechoic dots and linear arcs.

single movement while keeping bronchoscope as straight as possible. Two to three needle passes are sufficient for obtaining cytology specimen from the peripheral tumors.

BIBLIOGRAPHY AND FURTHER READING

1. Bilaçeroğlu S, Kumcuoğlu Z, Alper H, Osma E, Cağirici U, Günel O, et al. CT bronchus sign-guided bronchoscopic multiple diagnostic procedures in carcinomatous solitary pulmonary nodules and masses. Respiration. 1998;65(1):49-55.
2. Bonifazi M, Sediari M, Ferretti M, Poidomani G, Tramacere I, Mei F, et al. The role of the pulmonologist in rapid on-site cytologic evaluation of transbronchial needle aspiration: a prospective study. Chest. 2014;145(1):60-5.
3. Bonifazi M, Zuccatosta L, Trisolini R, Moja L, Gasparini S. Transbronchial needle aspiration: a systematic review on predictors of a successful aspirate. Respiration. 2013;86(2):123-34.
4. Caglayan B, Akturk UA, Fidan A, Salepci B, Ozdogan S, Sarac G, et al. Transbronchial needle aspiration in the diagnosis of endobronchial malignant lesions: a 3-year experience. Chest. 2005;128:704-8.
5. Chin R Jr, McCain TW, Lucia MA, Cappellari JO, Adair NE, Lovato JF, et al. Transbronchial needle aspiration in diagnosing and staging lung cancer: how many aspirates are needed? Am J Respir Crit Care Med. 2002;166(3):377-81.
6. Dasgupta A, Jain P, Minai OA, Sandur S, Meli Y, Arroliga AC, et al. Utility of transbronchial needle aspiration in the diagnosis of endobronchial lesions. Chest. 1999;115:1237-41.
7. Diacon AH, Schuurmans MM, Theron J, Brundyn K, Louw M, Wright CA, et al. Transbronchial needle aspirates: how many passes per target site? Eur Respir J. 2007;29(1):112-6.
8. Harrow EM, Abi-Saleh W, Blum J, Harkin T, Gasparini S, Addrizzo-Harris DJ, et al. The utility of transbronchial needle aspiration in the staging of bronchogenic carcinoma. Am J Respir Crit Care Med. 2000;161:601-7.
9. Holty JE, Kuschner WG, Gould MK. Accuracy of transbronchial needle aspiration for mediastinal staging of non-small cell lung cancer: a meta-analysis. Thorax. 2005;60(11):949-55.
10. Hsu LH, Liu CC, Ko JS. Education and experience improve the performance of transbronchial needle aspiration: a learning curve at a cancer center. Chest. 2004;125:532-40.
11. Mazzone P, Jain P, Arroliga AC, Matthay RA. Bronchoscopy and needle biopsy techniques for diagnosis and staging of lung cancer. Clin Chest Med. 2002;23:137-58.
12. Medford AR, Agrawal S, Free CM, Bennett JA. A prospective study of conventional transbronchial needle aspiration: performance and cost utility. Respiration. 2010;79(6):482-9.
13. Mehta AC, Cicenia J. ROSEs are read. Chest. 2014;145(1):7-9.
14. Mehta AC, Wang KP. Teaching conventional transbronchial needle aspiration. A continuum. Ann Am Thorac Soc. 2013;10(6):685-9.
15. Patel NM, Pohlman A, Husain A, Noth I, Hall JB, Kress JP. Conventional transbronchial needle aspiration decreases the rate of surgical sampling of intrathoracic lymphadenopathy. Chest. 2007;131(3):773-8.
16. Rusch VW, Asamura H, Watanabe H, Giroux DJ, Rami-Porta R, Goldstraw P, et al. The IASLC lung cancer staging project:

a proposal for a new international lymph node map in the forthcoming seventh edition of the TNM classification for lung cancer. J Thorac Oncol. 2009;4(5):568-77.

17. Shure D, Fedullo PF. Transbronchial needle aspiration in the diagnosis of submucosal and peribronchial bronchogenic carcinoma. Chest. 1985;88(1):49-51.
18. Trisolini R, Cancellieri A, Tinelli C, Paioli D, Scudeller L, Forti Parri SN, et al. Performance characteristics and predictors of yield from transbronchial needle aspiration in the diagnosis of peripheral pulmonary lesions. Respirology. 2011;16(7):1144-9.
19. Trisolini R, Lazzari Agli A, Cancellieri A, Poletti V, Candoli P, Paioli D, et al. Transbronchial needle aspiration improves the diagnostic yield of bronchoscopy in sarcoidosis. Sarcoidosis Vasc Diffuse Lung Dis. 2004;21:147-51.
20. Wang KP, Brower R, Haponik EF, Siegelman S. Flexible transbronchial needle aspiration for staging of bronchogenic carcinoma. Chest. 1983;84(5):571-6.
21. Wang KP, Haponik EF, Britt EJ, Khouri N, Erozan Y. Transbronchial needle aspiration of peripheral pulmonary nodules. Chest. 1984;86(6):819-23.
22. Yang H, Zhao H, Garfield DH, Teng J, Han B, Sun J. Endobronchial ultrasound-guided transbronchial needle aspiration in the diagnosis of non-lymph node thoracic lesions. Ann Thorac Med. 2013;8(1):14-21.
23. Yarmus L, Van der Kloot T, Lechtzin N, Napier M, Dressel D, Feller-Kopman D. A randomized prospective trial of the utility of rapid on-site evaluation of transbronchial needle aspirate specimens. J Bronchology Interv Pulmonol. 2011; 18(2):121-7.

Chapter

30

Bronchoalveolar Lavage

Simona Soresi, Claudio Sorino, Keith Meyer

OVERVIEW ON BRONCHOALVEOLAR LAVAGE

Bronchoalveolar lavage (BAL) is a mildly invasive technique used to obtain secretions and cells for diagnostic purposes from the peripheral airways and alveoli (Fig. 30.1). BAL has been reported to be a useful tool in addition to transbronchial biopsy for determining the etiology of pulmonary infiltrates, consolidation or solid lesions. It may help to establish a diagnosis in subjects with suspected immunologic, inflammatory, infectious or neoplastic lung disease, and it may provide useful information concerning disease activity in patients with interstitial lung disease (ILD). Box 30.1 lists the main indications for BAL.

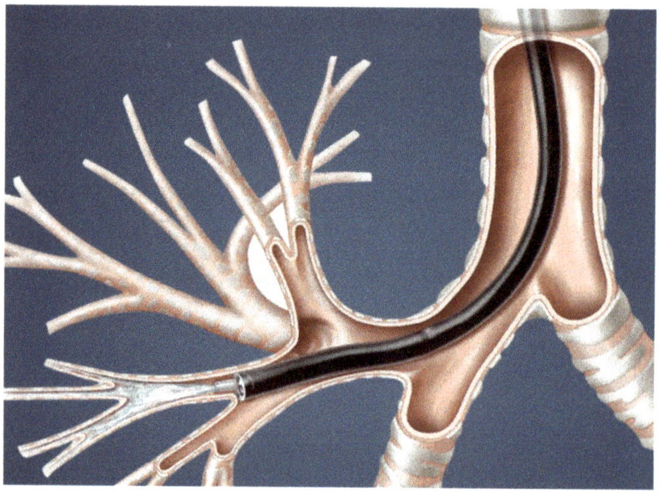

Fig. 30.1: Bronchoscope placement for performing bronchoalveolar lavage.
Courtesy: Olympus Europe SE & CO. KG.

Box 30.1: Main indications for bronchoalveolar lavage (BAL).

- Nonresolving, hospital-acquired, or ventilator-associated pneumonia
- Diffuse interstitial and/or alveolar lung infiltrates
- Suspected alveolar hemorrhage and related diseases (e.g. granulomatosis with polyangiitis)
- Infiltrates in an immunocompromised host
- Exclusion of diagnosable conditions by BAL
- Research purposes

Bronchoalveolar lavage can be performed simply and safely by wedging the distal end of a flexible fiberoptic bronchoscope in a segmental bronchus and instilling fluid (normal saline solution: 0.9% sodium chloride) that can reach the terminal bronchioles. Sequential aliquots of the instilled fluid are then retrieved, and the lavage fluid can then be analyzed to identify airspace cells and to detect and characterize inhaled particles, infectious organisms or various other BAL fluid constituents that may be present. Usually, lavaging the right middle lobe (RML) allows a greater amount of total fluid retrieval when compared to other areas of the lung, and using a handheld syringe to instill and aspirate lavage fluid aliquots can minimize airway trauma and damage to retrieved cells and may be preferable to using continuous negative pressure suction to retrieve instilled BAL fluid aliquots. The procedure of BAL has an excellent safety profile, but some precautions that can minimize risks for the patient and avoid potential complications deserve to be mentioned. Figure 30.2 is an exemplification of the procedure.

Normal saline solution is instilled into the peripheral alveolar airspaces through the working channel of a

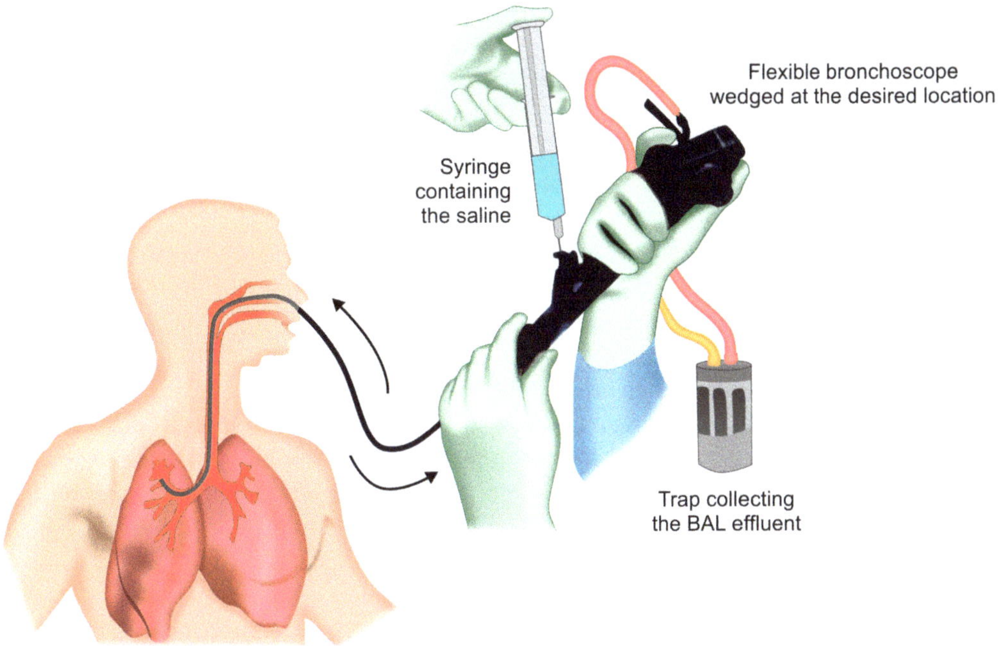

Fig. 30.2: Exemplification of bronchoalveolar lavage (BAL) and instruments used.

bronchoscope wedged into the selected bronchial segment. The solution is then retrieved by applying gentle suction to aspirate the lavage fluid.

The equipment required for bronchoalveolar lavage has been given in Box 30.2.

Box 30.2: Equipment required for bronchoalveolar lavage.

- Flexible bronchoscope
- Sterile collection trap
- Suction tubing
- Sterile physiological saline solution
- Vacuum source
- 60 mL syringe
- Optional three-way stopcock
- Local anesthetic (e.g. lidocaine 2%)

The first report of the use of bronchial irrigation with saline solution via a catheter through a bronchoscope was reported in 1927, but the term "bronchial lavage" was coined later and applied to the study of the human lung in the late 1960s and 1970s. The technique rapidly gained acceptance, and a large number of centers began to use BAL to obtain cells and proteins from the lower respiratory tract, which necessitated standardization of the method.

The British Thoracic Society (BTS) developed their first guidelines pertaining to the BAL procedure in 1993. Updates of the document were subsequently published with the main objective of reducing the risks of contaminating bronchoscopes, which could cause device-related iatrogenic infections. More recently the American Thoracic Society (ATS) provided a clinical practice guideline that updated previous statements and delineated the role of BAL in the diagnostic evaluation of patients with suspected ILD.

The optimal area of the lung in which to perform BAL is determined by the location and extent of the abnormalities noted on thoracic imaging, and recently obtained high-resolution computed tomographic (HRCT) imaging may be particularly useful for choosing the site in which to perform BAL when a diagnosis of ILD is suspected. When focal disease or lesions are observed, the optimal site for BAL is the bronchial segment that leads to the specific area of parenchymal abnormality. When diffuse disease is present, it may be preferable to direct the lavage to the RML or the lingula of the left upper lobe (LUL), as an adequate wedge position and optimal lavage fluid retrieval are more likely to be obtained in these areas.

Routine cytological evaluation can be performed to differentiate the types of inflammatory cells (nucleated immune cells) that are present. There is no agreement on whether the first recovered BAL should be analyzed separately from subsequently retrieved, pooled lavage fluid aliquots, and many centers pool all the retrieved aliquots for BAL analysis. However, the first retrieved lavage fluid aliquot typically has an increased number of epithelial cells and neutrophils, and some experts feel that this aliquot should be kept separate due to a tendency to represent more proximal airway secretions rather than a more distal alveolar sample. Therefore, some centers do not pool the first aliquot with subsequently retrieved aliquots when BAL analyses are performed for research studies. However, an analysis of the initially retrieved aliquot may be enriched for pathogens or malignant cells.

Specific criteria have been identified that indicate whether retrieved BAL fluid represents adequate sampling of airspace secretions that especially pertain to the evaluation of patients with suspected ILD. The presence of large numbers of epithelial cells suggests that sampling is suboptimal, especially if significant numbers of squamous epithelial cells are present, which suggest substantial aspiration of upper airway secretions into the lower respiratory tract. Similarly, when large amounts of mucopurulent secretions or blood are present, BAL analysis is likely to be difficult and potentially misleading, especially when accurate nucleated immune cell differential cell counts are needed.

The detection and quantitation of specific substances in the BAL may assist or guide the diagnosis in some instances. Specific examples include (1) an increased level of adenosine deaminase in a patient with tuberculosis or sarcoidosis; (2) the detection of a specific endotoxin in patients with invasive mechanical ventilation-associated pneumonia; (3) the presence of pneumococcal or *Legionella* antigens; (4) the detection of microbial nucleic acid sequences via polymerase chain reaction (PCR) technology (e.g. cytomegalovirus, *Pneumocystis jiroveci*, mycobacterial spp.); and (5) the presence of antigens that suggest the presence of fungal pathogens (e.g. galactomannan). Additionally, the quantitation and analysis of BAL-nucleated immune cells (e.g. total cell count, differential cell count) can provide useful information that supports the presence of inflammation and may detect cell differential patterns (e.g. lymphocytosis, neutrophilia, eosinophilia) that reflect and suggest specific types of inflammation, and, when combined with clinical and imaging data, can strongly implicate the potential presence of specific forms of ILD.

GENERAL RECOMMENDATIONS

- *Consent form*: Verbal and written consent should be provided by the patient or their guardian.
- *Position of the patient*: There are no studies comparing the effects of upright, semirecumbent, or supine position on BAL. Positioning should be determined according to the clinical situation affecting the patient and should be noted in the procedure report.
- *Bronchopulmonary segment lavaged in the lung*: The area of choice for the lavage is normally determined prior to the bronchoscopy according to chest X-ray or HRCT findings; performing BAL in the RML or lingula of the LUL provides easier access and usually provides a greater volume of fluid recovery versus other lung regions.
- *Total volume of normal saline instilled and aliquot for BAL*: A minimal total instilled volume of 100 mL and a standard protocol using 240 mL (4 × 60 mL aliquots) have been recommended by the European Respiratory Society (ERS). Excessive amounts of fluid instilled in a given segment, especially if lavage fluid retrieval is poor, may be more likely to cause complications such as post-bronchoscopy fever.
- *Use of suction*: Low pressure wall suction (< 60 mm Hg) has been recommended to prevent airway collapse that may occur when suction pressure is excessive, and high negative pressures may also compromise lavage fluid retrieval. Use of a handheld syringe rather than wall suction has the advantage of allowing the bronchoscopist to adjust suction pressure while visualizing the airway and avoiding airway collapse.

POSSIBLE COMPLICATIONS

The BAL procedure is generally considered to be quite safe, and it has been used widely for research purposes and clinical evaluation of patients with a diverse spectrum of disorders that ranges from asthma and chronic obstructive pulmonary disease (COPD) to ILD, infection, and lung transplantation.

The most commonly reported complication is fever within 24 hours following the procedure, and hypoxemia may also occur. These are almost always self-limited and have been linked to the use of larger total lavage volumes. Significant bleeding and pneumothorax are extremely rare when BAL is performed without an accompanying endoscopic lung biopsy.

SAFETY CONSIDERATIONS

- Adequate safety protocols should be utilized whenever bronchoscopy and BAL are performed to minimize the possibility of complications. A simple coagulation profile study [international normalized ratio (INR), platelet count, partial thromboplastin time] should be done to assess the risk of potential bleeding complications, and patients with kidney failure or significant renal impairment have an increased risk of bleeding despite a normal coagulation profile (e.g. normal INR).

- The bronchoscopist needs to be aware of and document the patient's use of anticoagulant (e.g. warfarin, heparin) or antiplatelet (e.g. clopidogrel, aspirin) medications and the presence of any medical conditions (e.g. uremia) that may increase the risk of bleeding.
- For patients who undergo the procedure and require sedation, an intravenous access route should be established.
- Heart rate, blood pressure and oxyhemoglobin saturation should be monitored continuously throughout the procedure.

MACROSCOPIC EXAMINATION OF BAL

The characteristics of airspace secretions visualized during the bronchoscopy as well as freshly retrieved BAL fluid may provide important clues that help clinicians differentiate among possible diagnoses. The presence of copious, mucopurulent yellowish or greenish secretions in the airways suggests bacterial infection. Thick and white secretions generally localized in the trachea or main bronchi suggest that fungal infection may be present. The color of the BAL fluid should be noted by the bronchoscopist, and the retrieved lavage fluid should have a clear appearance. Recovery of reddish fluid that appears progressively more hemorrhagic with the retrieval of sequential aliquots is pathognomonic of "diffuse alveolar hemorrhage". Recovery of milky or light tan and relatively opaque fluid that clears gradually over a relatively short period of time (e.g. 10–20 minutes) as particles settle out of the suspension with gravity and form a sediment in the bottom of a collection trap is highly suspicious for a diagnosis of pulmonary alveolar proteinosis (PAP), as shown in Flowchart 30.1.

CYTOLOGICAL EXAMINATION FROM BAL

- Cytopathology can be diagnostic when the causative organism cannot be identified, and direction can be given to further investigation by examination of the tissue reaction patterns. The three main types of reactions seen in lung infections are (1) necrosis, (2) inflammatory reactions and (3) epithelial changes with little inflammation; these patterns can act as clues to the diagnosis and help guide therapeutic interventions. This is particularly true among immunosuppressed patients. A recent comparison of the cytologic profile in controls (21 individuals without pulmonary diseases) and three different study groups [16 kidney transplant recipients (Group A), 14 dialysis patients (Group B) and 8 human immunodeficiency virus (HIV) positive patients (Group C) suspected of having pulmonary infections) showed that percentages of lymphocytes and neutrophils were significantly increased in all three patient groups as compared to controls. Moreover, the sensitivity of BAL cytology abnormalities was found to be significantly higher than microbial culture results (76% vs 31.5%) (*see* bibliography no. 36).
- The cytological analysis of BAL performed prospectively in mechanically ventilated patients with pneumonia (either community-acquired or hospital-acquired) showed that cytological changes consistent with alveolar damage (such as hemorrhage and desquamated type II pneumocytes) were detected more frequently than in BAL from patients without pneumonia. These elements had a high specificity for an infectious cause of pulmonary infiltrates, although specificity was low.
- The success rate of cytological examination of the BAL fluid in patients with primary or metastatic lung tumors varies considerably according to different authors. In a prospective study performed to establish the sensitivity of BAL in comparison with both transbronchial lung biopsy (TBB) and brushing, the sensitivity of the three methods was shown to be equal for primary as compared to metastatic tumors and for interstitial infiltrates as compared to coin lesions. Moreover, malignant cells were most frequently found in centrifuged BAL specimens. Therefore, BAL appears to be potentially useful in the evaluation of patients with suspected malignant interstitial or focal, rounded pulmonary infiltrates when these cannot be reached by forceps or brush or when TBB and brushing are contraindicated due to the presence of a hemorrhagic diathesis.
- Specific tumor markers, as carcinoembryonic antigen (CEA), squamous cell carcinoma (SCC) antigen, CYFRA 21-1, and neuron-specific enolase (NSE), have recently been found to be significantly elevated in the tumor-bearing lung as compared to cells from

Flowchart 30.1: Processing and laboratory analysis of diagnostic bronchoalveolar lavage.

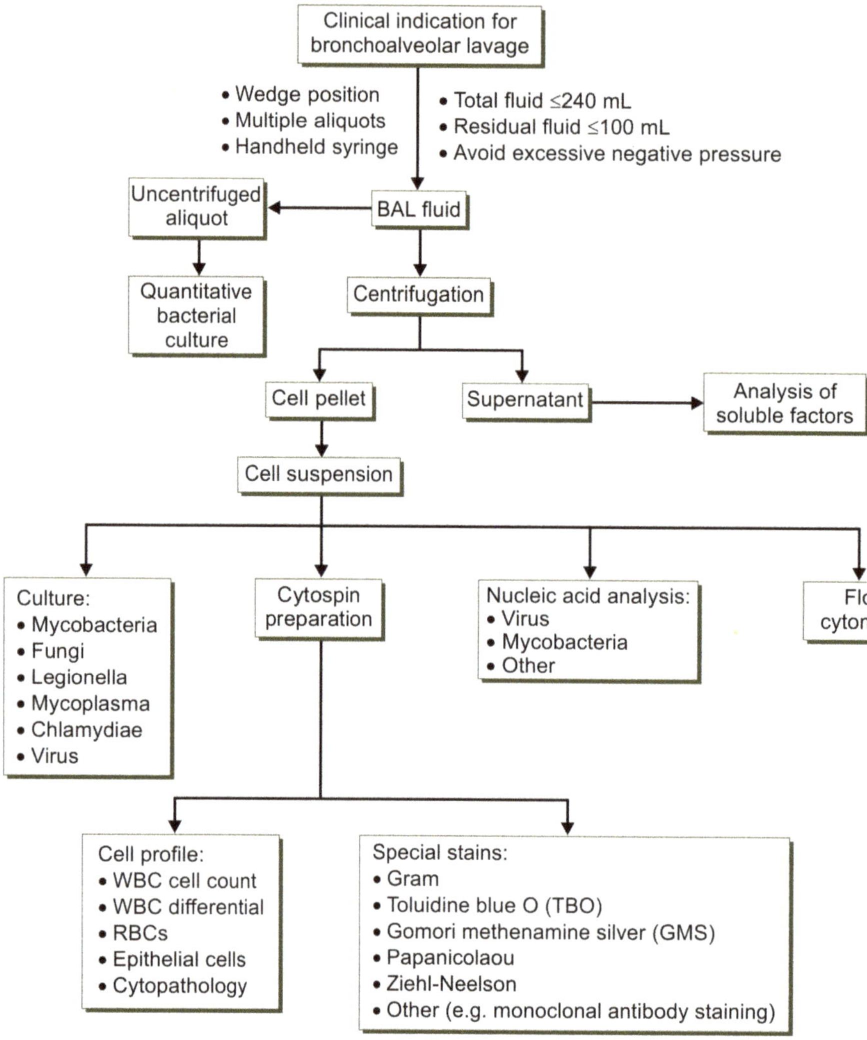

Source: Meyer KC. Bronchoalveolar lavage as a diagnostic tool. Semin Respir Crit Care Med. 2007;28(5):546-60. (Reprinted with permission from Thieme Medical Publishers and available at www.thieme.com.)

contralateral uninvolved and apparently healthy lungs in lung cancer patients or the lungs of patients with benign lung disease. Measurement of such markers in BAL may become important in the oncologic management of lung cancer patients.

- BAL cellular analysis may be a useful procedure in the diagnostic evaluation of individuals with suspected ILD who lack a confident usual interstitial pneumonia (UIP) pattern on HRCT imaging of the thorax. Although BAL-nucleated immune cell patterns (differential cell count) are nonspecific, the recognition of a predominantly inflammatory cellular pattern (increased lymphocytes, eosinophils and/or neutrophils) in the BAL cell differential profile frequently helps the clinician narrow the differential diagnosis of ILD. When BAL is performed in patients with suspected ILD, typical diagnostic studies include a differential cell count, microbiological studies (to screen for mycobacterial and fungal disease) and cytopathology. The presence of significantly increased numbers of specific nucleated immune cells in the BAL can often be correlated with an increased likelihood of certain types of ILD. Examples include pronounced BAL eosinophilia, which suggests the presence of eosinophilic pneumonia or a drug reaction, and BAL lymphocytosis, which can be seen in sarcoidosis, hypersensitivity pneumonitis, pneumotoxic drug reactions, or cellular nonspecific interstitial pneumonia (NSIP).

MICROBIOLOGY FROM BAL

Protocols for the microbiological analysis of BAL specimens in the microbiology laboratory have been in use since the early 1980s to identify the presence of bacterial infection or opportunistic infections, and BAL has been especially useful in the evaluation of immunocompromised patients or patients who are not able to expectorate secretions or have negative sputum cultures.

Although protocols tend to differ somewhat among various laboratory facilities, specimens are generally quantitatively cultured for bacteria on conventional agar media. All bacterial isolates that are greater than or equal to 10^3 colony forming units (CFU)/mL are usually speciated, and BAL bacterial isolates are generally considered significant if they contain greater than or equal to 10^4 CFU and less than or equal to 1% squamous epithelial cells are identified on Wright-stained slides.

After quantitative cultures have been prepared using appropriate media, the BAL specimen is centrifuged (at 1,500 g for 20 minutes at 4ºC) to obtain a pellet that is then resuspended and partitioned. A portion is plated for fungus (incubated at 30ºC in aerobic conditions for 4 weeks on Mycosel, Girasol, and Sabouraud's agar), and mycobacteria (at 37ºC in aerobic conditions for 6 weeks on Ogawa-Kudoh medium and thin layer agar). The other portion can be suspended in 4 mL of Hanks salt solution and cytocentrifuged at 1,500 rpm for 15 minutes (Cytospin III, Shandon Instruments, Sewickley, PA) after adjusting to 10^5 cells/mL. Slides can be then stained with Wright, Gram, Ziehl-Neelsen (ZN), modified Kinyoun and modified toluidine blue O (TBO).

Bronchoalveolar lavage samples can be used to diagnose viral respiratory infection by using real-time PCR assays, which far greater sensitivity than viral cultures. The epidemiology of respiratory viruses and their potential clinical impact when recovered in lower respiratory specimens has not been completely established in the hospital setting. In one hospital-based prospective cohort study, 299 symptomatic adult patients were enrolled and subjected to BAL, and the BAL specimens were analyzed via a PCR panel that could detect 17 different respiratory viruses. Coronaviruses (32.3%) were the most frequently detected virus followed by rhinovirus (22.6%), parainfluenza (19.5%), influenza (9.7%), respiratory syncytial virus (8.6%), human metapneumovirus (4.2%) and bocavirus (3.1%). Mixed model multivariate analysis showed that respiratory viral infections were associated with a lack of antibiotic treatment response and the absence of typical radiological infiltrates.

The impact of respiratory virus infections has been extensively studied among immunosuppressed patients. Lung transplant recipients are particularly susceptible to developing respiratory infections due to a combination of chronic immunosuppressive therapy as well as the direct exposure of the lung allograft to the ambient environment in the setting of impaired mucociliary clearance, disrupted lymphatic drainage and an impaired cough reflex. In addition to the direct effects of lower respiratory tract infection on morbidity and mortality, respiratory infections have been linked to chronic lung allograft dysfunction and bronchiolitis obliterans syndrome (BOS), which is a major cause of allograft loss and recipient death following initially successful lung transplantation. A recent review of the literature examining the clinical relationship between viral respiratory infection and graft complications showed a respiratory virus infection detection rate that ranged from 1.4% to 60%, and respiratory viruses were detected five times more frequently when respiratory symptoms were present.

The diagnosis of invasive pulmonary aspergillosis (IPA) can be very challenging. BAL fungal cultures are often negative even though *Aspergillus* infection is present, and cultures may not turn positive for days due to the slow growth of the fungus. The diagnosis of IPA in non-neutropenic, critically ill patients is difficult because signs and symptoms are nonspecific, and the initiation of additional diagnostic testing is often delayed because of low clinical suspicion for *Aspergillus* infection, although early diagnosis and prompt initiation of antifungal treatment could significantly improve the prognosis. Although histopathological evidence of IPA is defined as the diagnostic gold standard due to a very high tropism of aspergillus for blood vessels, transbronchial biopsy or surgical lung biopsy via minithoracotomy may not justify the risk of this invasive procedure in critically ill patients on mechanical ventilation or patients with a significant bleeding diathesis. Therefore, the diagnostic process must combine thoracic imaging results with the microbiological examination (direct microscopy and culture of sputum or BAL fluid). BAL has the highest sensitivity and specificity of various sampling techniques, and this can be increased by performing an *Aspergillus* colony count. Additionally, the probability of IPA is increased when multiple cultures reveal *Aspergillus* (5.9% if one culture is positive, 18.4% with two positive cultures and 38.2% with ≥ three cultures), but 61% of patients with confirmed IPA had only one positive culture, and only 18% of patients three or more positive.

Direct microscopic examination of a BAL specimen stained with specific fluorescent stain for chitin (a fungal cell wall component) is easy to perform, can be rapidly interpreted, and improves the sensitivity of fungus detection. Direct visualization of fungal hyphae makes it possible to discriminate between septate (e.g. *Aspergillus, Fusarium* and *Scedosporium*) and nonseptate (e.g. Mucorales) molds. A positive fungal culture allows identification and susceptibility testing to antifungal drugs, and the ability to culture a fungal isolate may allow sensitivity testing with antifungal agents.

None of these tests has enough sensitivity and specificity to definitely establish or rule out the diagnosis of IPA, but recently published studies have shown good sensitivity of the *Aspergillus* galactomannan (GM) antigen for the presence of *Aspergillus* infection. Because GM is a water-soluble carbohydrate, it can be detected and quantitated in BAL fluid. Although the Platelia enzyme-linked immunosorbent assay (ELISA) is not validated for detection of GM in this fluid, there is an increasing tendency to use these samples for diagnosis of IPA. In small clinical studies among patients with hematological malignancies and in solid organ transplant recipients, the sensitivity of the GM enzyme immunoassay (EIA) when applied to BAL ranged from 85% to 100% with a high index cut-off (> 1.5) to define positivity. However, there are several clinical circumstances that might influence the diagnostic performance of the GM antigen test in either serum or BAL fluid. These include (1) false-positive reactivity that can be caused by gastrointestinal translocation of fungal GM from contaminated food or drink that has been ingested, as demonstrated in small children and (2) the use of intravenous antibiotics (piperacillin-tazobactam and amoxicillin-clavulanic acid) which is associated with false-positive serum ELISA reactivity. Additionally, antifungal drug therapy can affect the release of GM antigens, and animal and human studies have shown decreased sensitivity of the GM assay when (prophylactic) antifungal drugs were being administered. Studies show that monitoring GM levels can be crucial to diagnose (and eventually monitor treatment outcome) correctly, and the GM assay should be performed twice weekly, preferably on receipt of the specimen.

Amplification of *Aspergillus* nucleic acid by PCR technology for the diagnosis of IPA is being increasingly studied, and it can be applied to BAL specimens as well as serum. However, experience is limited, and the utility and accuracy of such testing has not yet been clinically validated.

The utility of BAL in the diagnosis of fungal disease is best demonstrated in patients who have human immunodeficiency virus (HIV) infection with *Pneumocystis jiroveci* pneumonia (PJP). Although some experts advocate biopsy at the time of bronchoscopy, BAL alone has a sensitivity nearing 98% in these patients, especially when PCR is used to detect the presence of *Pneumocystis*. Unlike many other fungal pathogens, *Pneumocystis* cannot be cultured in the laboratory. Therefore, cytological examination remains the mainstay of diagnosis. Characteristic findings of *Pneumocystis* in BAL fluid include the presence of *Pneumocystis* cysts and clusters, foamy alveolar macrophages, foamy alveolar casts and activated T cells. There is higher detection sensitivity when commercialized fluorescein- or enzyme-labeled monoclonal or polyclonal antibodies are used on BAL fluid smears in addition to routine stains. Antibody tests are, however, more expensive and time-consuming. In addition, although immunofluorescent staining increases sensitivity, it is less specific than standard staining, resulting in a need to confirm the diagnosis with a second method. As experience with PCR increases, detection of *Pneumocystis* in BAL via PCR in combination with staining (e.g. TBO) of BAL specimens may become a preferred method for diagnosing PJP.

Histoplasmosis is the most common endemic mycosis in the United States, and *Histoplasma capsulatum* can cause various syndromes that range from asymptomatic infection with typical radiographic changes to fulminant respiratory failure. Histoplasmosis should be included in the differential diagnosis, particularly when patients live in an endemic area or travel to such areas. Although urine or serum antigen testing can be performed, these are often negative, and BAL remains an important means of diagnosis. Other fungi such as *Blastomyces dermatitidis* (endemic in the northeast and central US), *Coccidioides immitis* (endemic in the southwest US), or cryptococcus can also cause serious and life-threatening infections in immunocompetent or immunocompromised hosts and can be detected via BAL fluid analysis.

Bronchoalveolar lavage analysis should follow a protocol that includes several stains to detect *Histoplasma* or other fungal pathogens. Demonstration of the yeast inside of BAL phagocytes helps to differentiate *H. capsulatum* from *Pneumocystis* cysts and *Candida* species. Histopathologic examination of BAL specimens usually reveals the diagnosis within a few hours in those patients who have disseminated histoplasmosis. Histopathologic findings may be falsely negative, however, because of sampling error, a low number of organisms, or inexperienced cytologists who do not recognize the organism on prepared slides. As a result, the sensitivity of cytopathologic analysis of BAL for the presence of *H. capsulatum* varies among published studies, ranging from 40% to 85%. In addition, culture may require several weeks to isolate and correctly identify the organism. *Histoplasma* antigen testing performed on BAL samples can improve the sensitivity of BAL analysis, especially in concentrated specimens.

Bronchoalveolar lavage is an important adjunct to the diagnosis of pulmonary and disseminated fungal infections. Culture is the gold standard for diagnosis in many instances, but cytological and morphologic analysis is often diagnostic. Although newer molecular and antigen techniques may be applied to BAL samples, the role of such tests is yet to be defined for many pathogens.

EVOLVING AND FUTURE USES OF BAL FOR PATIENT MANAGEMENT AND CLINICAL RESEARCH

Bronchoalveolar lavage holds considerable promise as a modality that can provide useful information in the diagnosis and management of various lung disorders (respiratory tract infection, ILDs, bronchiectasis) and surveillance of the lung allograft in lung transplant recipients. Additionally, it can provide important information concerning lung immunology and the lung microbiome in both healthy individuals and in various lung disease states. Our knowledge of the lung microbiome is rapidly expanding and changing, and the ability to use new techniques has allowed the detection and quantitation of the diverse bacterial communities that inhabit the lung in patients with bronchiectasis [e.g. cystic fibrosis (CF) and non-CF bronchiectasis] as well as facilitating the characterization of the lung microbiome in other disorders such as asthma and COPD. Investigations in healthy subjects of varying age have shown that the immune profile in the lungs of elderly individuals varies significantly from that of young adults, and these changes may reflect evolving low-level inflammation in the aging lung as part of the normal aging process. As useful biomarkers and patterns of gene expression are identified that correlate with specific lung disorders, BAL may become very useful in differential diagnosis of ILDs and in monitoring responses to therapeutic interventions that may benefit these patients. BAL could also allow the detection of potential causes of lung injury and inflammation that may play an important role in the initiation, progression, or acute exacerbations of lung disease; a key example is the detection of bile acids or significantly increased pepsin levels in BAL that implicate gastroesophageal reflux and aspiration in patients with ILD [especially idiopathic pulmonary fibrosis (IPF)] or lung transplant recipients as causing or contributing to lung injury and dysfunction. Additionally, BAL is very useful for the surveillance of lung allografts to detect pathogens as well as detect immunologic changes that are characteristic of certain forms of chronic lung allograft dysfunction, as the information obtained can be used to direct specific, targeted therapies to prevent or treat lung allograft dysfunction in lung transplant recipients.

Key points of bronchoalveolar lavage have been given in Box 30.3.

Box 30.3: Bronchoalveolar lavage—key points.

- An appropriate imaging study (e.g. recently obtained HRCT in a patient with suspected ILD) should be used to select an optimal site for performing BAL
- BAL should be performed with the distal end of the bronchoscope wedged in a segmental bronchus
- Fluid retrieval is optimal if BAL is performed in the right middle lobe or lingula of the left upper lobe (e.g. when diffuse lung involvement is present on imaging studies)
- Excessive negative suction pressure should be avoided when instilled fluid is aspirated
- If fluid return from a segmental bronchus is poor and the retained BAL fluid volume exceeds 100 mL, instillation of additional saline aliquots in that segment should be avoided
- Total volume of retrieved BAL fluid should be ≥30% of the total instilled (a lower return may reflect suboptimal sampling of distal bronchoalveolar airspaces)
- Retrieved BAL fluid should be examined for color changes that provide important diagnostic clues (e.g. bloody discoloration that indicates hemorrhage, opaque with whitish color that suggests alveolar proteinosis)
- BAL processing and analysis should follow recommendations given in published guidelines
- BAL differential nucleated immune cell counts can provide useful information (e.g. evaluation of suspected ILD or infection), but a normal differential cell count does not rule out the presence of tissue inflammation
- Determination of lymphocyte subsets (e.g. CD4+/CD8+ ratio) should not be performed routinely, although the identification of cellular subsets may prove clinically useful in certain situations and for research purposes
- BAL by itself is rarely diagnostic; BAL analysis results must be interpreted in the context of the clinical presentation of the patient, thoracic imaging findings, and other laboratory testing

(HRCT: High-resolution computed tomography; ILD: Interstitial lung disease; BAL: Bronchoalveolar lavage).

BIBLIOGRAPHY AND FURTHER READING

1. Albera C, Mabritto I, Ghio P, Solidoro P, Marchetti L, Pozzi E. Adenosine deaminase activity and fibronectin levels in bronchoalveolar lavage fluid in sarcoidosis and tubercolosis. Sarcoidosis. 1993;10:18-25.
2. Baughman RP, Rennard SI. Bronchoalveolar lavage sampling and general approaches to correction for variability of dilution and lung permeability. Eur Respir J. 1999;9:28-31.
3. Bergeron A, Belle A, Sulahian A, Lacroix C, Chevret S, Raffoux E, et al. Contribution of galactomannan antigen detection in BAL to the diagnosis of invasive pulmonary aspergillosis in patients with hematologic malignancies. Chest. 2010;137(2):410-5.
4. Borensztajn K, Crestani B, Kolb M. Idiopathic pulmonary fibrosis: from epithelial injury to biomarkers—insights from the bench side. Respiration. 2013;86(6):441-52.
5. Bouza E, Guinea J, Peláez T, Pérez-Molina J, Alcalá L, Muñoz P. Workload due to Aspergillus fumigatus and significance of the organism in the microbiology laboratory of a general hospital. J Clin Microbiol. 2005;43:2075-9.
6. Bretagne S, Costa JM, Marmorat-Khuong A, Poron F, Cordonnier C, Vidaud M, et al. Detection of Aspergillus species DNA in bronchoalveolar lavage samples by competitive PCR. J Clin Microbiol. 1995;33:1164-8.
7. British Thoracic Society Bronchoscopy Guidelines Committee, a Subcommittee of Standards of Care Committee of British Thoracic Society. British Thoracic Society guidelines on diagnostic flexible bronchoscopy. Thorax. 2001;56 (Suppl 1):i1-21.
8. Chamberlain DW, Braude AC, Rebuck AS. A critical evaluation of bronchoalveolar lavage. Criteria for identifying unsatisfactory specimens. Acta Cytol. 1987;31:599-605.
9. Costabel U. Bronchoalveolar lavage: a standardized procedure or a technical dilemma? Eur Respir J. 1991;4:776-7.
10. Crystal RG, Reynolds HY, Kalica AR. Bronchoalveolar lavage. The report of an international conference. Chest. 1986;90:122-31.
11. Debeljak A, Mermolja M, Sorli J, Zupancic M, Zorman M, Remskar J. Bronchoalveolar lavage in the diagnosis of peripheral primary and secondary malignant lung tumors. Respiration. 1994;61(4):226-30.
12. Dickson RP, Erb-Downward JR, Prescott HC, Martinez FJ, Curtis JL, Lama VN, et al. Cell-associated bacteria in the human lung microbiome. Microbiome. 2014;2:28.
13. Dickson RP, Martinez FJ, Huffnagle GB. The role of the microbiome in exacerbations of chronic lung diseases. Lancet. 2014;384(9944):691-702.
14. Dransfield MT, Garver RI, Weill D. Standardized guidelines for surveillance bronchoscopy reduce complications in lung transplant recipients. J Heart Lung Transplant. 2004;23:110-4.
15. Garbino J, Gerbase MW, Wunderli W, Deffernez C, Thomas Y, Rochat T, et al. Lower respiratory viral illnesses: improved diagnosis by molecular methods and clinical impact. Am J Respir Crit Care Med. 2004;170:1197-203.
16. Garbino J, Soccal PM, Aubert JD, Rochat T, Meylan P, Thomas Y, et al. Respiratory viruses in bronchoalveolar lavage: a hospital-based cohort study in adults. Thorax. 2009; 64(5):399-404.
17. Goldstein RA, Rohatgi PK, Bergofsky EH, Block ER, Daniele RP, Dantzker DR, et al. Clinical role of bronchoalveolar lavage in adults with pulmonary disease. Am Rev Respir Dis. 1990;142:481-6.
18. Grigoriu B, Jacobs F, Beuzen F, El Khoury R, Axler O, Brivet FG, et al. Bronchoalveolar lavage cytological alveolar damage in patients with severe pneumonia. Crit Care. 2006;10(1):R2.
19. Gutierrez ME, Canton A, Connolly P, Zarnowski R, Wheat LJ. Detection of Histoplasma capsulatum antigen in Panamanian patients with disseminated histoplasmosis and AIDS. Clin Vaccine Immunol. 2008;15(4):681-3.
20. Harris B, Lowy FD, Stover DE, Arcasoy SM. Diagnostic bronchoscopy in solid-organ and hematopoietic stem cell transplantation. Ann Am Thorac Soc. 2013;10:39-49.
21. Harrison BD. Guidelines for care during bronchoscopy: British Thoracic Society. Thorax. 1993;48:584.
22. Hertz MI, Woodward ME, Gross CR, Swart M, Marcy TW, Bitterman PB. Safety of bronchoalveolar lavage in the critically ill, mechanically ventilated petient. Crit Care Med. 1991;19:1526-32.
23. Huang L, Morris A, Limper AH, Beck JM; ATS Pneumocystis Workshop Participants. An Official ATS Workshop summary: recent advances and future directions in Pneumocystis pneumonia (PCP). Proc Am Thorac Soc. 2006;3(8):655-64.
24. Huang YC, Bassett MA, Levin D, Montilla T, Ghio AJ. Acute phase reaction in healthy volunteers after bronchoscopy with lavage. Chest. 2006;129:1565-9.
25. Husain S, Paterson DL, Studer SM, Crespo M, Pilewski J, Durkin M, et al. Aspergillus galactomannan antigen in the bronchoalveolar lavage fluid for the diagnosis of invasive aspergillosis in lung transplant recipients. Transplantation. 2007;83(10):1330-6.
26. Ioachimescu OC, Stoller JK. Diffuse alveolar hemorrhage: diagnosing it and finding the cause. Cleve Clin J Med. 2008;75(4):258, 260, 264-5.
27. Jiménez P, Meneses M, Saldias F, Velásquez M. Pneumococcal antigen detection in bronchoalveolar lavage fluid from patient with pneumonia. Thorax. 1994;49:872-4.
28. Kahn FW, Jones JM. Analysis of bronchoalveolar lavage specimens from immunocompromised patients with a protocol applicable in the microbiology laboratory. J Clin Microbiol. 1988;26(6):1150-5.
29. Kennedy VE, Todd JL, Palmer SM. Bronchoalveolar lavage as a tool to predict, diagnose and understand bronchiolitis obliterans syndrome. Am J Transplant. 2013;13(3):552-61.
30. Kuypers J, Wright N, Ferrenberg J, Huang ML, Cent A, Corey L, et al. Comparison of real-time PCR assays with fluorescent-antibody assays for diagnosis of respiratory virus infections in children. J Clin Microbiol. 2006;44:2382-8.
31. Kvale PA. Bronchoscopic biopsies and bronchoalveolar lavage. Chest Surg Clin N Am. 1996;6:205-22.
32. Lautenschlager I, Lyytikainen O, Jokipii L, Jokipii A, Maiche A, Ruutu T, et al. Immunodetection of Pneumocystis

carinii in bronchoalveolar lavage specimens compared with methenamine silver stain. J Clin Microbiol. 1996;34(3): 728-30.
33. LiPuma JJ. Expanding our understanding of respiratory microbiota in cystic fibrosis. Ann Am Thorac Soc. 2014;11(7):1084-5.
34. Lu BS, Yu AD, Zhu X, Garrity ER Jr, Vigneswaran WT, Bhorade SM. Sequential gene expression profiling in lung transplant recipients with chronic rejection. Chest. 2006;130:847-54.
35. Menon LR, Divate S, Acharya VN, Mahashur AA, Natrajan G, Almeida AF. Utility of bronchoalveolar lavage in the diagnosis of pulmonary infections in immunosuppressed patients. J Assoc Physicians India. 2002;50:1110-4.
36. Meyer KC, Raghu G, Baughman RP, Brown KK, Costabel U, du Bois RM, et al, An Official American Thoracic Society Clinical Practice Guideline: the clinical utility of bronchoalveolar lavage cellular analysis in interstitial lung disease. Am J Respir Crit Care Med. 2012;185:1004-14.
37. Meyer KC, Raghu G, Verleden GM, Corris PA, Aurora P, Wilson KC, et al. An international ISHLT/ATS/ERS clinical practice guideline: diagnosis and management of bronchiolitis obliterans syndrome. Eur Respir J. 2014;44(6): 1479-503.
38. Meyer KC, Raghu G. Bronchoalveolar lavage for the evaluation of interstitial lung disease: is it clinically useful? Eur Respir J. 2011;38(4):761-9.
39. Meyer KC. Aging. Proc Am Thorac Soc. 2005;2(5):433-9.
40. Meyer KC. Bronchoalveolar lavage as a diagnostic tool. Semin Respir Crit Care Med. 2007;28:546-60.
41. Procop GW, Haddad S, Quinn J, Wilson ML, Henshaw NG, Reller LB, et al. Detection of Pneumocystis jiroveci in respiratory specimens by four staining methods. J Clin Microbiol. 2004;42:3333-5.
42. Pugin J, Auckenthaler R, Delaspre O, van Gessel E, Suter PM. Rapid diagnosis of Gram negative pneumonia by assay of endotoxin in bronchoalveolar lavage fluid. Thorax. 1992;47:547-9.
43. Rahman M, Lakshmi V, Patel M, et al. Comparison of fiberoptic bronchoscopy (FOB) in renal failure (RF) and non-renal failure patients. Chest. 2003;124:147S.
44. Reynolds HY, Newball HH. Analysis of proteins and respiratory cells obtained from human lungs by bronchial lavage. J Lab Clin Med. 1974;84:559-73.
45. Reynolds HY, Thompson RE. Pulmonary host defenses. I. Analysis of protein and lipids in bronchial secretions and antibody responses after vaccination with Pseudomonas aeruginosa. J Immunol. 1973;111:358-68.
46. Reynolds HY, Thompson RE. Pulmonary host defenses. II. Interaction of respiratory antibodies with Pseudomonas aeruginosa and alveolar macrophages. J Immunol. 1973;111:369-80.
47. Reynolds HY. Use of bronchoalveolar lavage in humans—past necessity and future imperative. Lung. 2000; 178:271-93.
48. Sanguinetti M, Posteraro B, Pagano L, Pagliari G, Fianchi L, Mele L, et al. Comparison of real-time PCR, conventional PCR, and galactomannan antigen detection by enzyme-linked immunosorbent assay using bronchoalveolar lavage fluid samples from hematology patients for diagnosis of invasive pulmonary aspergillosis. J Clin Microbiol. 2003;41:3922-5.
49. Savarino E, Carbone R, Marabotto E, Furnari M, Sconfienza L, Ghio M, et al. Gastro-oesophageal reflux and gastric aspiration in idiopathic pulmonary fibrosis patients. Eur Respir J. 2013;42(5):1322-31.
50. Selman M, Pardo A, Barrera L, Estrada A, Watson SR, Wilson K, et al. Gene expression profiles distinguish idiopathic pulmonary fibrosis from hypersensitivity pneumonitis. Am J Respir Crit Care Med. 2006;173:188-98.
51. Shah PL, Hansell D, Lawson PR, Reid KB, Morgan C. Pulmonary alveolar proteinosis: clinical aspects and current concepts on pathogenesis. Thorax. 2000;55:67-77.
52. Skladny H, Buchheidt D, Baust C, Krieg-Schneider F, Seifarth W, Leib-Mösch C, et al. Specific detection of Aspergillus species in blood and bronchoalveolar lavage samples of immunocompromised patients by two-step PCR. J Clin Microbiol. 1999;37:3865-71.
53. Stitt HL. Bronchial aspiration and irrigation with a hypertonic saline solution. J Med. 1927;5:112-7.
54. Thomson RB Jr. Laboratory diagnosis of respiratory infections. Curr Opin Infect Dis. 1999;12:115-9.
55. Thonhofer R, Maercker C, Popper HH. Expression of sarcoidosis related genes in lung lavage cells. Sarcoidosis Vasc Diffuse Lung Dis. 2002;19:59-65.
56. Vandewoude KH, Blot SI, Depuydt P, Benoit D, Temmerman W, Colardyn F, et al. Clinical relevance of Aspergillus isolation from respiratory tract samples in critically ill patients. Crit Care. 2006;10:R31.
57. Vu DL, Bridevaux PO, Aubert JD, Soccal PM, Kaiser L. Respiratory viruses in lung transplant recipients: a critical review and pooled analysis of clinical studies. Am J Transplant. 2011;11:1071-8.
58. Weiss SM, Hert RC, Gianola FJ, Clark JG, Crawford SW. Complications of fiberoptic bronchoscopy in thrombocytopenic patients. Chest. 1993;104:1025-8.
59. Wheat LJ, Connolly-Stringfield P, Williams B, Connolly K, Blair R, Bartlett M, et al. Diagnosis of histoplasmosis in patients with the acquired immunodeficiency syndrome by detection of Histoplasma capsulatum polysaccharide antigen in bronchoalveolar lavage fluid. Am Rev Respir Dis. 1992;145(6):1421-4.
60. Williams B, Fojtasek M, Connolly-Stringfield P, Wheat J. Diagnosis of histoplasmosis by antigen detection during an outbreak in Indianapolis, Ind. Arch Pathol Lab Med. 1994;118(12):1205-8.

Chapter

31

Thoracentesis

Claudio Sorino, Danai Khemasuwan, Anna Rosa Maspero, Atul C Mehta

OVERVIEW OF PLEURAL EFFUSION AND THORACENTESIS

The virtual space existing between the two pleural layers contains a small amount of fluid that lubricates the surface of visceral and the parietal pleura. The fluid facilitates the sliding of pleural surfaces on each other during movements of the lung and the thoracic cage. Normally, the pleural fluid is formed and removed slowly, at an equal rate, and has a lower protein concentration than lung and peripheral lymph. An excessive accumulation of fluid in the pleural space is called pleural effusion and indicates an imbalance between pleural fluid formation and/or drainage.

Table 31.1 represents common etiologies and mechanisms by which the pleural effusion is formed. Although many different conditions may provokea pleural effusion, the most common causes in adults are heart failure, malignancy, pneumonia, tuberculosis, and pulmonary embolism, whereas pneumonia is the leading etiology in children.

Thoracentesis or *pleural tap* is a minimally invasive procedure aimed at extracting fluid from the pleural space. Thoracentesis may have a diagnostic purpose (to understand the cause of pleural effusion) or a therapeutic purpose (to alleviate dyspnea caused by pleural effusions which compress the lung). It can be performed at the bedside through a needle that is inserted through the chest wall in between two ribs. If obtaining pleural fluid is difficult due to small size of the effusion or the presence of loculations, ultrasound-guided thoracentesis can be useful and minimizes the risk for iatrogenic pneumothorax.

Pleural fluid removed by thoracentesis undergoes chemical-physical, microbiological and cytological analyses.

Table 31.1: Causes and mechanisms leading to pleural effusions.

Etiologies	*Mechanisms*
Congestive heart failure	Increased hydrostatic pressure in pulmonary capillary pressure
Hypoalbuminemia	Decreased oncotic pressure in the microvascular circulation
Large atelectasis	Raised negative pressure in the pleural space
Trapped lung (separation of the pleural surfaces)	Decreased movement of fluid in the pleural space and inhibition of pleural lymphatic drainage
Pleural fibrosis	Obstruction of lymphatic drainage
Pleural malignancy and infection	Local production of inflammatory mediators, increased permeability of the microvascular circulation and leak of fluid and protein across the lung and visceral surface into pleural space
Chylothorax	Rupture or obstruction of the thoracic duct or its tributaries
Hemothorax	Injury to the chest with rupture of the visceral and parietal pleura and blood accumulation in the pleural cavity
Hepatic hydrothorax	Movement of ascitic fluid from the peritoneal space through either diaphragmatic lymphatics or diaphragmatic defects

INDICATIONS

Thoracentesis is indicated for the diagnostic purposes in all pleural effusions of unknown origin. It allows to evaluate the macroscopic features of the pleural fluid, to ascertain its transudative or exudative nature through biochemical analysis, and to perform other analyses useful in making the etiologic diagnosis, such as microbiological and cytological examination of the pleural fluid. Generally, diagnostic thoracentesis is not performed when the pleural effusion is small [i.e. < 1 cm height on lateral decubitus radiograph, ultrasound, or computed tomography (CT)] or when the diagnosis is clinically certain, such as in patients with heart failure or recent surgery. If there is evidence of heart failure, diagnostic thoracentesis is indicated only if any of the following atypical circumstances is present: (1) fever; (2) pleuritic chest pain; (3) unilateral effusion or considerable discrepancy in size between the left and right pleural effusion; (4) absence of cardiomegaly; or (5) lack of reduction in pleural effusion despite optimal management of heart failure.

Thoracentesis is also indicated for therapeutic purposes in massive pleural effusions resulting in breathlessness, respiratory failure, and/or shift of the mediastinum. Recurrent pleural effusions may require the placement of a chest tube to drain the pleural fluid and perform pleurodesis if no further diagnostic doubts exist.

Thoracentesis is an urgent procedure if there is the suspicion that the pleural space contains blood (hemothorax) or pus (empyema) since in such situations rapid tube thoracostomy is required.

RELATIVE CONTRAINDICATIONS

There are no absolute contraindications for thoracentesis. It is important to evaluate the risk/benefit ratio of each specific clinical circumstance. Relative contraindications include the following:

- Uncorrectable coagulopathy or active anticoagulant therapy with international normalized ratio (INR) greater than 1.6 or platelet count less than 25,000 cells/μL
- Skin or soft tissue infection at the intended site of puncture (e.g. chest wall cellulitis or abscess, burn, herpes zoster, etc.)
- Renal failure with serum creatinine greater than 6 mg/dL
- Uncooperative patient or inability to maintain adequate position

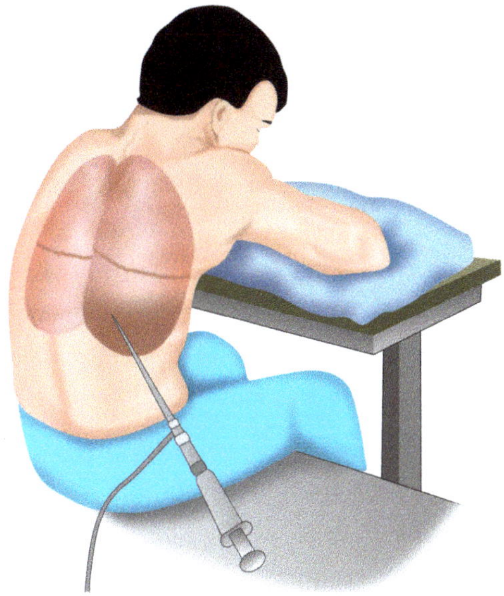

Fig. 31.1: Recommended position of the patient who undergoes thoracentesis.

- Lack of functioning contralateral lung (reduced respiratory reserve)
- Positive-pressure mechanical ventilation.

Several studies have shown an insignificantly higher risk for developing a pneumothorax following thoracentesis in patients receiving mechanical ventilation compared with nonmechanically ventilated patients. However, mechanically ventilated patients are at increased risk of developing tension physiology or persistent air leak (bronchopleural fistula) if a pneumothorax develops. Therefore, in such patients, thoracentesis should be avoided if the effusion is minimal or if a positive end-expiratory pressure (PEEP) cannot be suspended. Ultrasound guidance reduces the risk of pneumothorax after thoracentesis to less than 7%.

PATIENT PREPARATION AND POSITION

The patient who undergoes thoracentesis should assume a position as comfortable as possible, so that it can be maintained for the whole duration of the procedure (usually 10–15 minutes, unless if there is a large quantity of fluid to be drained).

Generally, the patient can sit on the bed, which is raised for the operator comfort. The feet may be resting on a stool. Both arms, or at least the arm on the side where the thoracentesis is performed, must be kept raised in order to broaden the intercostal spaces (Fig. 31.1).

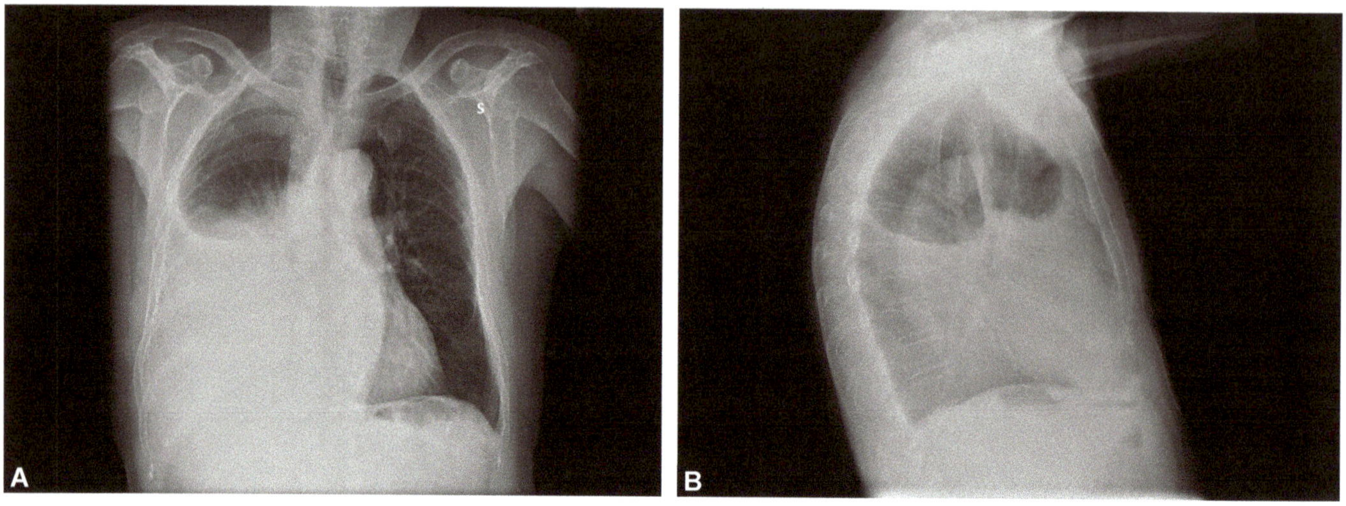

Figs. 31.2A and B: Chest X-ray revealing right pleural effusion: (A) Posteroanterior view. (B) Lateral view.

If the patient is unable to maintain this position, the back of the bed can be raised to a 45° angle and thoracentesis performed by inserting the needle along the mid or posterior axillary line.

PREPROCEDURE PLANNING

As with any other invasive procedure, it is necessary to inform the patient about the possible benefits and risks of the thoracentesis. Written consent needs to be obtained and attached to the clinical report and/or medical record.

Before the procedure, bedside ultrasonography should be performed to confirm the presence of pleural effusion, estimate its size, assess the presence of loculations, and identify the optimal site for the needle insertion (this can be marked on the patient's chest wall with a skin marker).

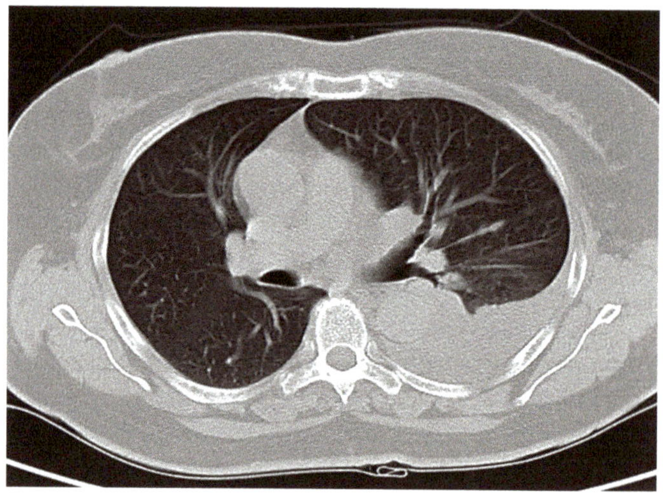

Fig. 31.3: Chest CT revealing left pleural effusion.

If transthoracic ultrasound is not available, the choice of the site where to insert the needle should be determined on the basis of radiological imaging (Figs. 31.2 and 31.3) and a careful physical examination of the thorax. In the area of chest wall corresponding to the pleural effusion, plexus dullness and reduced tactile vocal tremor can be appreciated. The puncture is usually performed at least one or two intercostal spaces below the disappearance of the vocal tremor, since the needle needs to be inserted below the level of the lungs, in the costodiaphragmatic recess. At the midclavicular line, the recess is between rib spaces 6 and 8, at the midaxillary line it is between 8 and 10, and at the paravertebral line between 10 and 12. The posterior approach is the most affordable because the posterior gutters are the site where the fluid tends to collect in the erect position and because the interspaces are wider in the back as compared to the front. It is preferred to perform thoracentesis along the Posterior axillary line or midscapular or somewhere in between (Fig. 31.4).

All materials needed for the procedure should be available near the patient. These include sterile drape, gauze pieces, gloves, disinfectant, local anesthetic agent (usually lidocaine 1% or 2% without epinephrine), 20 and 60 mL syringes, needles of various diameters and lengths, thoracentesis kit, test tubes for collecting the liquid to be sent to the analysis. If it is expected to remove a fair amount of pleural fluid, the operator should also have a collection bag or a container, a three-way valve (Fig. 31.5) and

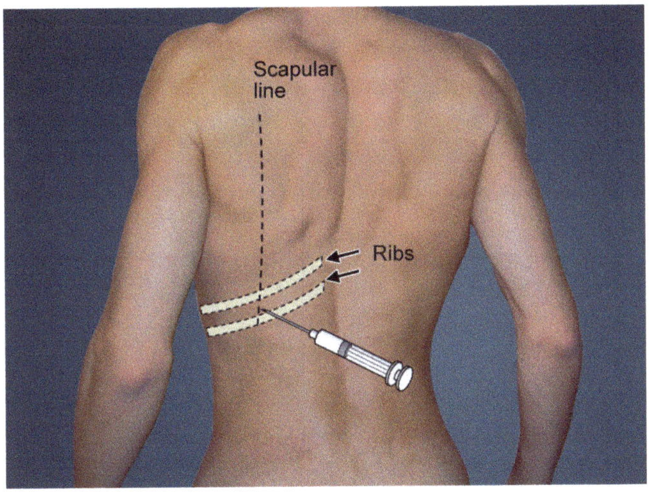

Fig. 31.4: Ideal site where to perform a thoracentesis.

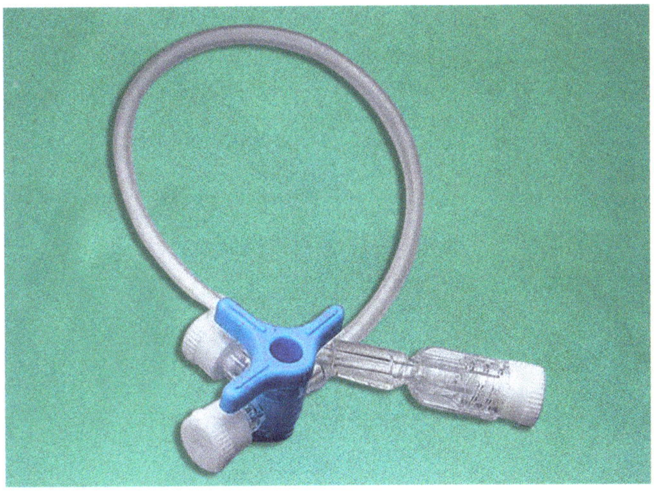

Fig. 31.5: Three-way valve.

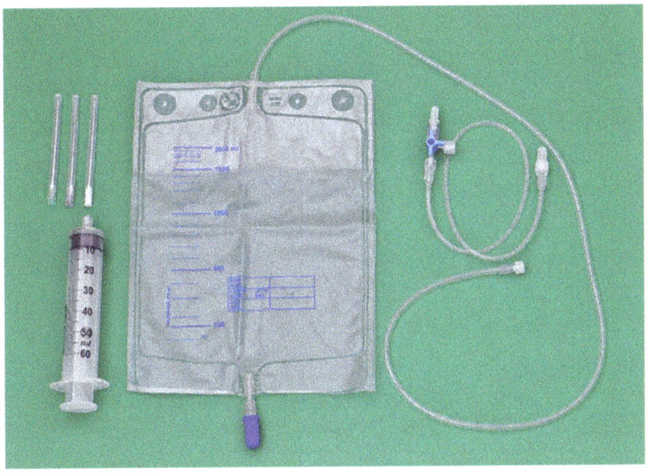

Fig. 31.6: Example of kit for thoracentesis.

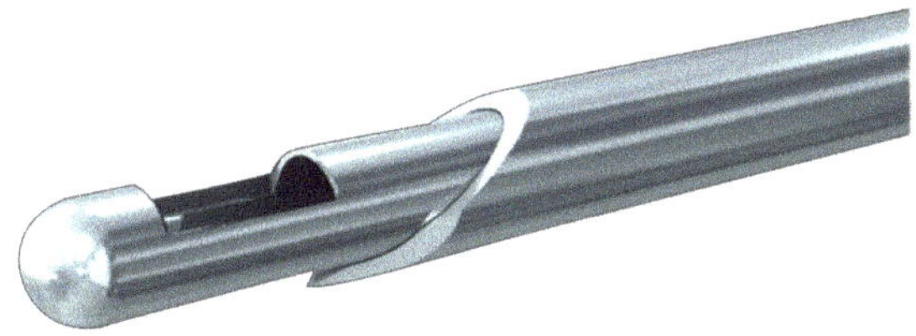

Fig. 31.7: Example of needle for thoracentesis with atraumatic retractable tip.

connecting pipes, usually included in the kit for thoracentesis (Fig. 31.6).

Several types of needles for thoracentesis exist. Most recently introduced needles have a spring-loaded core that is retracted when pressure is applied along the length of the needle, allowing penetration of the chest wall (Fig. 31.7). An entry into the pleural space is indicated by a "popping" sound from the spring-loaded valve system and sight of a visual indicator that show when the blunt core protrudes over the sharp needle tip to avoid the contact between visceral pleura and the sharp needle tip, thus preventing pneumothorax.

It is recommended that intravenous access is established prior to the procedure. Appropriate instructions to the patient, at the time of obtaining the consent, help avoid or minimize the administration of sedations and anxiolytics. Atropine should be available for the treatment of possible bradycardia from a vasovagal reaction.

HOW THE TEST IS PERFORMED

After identifying the anatomical site where to perform thoracentesis, it is necessary to make a thorough disinfection of the skin area, preferably with an iodophor- or chlorhexidine-containing antiseptic. The physician who performs the thoracentesis should wear sterile gloves, and from this moment on, everything that is not sterile can be touched only by assistants without sterile clothing.

The physician should fill a 10-mL syringe with the content of a vial of lidocaine 1% or 2% without epinephrine for local anesthesia. Then the upper margin of the rib should be identified by palpation (this can be difficult in obese patients) and the local anesthetic injected by a 21-gauge needle at consecutively deeper levels: into the subcutaneous tissue, the periosteum of the rib and the parietal pleura. The insertion of the needle in the pleural space over the upper margin of the rib ensures maximum distance from the intercostal neurovascular bundles (Fig. 31.8). The needle

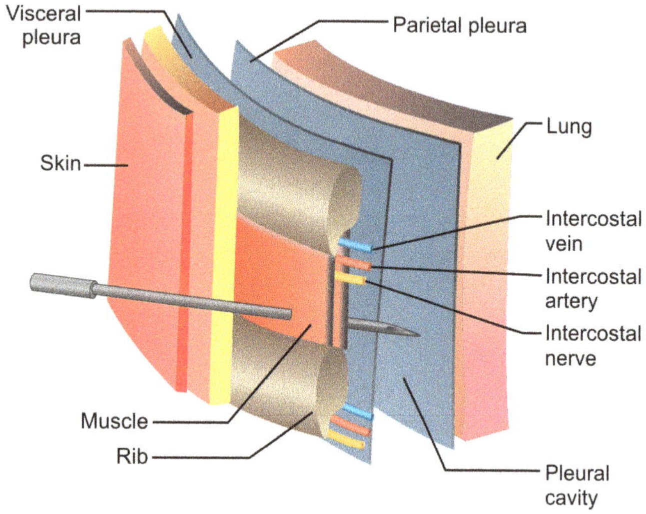

Fig. 31.8: Structures crossed by the needle during thoracentesis. To avoid injury of the intercostal neurovascular bundles, the needle should be inserted just above the upper margin of the rib.

should always be maintained perpendicular to the patient skin and advanced into the deeper layers of the chest wall while a negative pressure is created within the syringe by applying aspiration. This allows to understand when the needle reaches the pleural space (the pleural fluid comes into the syringe) and to assess inadvertent insertion into a blood vessel (leakage of bright red blood). Once the pleural fluid is aspirated, the needle can be retracted outside the pleural space. It is recommended not to inject more anesthetic when removing the needle, to prevent the spread of pleural diseases in the chest wall. If fluid cannot be obtained with a small-gauge needle, no attempts should be made at placing a large-bore thoracentesis needle or catheter.

Lidocaine has a short onset of action (within 2–5 minutes of injection) and its effects last up to 2 hours without epinephrine (3 hours with epinephrine). The most painful level after the skin is the parietal pleura, which should be infiltrated the most. Usually 5–6 mL of lidocaine 2% is enough to adequately anesthetize the puncture site.

While the operator waits a few minutes for the anesthetic to act, the kit for thoracentesis can be assembled. The needle should be attached to the pipe that leads to the three-way stopcock and then to the collection bag.

A 30- to 60-mL syringe can be connected to the three-way valve in order to collect the specimen to be analyzed. It is recommended to heparinize the syringe to prevent the aggregation of cells of the pleural fluid.

A few minutes after an injection of anesthesia, the large-bore needle for thoracentesis (or a catheter-over-needle system) can be inserted and the fluid aspirated under continuous application of suction by drawing back the plunger of the syringe. If a needle with a spring-loaded safety core is used, a "popping" sound is perceived when the needle reaches the pleural space. Successively, further fluid can be extracted simply by pressure difference between the pleural cavity and the collection bag.

If a catheter-over-needle system is used, it should be advanced another 1 cm after obtaining pleural fluid, in order to place the catheter with its maximum diameter in the pleural space; without advancing the needle, the catheter should be stripped into the pleural space, and the needle removed. The thoracentesis catheter should be then connected to the drainage tubing and collection bag. If a thoracentesis stopcock is available, it must be turned off to prevent air entry into the pleural space during such an operation.

RISKS AND POSSIBLE COMPLICATIONS

When the collapsed lung re-expands, the two pleural surfaces progressively become reopposed. If the visceral pleura with underlying lung comes in contact with the core of the neede, the latter may be retracted, leading to exposure of the sharp tip of the needle causing pneumothorax.

The risk is increased by coughing, since cough may lead to parting of the pleural surfaces followed by rapid apposition during subsequent inspiration. Complete drainage of fluid and the use of a sharp needle are other factors that may increase the risk of pneumothorax complicating the procedure.

Re-expansion pulmonary edema is a rare complication resulting from rapid emptying of air or liquid from the pleural cavity performed by either thoracentesis or chest tube drainage. Despite being infrequent, mortality may occur in up to 20% of cases and is attributed to the abrupt reduction in pleural pressure, especially as a result of extensive pneumothorax drainage or when there is long-term pulmonary collapse.

Pulmonary re-expansion edema may be considered an iatrogenic complication due to rapid emptying of the pleural cavity. The incidence referred is less than 1%, and mortality can reach up to 20%.

POST-PROCEDURE CARE

After removing the thoracentesis needle, the site of puncture should be covered with a simple dressing and controlled for bleeding or drainage. A physical examination of the chest should be performed. The auscultation with a stethoscope is particularly important, since if the breath sounds are bilaterally detected, it is very unlikely that a pneumothorax has occurred. A demise of tactile fremitus over the upper part of the aspirated hemithorax may be suggestive of a partial pneumothorax.

Chest radiography can be ordered after thoracentesis to document changes in the appearance of the lung fields, and to look for possible pneumothorax. Although commonly performed, it is not strictly necessary unless there is a clinical suspicion of pneumothorax. This can arise from the evidence of air outflow during the procedure or the appearance of symptoms such as dyspnea, cough, or chest pain. Vital signs with blood pressure and oxygen saturation should be assessed every 15 minutes until stable.

INTERPRETATION OF PLEURAL FLUID ANALYSIS

Pleural effusions are commonly distinguished into transudates and exudates on the basis of biochemical characteristics of the fluid, which reflect the physiologic mechanism of its formation.

Transudative effusions result from imbalances in hydrostatic and oncotic forces and have a low protein content. They may occur in a relatively small number of clinical conditions such as *heart failure* and *cirrhosis*. Less common causes include nephrotic syndrome, atelectasis, peritoneal dialysis, constrictive pericarditis, superior vena cava obstruction and urinothorax. If the physical-chemical examination of pleural fluid indicates a transudate, further diagnostic procedures are not necessary. A transudative effusion usually responds to treatment of the underlying condition (e.g. diuretic therapy).

Exudative effusions derive from the alteration of local factors that increase the permeability of the pleural surfaces and blood vessels, favoring the accumulation of pleural fluid. They have a relatively high protein content. Pneumonia, malignancy and thromboembolism account for most exudative effusions. Table 31.2 shows the most common criteria for classifying a pleural effusion as a transudate or exudates.

In patients with exudative effusion, further pleural fluid analyses should be performed on fluid obtained during the initial thoracentesis, including cell counts and differential, glucose, adenosine deaminase (ADA), and cytologic analysis.

To achieve an adequate white blood cell (WBC) count and differential cell count, it is necessary to prevent the pleural fluid clots by sending it in an anticoagulated tube.

Table 31.2: Light's criteria for distinguishing transudative from exudative pleural fluid. A single positive criterion is enough to classify the fluid as an exudate.

	Pleural/serum protein ratio	*Pleural/serum LDH ratio*	*Pleural LDH*
Transudate	≤ 0.5	≤ 0.6	≤ 200 U/L*
Exudate	> 0.5	> 0.6	> 200 U/L*

(LDH: Lactate dehydrogenase).
*Corresponding to two-thirds upper limit of normal serum level.

The finding of neutrophil-rich fluid suggests an acute process such as parapneumonic pleural effusion, whereas a predominance of lymphocytes raises the suspicion of a chronic process like cancer or tuberculosis.

Adenosine deaminase is an enzyme that plays an important role in lymphoid cell differentiation. A pleural fluid ADA level greater than 40 U/L (667 nkat/L) has a sensitivity of 90–100% and a specificity of 85–95% for the diagnosis of tuberculous pleurisy.

Bacterial cultures and pH should be tested if infection is a concern. A pleural effusion associated with pneumonia (parapneumonic effusion) is typically an inflammatory exudate with a predominance of polymorphonuclear leukocytes. A simple parapneumonic effusion may be complicated by bacterial invasion of the pleural space (empyema). This is characterized by an increase in lactic acid production with consequent development of a pleural fluid acidosis (pH < 7.20), associated with a rising pleural level of lactate dehydrogenase (LDH) (> 1,000 IU/L) due to leukocyte death and a falling glucose level (< 2.2 mmol/L) due to an increase of glucose metabolism. The abovementioned facts constitute the biochemical criteria for pleural infection. Pleural fluid pH is the most useful index predicting the need for chest tube drainage, highly recommended for pH values less than 7.2. Table 31.3 shows the most common characteristics of parapneumonic pleural effusions.

Pleural fluid sample for pH should be collected anaerobically, heparinized, and then assessed in a blood gas analyzer. Commercial local anesthetic solutions have an acidic pH to maximize their water solubility and chemical stability (that is why a burning sensation is felt during their administration). As a consequence, physicians should be aware that the anesthetic may depress measured pH if given in large amount or left in the same syringe used for its local administration.

Measurement of pleural fluid pH is unreliable when analyzed by pH litmus paper or a pH meter, and these should not be considered as acceptable alternatives to a blood gas analyzer.

Table 31.3: Common characteristics of parapneumonic pleural effusions.

	Simple parapneumonic effusion	*Complicated parapneumonic effusion*	*Empyema*
Macroscopic appearance	Clear fluid	Clear fluid or cloudy/turbid	Frank pus
pH	> 7.2	< 7.2	Not recommended
LDH	< 1,000 IU/L	> 1,000 IU/L	Not recommended
Glucose	< 1,000 IU/L	> 2.2 mmol/L	Not recommended
Culture or Gram stain	Negative	Sometime positive	Often positive
	Generally, resolves with antibiotics. The drainage of the pleural effusion can alleviate symptoms	Requires chest tube drainage	Requires chest tube drainage Does not require any additional biochemical tests on pleural fluid

(LDH: Lactate dehydrogenase).

It is not advisable to put frank pus through a blood gas analyzer. Furthermore, this is unnecessary since the aspiration of frank pus by thoracentesis already indicates the need for chest tube drainage of the effusion.

Cytologic analysis of pleural fluid is performed mainly for the purpose of trying malignant tumor cells.

BIBLIOGRAPHY AND FURTHER READING

1. Barnes TW, Morgenthaler TI, Olson EJ, Hesley GK, Decker PA, Ryu JH. Sonographically guided thoracentesis and rate of pneumothorax. J Clin Ultrasound. 2005;33:442-6.
2. Diacon AH, Brutsche MH, Solèr M. Accuracy of pleural puncture sites: a prospective comparison of clinical examination with ultrasound. Chest. 2003;123:436-41.
3. Duncan DR, Morgenthaler TI, Ryu JH, Daniels CE. Reducing iatrogenic risk in thoracentesis: establishing best practice via experiential training in a zero-risk environment. Chest. 2009;135:1315-20.
4. Du Rand I, Maskell N. Introduction and methods: British Thoracic Society Pleural Disease Guideline 2010. Thorax. 2010;65 (Suppl 2):ii1-3.
5. Eibenberger KL, Dock WI, Ammann ME, Dorffner R, Hörmann MF, Grabenwöger F. Quantification of pleural effusions: sonography versus radiography. Radiology. 1994;191:681-4.
6. Feller-Kopman D, Berkowitz D, Boiselle P, Ernst A. Large-volume thoracentesis and the risk of reexpansion pulmonary edema. Ann Thorac Surg. 2007;84:1656-61.
7. Gordon CE, Feller-Kopman D, Balk EM, Smetana GW. Pneumothorax following thoracentesis: a systematic review and meta-analysis. Arch Intern Med. 2010;170:332-9.
8. Havelock T, Teoh R, Laws D, Gleeson F; BTS Pleural Disease Guideline Group. Pleural procedures and thoracic ultrasound: British Thoracic Society Pleural Disease Guideline 2010. Thorax. 2010;65(Suppl 2):ii61-76.
9. Heidecker J, Huggins JT, Sahn SA, Doelken P. Pathophysiology of pneumothorax following ultrasound-guided thoracentesis. Chest. 2006;130:1173-84.
10. Huggins JT, Doelken P. Pleural manometry. Clin Chest Med. 2006;27:229-40.
11. Huggins JT, Sahn SA, Heidecker J, Ravenel JG, Doelken P. Characteristics of trapped lung: pleural fluid analysis, manometry, and air-contrast chest CT. Chest. 2007;131:-206-13.
12. Josephson T, Nordenskjold CA, Larsson J, Rosenberg LU, Kaijser M. Amount drained at ultrasound-guided thoracentesis and risk of pneumothorax. Acta Radiol. 2009;50:42-7.
13. Light RW. Clinical practice. Pleural effusion. N Engl J Med. 2002;346:1971-7.
14. Maskell NA, Butland RJ; Pleural Diseases Group, Standards of Care Committee, British Thoracic Society. BTS guidelines for the investigation of a unilateral pleural effusion in adults. Thorax. 2003;58 (Suppl 2):ii8-17.
15. Mayo PH, Goltz HR, Tafreshi M, Doelken P. Safety of ultrasound-guided thoracentesis in patients receiving mechanical ventilation. Chest. 2004;125:1059-62.
16. Suzuki S, Tanita T, Koike K, Fujimura S. Evidence of acute inflammatory response in reexpansion pulmonary edema. Chest. 1992;101:275-6.
17. Wrightson JM, Fysh E, Maskell NA, Lee YC. Risk reduction in pleural procedures: sonography, simulation and supervision. Curr Opin Pulm Med. 2010;16:340-50.
18. Wrightson JM, Helm EJ, Rahman NM, Gleeson FV, Davies RJ. Pleural procedures and pleuroscopy. Respirology. 2009;14:796-807.

Chapter

32

Mediastinoscopy

Massimo Guglielmetti, Angelo Maria Calati, Simona Maida, Daniele Trevisan, Claudio Sorino, Roberto Caronno

OVERVIEW OF MEDIASTINOSCOPY

The cervical mediastinoscopy technique, first described in 1959 by Carlens, is an invasive diagnostic technique used for the diagnosis of lesions located in the superior and middle mediastinum, pretracheal and paratracheal spaces, and subcarinal lymph nodes. This approach is generally used for diagnosis and staging of non-small cell lung cancers and small cell lung cancers, and sometimes for diagnosis of other mediastinal lymphadenopathies and mediastinal masses.

In the last decades, the technical refinements achieved using a video-assisted approach (video-mediastinoscopy) have contributed to increase the acceptance of the procedure because of improved magnification of the dissection field, which renders this operation more efficient and less risky.

MAIN INDICATIONS

The cervical mediastinoscopy is employed for diagnosis and staging in patients with potentially operable *non-small cell lung cancers*, to obtain histologic confirmation or exclusion of *mediastinal nodes involvement* (N2 or N3). The technique allows the access to the left and right paratracheal lymph nodes (levels 2R, 4R, 2L, 4L), the prevascular and retrotracheal nodes (3a and 3p) and the subcarinal nodes (level 7). The biopsies of the right paratracheal nodes (2R and 4R) are quite easy, while they are feasible but less easy in the left paratracheal (2L and 4L), prevascular (3a), retrotracheal (3p) and subcarinal (station 7) levels. The access to the aortopulmonary window (levels 5 and 6) is limited by the aorta and the left main stem bronchus, and it is much difficult. A modification of the technique proposed by Ginsberg is the so-called "extended cervical mediastinoscopy", which was conceived to reach these difficult sites, in particular the lymph nodes of the aortopulmonary window and the anterior prevascular mediastinal masses.

The advantages of video-mediastinoscopy are that the biopsies are almost always representative: the sensitivity is between 85% and 92%, and the specificity is about 100%. The disadvantages are that it is an invasive technique, general anesthesia is required, short hospitalization (1–2 days) is necessary, the application is limited to the superior mediastinum and subcarinal space, and complications are rare but they could be life-threatening.

Even if new technologies have been developed in the last decades, such as positron emission tomography (PET), endoscopic bronchial ultrasonography-guided transbronchial needle aspiration (EBUS-TBNA) and esophageal ultrasonography-guided fine-needle aspiration (EUS-FNA), the cervical mediastinoscopy remains the "gold standard" for the exploration of mediastinal lymph nodes. Anyway, the indications of mediastinoscopy are currently more precise and less extensive than some decades ago, and sometimes they are still a matter of debate.

SURGICAL TECHNIQUE

The patient is placed in the supine position. The general anesthesia is necessary. The endotracheal tube is armed to avoid the compression of the trachea during the exploration of the mediastinum. The surgeon is behind the head of the patient, and the assistant is on his right side. The video is in front of the surgeon, near the feet of the patient. An inflatable bag is placed under the shoulders to allow the hyperextension of the neck. The draping of the operating

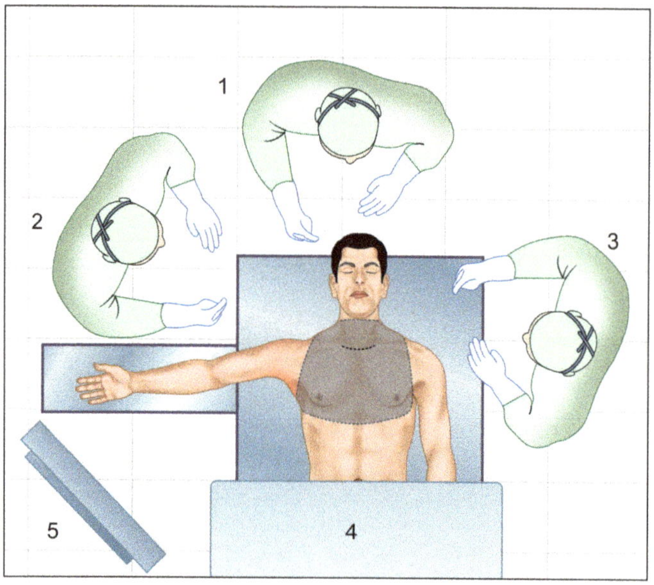

Fig. 32.1: The patient is lying in the operating room; the gray area is the operating field; the dotted line is the site of the skin incision above the sternal notch; the surgeon is indicated with the number 1, his assistant with the number 2, the nurse is the number 3; the table for the surgical instruments is indicated with the number 4, the video connected to the mediastinoscope is the number 5.

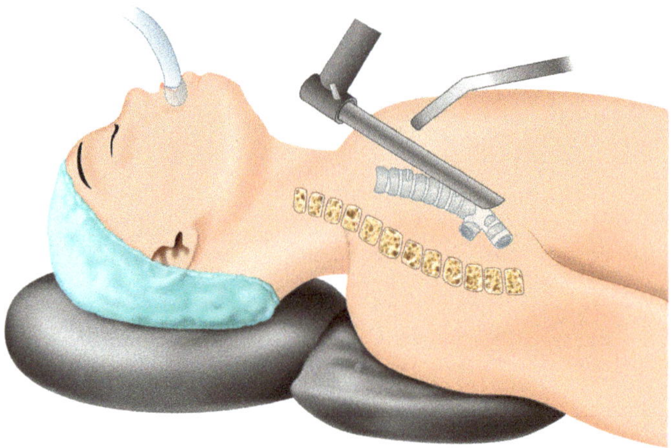

Fig. 32.2: The mediastinoscope has been inserted in the pretracheal space.

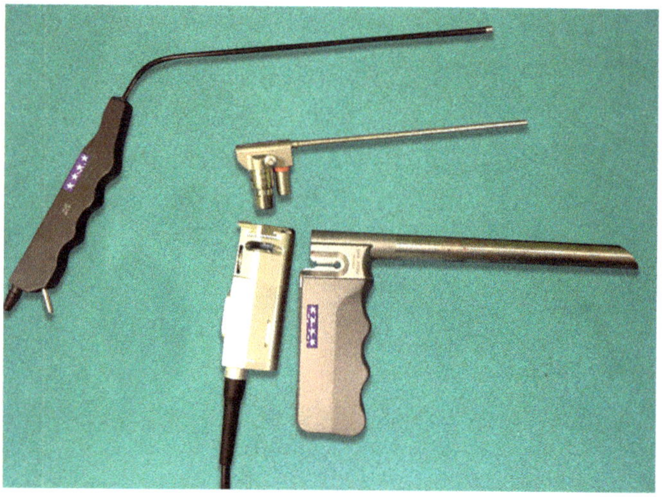

Fig. 32.3: The mediastinoscope is near the camera and the optical device which will be connected to it to make the video-mediastinoscope; the dissector is also a suction device and a cauterization instrument.

field with the surgical towels must include the neck and the chest from the chin to the subxiphoid region: even if an urgent median sternotomy is unlikely as a consequence of complications of mediastinoscopy, it could be necessary and the patient must be prepared (Figs. 32.1 and 32.2). For the same reason, a sternal saw, sternal and chest retractors must be prepared in the operating room. There are some surgical instruments that are specific for this procedure: a suction device which can also cauterize, scissors and grasps like those used in minimally invasive surgery, biopsy forceps. Nowadays the video-mediastinoscope has replaced the Carlens' instrument. It has a retractor device, an operative channel, and the camera and the light are connected inside (Fig. 32.3). The contribution of the video-surgery to the cervical mediastinoscopy is immense, because the images are larger and much more clear, so that the procedure is more efficacious and less dangerous.

The skin incision is horizontal in the lower part of the neck, 2 cm above the sternal notch, and the length of the incision is about 2–4 cm. The platysma is sectioned, the superficial median fascia of the neck is incised. The infrahyoid muscles are spread apart. The pretracheal fascia is incised and the finger of the surgeon can slide along the anterior surface of the trachea in an avascular plane. The mediastinoscope is inserted in the pretracheal space (Fig. 32.2). The dissection continues along that plane with the suction device; most of the dissection is blunt, sometimes adding the use of the cautery, so that the enlarged lymph nodes can be identified. Safety is maintained if the trachea is kept in view at all times. The node must be bluntly dissected, so that it is well recognized and delimited, and the surgeon is sure that it is a lymph node and the biopsy can be taken without risks to sample another anatomic structure, in particular a large vessel. Another strategy that reduces the risk of a vascular complication is the use of a needle to aspirate the nodes before biopsy. Biopsies of the selected nodes are taken under direct vision. Sometimes it is possible to excise the whole lymph node, but it is not essential. A frozen section of the biopsy is often performed, so the surgeon is sure that the sample is representative of the pathology. Sometimes a biopsy is taken for bacteriology and mycobacterium cultures. In some cases, it is useful to leave a thin drainage for little blood loss, then the incision is closed suturing the muscles and the skin.

The modified extended cervical mediastinoscopy was described by Ginsberg in 1987. It allows the surgeon to reach the prevascular space, and the thymic area, to biopsy mediastinal masses or lymph nodes in that site. With the same incision, the surgeon can also open the left mediastinal pleura between the brachiocephalic artery and the left common carotid artery to reach the aortopulmonary window and its lymph nodes. The skin incision is the same as in the cervical mediastinoscopy, and the dissection in made between the anterior surface of the left innominate vein and the posterior surface of the sternum; it allows to reach the level of the aortic arch at the origin of the innominate artery; the mediastinoscope is then passed by sliding it along the left anterolateral surface of the aortic arch until it reaches the aortopulmonary window. Anyway, this technique never gained wide acceptance because of its difficulties, and it is currently used only in few centers, and in special cases. Many authors consider this way too dangerous, and they prefer the anterior mediastinotomy or left thoracoscopy to reach those sites.

The anterior mediastinotomy was described by Chamberlain in 1966. It is a short anterior thoracotomy in the second intercostal space, using the video-mediastinoscope to reach the para-aortic region and sometimes the aortopulmonary window. The patient is in the supine position, in general anesthesia. An inflatable bag is placed under the lower part of the scapula. A video is in front of the surgeon. The instruments are the same of the cervical mediastinoscopy. The skin is incised at the second or third costal cartilage; the major pectoralis muscle is divaricated. A short tract of the cartilage is removed, and the mammary vessels are sutured and cut. The dissection is carried out without opening the pleura, if it is possible. A special care must be used not to injury the left phrenic nerve, which passes just anterior to the lung hilum. The biopsies of the lymph nodes are taken. A thin drainage is left for 24–48 hours and the incision is closed.

A special issue is represented by the repeat mediastinoscopy procedure. Some authors state that it is a reliable technique, but many other surgeons consider it difficult and dangerous: the natural plane that exists along the anterior wall of the trachea is absent due to scarring from the first mediastinoscopy performed and sometimes because of radiotherapy too; in this setting, the maneuvers become very risky and less efficacious, so repeat mediastinoscopy is controversial; the indications would be the staging of the mediastinum after induction therapies, to verify the utility to add surgery for the treatment of the pathology, but this issue is not addressed by randomized studies, and no clear guidelines can be drawn. Many controversies exist between the surgeons, and the procedure is not a standard nowadays.

RISKS AND POSSIBLE COMPLICATIONS

The mortality of the mediastinoscopy ranges between 0% and 1%. The complications are rare and they are usually not life-threatening, but because of the vital structures in the mediastinum, there remains a potential for severe and sometimes lethal injuries. The most dangerous complication is bleeding. A serious bleeding is rare, and it is usually related to a lesion of a bronchial artery in the subcarinal space or hypertrophic vessels of the enlarged lymph nodes. A gentle pressure with the anterior part of the mediastinoscope or the suction device is usually enough to control the bleeding; then the cautery can be applied to definitely stop the bleeding; if the bleeding continues, the surgeon can pack the mediastinum with a long narrow gauze; it usually stops the bleeding and must be left in place for some minutes (5–10 minutes), so that the vessel clots; then the gauze is removed: the bleeding is usually absent or modest and the site is cauterized additionally to obtain a better hemostasis.

If a major hemorrhage from a large vessel appears, a thoracotomy or sternotomy becomes necessary for direct surgical repair. A lesion of the bronchus or the trachea is promptly recognized; in this case, it is necessary to perform a thoracotomy to repair the lesion. If the lesion is very small, a drainage can be left in the mediastinum for some days, without the need to perform a thoracotomy. A damage of the esophagus is rare but it is difficult to be recognized. The immediate surgical repair has a good prognosis, while it is worse if a mediastinitis appears. A lesion of a recurrent nerve could occur, even if it is quite rare. It can be avoided if the use of the cautery is reduced as much as possible, in particular in the left tracheobronchial angle. The bilateral lesion of the recurrent nerves could cause the closure of the glottis, so that an emergency tracheotomy must be performed, but it is a very rare event, and it is almost always temporary.

DISCUSSION

The main indications of mediastinoscopy are the diagnosis and staging of lung cancer and the diagnosis of mediastinal neoplasms.

The guidelines of the European Society of Thoracic Surgeons (ESTS) try to give the recommendations about the indications and modality of realization of mediastinoscopy.

Regarding the staging of non-small cell lung cancer, the ESTS guidelines report important statements that are summarized hereafter.

A diameter larger than 1 cm in the short axis is generally considered as the standard criterion for a suspicious lymph node using the computed tomography (CT) scan.

Due to the high negative predictive value of PET scan, mediastinoscopy can generally be omitted in patients with clinical stage I non-small cell lung cancer with negative mediastinal PET images. This rule should be dealt with caution in case of patients with central tumors, central hilar N1 lymphadenopathy on CT scan, bronchioloalveolar carcinomas or in all the situations with low glucose PET uptake in the primary tumor and mediastinal PET negative lymph nodes larger than 15 mm on CT scan.

The positive predictive value of PET scan is only 79%, so in case of positive mediastinal PET, tissue confirmation is still needed. The literature available studies show an increased diagnostic accuracy of integrated PET-CT scan compared to PET alone.

Mediastinoscopy remains the "gold standard" for invasive staging of patients with potentially operable lung cancer.

There is no internationally accepted recommendation on how many lymph node mediastinal stations should be examined during the cervical mediastinoscopy.

The American Thoracic Society stated that all reachable nodal stations should be explored; so right and left superior and inferior paratracheal nodes (2R, 2L, 4R, 4L), right and left tracheobronchial nodes (10R and 10L) and subcarinal nodes (level 7) should be biopsied. The Society also recommend to perform the left anterior mediastinotomy to explore the subaortic pulmonary window (levels 5 and 6) in patients with left lung tumors and suspicious nodes.

Detterbeck and colleagues stated that the ideal exploration would include at least one node from the right and the left superior and inferior paratracheal nodes and the subcarinal station, unless more nodes are present.

Smulders and coworkers suggest that the minimally acceptable exploration includes biopsy of nodes from inferior paratracheal stations on both sides, and from subcarinal station.

The ESTS guidelines recommend to systematically explore and biopsy the right and left lower paratracheal nodes and the subcarinal nodes; additionally, if present, the upper paratracheal nodes should be sampled and biopsied.

In a recent review, the sensitivity of cervical mediastinoscopy varied between 72% and 89%.

Stations 5 and 6 cannot be reached by the standard cervical mediastinoscopy, so they should be explored by the "extended cervical mediastinoscopy" (proposed by Ginsberg), left anterior mediastinotomy or left thoracoscopy, when they are suspected to be involved by the tumor.

Thoracoscopy can also be used for levels 8 and 9 (paraesophageal and pulmonary ligament nodes).

Some recent reviews compared the accuracy of mediastinoscopy with less invasive techniques.

The transbronchial needle aspiration (TBNA) showed a sensitivity of 76% with false-negative rate of 29% in clinical N2 disease. So it could be used as a preliminary diagnostic test, complemented with the surgical staging in negative cases (ESTS guidelines). Its accuracy can be improved by guidance with endoscopic ultrasonography (EBUS-TBNA). Additionally the hilar stations (level 10) and the intrapulmonary nodal stations (levels 11, 12, and 13) can be biopsied with TBNA.

Esophageal ultrasound-guided fine-needle aspiration is mainly suitable for the assessment of lymph nodes in the posterior part of levels 4, 5, and 7, and the inferior mediastinum (levels 8 and 9). A review of the literature reported a pooled sensitivity of 88%, and a specificity of 91%, but most of the studies were performed in patients with a high suspicion of N2-N3 disease. It is generally accepted that endoscopic techniques (both EBUS-TBNA and EUS-FNA) are suitable to provide histologic proof of suspicious mediastinal nodes but cannot be used to exclude mediastinal lymph node disease because of the low negative predictive value.

The transthoracic needle aspiration (TTNA) is performed with CT guidance, and it can be used in patients with enlarged or bulky mediastinal lymph nodes. Almost all mediastinal nodal stations are accessible with this technique by anterior or posterior approach, but only in selected cases, because the other techniques are usually more efficacious and less risky.

The invasive staging can be omitted in patients with stage I non-small cell lung cancer and negative mediastinal PET images. Invasive staging is indicated in low PET uptake tumors with lymph nodes larger than 16 mm on CT scan.

PET positive mediastinal nodes should be histologically or cytologically confirmed.

At least one ipsilateral, one contralateral and the subcarinal nodes should be biopsied, and ideally all accessible lymph node stations.

BIBLIOGRAPHY AND FURTHER READING

1. Bisson A. Chirurgia diagnostica del mediastino: mediastinoscopia e mediastinotomia. In: Collectif (Ed). Encyclopédie médico-chirurgicale. Paris: Elsevier; 1996.
2. Carlens E. Mediastinoscopy: a method for inspection and tissue biopsy in the superior mediastinum. Dis Chest. 1959;36:343-52.
3. De Leyn P, Lardinois D, Van Schil PE, Rami-Porta R, Passlick B, Zielinski M, et al. ESTS guidelines for preoperative lymph node staging for non-small cell lung cancer. Eur J Cardiothorac Surg. 2007;32:1-8.
4. Detterbeck FC, Jones DR, Parker LA. Intrathoracic staging. In: Detterbeck FC, Rivera MP, Socinki M, Rosenman J (Eds). Diagnosis and Treatment of Lung Cancer: An Evidence-Based Guide for the Practicing Clinician. Philadelphia: WB Saunders; 2001. pp. 73-93.
5. Ginsberg RJ, Rice TW, Goldberg M, Waters PF, Schmocker BJ. Extended cervical mediastinoscopy. A single staging procedure for bronchogenic carcinoma of the left upper lobe. J Thorac Cardiovasc Surg. 1987;94:673-8.
6. Lardinois D, Schallberger A, Betticher D, Ris HB. Postinduction video-mediastinoscopy is as accurate and safe as video-mediastinoscopy in patients without pretreatment for potentially operable non-small cell lung cancer. Ann Thorac Surg. 2003;75:1102-6.
7. Lardinois D, Weder W. Diagnostic strategies in mediastinal mass. In: Patterson GA, Pearson FG, Cooper JD, Deslauriers J, Lerut AEMR, Luketich JD, Rice TW (Eds). Pearson's Thoracic and Esophageal Surgery, 3rd edition. New York: Churchill Livingstone; 2008. pp. 1506-20.
8. Marcheix B, Brouchet L, Renaud C, Berjaud J, Dahan M. Mediastinoscopia. In: Collectif (Ed). Encyclopédie médico-chirurgicale. Paris: Elsevier; 2004.
9. McNeill TM, Chamberlain JM. Diagnostic anterior mediastinotomy. Ann Thorac Surg. 1966 Jul; 2(4):532-9.
10. Meyers BF, Lerut T. Mediastinoscopy. In: Patterson GA, Pearson FG, Cooper JD, Deslauriers J, Lerut AEMR, Luketich JD, Rice TW (Eds). Pearson's Thoracic and Esophageal Surgery, 3rd edition. Churchill Livingstone; 2008. pp. 102-8.
11. Smulders SA, Smeenk FW, Janssen-Heijnen ML, Wielders PL, de Munck DR, Postmus PE. Surgical mediastinal staging in daily practice. Lung Cancer. 2005;47:243-51.
12. Tisi GM, Friedman PH, Peters RM, Pearson FG, Carr D, Lee RE, et al. American Thoracic Society. Medical section of the American Lung Association. Clinical staging of primary lung cancer. Am Rev Respir Dis. 1983;127:659-64.
13. Toloza EM, Harpole L, Detterbeck F, McCrory DC. Invasive staging of non-small cell lung cancer: a review of the current evidence. Chest. 2003;123:157S-66S.

Chapter 33

Video-Assisted Thoracic Surgery as a Diagnostic Tool

Angelo Maria Calati, Massimo Guglielmetti, Claudio Sorino, Roberto Caronno

BACKGROUND

Thoracoscopy has a high diagnostic yield (higher than 90% according to the majority of studies). Even if it is a more invasive procedure compared with image-guided pleural biopsy, thoracoscopy has the advantage to allow a therapeutic intervention in the same session as the diagnostic biopsy of the pleura. Thoracic surgery that does not use a formal thoracotomy incision. It has been used in diagnosis and therapy of thoracic diseases since the reports of the Swedish internist HC Jacobaeus in 1922. The technique had strong improvements and large employment only in 1990s, due to the technological improvement and the subsequent daily performing of laparoscopic surgery. In this chapter, we will address only the diagnostic applications of VATS.

INDICATIONS AND CONTRAINDICATIONS

Video-assisted thoracic surgery can be effective for pleural biopsies, complete evacuation of pleural effusions and hemothorax, even post-traumatic, talc poudrage for palliative treatment of malignant effusions, thoracic denervations (sympathectomy, splanchnicectomy), mediastinal biopsies (masses, lymphadenopathies), excision of lung nodules, and lung biopsy. VATS have many therapeutic applications, including major pulmonary resections, especially lobectomies, resection of peripheral pulmonary nodule, treatment of recurrent pneumothorax, management of loculated empyema, etc.

Thoracoscopy is recommended in patients with large and/or recurrent pleural effusions of unknown cause, to obtain drainage and pleurodesis, to direct observe the pleural cavity, and to perform biopsy of the pleura. Moreover, it is the procedure of choice when imaging (mainly CT scan) does not show clear target lesion and when the analysis of pleural fluid removed by thoracentesis is not diagnostic.

Indeed, in about 20% of pleural effusions, the cause remains unknown after nonsurgical techniques. In such situations, thoracoscopy has a high diagnostic yield (higher the 90% according to the majority of studies).

VATS allows for all the pleural surface (mediastinal, diaphragmatic, and visceral) to be fully visualized and accessible for biopsy.

Although it is a more invasive procedure compared with image-guided pleural biopsy, thoracoscopy has the advantage to allow a therapeutic intervention in the same session as the diagnostic biopsy of the pleura. Moreover, VATS has been shown to be an accurate method for identifying diaphragmatic injuries after penetrating thoraco-abdominal trauma.

The procedure also allows the surgeon to diagnose less common causes of undetermined pleural effusion, such as peritoneal fistulas associated with peritoneal dialysis, and to locate and repair the source of persistent chylothorax. Before performing a VATS, the physician should take into account the expected benefits from the procedure. Particular attention should be paid to debilitated patients who can not be subjected to any treatment after the definition of a pleural disease.

Absolute contraindications to VATS include the following:

- Clinical instability or shock
- Extensive adhesions obliterating the pleural space
- Prior talc pleurodesis.

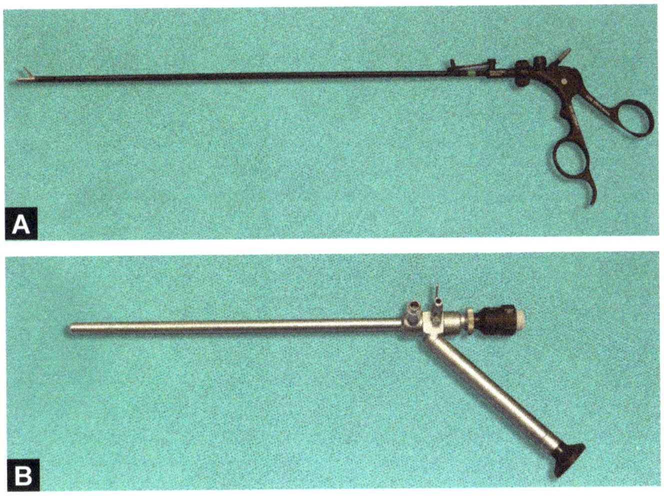

Figs. 33.1: Single-access (coaxial) thoracoscope (A) with biopsy forceps (B).

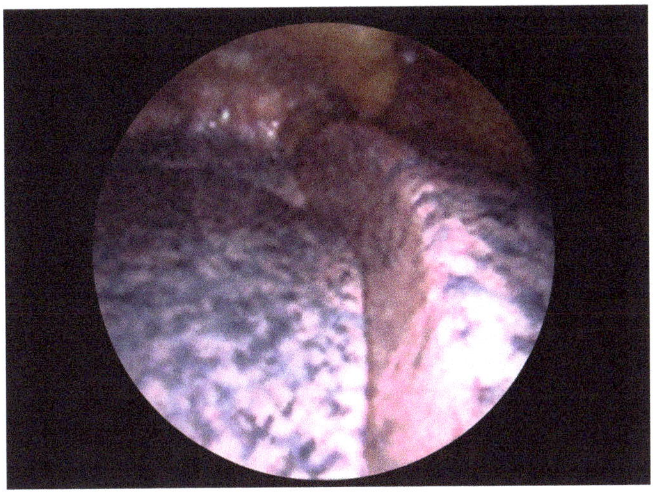

Fig. 33.2: Thoracoscopic appearance of a pleural carcinomatosis (malignant mesothelioma).

Relative contraindications include the following:

- Difficulty to tolerate single lung ventilation
- Previous thoracotomies
- Extensive pleural diseases
- Coagulation disturbances
- Prior radiation treatment for thoracic malignancy.

PROCEDURE

Simplest VATS procedures can be performed in local anesthesia, but more often they require general anesthesia with double-lumen ventilation that allows ventilatory exclusion of the lung, and thus a well-equipped operating room. Disposition of the surgical team depends on the habits of the operators; most often 1st and 2nd surgeon stay at the same side of the patient, who lies in lateral decubitus (obviously exposing the side of the pathology). The video camera introduced in the pleural space reproduces images with approximately 5x magnification on one or two screens visible to all the components of the team.

Pleural biopsies, toilette of effusions, talc poudrage can be performed safely and effectively with single-access VATS. This technique requires a coaxial thoracoscope (Figs. 33.1A).

A small (1–1.5 cm) incision allows the access to the pleural space, introducing a standard trocar after ventilatory exclusion of the lung. After the evacuation of the effusion, if present, the thoracoscope is introduced. The optical device (0–5°) is coaxial in the instrument. The pleural space can so be explored. Figure 33.2 shows the thoracoscopic appearance of a pleural carcinomatosis.

Through the thoracoscope, biopsy forceps and other instruments (Fig. 33.1B) can be introduced. The diameter of the instrument limits the degree of movements of the instrument. As a consequence, if possible the surgeon should perform the access in front of the lesion(s), almost always defined not only by standard chest X-ray but by CT scan too. In case of massive pleural effusion without lesions at the CT scan, the surgeon must bear in mind that there can be the chance of pleural nodules in posterior and inferior part of the pleural space. So, with patient in lateral decubitus, the access will be more often anterior, i.e. through mammary line or anterior axillary line, with the surgeon in front of it, and the main screen behind the back of the patient. A pleural biopsy during VATS is shown in Figure 33.3.

Hemostasis, if necessary, can be performed by electrocoagulation and/or hemostatic gauzes and devices. Through the thoracoscope, talc poudrage can be performed easily and safely. This is a palliative treatment of malignant pleural effusion (talc-induced pleurodesis reduces or eliminates the effusion) and it seems more effective if performed in VATS rather than with talc slurry introduced through a pleural drainage.

Excision of a lung nodule by VATS could be a diagnostic and therapeutic procedure at the same time. This usually requires two or, more often, three small incisions that allow the positioning of the trocars and the camera. The trocars are in line with the right hand of the surgeon, with his/her eyes (the camera, holden by the 2nd surgeon), and with his left hand, so they must be placed as a triangle. A 30-degree camera allows better visualization. It is important not to

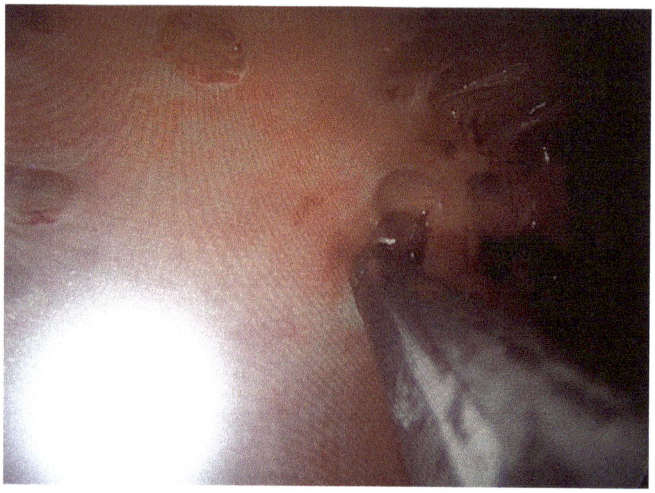

Fig. 33.3: Thoracoscopic pleural biopsy (malignant mesothelioma).

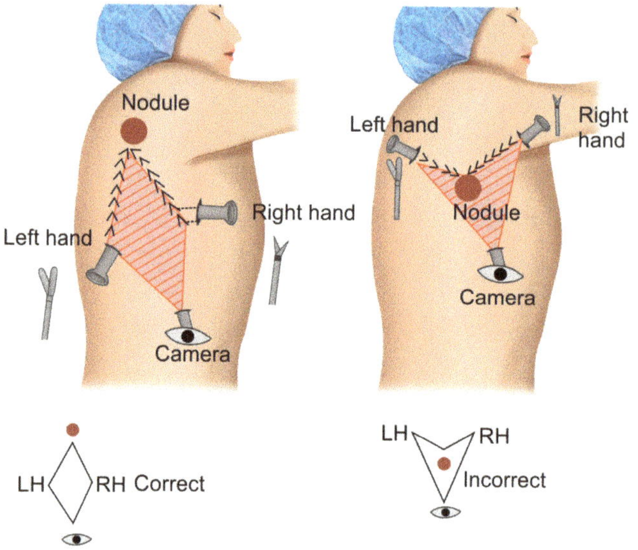

Fig. 33.4: Positioning of the thoracoscopic accesses.

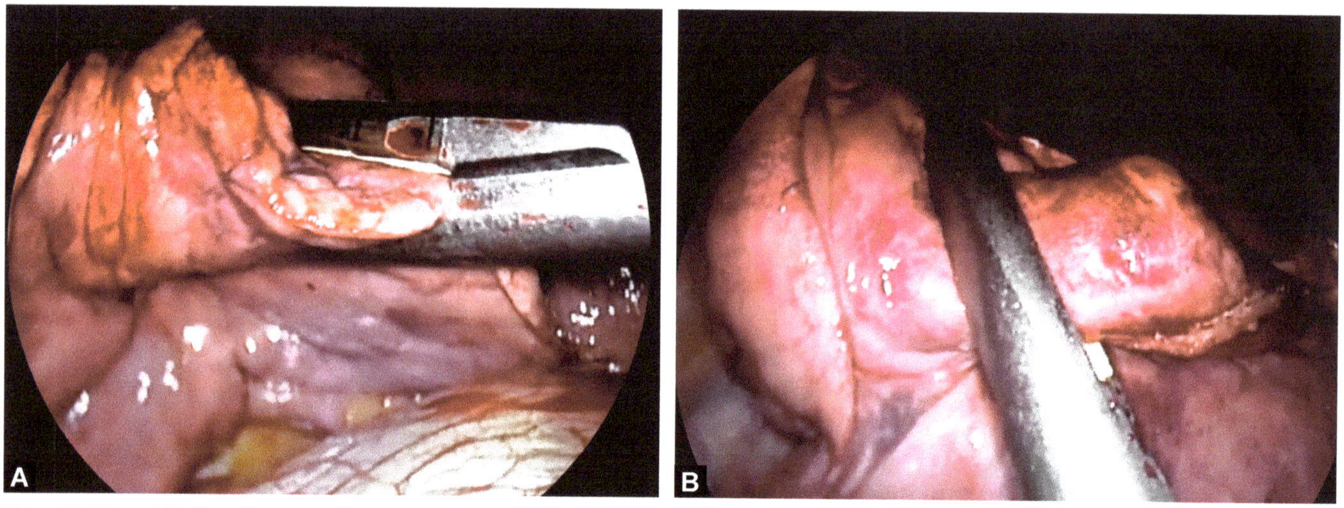

Figs. 33.5A and B: Excisional biopsy of a pulmonary nodule: (A) 1st endoscopic suture and section. (B) 2nd endoscopic suture and section.

place the trocars too close to each other, in order to avoid conflicts between the instruments, and to have the site of the lung biopsy distal to the three trocars. As shown in Figure 33.4, ideally the three access sites (two trocars and the camera) and the skin projection of the nodule should draw a rhombus.

If the site of the excision is proximal, maneuvers become very difficult, requiring "reverse" movements, as looking at a mirror.

The introduction of devices for endoscopic sutures made pulmonary resections safe and simple. Hemostasis and aerostasis are usually satisfying and do not require further maneuvers or devices. Figures 33.5A and B show a peripheral (transegmentary) resection for excisional biopsy of a lung nodule.

The extraction of the specimen requires a plastic bag to avoid neoplastic or microbiological contamination of the incision (Fig. 33.6).

Talc poudrage through a single-access diagnostic VATS brings often to high daily volumes of pleural effusion, so the drainage must not be removed, often for more days than for a three-access resection of a lung nodule.

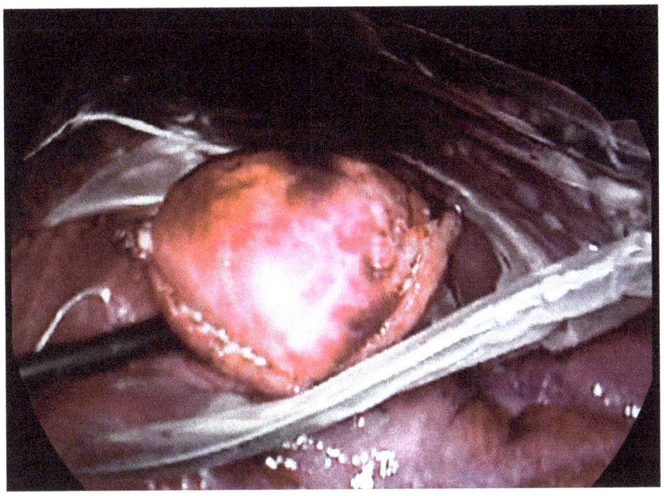

Fig. 33.6: Excisional biopsy of a pulmonary nodule: extraction of the specimen with plastic bag.

Postoperative pain is easily treated and the patient should be mobilized the same day of the operation. Both in single- and multiple-access VATS, the hospital stay is determined by how long the pleural drainage has to be held in place.

BIBLIOGRAPHY AND FURTHER READING

1. Adams RF, Gleeson FV. Percutaneous image-guided cutting needle biopsy of the pleura in the diagnosis of malignant mesothelioma. Chest. 2001;120:1798-802.
2. Ahmed N, Jones D. Video-assisted thoracic surgery: state of the art in trauma care. Injury. 2004 May;35(5):479-89.
3. Antunes G, Neville E, Duffy J, Ali N, Pleural Diseases Group, Standards of Care Committee, British Thoracic Society BTS guidelines for the management of malignant pleural effusions. Thorax. 2003;58(Suppl 2):1129-38.
4. Brodsky JB. Cohen E. Video-assisted thoracoscopic surgery. Current Opinion in Anaesthesiology. 2000;13(1):41-45.
5. Freeman RK, Al-Dossari G, Hutcheson KA, et al. Indications for using video-assisted thoracoscopic surgery to diagnose diaphragmatic injuries after penetrating chest trauma. Ann Thorac Surg. 2001 Aug;72(2):342-7.
6. Landreneau RJ, Mack MJ, Hazelrigg SR, et al. Video-assisted thoracic surgery: basic technical concepts and intercostal approach strategies. The Annals of Thoracic Surgery. 1992;54(4):800-807
7. Maskell NA, Butland RJ, Pleural Diseases Group, Standards of Care Committee, British Thoracic Society BTS guidelines for the investigation of a unilateral pleural effusion in adults. Thorax. 2003;58(Suppl 2):118-7.
8. Medford ARL, Awan YM, Marchbank A, et al. Diagnostic and therapeutic performance of video-assisted thoracoscopic surgery (Vats) in investigation and management of pleural exudates. Ann R Coll Surg Engl. 2008 Oct;90(7):579-600.
9. Yim APC, Sihoe ADL. Video-assisted Thoracic Surgery as a Diagnostic Tool. In: Shields TW, LoCicero J, Reed CE, Feins RH, General Thoracic Surgery, Volume 1, Lippincott Williams & Wilkins, 2009.

Chapter

34

Endobronchial Ultrasound

Sixto Arias, Hans Lee, Ricardo Ortiz, David Feller-Kopman, Lonny Brett Yarmus, Claudio Sorino, Kazuhiro Yasufuku

OVERVIEW OF ENDOBRONCHIAL ULTRASOUND

Miniaturization of endoscopic ultrasound (EUS) technology and its combination with bronchoscopy in a hybrid bronchoscope constituted a breakthrough in the evaluation of lesions beyond the limits of the airways walls. Endobronchial ultrasound (EBUS) is a bronchoscopic technique that uses ultrasound to visualize structures contiguous with the airways. There are two types of EBUS probes currently available: (1) *radial* and (2) *curvilinear*. The introduction of radial probe-EBUS (RP-EBUS) and its 20-MHz probe (diameter of 2.5 mm) (Fig. 34.1) enabled detailed 360° images with a penetration of 5 cm. Curvilinear ultrasound probes (7.5 MHz) (Fig. 34.2), located at the distal end of the bronchoscope, enabled full ultrasonic visualization of the needle when inserted into the target lesion for real-time EBUS-guided transbronchial needle aspiration (EBUS-TBNA) using the convex probe EBUS (CP-EBUS). The live-imaging capability of EBUS allows for a more objective, less operator dependent, sampling technique than conventional transbronchial needle aspiration (C-TBNA). Originally popularized by Wang in the 1980s, TBNA is a biopsy technique used during bronchoscopy that involves passing a needle-containing catheter through the airway wall into lymph nodes or masses to obtain samples for cytopathologic analysis (*see* Chapter 29 for further details on C-TBNA). It has been shown to be effective in both the

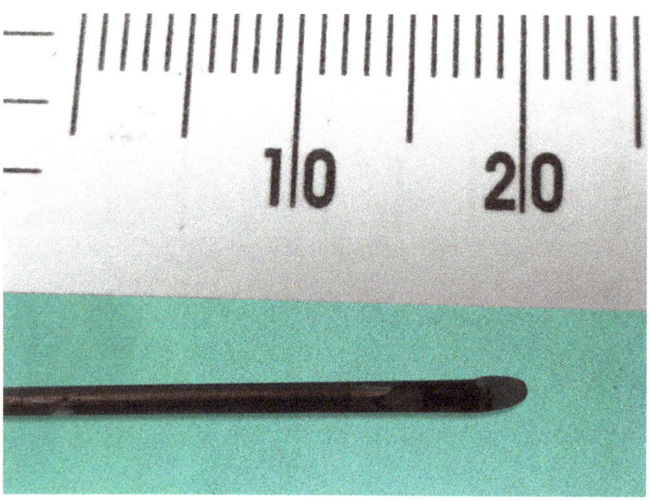

Fig. 34.1: Olympus radial endobronchial ultrasound (20-MHz probe UM-S20-20R).

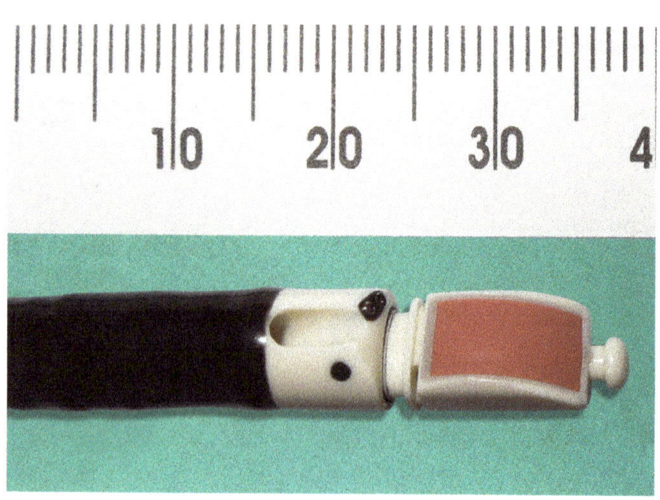

Fig. 34.2: Olympus curvilinear ultrasound probe (7.5 MHz).

diagnosing and staging of lung cancer. The procedure is minimally invasive, safe, less costly than mediastinoscopy, and has been shown to preclude surgery in up to almost one-third of patients with lung cancer. The procedure is now routinely performed for mediastinal staging and is recommended as a first-line intervention. Literature reported values for sensitivity range from 46% to 97%.

Endobronchial ultrasound-guided TBNA was initially performed by inserting a radial ultrasound probe through the working channel of the bronchoscope, identifying the target, and then removing the probe and performing TBNA. Although this was not a true "real-time" guidance technique, EBUS significantly improved the yield of TBNA.

In 2003, Krasnik et al. sampled 15 lesions using a prototype ultrasonic bronchoscope [Olympus (XBF-UC40P, Tokyo, Japan)]. The instrument had a small curved array transducer located at the distal end and a 2 mm working channel. This bronchoscope allowed for simultaneous direct transducer contact with the airways and biopsy, thus allowing for real-time visualization of the target lesions during TBNA. The bronchoscopies were performed under general anesthesia and the aspirated material obtained from the different lesions was diagnostic in all cases. Since then the number of publications increased significantly demonstrating its benefits in patients that need mediastinal staging.

Endobronchial ultrasound-guided transbronchial needle aspiration is a safe, minimally invasive procedure with a high diagnostic value for the diagnosis and staging of lung cancer. A thorough understanding of mediastinal anatomy is essential to accurately stage the mediastinum. Determination of mediastinal and hilar metastasis influences decisions about the appropriateness of surgery, radiation and systemic therapy. EBUS-TBNA also plays an important role in the diagnosis of lymphoma and sarcoidosis.

TECHNOLOGY

The introduction of flexible bronchoscopy by Ikeda in 1966 accelerated the development of instruments and techniques with diagnostic and therapeutic implications. This advance in technology and the miniaturization of EUS eventually led to the first flexible ultrasonic bronchoscope, developed by Olympus. Today, the commercially available instrument by Olympus (BF-UC180F, Tokyo, Japan) (Fig. 34.3) has an outer diameter of 6.9 mm and a working length of 600 mm. The angulation range of the distal end of the endoscope is 120° upward and 90° downward. The instrument has a small curved linear array electronic

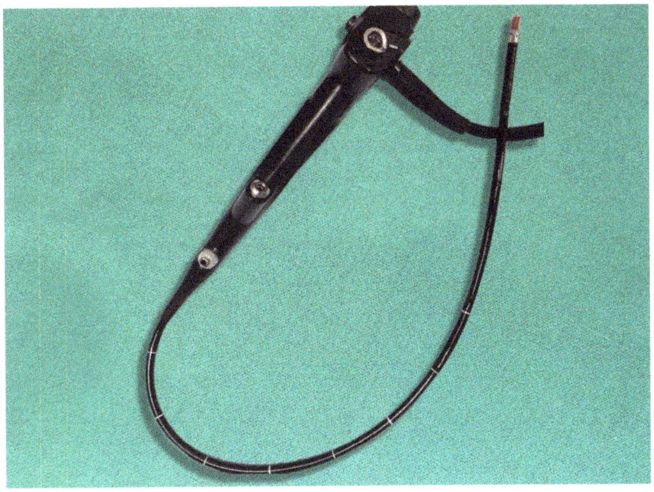

Fig. 34.3: Olympus (BF-UC180F) endobronchial ultrasound (EBUS) scope.

transducer with a length of 10 mm, located at the distal end of the endoscope in front of a 35° oblique forward viewing fiberoptic lens (angle of view 80°). The diameter of the distal end of the endoscope with the transducer is 6.9 mm, and the endoscope has a working channel of 2.2 mm. The ultrasonic quad-frequencies (5, 7.5, 10, and 12 MHz) allow for different depths of penetration. The scanning direction is parallel to the longitudinal axis of the endoscope with a scanning angle of 50°. The charge-coupled device (CCD) is built in the control section. The Fuji EBUS scope (Fujifilm, Japan, EB-530US) (Fig. 34.4) is a flexible multifrequency (5–12 MHz) ultrasonic bronchoscope. The scope has a CCD image chip technology with two light guides. The outer diameter of the insertion tube and the tip are 6.3 mm and 6.7 mm. It provides a 120° field of view at a 10° forward oblique angle. The Pentax EB-1970UK EBUS scope provides a 75° ultrasound angle and a 2.0 mm working channel. The Olympus 19-, 21-, and 22-gauge EBUS needle and the WANG° MW319, SW221 needle (ConMed, USA) could be used for TBNA with this scope. A disposable latex balloon placed over the ultrasound probe is filled with saline to reduce the air interface and facilitate imagining acquisition (Fig. 34.5)

The EBUS bronchoscope requires a specialized needle to perform the procedure. Disposable 19-, 21-, or 22-gauge dedicated EBUS-TBNA needles with a total length of 40 mm (Olympus ViziShot®) and 22- to 25-gauge with 50 mm length (COOK Medical EchoTip) are commercially available. The ultrasonographic images acquired with the convex probe are transmitted and processed by a central ultrasound unit that allows the use of different applications

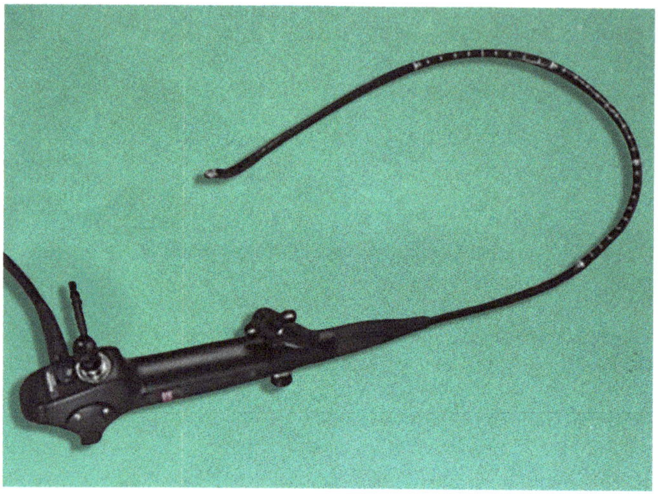

Fig. 34.4: Fuji (EB-530US) EBUS scope.

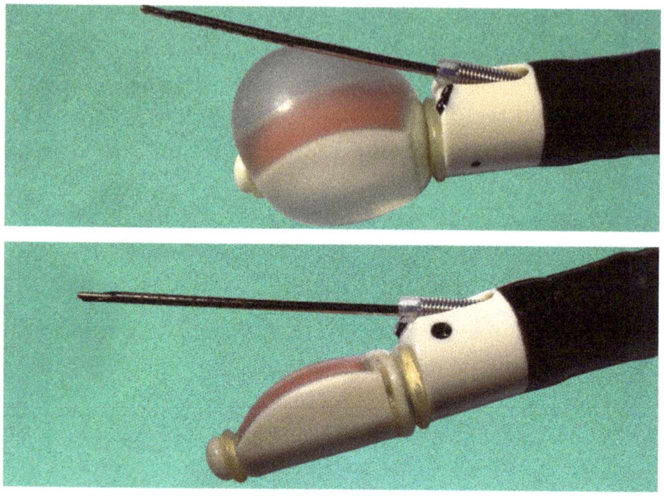

Fig. 34.5: Olympus curvilinear probe, saline filled balloon/empty and biopsy needle.

like color Doppler, calipers, measurements of the lesion, labels, gain adjustment, etc. Image artifacts are commonly encountered during ultrasonography, frequent ones includes reverberation and attenuation. Reverberation appears as multiple equidistantly spaced linear reflections. Acoustic shadow artifacts result from reduced amplitude caused by intervening structures with high attenuation.

INDICATIONS

Initial data examining the yield of EBUS-TBNA primarily concentrated on lung cancer. Due to the fact identifying nodule metastasis is one of the most important factors establishing prognosis and determines the ideal therapy, EBUS is an ideal modality to sample the mediastinum. Other studies have examined the utility of EBUS-TBNA for the diagnosis of sarcoidosis and lymphoma. Several studies reviewed here have shown that EBUS-TBNA may be the preferred diagnostic modality for the investigation of pulmonary sarcoidosis. One study showed a sensitivity of 85% for the diagnosis of sarcoidosis using EBUS-TBNA as a first-line diagnostic test. Tremblay and colleagues completed a randomized trial examining the diagnostic efficacy of EBUS-TBNA versus standard TBNA in sarcoidosis and found an increase in diagnostic yield of 83% versus 54% and an increase in sensitivity of 83% versus 61%. Recently, Moonim et al. prospectively studied 2,256 patients and reported a sensitivity, specificity, positive predictive value (PPV), negative predictive value (NPV) and accuracy of EBUS-TBNA in the diagnosis of mediastinal lymphoma of 89%, 97%, 98%, 83%, and 91%, respectively.

TECHNIQUE

Endobronchial ultrasound-guided transbronchial needle aspiration is an extension of conventional TBNA. It is an ambulatory procedure that is performed under moderate or deep sedation. Laryngo-tracheo-bronchial topical anesthesia reduces the cough reflex and the need of higher doses of intravenous sedatives. Amide-based local anesthetics like lidocaine administered up to a total dose of 3–4 mg/kg can be atomized in the airway mucosa for this purpose. The EBUS scope can be introduced nasally or orally, but the oral route is preferred due to the dimension of the distal end of the scope. If endotracheal intubation is required to perform the procedure, an endotracheal tube (ETT) equal or larger than size 8 is recommended. A laryngeal mask airway (LMA) is a safe, effective and useful modality during EBUS bronchoscopy and is an excellent alternative to endotracheal intubation. It is recommend a rapid survey of the tracheobronchial tree anatomy with a white light bronchoscope prior to EBUS bronchoscopy. Visualization of an endoscopic view of the larynx using the Olympus/Pentax EBUS scopes requires downward flexion to correct for the 35° forward oblique angle. This maneuver is obviated with the use of the 10° forward oblique angle Fuji EBUS systems. Once the trachea is intubated with the EBUS bronchoscope, it is positioned in the area of interest and the tip flexed against the airway wall to obtain an ultrasonographic view. At this point, the latex balloon is filled if maximum contact with the airway wall was not achieved with simple flexion of the tip. Adequate preprocedure study of the computed tomography (CT) of the chest, familiarization with the endobronchial

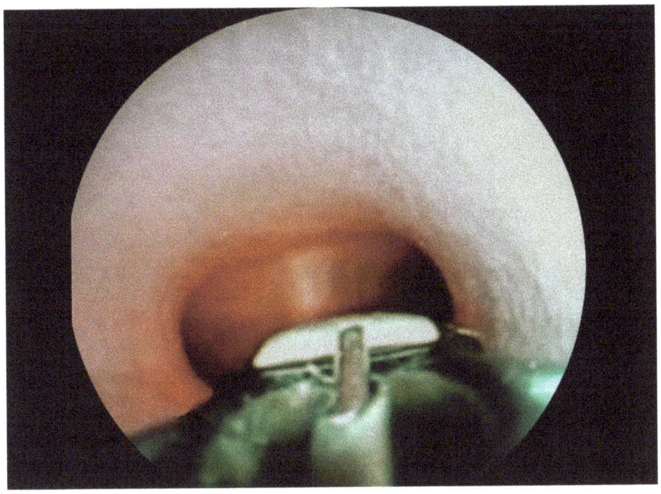

Fig. 34.6: Endobronchial ultrasound (EBUS) optical view of the airways (Fuji EB-530US).

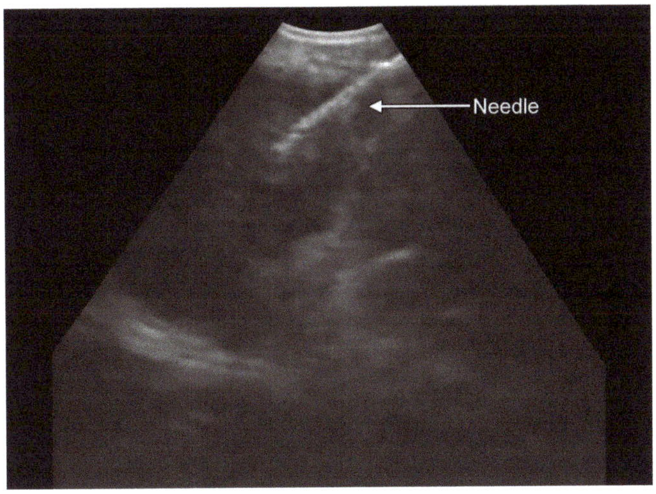

Fig. 34.7: Ultrasonographic view. Biopsy needle inside the target.

anatomy and ultrasonographic identification of the vascular landmarks are essential to target each nodal station defined by the International Association for the Study of Lung cancer (IASLC) lymph node map. Ultrasonographic lymph node features have been evaluated as a predictor of malignancy. Size and shape appears to predict metastasis, but absence of those features should not preclude the node from biopsy. Large nodes may be benign and small nodes (< 15 mm) may contain metastases in up to 20% of cases.

Once the puncture site is identified the needle is introduced through the working channel and locked in place. The needle sheath is adjusted so the tip can be visualized in the endoscopic view (Fig. 34.6) The location of the target lesion is verified in the ultrasonographic view, avoiding the airway cartilage, and then the needle adjuster is set at the appropriate length based on the lesion size and desired depth. The needle is deployed and advanced in the lymph node/lesion (Fig. 34.7), the stylet is removed and suction can be applied connecting a syringe to the distal luer-lock tip of the needle, although one study found that negative pressure did not increase yield. However, most centers continue to use suction routinely while more evidence is generated. The lesion is sampled by moving the needle back and forth, suction is discontinued, the needle is retrieved into the sheath, and the dedicated EBUS-TBNA needle is completely removed from the bronchoscope.

For mediastinal staging of non-small cell lung cancer (NSCLC), three needle aspirations per node are recommended for optimal diagnostic yield and four for molecular profiling pathologic differentiation. In terms of needle size, there is no significant difference in the diagnostic yield between the 21- and 22-gauge needles, but it appears that the histological structure is better preserved with the 21-gauge needles and likely provides more cellularity for molecular marker analysis.

Specimen handling and preparation is a critical step for best results. In centers with rapid on-site evaluation (ROSE), the cytopathologist takes the first few drops of the sample to prepare a slide using a modified Romanowsky stain know as Diff-Quik and provides a real-time assessment to the bronchoscopist. The remaining material is placed in saline or Cytolyt for later centrifugation and conventional cell block preparation. Alternatively, the sample is pushed out the needle using the wire stylet, onto a piece of filter paper to build up a cone-shaped coagulum; a technique known as "tissue coagulum clot" cell block (TCC-CB) method. The coagulum is then processed as a cell block.

MEDIASTINAL AND HILAR LYMPH NODES

With the exception of stations 3a, 5, 6, 8, and 9, all the other mediastinal and hilar lymph node stations are accessible by EBUS-TBNA through the airway (Fig. 34.8).

Station 7

The lymph nodes are located between the left and right main bronchus, and an ultrasonographic view can be obtained either from the right or the left of the main carina. The bronchoscope can be placed against the medial wall of the right main bronchus approximately at the level of the right upper lobe bronchus.

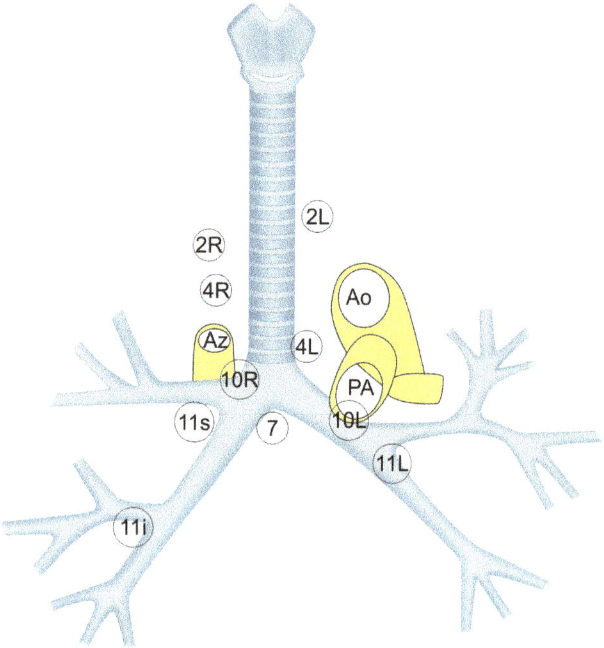

Fig. 34.8: Modified IASLC lymph node map. (PA: Pulmonary artery, Ao: Aorta, AZ, Azygos vein, L: Left, R: Right, s: Superior, i: Inferior. *Courtesy*: Eduardo Arias.

Station 11R

In between the right upper lobe bronchus and the bronchus intermedius (BI) and more distal in the anterolateral aspect of the BI resides the nodes for this station. To access the node, advance the scope to the level of the BI turn to the 2–4 o'clock position and scan from the distal BI to the level of the right first secondary carina (RC1) without entering the upper lobe bronchus.

Station 10R

Lymph nodes for this station are identified in the right main bronchus, at the 2–3 o'clock position, proximal to the right upper lobe entrance, in the ultrasonographic view distal to the azygos vein.

Station 4R

In the trachea, just proximal to the main carina, at the 2 o'clock position behind the superior vena cava and proximal to the azygos vein is this station. The cephalic limit is defined by the caudal border of the brachiocephalic vein. Very often nodes for this station are located closer to the midline, in the pretracheal region behind the ascending aorta, in such cases turn the scope toward the 12 o'clock position.

Station 2R

In the trachea at the 2–3 o'clock position, cephalic to the brachiocephalic vein is station 2R.

Station 11L

Interlobar nodes are located between the left upper lobe and the left lower lobe bronchus in proximity to the interlobar pulmonary artery. Place the scope at the 2 o'clock position slightly distal to the secondary carina (LC2).

Station 10L

In the distal portion of the left main bronchus toward the secondary carina (LC2), at 11 o'clock position distal to the upper border of the main pulmonary artery.

Station 4L

In the lateral trachea, close to the junction of the trachea and the left main bronchus, at the 9 o'clock position. Station 4L is defined by the cephalic border of the aortic arch to the upper border of the left main pulmonary artery and lateral to the ligamentum arteriosum.

Station 2L

In the mid trachea at the 9 o'clock position and proximal to the upper border of the aortic arch without crossing the left border of the trachea that defines left from right as determined by the IASLC.

When performing EBUS-TBNA for the diagnosis or staging of lung cancer, examination should begin with sampling N3 nodes, follow by N2 and N1 if necessary. The procedure may be terminated at the highest stage if ROSE is utilized confirming malignant cells.

EBUS AND LUNG CANCER

Lung cancer remains the leading cause of cancer deaths in the United States. Each year in the United States over 200,000 people are diagnosed with lung cancer, and 160,000 die of this disease. Lung cancer represents 14% of all invasive cancers diagnosed each year and 28% of all cancer deaths in the United States. It is estimated that over 90% of all lung cancer deaths in the United States each year are directly caused by tobacco abuse. More than half of lung cancers have distant metastasis at the time of diagnosis. Prognostic data, including response to treatment and survival as well as guidance for treatment management, has all been closely linked with staging of the disease. The staging of NSCLC is defined by the tumor, node, metastasis (TNM) system. NSCLC is staged clinically and pathologically. The clinical stage is based upon the patient's examination, radiographic evaluations and prior tissue sampling. Noninvasive staging techniques use radiologic procedures like CT and positron emission tomography (PET) scans. PET scanning offers a sensitivity of 80% with a specificity of around 90%. Sensitivities and NPV for PET scan and mediastinoscopy are comparable; however, the PPV and specificity are lower (sensitivity ~80%, NPV ~90%). PPV of the PET scan is only 79%; therefore, tissue confirmation is needed in cases of PET-avid mediastinal nodes.

The pathologic stage is defined by the histopathologic data obtained after the primary tumor is resected or pathologic confirmation of the most advanced site of disease is obtained. It has been shown that up to 24% of patients are clinically overstaged and 20% are understaged when compared to pathologic data. Determination of the N component of the TNM system requires an accurate assessment of the mediastinal lymph nodes.

Endobronchial ultrasound has made a significant impact on the practice and yield of diagnostic testing for mediastinal staging of lung cancer. Overall, EBUS-TBNA showed a median sensitivity of 89%, with values ranging from 46% to 97% and a median NPV of 91% as reported on a recent systematic review that included 2,756 patients. In a study by Herth et al., with 572 lymph nodes in 500 patients, EBUS-TBNA was shown to have a diagnostic yield of 94%. The biopsy specimens were taken from multiple nodal stations including hilar and mediastinal areas. Lymph nodes in region 2L (40 nodes), 2R (53 nodes), 3 (35 nodes), 4R (86 nodes), 4L (77 nodes), 7 (127 nodes), 10R (38 nodes), 10L (43 nodes), 11R (40 nodes), and 11L (33 nodes) were all sampled with a pooled sensitivity of 94%, a specificity of 100% and a PPV of 100% calculated per patient.

There have also been studies which use EBUS to evaluate the radiologically normal mediastinum. A hundred patients with NSCLC and a chest CT with no mediastinal (lymphadenopathy > 10 mm) underwent EBUS-TBNA of all identifiable nodes and then subsequent surgical staging with mediastinoscopy or thoracotomy. Cancer was found by EBUS in 19 patients and missed in 2. These 19 patients were subsequently upstaged from N0 to N1 in 3 patients, N2 in 13 patients and N3 in 3 patients. These results in conjunction with a sensitivity of 92%, specificity of 100% and NPV of 96% in this study suggest that EBUS could aid in avoiding surgery in 17% of patients who, the literature suggests, would not benefit from surgical resection at that time. It is important to recognize the limitation of EBUS-TBNA in that a nondiagnostic examination will not be considered a negative test. If a nondiagnostic result is obtained, confirmatory tissue is required.

Herth et al. evaluated 124 patients with stage IIIa-N2 NSCLC who received induction chemotherapy. Post therapy CT scanning revealed 58 patients with stable disease and 66 patients with a partial response. These patients then underwent an EBUS-TBNA followed by a thoracotomy with lymph node dissection. The EBUS results showed 89 patients (72%) with persistent disease. Out of the 35 patients who had a nondiagnostic EBUS and underwent thoracotomy, 25 had residual disease by thoracotomy with a sensitivity of 76%, specificity of 100%, PPV of 100% and a NPV of 20%. Although the procedure has great promise for restaging all negative result findings should be referred for surgical restaging.

Endobronchial ultrasound-guided transbronchial needle aspiration is limited to sampling targets adjacent to the airway. The subaortic stations 5, 6 and paraesophageal stations 8 and 9 are not accessible by EBUS. When combined with esophageal EUS, most of the mediastinal stations can be reached with the exception of 5 and 6. By combining both technologies during the same procedure studies have shown a sensitivity of 93% and a NPV of 97%. We recommend starting with EUS, because if the left adrenal gland is compromised, it would preclude the need of further staging.

POSSIBLE COMPLICATIONS

Serious complications after EBUS-TBNA are rare. Bleeding, infection (mediastinitis, pneumonia, pericarditis, cyst infection, and sepsis), pneumothorax and pneumomediastinum have been reported. Data from the American College of Chest Physicians Quality Improvement Registry, Evaluation and Education (AQuIRE), which prospectively enrolled 1,317 patients, reported complications in 19 (1.44%; 95% CI, 0.87–2.24%). Complication rates for pneumothorax, sustained hypoxia, and bleeding were 0.53%, 0.3%, and 0.2%, respectively.

BIBLIOGRAPHY AND FURTHER READING

1. Casal RF, Staerkel GA, Ost D, Almeida FA, Uzbeck MH, Eapen GA, et al. Randomized clinical trial of endobronchial ultrasound needle biopsy with and without aspiration. Chest. 2012;142(3):568-73.

2. Dasgupta A, Mehta AC. Transbronchial needle aspiration. An underused diagnostic technique. Clin Chest Med. 1999;20(1):39-51.
3. De Leyn P, Vansteenkiste J, Cuypers P, Deneffe G, Van Raemdonck D, Coosemans W, et al. Role of cervical mediastinoscopy in staging of non-small cell lung cancer without enlarged mediastinal lymph nodes on CT scan. Eur J Cardiothorac Surg. 1997;12(5):706-12.
4. D'Cunha J, Herndon JE 2nd, Herzan DL, Patterson GA, Kohman LJ, Harpole DH, et al. Poor correspondence between clinical and pathologic staging in stage 1 non-small cell lung cancer: results from CALGB 9761, a prospective trial. Lung Cancer. 2005;48(2):241-6.
5. Eapen GA, Shah AM, Lei X, Jimenez CA, Morice RC, Yarmus L, et al. Complications, consequences, and practice patterns of endobronchial ultrasound-guided transbronchial needle aspiration: results of the AQuIRE registry. Chest. 2013;143(4):1044-53.
6. Ernst A, Anantham D, Eberhardt R, Krasnik M, Herth FJ. Diagnosis of mediastinal adenopathy-real-time endobronchial ultrasound guided needle aspiration versus mediastinoscopy. J Thorac Oncol. 2008;3(6):577-82.
7. Fujiwara T, Yasufuku K, Nakajima T, Chiyo M, Yoshida S, Suzuki M, et al. The utility of sonographic features during endobronchial ultrasound-guided transbronchial needle aspiration for lymph node staging in patients with lung cancer: a standard endobronchial ultrasound image classification system. Chest. 2010;138(3):641-7.
8. Garwood S, Judson MA, Silvestri G, Hoda R, Fraig M, Doelken P. Endobronchial ultrasound for the diagnosis of pulmonary sarcoidosis. Chest. 2007;132(4):1298-304.
9. Harrow EM, Abi-Saleh W, Blum J, Harkin T, Gasparini S, Addrizzo-Harris DJ, et al. The utility of transbronchial needle aspiration in the staging of bronchogenic carcinoma. Am J Respir Crit Care Med. 2000;161(2 Pt 1):601-7.
10. Hecht SS. Tobacco smoke carcinogens and lung cancer. J Natl Cancer Inst. 1999;91(14):1194-210.
11. Herth FJ, Annema JT, Eberhardt R, Yasufuku K, Ernst A, Krasnik M, et al. Endobronchial ultrasound with transbronchial needle aspiration for restaging the mediastinum in lung cancer. J Clin Oncol. 2008;26(20):3346-50.
12. Herth FJ, Eberhardt R, Vilmann P, Krasnik M, Ernst A. Real-time endobronchial ultrasound guided transbronchial needle aspiration for sampling mediastinal lymph nodes. Thorax. 2006;61(9):795-8.
13. Herth FJ, Ernst A, Eberhardt R, Vilmann P, Dienemann H, Krasnik M. Endobronchial ultrasound-guided transbronchial needle aspiration of lymph nodes in the radiologically normal mediastinum. Eur Respir J. 2006;28(5):910-4.
14. Howlader N, Noone AM, Krapcho M, et al. SEER cancer statistics review, 1975-2010. (2013). National Cancer Institute, Bethesda (MD). [online] Available from http://seer.cancer.gov.ezproxy.welch.jhmi.edu/csr/1975_2010/. [Accessed January, 2016].
15. Ikeda S. The flexible broncho fiberscope. Keio J Med. 1968;17:1-16.
16. Kennedy MP, Jimenez CA, Bruzzi JF, Mhatre AD, Lei X, Giles FJ, et al. Endobronchial ultrasound-guided transbronchial needle aspiration in the diagnosis of lymphoma. Thorax. 2008;63(4):360-5.
17. Krasnik M, Vilmann P, Larsen SS, Jacobsen GK. Preliminary experience with a new method of endoscopic transbronchial real-time ultrasound-guided biopsy for diagnosis of mediastinal and hilar lesions. Thorax. 2003;58(12):1083-6.
18. Lee HS, Lee GK, Lee HS, Kim MS, Lee JM, Kim HY, et al. Real-time endobronchial ultrasound-guided transbronchial needle aspiration in mediastinal staging of non-small cell lung cancer: how many aspirations per target lymph node station? Chest. 2008;134(2):368-74.
19. Moonim MT, Breen R, Fields PA, Santis G. Diagnosis and subtyping of de novo and relapsed mediastinal lymphomas by endobronchial ultrasound needle aspiration. Am J Respir Crit Care Med. 2013;188(10):1216-23.
20. Nakajima T, Yasufuku K, Takahashi R, Shingyoji M, Hirata T, Itami M, et al. Comparison of 21-gauge and 22-gauge aspiration needle during endobronchial ultrasound-guided transbronchial needle aspiration. Respirology. 2011;16(1):90-4.
21. Ortiz R, Hayes M, Arias S, Lee HJ, Feller-Kopman D, Yarmus L. Pneumomediastinum and pneumopericardium after endobronchial ultrasound-guided transbronchial needle aspiration. Ann Am Thorac Soc. 2014;11(4):680-1.
22. Pieterman RM, van Putten JW, Meuzelaar JJ, Mooyaart EL, Vaalburg W, Koëter GH, et al. Preoperative staging of non-small-cell lung cancer with positron-emission tomography. N Engl J Med. 2000;343(4):254-61.
23. Silvestri GA, Gonzalez AV, Jantz MA, Margolis ML, Gould MK, Tanoue LT, et al. Methods for staging non-small cell lung cancer: Diagnosis and management of lung cancer, 3rd ed: American College of Chest Physicians evidence-based clinical practice guidelines. Chest. 2013;143(5 Suppl):e211S-50S.
24. Tremblay A, Stather DR, Maceachern P, Khalil M, Field SK. A randomized controlled trial of standard vs endobronchial ultrasonography-guided transbronchial needle aspiration in patients with suspected sarcoidosis. Chest. 2009;136(2):340-6.
25. US Cancer Statistics Working Group. United States cancer statistics: 1999-2010 incidence and mortality web-based report. US Department of Health and Human Services, Centers for Disease Control and Prevention and National Cancer Institute, Atlanta (GA); 2013.
26. Wallace MB, Pascual JM, Raimondo M, Woodward TA, McComb BL, Crook JE, et al. Minimally invasive endoscopic staging of suspected lung cancer. JAMA. 2008;299(5):540-6.
27. Wang KP, Brower R, Haponik EF, Siegelman S. Flexible transbronchial needle aspiration for staging of bronchogenic carcinoma. Chest. 1983;84(5):571-6.
28. Wang KP, Marsh BR, Summer WR, Terry PB, Erozan YS, Baker RR. Transbronchial needle aspiration for diagnosis of lung cancer. Chest. 1981;80(1):48-50.

29. Wang KP, Terry PB. Transbronchial needle aspiration in the diagnosis and staging of bronchogenic carcinoma. Am Rev Respir Dis. 1983;127(3):344-7.
30. Wong M, Yasufuku K, Nakajima T, Herth FJ, Sekine Y, Shibuya K, et al. Endobronchial ultrasound: new insight for the diagnosis of sarcoidosis. Eur Respir J. 2007;29(6): 1182-6.
31. Yarmus L, Akulian J, Gilbert C, Feller-Kopman D, Lee HJ, Zarogoulidis P, et al. Optimizing endobronchial ultrasound for molecular analysis. How many passes are needed? Ann Am Thorac Soc. 2013;10(6):636-43.
32. Yung RC, Otell S, Illei P, Clark DP, Feller-Kopman D, Yarmus L, et al. Improvement of cellularity on cell block preparations using the so-called tissue coagulum clot method during endobronchial ultrasound-guided transbronchial fine-needle aspiration. Cancer Cytopathol. 2012;120(3):185-95.
33. Zielinski M, Szlubowski A, Kołodziej M, Orzechowski S, Laczynska E, Pankowski J, et al. Comparison of endobronchial ultrasound and/or endoesophageal ultrasound with transcervical extended mediastinal lymphadenectomy for staging and restaging of non-small-cell lung cancer. J Thorac Oncol. 2013;8(5):630-6.

Index

Page numbers followed by *f* refer to figure and *t* refer to table.

D

E

F

G

H

I

K

L

M

S

T

U

V

W

X

Z

www.ingramcontent.com/pod-product-compliance
Lightning Source LLC
LaVergne TN
LVHW070904300926
849162LV00011B/1851
9789386056009